Progress in
Neutron Capture Therapy
for Cancer

Progress in
Neutron Capture Therapy
for Cancer

Edited by

Barry J. Allen

Australian Nuclear Science and Technology Organisation
Menai, New South Wales, Australia

Douglas E. Moore

University of Sydney
Sydney, New South Wales, Australia

and

Baiba V. Harrington

Australian Nuclear Science and Technology Organisation
Menai, New South Wales, Australia

SPRINGER SCIENCE+BUSINESS MEDIA, LLC

Library of Congress Cataloging-in-Publication Data

Progress in neutron capture therapy for cancer / edited by Barry J.
  Allen, Douglas E. Moore, and Baiba V. Harrington.
      p.   cm.
    Proceedings of the Fourth International Symposium on Neutron
  Capture Therapy for Cancer, held December 4-7, in Sydney, Australia.
    Includes bibliographical references and index.
    ISBN 978-0-306-44104-2   ISBN 978-1-4615-3384-9 (eBook)
    DOI 10.1007/978-1-4615-3384-9
    1. Boron-neutron capture therapy--Congresses. 2. Cancer-
  -Radiotherapy--Congresses.   I. Allen, B. J. II. Moore, Douglas E.,
  1938-   . III. Harrington, Baiba V. IV. International Symposium on
  Neutron Capture Therapy for Cancer (4th : 1990 : Sydney, Australia)
    [DNLM. 1. Neoplasms--therapy--congresses. 2. Neutrons-
  -therapeutic use--congresses.   QZ 269 P9655]
  RC271.R3P755 1992
  616.99'40642--dc20
  DNLM/DLC
  for Library of Congress   91-45564
                                                                CIP

Proceedings of the Fourth International Symposium on Neutron Capture
Therapy for Cancer, held December 4-7, 1990, in Sydney, Australia

ISBN 978-0-306-44104-2

© 1992 Springer Science+Business Media New York
Originally published by Plenum Press, New York in 1992

SYMPOSIUM ORGANISATION AND SPONSORS

HOSTS: International Society for Neutron Capture Therapy

Australian Nuclear Science & Technology Organisation

The University of Sydney

AUSPICES: International Union Against Cancer (UICC)

SPONSORS: Australian Cancer Society

Sydney Melanoma Foundation

Australian Nuclear Science & Technology Organisation

Qantas

Ansett

General Atomics

Energy Resources Australia

Peter MacCallum Cancer Institute

U.S. Department of Energy

Department of Industry, Technology and Commerce

Callery Chemical Company

NATIONAL ADVISORY COMMITTEE

Barry Allen - Ansto: Chair
David Barkla - Monash University
Alan Coates - Royal Prince Alfred Hospital
Peter Hersey - Royal Newcastle Hospital
Robert Jones - Prince of Wales Childrens Hospital
Andrew Kaye - Royal Melbourne Hospital
Hedy Mameghan - Prince of Wales Hospital
Roger Martin - Peter MacCallum Cancer Institute
Doug Moore - University of Sydney
Peter Parsons - Queensland Institute of Medical Research
Dace Shugg - Tasmania Cancer Registry
Martin Tattersall - University of Sydney
Rod Withers - Prince of Wales Hospital

INTERNATIONAL ADVISORY COMMITTEE

Barry Allen - Ansto, Australia: Convenor
Christopher Adams - Oxford, UK
Rolf F Barth - Ohio State University, USA
Gordon L Brownell - Massachusetts General Hospital, USA
Robert Brugger - University of Missouri, Columbia, USA
Geoffrey Constantine - Harwell, UK
Ron Dorn III - Mountain Tumour Institute, Idaho, USA
Frank Ellis - Oxford, UK
Ralph Fairchild - Brookhaven National Laboratory, USA
Heinz Fankhauser - Centre Hospitalier, Lausanne, Switzerland
Ludwig E Feinendegen, Julich, FRG
Detlef Gabel - University of Bremen, FRG
Merle Griebenow - Idaho Nuclear Engineering Laboratory, USA
Otto Harling - Massachussetts Institute of Technolgy, USA
Hiroshi Hatanaka - Teikyo University, Japan
John Hopewell - Churchill Hospital, UK
William E Hunt - Ohio State University, USA
Steve Kahl - University of California, San Francisco, USA
Keiji Kanda - Kyoto University, Japan
Börje Larsson - Gustaf Werner Institute, Sweden
Yutaka Mishima - Kobe University School of Medicine, Japan
John L Russell - Atlanta, USA
Tadashi Sato - Atomic Energy Research Laboratory, Japan
Toshikazu Shibata - Kyoto University, Japan
Albert Soloway - Ohio State University, USA
William H Sweet - Massachusetts General Hospital, USA
Akira Takeuchi - University of Tokyo, Japan
Robert Zamenhof - Tufts New England Medical Centre, USA

SECRETARIAT

Tonina Jerez - Conference and Proceeding
Cynthia Allen - Partner's Program

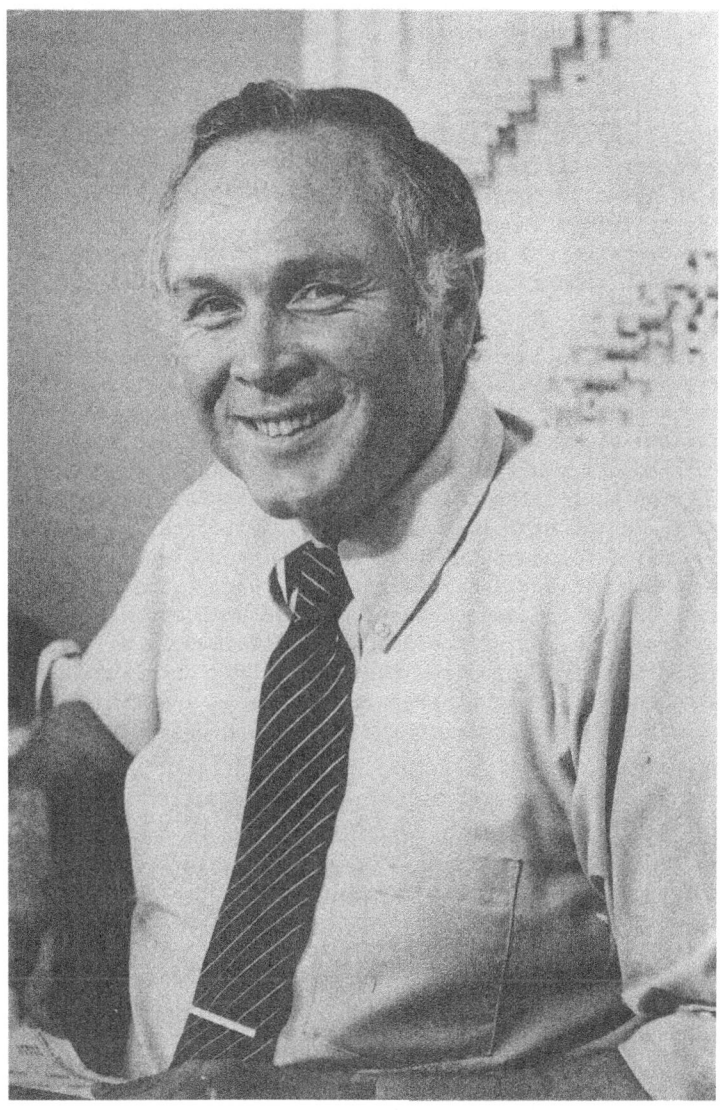

RALPH GRANDISON FAIRCHILD
(1935-1990)

Boron Neutron Capture Therapy lost a powerful advocate and contributor with the premature and untimely passing of Ralph G. Fairchild on December 18, 1990. The impact was particularly severe because he had just attended the Fourth International Symposium on Neutron Capture Therapy where he was an active participant in most of the sessions and other functions.

Ralph graduated with a B.S. in Physics from St. Lawrence University in 1958, and M.S. in Nuclear Engineering from Cornell University in 1961, and a Ph.D. from Adelphi University in 1975. He began his affiliation with Brookhaven National Laboratory in 1961 as a Medical Physicist in the Medical Department and it was then that he began his BNCT-related experimentation with foresight and determination. In 1965, Ralph initiated experiments on an epithermal neutron beam which, by allowing deeper penetration in tissue, overcame a principal problem associated with the use of thermal neutrons. Thus, more than any other scientist in the United States, he kept the possibility of BNCT alive during some very lean decades.

He was the first to describe the physical dosimetry and radiobiological characteristics of californium-252 brachytherapy sources. Additionally, he contributed to the development of ^{125}I plaques for the treatment of ocular melanoma. He evaluated numerous melanaffinic agents for their utility in the treatment of malignant melanoma, and identified radiolabelled thouracil as one of the most significant biomolecules for use in both diagnosis and therapy.

Fairchild was a firm believer that cancer radiotherapy would best be improved through the utilization of binary systems involving the exploitation of the cell's own physiological requirements to permit the uptake of various biomolecules carrying target atoms, followed by the activation of these atoms with radiation. In addition to BNCT, Ralph postulated Photon Activation Therapy (PAT) as another binary system for the treatment of malignant brain tumours. In a theoretical paper in 1982, he proposed the use of iododeoxyuridine (IdUrd) incorporated in tumour cell DNA and its subsequent activation with photons above the K absorption edge of iodine to induce a photoelectric effect and concomitant Auger cascades. He identified samarium-145 as the isotope with the most suitable energy for inducing this effect, and proposed the interstitial implantation of these radioactive sources via brachytherapy techniques. Initial clinical trials with PAT are currently underway at the Ohio State University.

Many of us who have had the privilege of knowing Ralph well will remember the unusual and admirable qualities that he possessed. In addition to a wonderful sense of humour, his quiet, humble, gentle and unassuming manner concealed an intense energy and drive for work. His deep-thinking and incisive mind, coupled with curiosity, a keen power of observation for scientific facts and a genuine love for science distinguished his person. His enthusiasm was infectious. Many of Ralph Fairchild's activities were given unselfishly to the interest of others, to colleagues in science, to teaching, and to his research collaborators.

He has been recognized internationally by his collaborators as the undisputed leader in the field of BNCT. He has been referred to as the intellectual glue which bonded the efforts of BNCT investigators throughout America. His collaborators describe him as open minded, honest, self-critical and, more importantly, as someone who was sincerely and genuinely interested in each of their research endeavours. Ralph's breadth of knowledge was always available for others to utilize. Working with him meant not only a symbiotic relationship, but a synergistic one as well.

He will always be remembered as a good friend, an excellent and dedicated scientist, and as the leading contributor to the scientific body of knowledge in the field of Neutron Capture Therapy. He has spawned a generation of friends and scientists to whom he has given the task of carrying out his dream.

Victor P. Bond
Brookhaven National Laboratory

PREFACE

Despite the many advances made in the diagnosis and therapy of cancer, the
mortality rate is still about half that of the incidence rate. However,
the odds are not evenly distributed. Prognosis for some cancers is good,
but for others, few patients will survive 12 months. This latter group of
cancers is characterised by a proclivity to disseminate malignant cells in
the host organ. The degree of surgery possible may be limited by the
critical nature of the organ, and chemotherapy and radiotherapy are of
palliative value only. In some cases systemic metastases occur, but in
other cases, failure to achieve local control results in death. First among
these cancers are the high grade brain tumours, astrocytoma 3,4 and
glioblastoma multiforme. Local control of these tumours should lead to
cure. Other cancers melanoma metastatic to the brain, for which a useful
palliative therapy is not yet available, and pancreatic cancer for which
localised control at an early stage could bring about improved prognosis.
Patients with these cancers have little grounds for hope. Our primary
objective is to reverse this situation with Neutron Capture Therapy (NCT).
The purpose of this fourth symposium is to hasten the day whereby patients
with these cancers can reasonably hope for substantial remissions.

The first symposium on NCT was held in Boston in 1983, followed by Tokyo in
1985 and Bremen, Germany in 1988. A tradition of multidisciplinary papers
presented in plenary sessions has been established and is continued in this
symposium. Indeed many members of the International Advisory Committee were
particularly emphatic about this feature. It is the multidisciplinary
nature of NCT that sets this field somewhat apart from other research
areas.

The rapid growth in activity in NCT in recent years is mirrored by the
large number of submitted abstracts for this symposium. Over 150
participants from the USA, Japan, Europe and Australia presented more than
160 papers on aspects of physics, chemistry, biology and clinical oncology
in Neutron Capture Therapy. For the first time it was necessary to
introduce both parallel and poster sessions. The International Union
Against Cancer (UICC) granted auspices to the symposium, which was held at
the University of Sydney.

All papers published in these proceedings have been subject to review by
at least two referees, and in many cases the papers have been substantially
revised by the authors. In some cases controversy over results or
interpretation remains, and must be resolved by further research. In other
cases, the reviewing has been tempered because of the restricted page
allocation, submission deadlines and requirements for balanced reporting.
After all, these are conference proceedings and completeness is an
important issue. These proceedings therefore represent a snapshot of NCT
research around the world.

Binary Therapies

The binary therapy concept is one new approach whereby enhanced tumour specificity is achieved by the synergistic action of two different modalities. One example is photodynamic therapy, where a laser beam activates a non-toxic photosensitive compound to create a local chemical toxicity. This is being investigated in the intraoperative treatment of high grade brain tumours and some other cancers. However, this method is restricted by the limited penetration of the laser light through tissue. Another example is NCT, where non-toxic boron compounds are taken up by cancer cells and the boron is subsequently activated in situ by an incident neutron beam, causing a nuclear reaction with energy release being localised to the target and nearest neighbour cells. Thus individual cancer cells can be killed in the midst of normal cells with minimal damage to the host tissue if boron is selectively taken up by the cancer cells.

The implementation of this procedure is not necessarily straightforward but, as illustrated by many papers presented at the symposium, much progress has been made in recent years. Of particular interest were papers describing the new epithermal neutron beams, the rapidly growing European Collaboration and the extensive Washington State University (WSU) dog studies.

Animal studies show that NCT can achieve local control of melanoma xenografts in nude mice, brain tumours in rats, ocular melanoma in rabbits, spontaneous brain tumours in dogs and cutaneous melanoma and glioblastoma in human patients. These results and their significance are considered in more detail in the following discussion.

Thermal NCT for glioblastoma

To date, over 100 high-grade brain tumour patients have been treated by intra-operative NCT by Prof Hiroshi Hatanaka in Japan. The open tumour bed is irradiated by a thermal neutron beam after intracarotid injection of borocaptate (BSH). With the exception of grade 3,4 tumours in the cerebral mantle, 5-year patient survival is comparable to Hatanaka's own conventional treatment series, which in turn is similar to that obtained at other centres, ie 2-3% survival at 5 years. However, a dramatic difference is observed for tumours within 6 cm of the cortical surface. For the 12 patients in this group, seven have survived to 5 years. Only in this group has the weakly penetrating thermal neutron beam delivered an adequate dose to the deeper region of the tumour.

Since about one third of grade 3,4 gliomas occur in the cerebral mantle, a randomised trial of NCT seems warranted on the basis of Hatanaka's results.

Thermal NCT for subcutaneous melanoma

The Kobe group, led by Prof Yutaka Mishima, has pioneered the use of boronophenylalanine (BPA) in the treatment of subcutaneous melanoma by NCT. For these cases, the thermal neutron beam is ideal, as the maximum dose is at the surface. Yet, skin effects are limited to erythema and dry desquamation because of the low uptake of BPA by the skin. Complete local eradication of subungual or acral lentiginous melanoma has been achieved in 5 cases.

Epithermal NCT

An epithermal neutron beam which can penetrate up to 10-cm depth is
required to treat deep-seated lesions with NCT. Epithermal beams are now
available at BNL and Massachusetts Institute of Technology (MIT) in the
US, under test at the Joint Research Council (JRC) reactor at Petten in
The Netherlands and under consideration at the Idaho National Engineering
Laboratory, US and Ansto in Australia. These beams would potentially allow
treatment of high grade brain tumours by fractionated bilateral
irradiations of the head. The therapeutic ratio is the dose to the tumour
relative to the maximum dose to normal tissue. Values of 2-3 for this
ratio could be achieved across the whole brain if boron concentrations of
30 ppm are obtained in the tumour concomitantly with 3 ppm in normal
tissue.

Epithermal NCT in a spontaneous dog brain tumour model

Dogs with naturally occurring cerebral tumours have been irradiated with
epithermal neutrons at the BNL reactor after intravenous administration of
BSH. Blood boron concentration was about 25 ppm during the irradiation and
tumour to blood ratios were less than one. However tumour to normal brain
tissue ratios range up to 15. Nine dogs with contrast enhancing lesions in
CT scans were treated by NCT with detailed post-treatment
examinations. Some dogs have now survived in excess of 12 months.

Ocular melanoma in rabbits

An ocular melanoma model in the rabbit has been developed at BNL, where Dr
Jeff Coderre has demonstrated complete eradication of the implanted
melanoma in 10 of 13 NCT cases for an estimated therapeutic ratio of 3. A
BPA slurry was digested by the rabbits prior to thermal neutron
irradiation of the eye. Cataracts developed in all cases.

Rat Glioma model

Two reports of complete control of implanted brain tumours in the rat
glioma model also came from BNL. Using BPA, Coderre demonstrated long
term survival (150 days) in 7 of 16 rats with no survivors in the thermal
neutron control group (i.e no BPA injection) or unirradiated groups. Dr
Darryl Joel used the disulfide dodecaborane dimer with continuous tail-vein
infusion over 3 days, followed by neutron irradiation of the implanted
intracerebral gliosarcoma in rats. Untreated rats had a median
post-inoculation survival of 21 days, the boron free neutron controls
survived 26 days, and rats treated by NCT survived 60 days. Two of 12
animals lived more than one year. At a higher neutron dose, 6 of 10
animals remain alive more than 10 months after NCT.

Melanoma xenografts in nude mice

In the subcutaneous melanoma xenograft model, tumour growth rather than
survival is the endpoint as subcutaneous melanomas in this model are not
of themselves lethal. Harding-Passey melanoma cells were injected
subcutaneously in the thigh of nude mice. Two weeks later the mice
received an intraperitoneal injection of BPA, the melanomas were
irradiated with thermal neutrons and the subsequent growth rate monitored
and compared with the boron free neutrons group and unirradiated controls.
Dr Barry Allen of Ansto reported local control in 6 of 8 mice over 300
days, whereas only a 3 week growth delay was observed in mice treated by
neutron irradiation alone.

These results, together with the pharmacokinetic data now available for many different models, including patients, demonstrate the potential value of NCT. Nevertheless, the inability to achieve therapeutic boron concentrations in all cancer cells is the probable cause of the failure to achieve complete local control.

Research Awards

On behalf of the symposium sponsors, awards were made to scientists on the basis of their research contributions to the conference. Members of the executive board of the International Society for NCT and the Organising Committees were excluded. The Australian Cancer Society Award went to Dr Heinz Fankhauser, a neurosurgeon from Switzerland, for his study of the uptake of borocaptate sodium in brain tumour patients prior to surgery. These studies are providing the essential information needed to determine absorbed dose for clinical trials. The second recipient was Dr Pat Gavin, Veterinarian, Washington State University, for his extensive studies of the pharmacokinetics of borocaptate sodium in dogs with naturally occurring tumours and for demonstrating the efficacy of NCT in this animal model.

The Sydney Melanoma Foundation Award was presented to Dr Jeff Coderre, Brookhaven National Laboratory, for the successful treatment of ocular melanoma in rabbits by NCT.

The Callery Chemical Company Award went to Dr Stephen Kahl, a boron chemist from the University of California San Francisco and Dr John Hill, University of Melbourne, for the synthesis of the boron-porphyrin compound BOPP and the demonstration of highly specific uptakes by glioma cells in the rat brain glioma model. Tumour to normal brain tissue ratios of 300:1 were observed, and BOPP was detected in individual glioma cells separated from the tumour. This class of compound suggests a role for photodynamic therapy as an adjunct to NCT.

The General Atomics Award went to Dr Floyd Wheeler, of the Idaho National Engineering Laboratory, for studies of the physics of filtered neutron beams and dosimetry, while Prof Hiroshi Fukuda from Tohoku University received the Energy Resources of Australia Award for studies of normal tissue tolerance to NCT.

Round Table Debate

A feature of the symposium was the round table debate between Australian cancer specialists and a panel of international experts in NCT. The role of NCT in the control of locally incurable cancer was identified, but caution was urged with regard to clinical trials. NCT was regarded as a knife, albeit exceptionally sharp, and demonstration of the value of improved local control rather than cure should be the goal.

The need to eliminate every clonogenic cell was discussed. Whether this would ever be achievable by NCT is by no means certain. Boron is taken up in varying amounts by cells, depending on many factors such as tumour morphology and cell metabolism. Statistically, if the cell concentrations of boron were uniform, a very small number of cells would still be free of neutron capture reactions. Yet there is ample evidence in many models that tumours can be eradicated by NCT. Small tumours take up boron compounds more readily than larger tumours which have hypoxic and necrotic regions; cell killing by NCT may therefore be more efficacious in the former. However, standard external beam radiotherapy also fails to kill every clonogenic cell, and the question to be answered, ultimately by clinical trials, is whether NCT can do a better job.

Clinical Trials

Although more experimental work needs to be done the question of when to
commence further clinical trials was considered. Current therapy for high
grade brain tumours is palliative only, and a trial would soon determine
if NCT was advantageous. However, the risk to the future of NCT was
thought to take precedence over premature clinical trials which, if deemed
a failure, might also impede further development in the field.
Should trials be delayed until more highly tumour specific boron-
containing porphyrins are tested and approved for use? This was not the
consensus. Current compounds are expected to give therapeutic ratios of
2-3 across the brain and this is more than enough to investigate efficacy.
Nonetheless, vigorous development of new boron chemicals should continue.

Should NCT be incorporated into a radiotherapy protocol? This would be a
safe way to introduce NCT, by replacing 5 fractions of radiotherapy with
one NCT exposure. However, large numbers of patients might be required to
discern a significant improvement in prognosis.

Is an experimental therapy a better choice for patients than therapy known
to be of limited benefit for most patients? We do know how to limit dose
to normal tissue so toxicity to normal tissues should not be worse than
that achieved with conventional therapy. Should Hatanaka's results for
cerebral mantle tumours be confirmed in the forthcoming epithermal beam
trials for brain tumours at all sites, then a major advance in the
treatment of these cancers would have been achieved. But even without the
Hatanaka data, the results reported at the Fourth Symposium provide strong
and independent support for the potential of NCT to improve control in
localised tumours with poor prognoses.

Barry J. Allen
President, International Society for
Neutron Capture Therapy, 1988-1990

OPENING ADDRESS

Two years ago at the third international symposium on Neutron Capture Therapy in Bremen, Detlef Gabel related the fable of the four musicians of Bremen. These were the donkey, dog, cat and rooster. The musicians received little recognition until they played in concert. By analogy, the physicist, chemist, biologist and clinician must work together to overcome incurable cancer by NCT.

Now long ago in the dreamtime of the Australian aborigine, this problem was foreseen and solved. Unlike the European solution, where three placental animals must play to the tune of the rooster, the Australian solution was to invent the platypus.

The platypus is like the physicist, as busy as a beaver; in fact it has the tail of a beaver. It is also like the chemist because it synthesizes toxic chemicals for the venom in the spur of each hind leg. But it is the biologist's nightmare. The platypus lays eggs but suckles its young in a make-shift pouch. Moreover, it has a single ovary and is a monotreme, both very bird like properties. Finally, the platypus is noted for its bill, as is the clinician. This bill is both tough and electro-sensitive. Maybe it could take Mastercard too!

Thus the uniquely Australian solution is to combine all the requirements of the Bremen quartet into a singlet. Where many countries combine in Europe to form an NCT team, and many laboratories in the USA and Japan compete for NCT funds, in Australia it is Lucas Heights, with its Moata and HIFAR reactors, which is the natural centre to coordinate the first phase of NCT.

This symposium brings together the Bremen musicians, the Japanese crane, the great American bison and the Australian platypus. This week we shall all play in concert for the progress of NCT and the betterment of mankind.

Barry J. Allen
Convener, Fourth International Symposium On
Neutron Capture Therapy for Cancer

THE UNITED STATES DEPARTMENT OF ENERGY PROGRAM IN NEUTRON CAPTURE THERAPY

First, I would like to thank Dr Allen and his associates for having made the splendid arrangements for the symposium.

The United States involvement in Neutron Capture Therapy began in the 1950's as a cooperative program between the Brookhaven National Laboratory, the Massachusetts General Hospital and the Massachusetts Institute of Technology (MIT). Drs Sweet and Brownell, who were the prime movers in those studies, are present at this symposium.

The first clinical trials were performed at the Brookhaven Graphite reactor using a thermal neutron beam with B-10 sodium tetraborate or B-10 sodium pentaborate. Later, the Medical Research Reactor and the MIT reactor became available for these studies. The early clinical results, however, were disappointing, and the efforts shifted from clinical trials to more basic studies directed to finding alternative compounds and to improvement of the neutron beam. These studies continued at a rather modest level for many years during which it was recognized that an epithermal rather than a thermal neutron beam would be needed to provide the penetration required for treating the dee
per lesions, and Dr Soloway, who is also among those present today, the BSH compound (mercapto undecahydrododecaborate) that has been used in most of the more recent studies.

The clinical trials conducted by Dr Hatanaka in Japan have used the BSH compound. Dr Hatanaka's promising results stimulated a revival of interest in neutron capture therapy, and the support for work in this field has increased considerably. The Department of Energy currently supports work related to neutron capture therapy at the Idaho National Engineering Laboratory, Brookhaven National Laboratory, Ohio State University, the State University of New York at Stony Brook, the Massachusetts General Hospital, the Massachusetts Institute of Technology, Tufts-New England Medical Centre, and the University of Tennessee. Speakers representing these institutions will be presenting details of the program. With the very recent increased funding provided by Congress for the conversion of the Power Burst Facility at the Idaho National Engineering Laboratory, it can be expected that efforts in neutron capture therapy will continue to expand. We are of course deeply interested in the progress that is being made in other countries, and look forward to hearing about your plans and developments during this week's meetings.

Again, thanks to Dr Allen and his associates for the tremendous effort they have put into making this symposium possible.

James S. Robertson
United States Department of Energy

CONTENTS

PROJECTS REVIEWS

REACTOR NEUTRON SOURCES

ACCELERATOR NEUTRON SOURCES

BORON CHEMISTRY - BPA

BORON MACROMOLECULES

BORON ANALYSIS IN BIOLOGICAL SAMPLES

RADIOBIOLOGY

PRECLINICAL ANIMAL STUDIES

ACUTE AND LATE EFFECTS IN NORMAL TISSUES

BORON BIODISTRIBUTIONS IN GLIOMA PATIENTS

CLINICAL STUDIES OF CANCERS WITH POOR PROGNOSES

AN OPTIMIZED EPITHERMAL NEUTRON BEAM FOR NEUTRON CAPTURE THERAPY (NCT)

AT THE BROOKHAVEN MEDICAL RESEARCH REACTOR (BMRR)

R.G. Fairchild[1], V. Benary[1,6], J. Kalef-Ezra[1,2], S.K. Saraf[1], R.M. Brugger[4],
A. Shih[4], R.A. Gahbauer,[3] J.H. Goodman[3], B.H. Laster[1,5], J. Gajewski[5], E.B. Ramsay[5],
L.E. Reinstein[5], S. Fiarman[1], and Y. Kamen[1]

[1]Medical Department, Brookhaven National Laboratory, Upton, NY 11973, U.S.A.
[2]University of Ioannina, Ioannina, Greece
[3]Ohio State University Hospital, Ohio State University, Columbus, OH 43210, U.S.A.
[4]University of Missouri, Columbia, MO 65211, U.S.A.
[5]State University of New York, Stony Brook, NY 11794, U.S.A.
[6]Tel Aviv University, Tel Aviv, Israel

INTRODUCTION

The first clinical trials of NCT were initiated at Brookhaven in 1951, using the Brookhaven Graphite Research Reactor (BGRR). Subsequently, the Brookhaven Medical Research Reactor (BMRR) was built primarily for clinical applications of NCT, with an improved beam extraction facility providing flexibility for future development of filters/moderators for NCT. This flexibility was exploited to provide an optimized epithermal neutron beam which was recently installed and tested in the east irradiation facility (shutter) of the BMRR.

The new epithermal neutron beam was implemented using an Al_2O_3 moderator or "Spectrum Shifter" which was designed, installed and tested in collaboration with associates at Idaho National Engineering Laboratory (INEL). The resultant beam is "optimized" in that the fast neutron and γ contaminations have been reduced to acceptable values (less than a few % of maximum normal tissue dose), while the epithermal neutron flux density of 1.8×10^9 n/cm^2-sec allows NCT to be carried out in 30 min in a single application (1). It is, however, anticipated that clinical applications of NCT will be carried out in ~4 fractions (~15 min each, with bilateral irradiations), as recommended by an international committee convened to recommend the best approach to clinical trials (2). Biological parameters have been determined for the above beam, as described below. It is expected that sufficient data will be accumulated in ongoing phase I clinical trials with BSH and BPA, to allow a decision to be made about the advisability of initiating therapy trials in humans, in ~12-24 months.

BMRR EPITHERMAL BEAM

Facility and Beam Parameters. A cross section of the epithermal neutron beam facility, installed at the BMRR is shown in Ref. 3; the point of irradiation is 169 cm from the core center, with 65.4 cm of Al_2O_3 and 11.4 cm of Bi plus 2 thin sheets of Cd forming the filter/moderator in the movable shutter assembly. Beam parameters are summarized in Table 1 (1). The components of the biologically effective dose from the mixed field in a tissue equivalent cylinder (16.6 x 23 cm) and the dose to tissues containing 3 to 30 μg ^{10}B/g are given in Ref. 1 and 3. From these data it is possible to derive a dose distribution for bilateral irradiations, as in Fig. 1. From the above figures, conclusions can be drawn:

1. As has been prescribed by advisory panels on NCT, bilateral irradiations provide a uniform dose distribution throughout a human head, and should be used for treatment of deep seated tumors.

2. The current beam is "optimized" in that further reduction in the fast neutron or γ contamination in the incident beam would not significantly increase therapeutic gain (TG) (1,3).

Whole Body Dose. Measurements of absorbed dose to tissue were made along the wall (biological shield) at the center, and at 10, 35, 50 and 60 cm from the center of the epithermal neutron

Table 1. Summary of Beam Parameters for Current Optimized Epithermal-Neutron Beam (65.4 cm Al_2O_3 and Al plus 11.4 cm Bi) - Beam Size 10" x 10"

Power	3 MW
Epithermal-neutron flux density[*] (n/cm^2-s)	1.8×10^9
Fast-neutron flux density (n/cm^2-s)[**]	$\sim 1 \times 10^8$
Thermal-neutron flux density (peak at ~2-cm depth in phantom; n/cm^2-s)	2.8×10^9 (no added filtration) 2.5×10^9 (0.5-mm Cd added) 1.9×10^9 (1.0-mm ^6Li added)
Absorbed dose from fast neutrons free in air	4.5 rad/min
Absorbed dose from gammas, free in air	1.2 rad/min
Fast-neutron dose per epithermal neutron	4.2×10^{-11} rad/(n-cm^2)
Gamma dose per epithermal neutron	1.12×10^{-11} rad/(n-cm^2)
Fast-neutron dose per thermal neutron (no added filtration)	2.7×10^{-11} rad/(n-cm^2)

[*]Measured at center of irradiation port face; 0.4 to 10,000 eV
[**]Measured at center of irradiation port face; E>10 keV

beam facility. Values for "no shielding" were obtained at these locations. More measurements, with 2.54 cm for added shielding (LiOH, lithiated polyethylene or boronated polyethylene) were made in these same positions to evaluate the effects of such shielding. The measured values of absorbed dose in air at the facility wall surface indicate that whole body doses will be significantly reduced. It is clear that whole body dose for therapeutic irradiations in a 10" x 10" beam will be less than 20 rads, and thus not constitute a health hazard. This was verified by dog irradiations carried out by INEL and associates (both for tumor therapy of spontaneous brain tumors and for normal tissue tolerance studies) where the (normal) CNS was identified as the critical (limiting) tissue in these studies (4,5). The above is in contradiction to statements made by others, suggesting that "...neutron leakage through the present Brookhaven reactor biological shielding could be lethal to the patient from whole body dose before the tumor is destroyed" (6).

Subsequent to the above studies, 2.54 cm of ^6Li enriched lithiated polyethylene were added to the facility wall surrounding the 10 x 10 in. port, so that lower values should now be obtained.

COMPARISON OF EPITHERMAL NEUTRON BEAMS

A comparison of the various epithermal neutron beams proposed for NCT and available in the literature, is shown in Table 2, on the basis of "in air" parameters. It is evident that the D_2O moderated

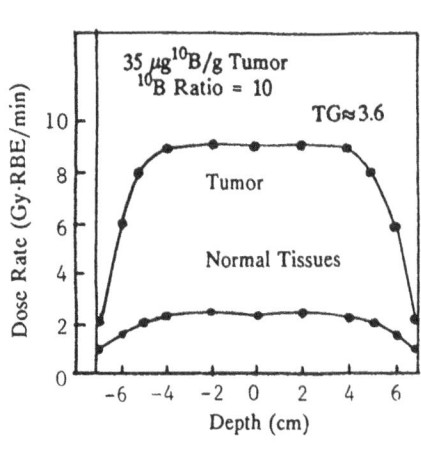

Fig. 1 BILATERAL IRRADIATION

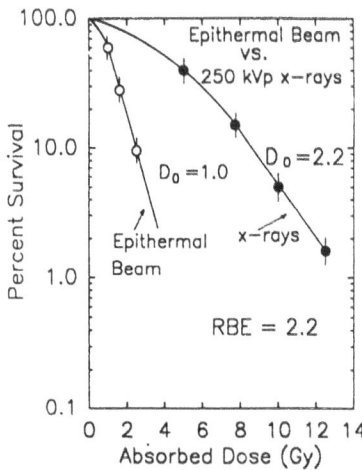

Fig. 2 CELL SURVIVAL

Table 2. Beam Parameters Measured or Calculated "In Air" for Various Epithermal Neutron Beams

Beam	Measurement or calculation	Epithermal neutron flux density (n/cm^2-sec)	Rad in Air/epithermal neutron (10^{-11} rad/neutron/cm^2) Neutrons	Gammas	Reference
BMRR (Al$_2$O$_3$ moderator)	M	1.8×10^9	4.2	1.1	
Harwell/Pluto (Fe filter)	M	2×10^7	29.0	4.2	1
BMRR* (D$_2$O moderator)	M	1.1×10^{10}	27.0	3.2	1
Georgia Tech* Research Reactor (Al-S filter)	M	6.9×10^7	14.8	27.0	1
MITR (Al-S moderator)	M	2.6×10^8	~24	?	23
HFR, Petten (Al-S-Ar moderator)	C	1.1×10^9	7.8	1.7	13
PBF (20 MW) (Al-D$_2$O)	C	10×10^9	2	1	14,15
MURR II (10 MW) (Al$_2$O$_3$)	C	7.9×10^9	2.8	0.3	16

beam developed at the BMRR in 1965, and the Fe filtered beam recently studied at Harwell are unfit for human use due to the high fast neutron dose (1). It should be noted that the University of Missouri Reactor at Columbia (MURR II), is as good as any reactor proposed to date, with respect to high intensity and purity; in addition, it can be easily modified for clinical applications at minimal cost (16).

RADIOBIOLOGICAL PARAMETERS

$^{10}B(n,\alpha)^7Li$ and $^{14}N(n,p)^{14}C$ Reaction. The RBE of the $^{10}B(n,\alpha)^7Li$ reaction were determined to be ~2.5 for uniformly distributed boron in the form of H$_3$BO$_3$ (7). Further calculations and studies showed that the "RBE" of any boron compound will be strongly dependent upon intra (or extra) cellular distribution (8); an experimental technique was devised to evaluate the intracellular distribution of "unknown" compounds (9). The RBE for the $^{14}N(n,p)^{14}C$ reaction was determined to be ~2.0 (7).

Fast neutrons. The RBE of fast (and epithermal) neutrons was measured with hamster V-79 cells irradiated in air at the "point of irradiation" (center of the bare port face) in Fig. 1. The RBE of ~2.2 was determined by comparison of D$_0$ values obtained with the neutrons, and 250 kV$_p$ x-rays as shown in Fig. 2 (10). It is of interest to note that while ~95% of the neutrons are in the epithermal range (0.5 eV to 10 keV) only ~15% of the H recoil dose comes from these neutrons, while the bulk of the dose comes from neutrons with energies of a few hundred keV. Thus, there are no untoward biological effects resulting from utilization of predominantly epithermal neutron beams.

Normal Tissue Tolerance. Dog irradiations being carried out by P. Gavin and associates at the BMRR epithermal neutron beam are designed to determine the limiting or "critical" tissue for head irradiations, in anticipation of treating brain tumors with BSH. Following irradiations of normal dogs with a 5 x 10 cm field, post administration of BSH, it was found (4,5) that:

    a. The highest physical dose occurred at ~3 cm;

    b. Severe neurological disease was observed at doses (to blood) exceeding 38 Gy;

It was concluded that:

    c. "... it is clear that the radiation changes (in normal brain) are from direct endothelial damage." and that

    d. "The dose distribution for the various components is driven mainly by the tissue boron concentration.

    e. Endothelium (in normal brain) was identified as the "critical tissue" (4).

From the above, it can be concluded that CNS should be the critical tissue for NCT irradiation with a 5 x 10 cm field, or larger, as the relative contribution from the $^{10}B(n,\alpha)^7Li$ reaction will increase as field size increases. It is anticipated that a 10 x 10 cm field (or larger) will be employed in clinical trials. It is important to note that, since a single acute exposure of ~2000 rads from photons would be

Table 3. Evaluation of BBB Integrity Following BNCT

Treatment	Group					
	t(h)	I	t(h)	II	t(h)	III
BSH	0	+	0	+	0	+
BMRR (2.1×10^{13} n/cm^2)	1	+		-		-
BSH	24	+	24	+		-
^{10}B in blood	25	12.2 ± 1.8	25	8.8 ± 1.0	1	12.1 ± 0.7
(number of mice)		(10)		(10)		(11)
^{10}B in brain	25	0.1 ± 0.0	25	0.1 ± 0.1	1	0.2 ± 0.1
(number of mice)		(9)		(8)		(8)

expected to produce necrosis in normal brain, it is evident that at least with BSH, there is a significant geometrical protection factor as predicted by Rydin et al., resulting from irradiation of endothelial cells from within the blood vessel only (11). Using numbers provided above, i.e., tolerance ≈ 2000 rads, blood dose from boron ~3800 rads, RBE (for uniform ^{10}B distribution) ~2.5, this protection factor would be ~4. While further refinement of the data is required, it is evident that such a geometrical protection exists, and is no doubt in part responsible for the efficacy reported by Joel et al. in the treatment of an intracranial rat tumor with BSSB (12).

Fractionation and the Blood Brain Barrier (BBB). There has been considerable concern on the part of some investigators regarding the possibility of breakdown of the BBB following fractionated irradiations in BNCT. Review papers have indicated that this possibility is somewhat remote with respect to the parameters encountered in BNCT (17). Experiments were recently performed in our laboratory in which possible breakdown of the BBB was evaluated in mice following delivery of 2.1×10^{13} n/cm^2, or 2100 rads (5250 rads x RBE) to the blood from the ^{10}B(n,α)^{7}Li reaction produced by BSH (18). This dose was obtained by irradiating mice ~70 min after administration of BSH, such that the blood concentration at the time of irradiation was ~12 μg ^{10}B/g. It is anticipated that BNCT will be carried out with a maximum fluence of ~5 x 10^{12} n/cm^2, and surely no more than 10^{13} n/cm^2 (1). With 4 fractions, the maximum fluence per fraction would be $\leq$2.5 x 10^{12}; thus, the current experiment involved the delivery of ~10x more thermal neutron fluence than would be encountered clinically (in a single fraction). Assessment of the BBB integrity was made by measuring ^{10}B concentration in normal brain at 24 hours following irradiation and the second application of BSH. Neutron autoradiographic techniques were used for this evaluation, with a sensitivity of 0.1 μg ^{10}B/g (22). Results are shown in Table 3.

Clearly there was no leakage of ^{10}B across the BBB of normal (irradiated) brain, indicating that in BNCT the integrity of the BBB would be retained in fractionated regimens (18).

TREATMENT PLANNING AND ISODOSE CHARTS

Given the availability of an optimized epithermal neutron beam, whose radiobiological parameters have been documented, it is necessary to develop a treatment planning capability. Upon successful completion of phase I clinical trials (distribution studies) with a boronated compound showing promising pharmacokinetic characteristics, therapy trials can then be initiated.

The consensus is that MCNP calculations are best suited for such evaluations. The distribution of the various beam components down the central axis of a TE cylindrical phantom have been calculated for an incident 2 keV beam. Such a standard geometry can be used for intercomparison between laboratories. Similar distributions were calculated for the BMRR epithermal beam (19). Isodose charts for each beam component were constructed from these data, using a program developed by two of us (RMB and AS). For example, an isodose chart for thermal neutrons is shown in Fig. 3. Similar charts are available for each component, with and without RBE, as desired. Additionally, 3-D plots are also available as is indicated in Fig. 4, for thermal neutrons.

COMPOUND DEVELOPMENT

As documented in papers presented at this Symposium, biological efficacy has been demonstrated for BSSB and BPA in an intracranial rat glioma. It is somewhat troubling that, although BSSB and BPA as well as boronated porphyrins demonstrate significantly greater biological efficacy than does BSH, both *in vitro* and *in vivo* (9,20), the latter compound is nevertheless being prepared for clinical trials both in the US and Europe.

It is our opinion that the full potential of NCT will be realized upon the exploitation of boronated

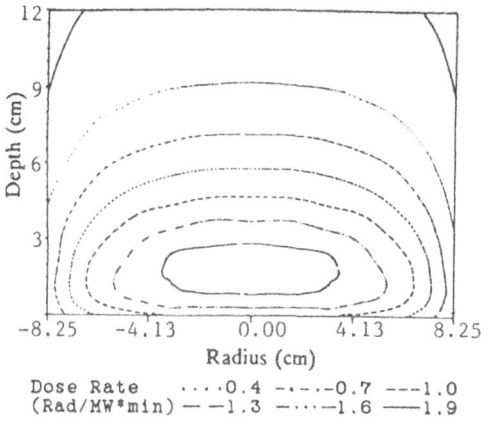

Dose Rate ····0.4 —·—·−0.7 −−−1.0
(Rad/MW*min) −−1.3 −···−1.6 −−−1.9

Fig. 3. THERMAL NEUTRON DOSE

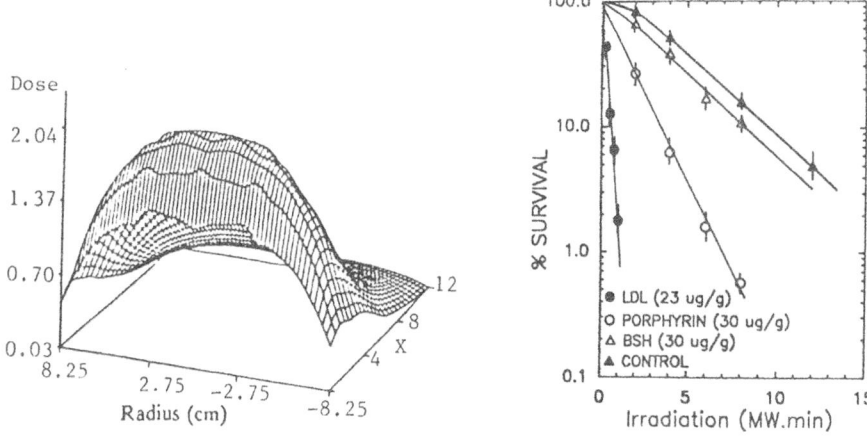

LDL (23 ug/g)
PORPHYRIN (30 ug/g)
BSH (30 ug/g)
CONTROL

Fig. 4. THERMAL NEUTRON DOSE   Fig. 5. CELL SURVIVAL

biomolecules showing selective and long term binding to tumor cells. Such characteristics will enable normal tissue to clear, and permit the superposition of boron concentration and distribution, following compound administration, to be of benefit in fractionated therapy.

While BSH, BSSB and BPA all demonstrated transient association with tumor, compounds are available which demonstrate high uptake and long term binding to tumor cells. In Fig. 5 the *in vitro* response to thermal neutrons of cells incubated in the presence of a boronated porphyrin (BOPP), and a boronated low density lipoprotein (B-LDL) is compared to BSH (cells washed before irradiation in boron-free medium, to reveal the effects of bound boron only). Figure 5 illustrates that the porphyrin (BOPP) is ~10x more effective than BSH, and that the B-LDL is ~10x more effective than BOPP (20,21). Clearly, significant increases in therapeutic gain will be best accomplished through the exploitation of such compounds.

ACKNOWLEDGMENTS

This research was carried out under the auspices of the U.S. Department of Energy under Contract No. DE-ACO2-76CH00016, and National Institute of Health, Grant No. CA37961.

REFERENCES

1.   Fairchild, R.G., Saraf, S.K., Kalef-Ezra, J., and Laster, B.H.   Comparison of measured parameters from a 24 keV and a broad spectrum epithermal neutron beam for neutron capture therapy (NCT): An identification of consequential parameters. *Med. Phys.* 17, 1045-1052 (1990).

5

2. Fairchild, R.G., Bond, V.P., and Woodhead, A., Eds. *Clinical Aspects of Neutron Capture Therapy.* Basic Sciences Series, Vol. 50, Plenum Press, New York (1989).

3. Fairchild, R.G., Kalef-Ezra, J., Saraf, S.K., Fiarman, S., Ramsay, E., Wielopolski, L., Laster, B., and Wheeler, F. Installation and testing of an optimized epithermal neutron beam at the Brookhaven Medical Research Reactor. *Proc. of Workshop on Neutron Beam Design, Development and Performance for Neutron Capture Therapy.* O.K. Harling, J.A. Bernard, and R.G. Zamenhof, Eds. Pg. 185-200, Vol. 54 Basic Life Sciences. Plenum Press, New York (1990).

4. Gavin, P.R., DeHaan, C.E., Kraft, S.L., and Moore, M.P. Dosimetric considerations: Radiation tolerance of the normal canine brain following boron neutron capture therapy. *Proc. Radiation Research Meeting,* New Orleans, 1990.

5. DeHaan, C.E., Gavin, P.R., Kraft, S.L., and Leathers, C.W. The effects of boron neutron capture therapy on the normal canine brain: Gross and histological observations. *Proc. Rad. Res. Meeting,* New Orleans, 1990.

6. Sen. J. McClure: Letter to Adm. J. Watkins, Aug. 22, 1990.

7. Gabel, D., Fairchild, R.G., Borner, H.G., and Larsson, B. The relative biological effectiveness in V79 Chinese hamster cells of the neutron capture reactions in boron and nitrogen. *Radiat. Res.* 98, 307-316 (1984).

8. Gabel, D., Foster, S., and Fairchild, R.G. The Monte-Carlo simulation of the biological effect of the $^{10}B(n,\alpha)^{7}Li$ reaction in cells and tissue and its implication for boron neutron capture therapy. *Radiat. Res.* 111, 14-25 (1987).

9. Fairchild, R.G., Kahl, S.B., Laster, B.H., Kalef-Ezra, J., and Popenoe, E.A. *In vitro* determination of uptake, retention, distribution, biological efficacy and toxicity of boronated compounds for neutron capture therapy: A comparison of porphyrins with sulfhydryl boron hydrides. *Cancer Res.* 50, 4860-4865 (1990).

10. Fairchild, R.G., Laster, B.H., and Kalef-Ezra, J. RBE of fast and epithermal neutrons at the BMRR epithermal neutron beam. In preparation.

11. Rydin, R.A., Deutsch, O.L., and Murray, B.W. *Phys. Med. Biol.* 21, 134-138 (1976).

12. Joel, D.D., Fairchild, R.G.,, Laissue, J.A., Saraf, S.K., Kalef-Ezra, J.A., and Slatkin, D.N. Boron Neutron Capture of intracellular rat gliosarcoma. *Proc. Nat. Acad. Sci.* In press (Dec. 1990).

13. Gabel, D. Goals of the European Collaboration on BNCT. (This Conference).

14. Fairchild, R.G., Kalef-Ezra, J., Fiarman, S., and Wheeler, F. Physics aspects of boron neutron capture therapy: Epithermal neutron beam optimization. *Proceedings of 1988 International Reactor Physics Conference,* Jackson Hole, Wyoming. Sept. 18-21, Vol. II, pp. 423-432 (1988).

15. Parsons, D.K., Wheeler, F.J., Rushton, B.C., and Nigg, D.W. Neutronic design of the INEL facility for BNCT clinical trials. *Proceedings of 1988 International Reactor Physics Conference,* Jackson Hole, Wyoming. Sept. 18-21, Vol. II, pp. 433-442 (1988).

16. Brugger, R.M., and Shih, J.A. Personal communication.

17. Gregoire, V., Keyeux, A., and Wambersie, A. Blood-brain barrier impairment after irradiation: Implication in BNCT. *Clinical Aspects of NCT,* R. Fairchild, V. Bond and A. Woodhead, Eds. Basic Life Sciences, Vol. 50, pp 299-310. Plenum Press, New York (1989).

18. Kalef-Ezra, J., Laster, B.H., and Fairchild, R.G. Integrity of the blood brain barrier following fractionated BNCT. In preparation.

19. Gajewski, J., Ramsay, E.B., Reinstein, L.E., Saraf, S., and Fairchild, R.G. Monte Carlo calculations results for the epithermal neutron beam at the Medical Reactor. (This Conference).

20. Laster, B.H., Kahl, S.B., Koo, M.-S., and Fairchild, R.G. Biological efficacy of a boronated porphyrin for neutron capture therapy in a murine tumor. Submitted.

21. Laster, B.H., Kahl, S.B., Popenoe, E.A., and Fairchild, R.G. Biological efficacy of boronated low density lipoproteins (LDL) for Neutron Capture Therapy (NCT) as measured in cell culture. Submitted.

22. Gabel, D., Holstein, H., Larsson, B., Gille, L., Eriksson, C., Sacker, D., Som, P., and Fairchild, R.G. Quantitative Neutron Capture radiography for studying the biodistribution of boron-containing compounds. *Cancer Res.* 47, 5451-5454 (1987).

23. Choi, JR., Zamenhof, R.G., Yanch, J.C., Rogus, R., and Harling, O.K. Performance of the currently available epithermal neutron beam at the Massachusetts Institute of Technology Research Reactor (MITRII). This symposium.

THE PETTEN BNCT PROJECT

R.L.Moss[1], F.Stecher-Rasmussen[2], R.Huiskamp[2], L.Dewit[3]
and B.Mijnheer[3]

[1]Commission of the European Communities, Joint Research
 Centre, Petten, The Netherlands
[2]Netherlands Energy Research Foundation ECN, Petten
 The Netherlands
[3]Netherlands Cancer Institute, Amsterdam, The Netherlands

INTRODUCTION

The revival of BNCT over the last decade, stimulated the formation in
1987 of the European Collaboration group on BNCT. The multi-disciplinary
nature of BNCT has drawn together groups of researchers from many
European institutes who are now collaborating in an effort to achieve the
implementation of BNCT in Europe at the earliest possible date. To accomplish this, it was well recognised that of the two basic preconditions
for successful BNCT, namely: i) the accumulation of enough boron in the
tumour cells with sufficient clearance of the surrounding tissues and ii)
the delivery of enough thermal neutrons at the tumour site to give rise
to a sufficient number of capture events; it was the latter, with respect
to identifying a suitable neutron source in Europe, that needed the most
attention from the Collaboration group. The former condition had to some
extent been resolved with the use of BSH, for example, and the development of other potentially promising compounds. For the latter condition,
the neutron source had to have not only the special prerequisite nuclear
and geometric characteristics, but also the financial resources and expertise to realise a facility. It was for this reason (but not the only),
that the High Flux Materials Testing Reactor (HFR) at Petten became involved in the European BNCT project.

The paper here summarises the evolution of BNCT at Petten, the
various activities of the Petten BNCT group, its role within the European
Collaboration group, and most importantly, the achievement within 3 years
to install an epithermal neutron beam at the HFR for BNCT applications. A
summary is also given of the tasks ahead prior to the first clinical trials which are now planned for 1992.

THE EUROPEAN COLLABORATION GROUP ON BNCT

The European Collaboration group, formed in 1987, receives financial
support in the form of a Concerted Action (CA) from the Commission of the
European Communities' Medical and Health Research programme in Brussels.
This enables through direct financial support, regular meetings to be

held, and personnel and material to be exchanged between countries and institutes. The activities of the CA[1] are coordinated by the project leader, Prof.Detlef Gabel and his Project Management group, which consists of representatives from all the disciplines in BNCT. Meetings in the sub-group areas of radiobiology, chemistry, physics and clinical applications, are now held on a frequent basis. It is apparent that the relatively rapid progress on BNCT in Europe, and especially at Petten, owes greatly to this collaboration.

THE PETTEN BNCT GROUP

The local activities at Petten are managed by the Joint Research Centre of the Commission of the European Communities, the owners of the HFR. The activities are coordinated by a so-called Petten BNCT group, consisting of members of the Physics Department at the neighbouring Netherlands Energy Research Foundation (ECN) Petten and the Department of Radiotherapy at the Netherlands Cancer Institute (NKI) in Amsterdam. The group has been extended to include expertise in radiobiology (ECN and NKI) and neurosurgery (University Hospital, Leiden). The Petten work forms an important and integral part of the European Collaboration group. The European group has given the development of BNCT at Petten, and in particular the treatment of glioblastoma, its highest priority. The complementary work within the European group, for example on pharmacokinetics in patients, boron compound development, dosimetry development and supporting radiobiological work, will be used in providing the necessary data to obtain permission to start clinical trials at Petten.

THE HIGH FLUX REACTOR AND BEAM TUBE HB11

Over the last 25 years, the HFR has been used predominately for irradiation testing of materials and nuclear fuel for the European civil nuclear power programme. The reactor operates at 45MW and is cooled and moderated by light water.[2] The standard core configuration consists of 33 fuel assemblies, 6 control rods, 16 beryllium reflector elements and 17 free positions for experimental facilities. The reactor is also equipped with 12 horizontal beam tubes, used mainly for nuclear physics and solid state physics research.

It is well known in the nuclear materials testing community that the HFR is a powerful machine, being very versatile and having a policy of continuous maintenance and major upgrading of aging components, including for example, the renewal 4 years ago of the complete reactor vessel. In comparison with other similar facilities in Europe, the HFR is effectively a new reactor.

With respect to BNCT, an adequate source of neutrons can only be acquired from a high flux reactor through a large diameter beam tube, that itself faces a large source area of the reactor. The beam tube arrangement, HB11/12, satisfies these physical requirements. In addition, the exit side of the beam has a large working area for developing an irradiation room. Furthermore, the facility faces the reactor building's emergency exit, giving in effect, unhindered access. An overview of the planned lay-out is shown in Fig.1.

PRE-STUDIES FOR THE APPLICATION OF BNCT AT THE HFR

Prior to designing the required epithermal neutron beam at HB11, two pre-studies were performed. The first, carried out in October 1988, measured and confirmed the favourable nuclear characteristics at the source plane of the reactor at the front end of beam tube.[3] The second, carried out in September 1989, aimed at providing confidence in the design methods. One of the smaller beam tubes, HB7, was used where a series of nuclear measurements were performed using various combinations of filter components including aluminium, liquid argon, titanium, cadmium, sulphur and boron. In addition, to assess if the beam quality could be improved even further, the periphery beryllium elements in the reactor core adjacent to the beam tube, were exchanged for aluminium plugs and/or a reactor fuel element. The work concluded that the neutron fluence rate measurements were in good agreement with the calculations.[4]

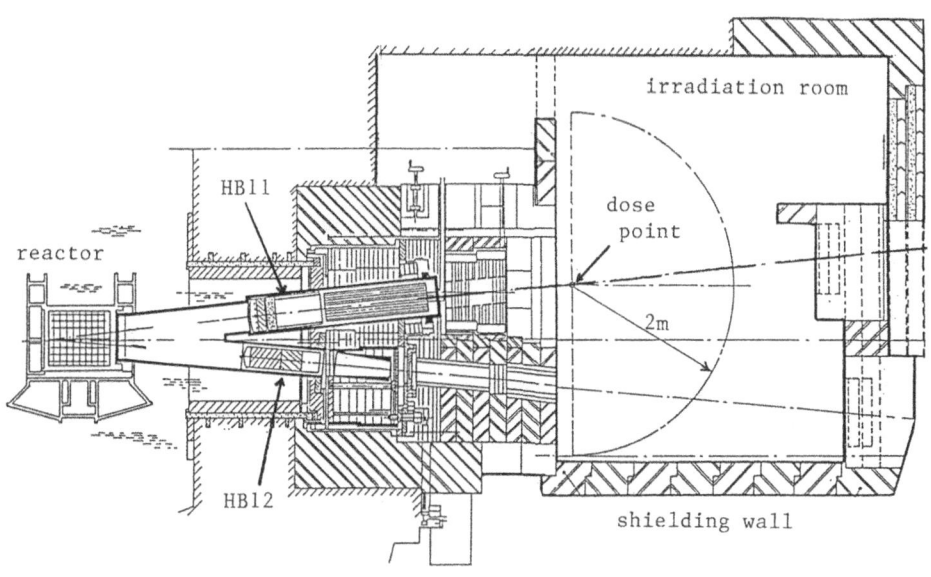

Fig 1 . Overview of the planned lay-out at HB11

DESIGN OF THE BNCT FACILITY AT HB11

The design goals, as agreed upon by the Project Management group of the European BNCT group, were :

    o neutron flux $> 1.0 \times 10^9$ neutrons / cm^2 s
                                    (at the therapy position),

    o average neutron dose $< 8.0 \times 10^{-11}$ rads cm^2/ neutron,
       (or mean neutron energy < 8.0 keV),

and   o gamma dose rate < 50 cGy / hr

The requirements were chosen to enable a treatment to be completed in a reasonable time (< 1 hour), probably in 6 fractions (≈ 10 min. each). The average neutron dose can been re-interpreted using the ICRU neutron dose function (ie. 10^{-11} rads cm^2/neutron ≈ 1 keV) to produce a mean energy in keV's. This is considered a very good indication of the quality of the beam and reflects the fast neutron contamination in the beam. The incident gamma dose rate must be sufficiently small as not to dominate the total (incident + induced) gamma dose rate at the tumour site.

The design of the facility was performed jointly between the Petten group and groups at AEA Harwell (UK) and JRC Ispra (Italy). The calculations (see Watkins, these proceedings) were performed using the Monte Carlo code, MCNP[5]. Literally hundreds of combinations of filter materials and sizes were analysed. The following combination was finally chosen :

15cm Al; 5cm S; 1cm Ti; 0.1cm Cd; and 150cm liquid Ar,

giving a predominately epithermal neutron beam that satisfies all the above criteria.

The various components, including the above filter materials, a new main beam shutter, an emergency beam shutter and new shielding blocks, were all installed in August, this year (1990). For more detail on the construction and installation features, see Moss, these proceedings.

EXPERIMENTAL PROGRAMME LEADING TO CLINICAL APPLICATIONS

Before clinical trials may begin, a series of experimental and computational work is foreseen, and indeed is required. A summary of the activities is given in the planning chart below.

Year	1990		1991				1992			
Item \ (quarter)	3	4	1	2	3	4	1	2	3	4
HB11 tests										
metrology - low power		▬								
metrology - full power			■							
commissioning & test			▬							
radiobiology										
cell culture + phantom				▬▬▬▬▬						
healthy tissue (dogs)				▬▬▬▬▬▬						
dosimetry development			▬▬▬▬▬▬▬▬▬▬▬▬							
therapy										
treatment planning				▬▬▬▬▬▬						
clinical trials										▬

Following the installation in the summer, the first nuclear measurements at low reactor power (300kW) were recently performed in November. The results are pending. Following a commissioning and testing period to satisfy the local safety requirements, further measurements are foreseen at full reactor power (45MW), when the beam will be fully characterised. With a fully operational facility, the radiobiological programme can begin. Various institutes will be involved, including JRC Petten, ECN Petten, NKI Amsterdam, AEA Harwell UK and Bremen University FRG. In vitro experiments will be performed using V79 Chinese hamster cells to biologically characterise the beam (see Huiskamp, these proceedings). In vivo experiments using mice have already been carried out to study the uptake of boronated compounds in different tumour types (see Gregoire, these proceedings). Irradiation experiments on mice to investigate the therapeutic gain of BNCT are also foreseen (see Huiskamp, these proceedings). These will be performed on the thermal neutron beam at the low flux facility at Petten. Available boron detection techniques at

Petten that will be utilised include ICP-AES and prompt gamma ray spectroscopy (see Stecher-Rasmussen, these proceedings).

Before the summer period (1991), a relatively large project using dogs (beagles) to determine the healthy tissue tolerance of the Petten beam will be started. It is considered that the tissue at most risk is not the skin but the normal brain. The dogs will be given different quantities of BSH and irradiated with graded doses of epithermal neutrons (see Huiskamp, these proceedings). The endpoint in the studies will be non-lethal vascular damage to the nervous system as measured by gadolinium-DTPA contrast enhanced magnetic resonance imaging (MRI) detectable brain lesions[6]. Besides MRI, other parameters will be investigated such as skin reactions, cellular blood count, blood chemistry, cerebrospinal fluid analysis, urine analysis and a total necropsy. The studies will be performed in close collaboration with Washington State University (Prof. P.Gavin). In addition, split dose studies (2 fractions) to evaluate the effect of low LET repair and possible damage to the blood-brain-barrier, will be carried out.

THE PROPOSED CLINICAL FACILITY

Apart from the above nuclear requirements that were implemented through astute physics and engineering design, the working area around the beam exit will be extended to produce a treatment room of dimensions 3 x 3.5 m and 2 m in height. This gives sufficient space to allow the head of the patient to be irradiated from two laterally opposing directions. In addition, the working area outside the shielded area of the treatment room is sufficient for placing instrumentation for medical observation purposes. Access to the facility from outside, fortuitously coincides with the reactor building's emergency exit which gives access without hinderance to normal reactor operations. An artists impression showing an overview of the treatment room, beam tube and reactor vessel is shown below.

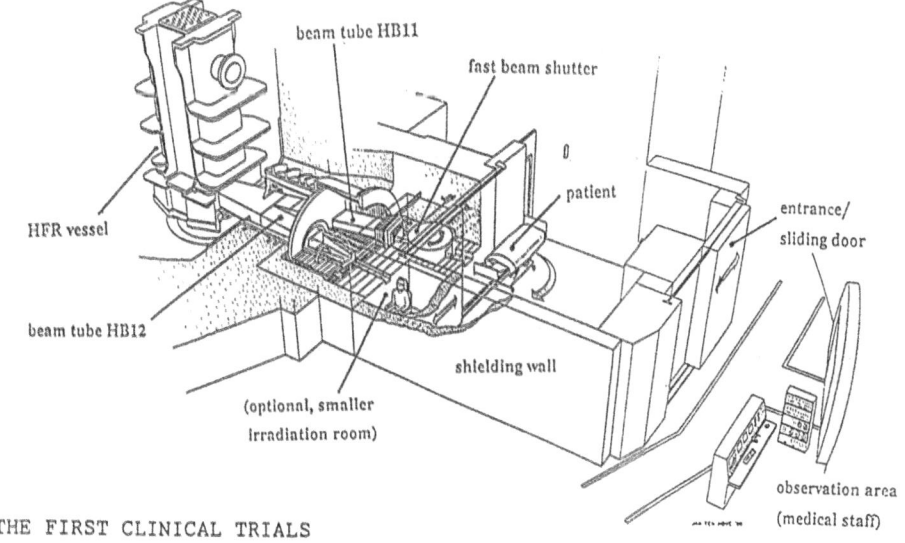

THE FIRST CLINICAL TRIALS

The start of clinical trials are presently planned for the latter half of 1992. The clinical pilot studies (see Dewit, these proceedings) include : pharmacokinetic studies with BSH in human patients, which have already started with hospitals at Bremen, Lausanne and Uppsala participating; fractionated pharmacokinetic studies to investigate, after repeated administration of BSH, if a modified fractionation schedule is needed; the development of a treatment planning scheme combining experimental results from phantom irradiations, computational work using MCNP and graphics packages, and the provision of patient data on tumour size and site; and lastly, the start of post-operative BNCT treatment of glioblastoma patients.

CONCLUDING REMARKS

Following the formation of both the European Collaboration group and the Petten BNCT group, the relatively rapid progress towards the implementation of BNCT at Petten owes greatly to the catalytic effect of these well-coordinated, multi-national, multi-disciplinary, groups. The apparent physical and geometric advantages of the HFR at Petten have been fully exploited, culminating recently in the installion of the epithermal neutron beam at beam tube HB11.

During the next 2 years, an extensive programme of experimental work should make it possible, providing no unforeseen problems arise, for the first clinical trials in Europe to start at Petten during 1992.

ACKNOWLEDGEMENTS

The funding of the European Collaboration group on BNCT and the main funding for the Petten facility are provided by the Medical Health and Research Programme of the Commission of the European Communities.

REFERENCES

1. Gabel,D., "Approach to Boron Neutron Capture Therapy in Europe: Goals of a European Collaboration on Boron Neutron Capture Therapy", Proc. 2nd. Eur. Particle Accelerator Conf., Nice, (1990)

2. Röttger,H. et al.,"High Flux Materials Testing Reactor Petten, Characteristics of the Facilities and Standard Irradiation Devices", Report", EUR 5700 EN, (1986/87).

3. Moss, R.L., "Progress towards Boron Neutron Capture Therapy at the High Flux Reactor Petten", Neutron Beam Design, Development and Performance for Neutron Capture Therapy, Basic Life Sciences, Vol.54, Plenum Press, (1990).

4. Constantine,G., Watkins,P.R.D., Perks,C., Dellafield,H., Ross,D., Voorbraak,W., Paardekooper,A., Freudenreich,W., Stecher-Rasmussen,F., Moss,R.L., "Progress in neutron beam development at the HFR Petten (Feasibility study for a BNCT facility)", Proc. 7th ASTM-EURATOM Symposium on Reactor Dosimetry, August 1990, Strasbourg, France.

5. Breimeister, J.F.(Ed), "MCNP - A General Monte Carlo Code for Neutron and Photon Transport", LA-7596-M, Rev.2.

6. Gavin,P.R., Kraft,S.L., Wendling,L.R. and Miller,D.L., "Canine spontaneous brain tumors - a large animal model for BNCT", Strahlenther. Onkol. 165 (1989).

THE IDAHO POWER BURST FACILITY/BORON NEUTRON CAPTURE

THERAPY (PBF/BNCT) PROGRAM OVERVIEW

Ronald V. Dorn III,[1,2] Merle L. Griebenow, Arlene L. Ackermann, Lowell G. Miller,[1] Patrick R. Gavin,[3] David L. Miller, Floyd J. Wheeler, Kenneth M. Bradshaw,[1] Todd L. Richards,[4] Daniel E. Wessol, Yale D. Harker, David W. Nigg, Peter D. Randolph, and William F. Bauer[1]

[1]PBF/BNCT Research Programs, Idaho National Engineering Laboratory, Idaho Falls, ID
[2]Mountain States Tumor Institute, Boise, ID
[3]College of Veterinary Medicine, Washington State University, Pullman, WA
[4]Imaging Research Laboratory, University of Washington, Seattle, WA

INTRODUCTION

The Power Burst Facility/Boron Neutron Capture Therapy (PBF/BNCT) Program has been funded since 1988 to evaluate brain tumor treatment using $Na_2B_{12}H_{11}SH$ (borocaptate sodium or BSH) and epithermal neutrons. The PBF/BNCT Program pursues this goal as a comprehensive, multidisciplinary, multiorganizational endeavor applying modern program management techniques. The initial focus was to: (1) establish a representative large animal model and (2) develop the generic analytical and measurement capabilities required to control treatment repeatability and determine critical treatment parameters independent of tumor type and body location. This paper will identify the PBF/BNCT Program elements and summarize the status of some of the developed capabilities.

ORGANIZATIONAL STRUCTURE

The PBF/BNCT Program is structured with a number of interconnected, parallel research projects and core components (Figures 1 and 2). The various tasks (Figure 3) within the individual projects use the expertise of a number of organizations from coast to coast in the United States (Figure 4) resulting in a program of truly national scope. There is extensive interaction of the PBF/BNCT Program with many other BNCT research endeavors both within and outside the United States. Projects and tasks within the Program will be reviewed with respect to: (1) goal and rationale and (2) results and current status.

GROSS BORON ANALYSIS (Project 1, Task 1)

Comprehensive investigation of BNCT, whether at the biological level or clinical level, requires boron content analysis of multiple biological (tissue and blood) samples to fully characterize differential boron concentration and distribution. The necessity for a rapid, reproducible technique to accomplish this task (without the requirement for a reactor) is addressed in this task. Inductively coupled plasma-atomic emission spectroscopy (ICP-AES) has been developed as the reference procedure for this task. Once developed, the ICP-AES technique has been refined, increasing the sensitivity and throughput, and has been used to analyze thousands of biological samples in support of the PBF/BNCT Program. This technology has been recognized as a valuable resource and international standard by the BNCT research community.[2,3]

ANALYTICAL METHODOLOGIES DEVELOPMENT FOR BORON COMPOUND PURITY (Project 1, Task 2)

Prior to the institution of the PBF/BNCT Program, it was recognized that BNCT research with the BSH compound would require the ability to determine compound purity to allow reproducibility of experimental data. Previous work with this compound did not include purity/consistency analyses, resulting in a level of uncertainty in the results. Boron compound purity analysis procedures have been developed and transferred to the boron drug (BSH) manufacturer for use in their quality control procedures. In addition, the technology was included in the U.S. Food and Drug Administration (FDA) Investigational New Drug (IND) application submitted by Ohio State University researchers to allow the use of BSH in clinical studies.

SUBCELLULAR BORON DISTRIBUTION (Project 1, Task 4)

The efficiency of, indeed the success of, BNCT lies in the uptake of the boron compound into the malignant tumor cell. Knowledge of boron concentration at the macroscopic level, while important, must be supplemented by information concerning boron concentration and location at the cellular and subcellular level to allow for determination of BNCT efficacy and precise microdosimetry. Secondary Ion Microscopy (SIMS) has been demonstrated to have the capability of quantifying intra- and intercellular boron. Tissue acquisition and preparation procedures have been qualified and the technology is now being transferred to an analytical support laboratory for routine use in biological samples. Research continues into other technologies that may allow more rapid and precise determination of boron at the cellular level.[1]

NONINVASIVE BORON QUANTIFICATION (Project 1, Task 5)

The _routine_ clinical (and even experimental) application of BNCT clearly must involve the ability to assess the presence and concentration of the boron compound within the tissues of interest in a noninvasive fashion. Development of this technology was felt to be necessary in support of animal pharmacokinetic studies, proposed human pharmacokinetic studies, and hopefully, to accommodate patient screening for treatment suitability. With the acknowledgement of this requirement, PBF/BNCT Program researchers focused on Magnetic Resonance Imaging and Spectroscopy (MRI/S). Analysis of the problem indicated specific requirements: (1) hardware modification of the standard clinical MRI system in the areas of radiofrequency (RF) subsystem changes for 20.5 Mhz (^{11}B) and 6.86 MHz (^{10}B), and RF coil development; and (2) software development for short T2 (approximately 600 microseconds) to allow whole-head boron MR spectroscopy and two- and three-dimensional chemical shift imaging (CSI). The technology has now been developed and demonstrated in the following studies:

1. Whole-head boron MR spectroscopy has been successfully performed and correlated with tissue-sample ICP-AES analysis (in the large-animal model system) permitting noninvasive BSH pharmacokinetic studies, and

2. Successful CSI imaging has been correlated with standard proton anatomical images showing boron concentration location in two- and three-dimensions.

Research continues in both hardware and software areas to develop more rapid data acquisition and finer detail.[4,5,15]

ANALYTICAL RADIATION TRANSPORT AND INTERACTION MODELING (Project 1, Task 7)

BNCT is certainly the most complicated form of radiation therapy ever delivered to biological systems. The total radiation dose is a combina-

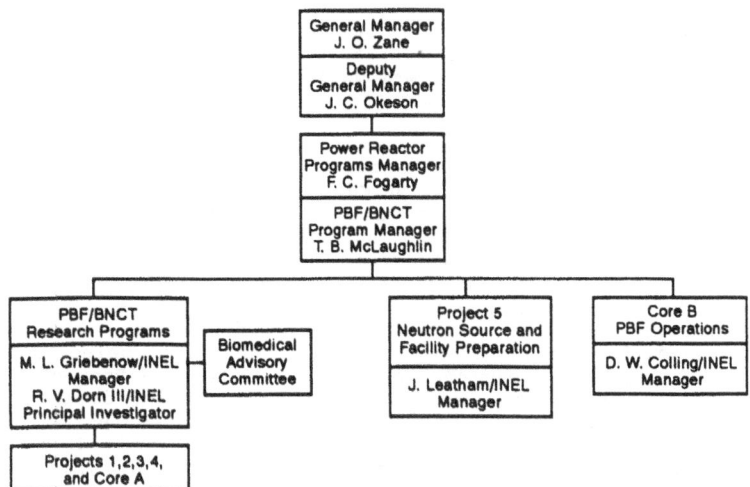

Figure 1. EG&G Idaho, Inc. PBF/BNCT Program organization.

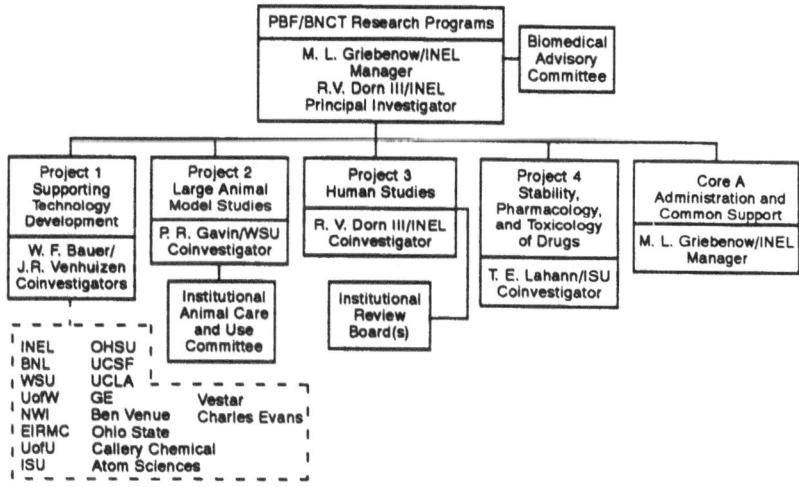

Figure 2. PBF/BNCT Research Programs organization.

tion of a mixed beam of incident radiations (thermal neutrons, epithermal neutrons, fast neutrons, gamma rays) plus the variety of radiations produced by the boron capture event (lithium ion, alpha particle, gamma rays) and capture events with other elements such as nitrogen and hydrogen. In addition, the mix of incident radiations varies considerably depending on the particular reactor source and filter used; the boron capture component (as a percentage of the total radiation dose) varies according to the boron concentration at the time of the irradiation. Finally, expected cell lethality will be greatly affected by the intracellular location of the boron and the resultant microdosimetry. As a consequence, the radiation dose-modeling tool needed for BNCT must be far more complex and rigorous than that used for more conventional types of irradiation.

The considerable effort to develop such a capability with the PBF/BNCT Program has successfully produced a true three-dimensional, dose-distribution tool that has been validated against measurements. This Monte-Carlo-based system has been successfully used in support of the PBF/BNCT Program effort (in conjunction with Core A and Project 1, Task 6) to design, install, and characterize the epithermal-neutron beam "filter" at the Brookhaven Medical Research Reactor (BMRR). In addition, it is now being routinely used to calculate and predict total and component radiation doses for the large animal model irradiations being conducted by the PBF/BNCT Program's research team at the BMRR (see Project 2 below). Current research activities within this task are being directed toward: (1) a parallel, deterministic, three-dimensional, dose-distribution tool, (2) increasing computational speed and efficiency, and (3) interfacing this computational tool with three-dimensional anatomical information and display. The three-dimensional, anatomical, display software, with reconstruction from computed tomography (CT) or MRI scans, has been developed under subcontract with the University of Utah.[13,16-21]

LARGE ANIMAL MODEL STUDIES (Project 2)

At the onset of the PBF/BNCT Program, it was determined that a large animal model using spontaneous tumors was required to fully investigate epithermal-based BNCT: (1) to provide sufficient tissue mass to thermalize the epithermal neutrons, without delivering excessive whole-body radiation doses, (2) the dosimetry of epithermal-based BNCT of deep-seated tumors is very different from thermal BNCT of surface tumors, (3) epithermal (as opposed to thermal) BNCT will be required if BNCT is to become a significant treatment modality for large numbers of human tumors, and (4) a spontaneous tumor with its in-vivo blood supply is a far better model for the assessment of boron compound adequacy than are implantable tumors or tissue culture.

Project 2, under the direction of Dr. Patrick R. Gavin at the College of Veterinary Medicine at Washington State University, has successfully pioneered the use of the spontaneous brain tumor dog model for the study of epithermal BNCT and has achieved the following accomplishments:[6,10,11,14]

1. The spontaneous canine brain tumor recruitment network is operational, accruing 1-2 subjects a month.

2. Canine, intravenous-administration, BSH kinetics have been established showing therapeutic tumor concentrations, low normal-brain parenchyma concentration, and blood, scalp, retina, and tongue concentrations equivalent to tumor concentration.

3. Plasmapheresis has been shown to reduce blood-brain concentration by approximately 30% with no commensurate reduction in tissue or tumor-boron content.

4. Twelve (12) tumor dogs have been treated with single-dose epithermal BNCT with remarkably rapid tumor response and encouraging tumor control (longest survival now 13 months) with 14.5-29 ppm ^{10}B in blood, and 16.5-22 Gy maximum total dose.

Of perhaps greater importance, initial canine, gross dose-tolerance studies have been completed (with the BMRR reactor) showing:[7,9,12] (1)

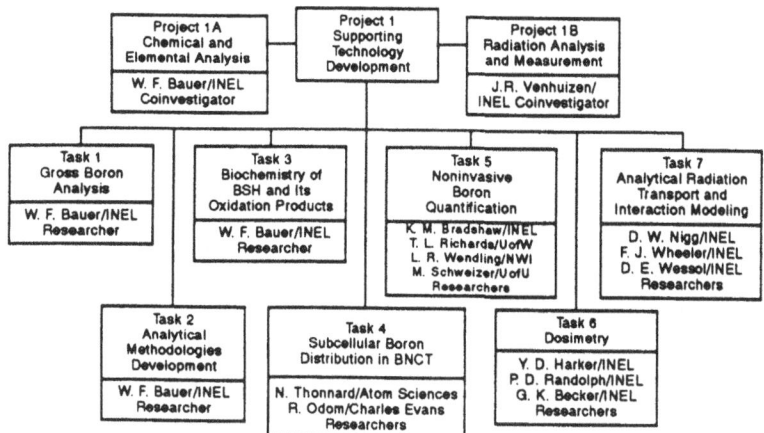

Figure 3. PBF/BNCT Research Programs Project 1 organization.

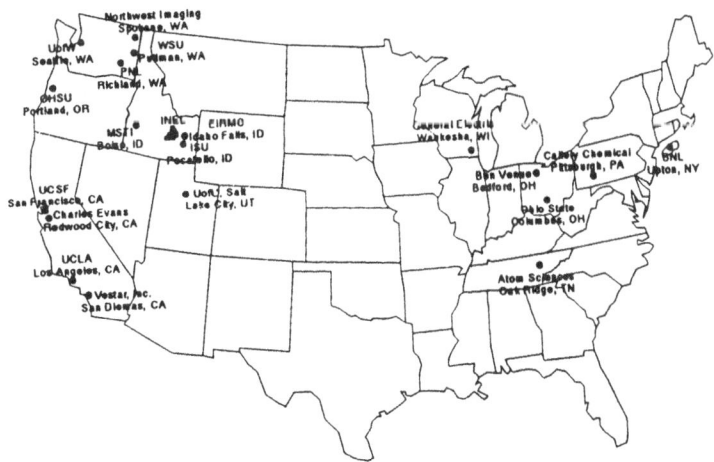

Figure 4. PBF/BNCT Program participating organizations.

radiation (beam only) scalp tolerance between 10 and 15 Gy, (2) 25 ppm ^{10}B interbrain tolerance of 21 $\pm$ 2 Gy, (3) 50 ppm ^{10}B interbrain tolerance of 28 $\pm$ 2 Gy, and (4) significant normal, interbrain vascular endothelium and skin/muscle dose sparing from the boron-capture reaction.

Further, and of critical importance, the canine dose-tolerance studies have demonstrated that the relative biological effectiveness (RBE) of the fast-neutron beam contaminant is approximately 4-6 (unpublished data), emphasizing the vital need to reduce the amount of this contaminant in epithermal beams intended for use in human clinical trials.

DISCUSSION AND FUTURE DIRECTIONS

During the three years since its initial activation and funding, the PBF/BNCT Program's research has demonstrated the efficacy of a comprehensive, multidisciplinary, multiorganizational program applying modern program management techniques. Significant advances have been made in multiple areas, helping to bring the BNCT research community closer to the realization of large clinical trials. Extensive cooperation with the other exciting international and U.S. BNCT research programs further contributes to this progress.

Expansion of the PBF/BNCT Program is currently taking place in: (1) a comprehensive, parallel PBF/BNCT Program for melanoma is being activated that will also use a spontaneous canine tumor model (oral melanoma), and will establish additional mechanisms for screening promising new boron compounds,[8] and (2) funding has been received for and work begun on modifying the Power Burst Facility (PBF) reactor for use in future BNCT research. The availability of this resource will permit expanded epithermal- and thermal-BNCT research, efficient studies of fractionation vs single dose, dose-rate studies, and design-requirement information for future BNCT radiation sources -- in short, a valuable addition to the international resources available for BNCT research.

REFERENCES

1. Ausserer, W. A., "Quantitative Imaging of Boron, Calcium, Magnesium, Potassium, and Sodium Distributions in Cultured Cells with Ion Microscopy," Analytical Chemistry 61: (24) 2690-2695 (1988).

2. Bauer, W. F., et al., "Flow Injection for Sample Introduction into Inductively Coupled Plasmas for the Determination of Boron in Biological Samples," Fourth International Symposium on Neutron Capture Therapy for Cancer, Sydney, New South Wales, Australia, December 4-7, 1990.

3. Bauer, W. F., et al., "Comparison of Digestion Procedures Used for the Determination of Boron in Animal Tissues by Inductively Coupled Plasma-Atomic Emission Spectroscopy," Analytical Chemistry (submitted for publication April 1989).

4. Bradshaw, K. M., et al., "Interactions Between Boron Containing Compounds and Serum Albumin Observed by Nuclear Magnetic Resonance," fourth International Symposium on Neutron Capture Therapy for Cancer, Sydney, New South Wales, Australia, December 4-7, 1990.

5. Bradshaw, K. M., et al., "In-Vivo Pharmacokinetic Evaluation of Boron Compounds Using Magnetic Resonance Spectroscopy and Imaging," Fourth International Symposium on Neutron Capture Therapy for Cancer, Sydney, New South Wales, Australia, December 4-7, 1990.

6. DeHaan, C. E., et al., "The Response of Spontaneously-Occurring Canine Brain Tumors to BNCT Using CT and MRI," (oral presentation) American College of Veterinary Radiology Meeting, Chicago, IL, April 1990.

7. DeHaan, C. E., at al., "Acute and Late Reactions Following Epithermal-Neutron Irradiation of the Normal Canine Brain," Fourth International Symposium on Neutron Capture Therapy for Cancer, Sydney, New South Wales, Australia, December 4-7, 1990.

8. Gavin, P. R., et al., "Spontaneous Canine Oral Melanoma: A Large Animal Model for BNCT," _Fourth International Symposium on Neutron Capture Therapy for Cancer, Sydney, New South Wales, Australia, December 4-7, 1990._

9. Gavin, P. R., et al., "Regional and Total Body Dose Following BNCT Epithermal Head Irradiation: Biologic and Dosimetric Evaluation," _Fourth International Symposium on Neutron Capture Therapy for Cancer, Sydney, New South Wales, Australia, December 4-7, 1990._

10. Gavin, P. R., et al., A Large Animal Model for Boron Neutron Capture Therapy," _Fourth International Symposium on Neutron Capture Therapy for Cancer, Sydney, New South Wales, Australia, December 4-7, 1990._

11. Gavin, P. R., et al., "The Magnetic Resonance and Computed Tomographic Features of Canine Brain Tumors Following Boron Neutron Capture Therapy," _American Society of Therapeutic Radiology and Oncology Annual Meeting, Miami, FL, October 1990._

12. Gavin, P. R., et al., "Acute and Late Reactions Following Boron Neutron Capture Epithermal-Neutron Therapy in Dogs with Spontaneous Brain Tumors," _Fourth International Symposium on Neutron Capture Therapy for Cancer, Sydney, New South Wales, Australia, December 4-7, 1990._

13. Harker, Y. D., et al., "Spectral Characterization of the Epithermal-Neutron Beam at the Brookhaven Medical Research Reactor (BMRR)," _1990 ANS Meeting, Nashville, TN, August 1990._

14. Kraft, S. L., et al., "The Biodistribution of Boron in Canine Spontaneous Intracranial Tumors Following Borocaptate Sodium Infusion," _Fourth International Symposium on Neutron Capture Therapy for Cancer, Sydney, New South Wales, Australia, December 4-7, 1990._

15. Madden, D. M., et al., "A Demonstration of Three-Dimensional Radiation Transport Theory Dose Distribution Analysis for Boron Neutron Capture Therapy," _Medical Physics Journal_ (submitted May 1990).

16. Nigg, D. W., et al., "A Demonstration of Three-Dimensional Radiation Transport Theory Dose Distribution Analysis for Boron Neutron Capture Therapy," _Medical Physics Journal_ (submitted May 1990).

17. Nigg, D. W., et al., "Characterization of the BMRR and PBF Epithermal-Neutron Beam in Phantom Using Three-Dimensional Deterministic Radiation Transport Theory," _Fourth International Symposium on Neutron Capture Therapy for Cancer, Sydney, New South Wales, Australia, December 4-7, 1990._

18. Wessol, D. E., et al., "Interactive Generation of 3-D, B-Spline Objects from Planar Image Data for Multidimensional Analysis," (oral presentation/poster) _Society of Exploration Geophysicists, San Francisco, CA, 1990._

19. Wheeler, F. J., "Beyond the Epithermal-Neutron Beam: The Analytical Physicist's Role," _Fourth International Symposium on Neutron Capture Therapy for Cancer, Sydney, New South Wales, Australia, December 4-7, 1990._

20. Wheeler, F. J., et al., "Analytical Dosimetry for Spontaneous-Tumor Dogs Receiving BNCT," _Fourth International Symposium on Neutron Capture Therapy for Cancer, Sydney, New South Wales, Australia, December 4-7, 1990._

21. Wheeler, F. J., et al., "Dose Prediction Models for Canine Brain Irradiations for Boron Neutron Capture Therapy Research," _American Society of Therapeutic Radiology and Oncology Annual Meeting, Miami, FL, 1990._

THE NEUTRON CAPTURE THERAPY RESEARCH PROGRAM AT NEW ENGLAND MEDICAL CENTER AND THE MASSACHUSETTS INSTITUTE OF TECHNOLOGY

R.Zamenhof[1], H.Madoc-Jones[1], O.Harling[2], D.Wazer[1], S.Saris[1], J.Yanch[2], G.Solares[1], G.Rogers[3]

[1]Tufts University School of Medicine and New England Medical Center Hospitals, Boston, MA 02111, USA
[2]Massachusetts Institute of Technology, Cambridge, MA 02139, USA
[3]Boston University School of Medicine, Boston, MA 02118, USA

INTRODUCTION

The T-NEMC/MIT program in neutron capture therapy (NCT) is a collaborative research endeavor between T-NEMC (one of the principal tertiary care teaching hospitals in the Boston area) and the Nuclear Reactor Laboratory at MIT, where the MIT Research Reactor, MITR-II, is located. The program has been federally funded since 1987 by the U.S. Department of Energy, and a recent renewal continues funding through 1993. This paper will briefly review the program's accomplishments over the past 3-4 years.

IDEAL NEUTRON BEAM STUDIES BY MONTE CARLO SIMULATION

To gain a better intuitive understanding of the parameters relating to the optimization of neutron beams for NCT, we have carried out a number of monoenergetic neutron beam Monte Carlo simulations using the MCNP code. Using figures of merit such as "advantage depth" (AD) and "advantage ratio" (AR), previously devised as an aid to neutron beam design[1,2], we have shown that a wide range of epithermal neutron beam energies may be quite acceptable for NCT[1]. This provided some confidence to the use of aluminum and sulphur resonance scattering filters which we proposed for the design of a practical epithermal neutron beam at MITR-II. Figure 1 shows a parametric plot of AD and AR figures of merit for ideal beams of various energies. It can be seen that neutron energies approximately in the range of 1 eV-20 keV show favorable combinations of AD and AR.

EPITHERMAL NEUTRON BEAM DESIGN & CONSTRUCTION AT MITR-II

Figure 2 shows a cutaway illustration of the MIT Research Reactor, MITR-II, showing the design and location of the Medical Therapy Facility. The neutron beam exiting the collimator in the ceiling of the facility was originally the thermal beam that was used in the unsuccessful NCT clinical trials in the early 1960's. We have redesigned the beam line to produce a high quality epithermal neutron beam using the composite resonance scattering filter approach[2,3]. Figure 3 shows the components of the currently installed filter which was designed using a combination of Monte Carlo simulation and experimental measurements. The design is such that it is feasible to switch between the epithermal and the original thermal neutron beams in less than one day.

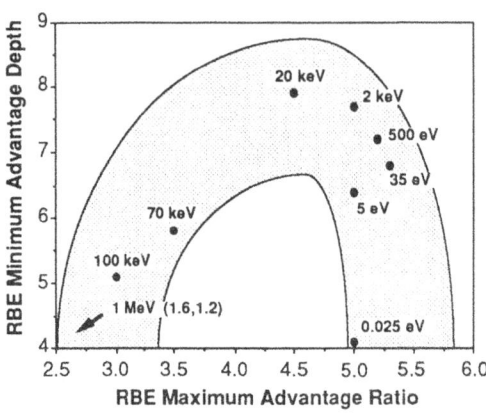

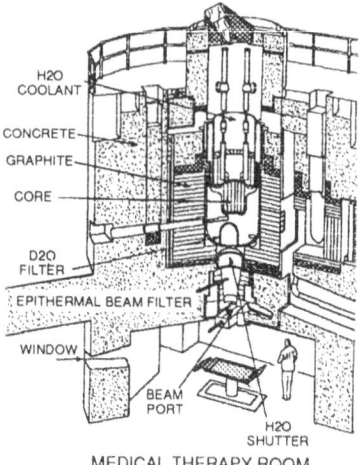

Fig. 1. Parametric representation of the figures of merit AD and AR for a
number of ideal neutron beams characterized using Monte Carlo simulation.

Fig. 2 Line Drawing of the MIT Research
Reactor, MITR-II, showing the location of the specially designed and
constructed Medical Therapy Facility.

DOSIMETRIC CHARACTERIZATION OF THE MITR-II EPITHERMAL NEUTRON BEAM

Dosimetry of the epithermal beam at MITR-II has been carried out using activation foils and paired tissue-equivalent/graphite ionization chambers[2,3]. Measurements have been done in a variety of phantoms, the current one being a water filled ellipsoidal head phantom. Figure 4 shows the central axis dose/depth characterization of the epithermal beam in the current phantom[3]. Unless stated otherwise, the RBE's used were: 2.3 for the ^{10}B dose, 1.6 for neutron dose, and 1.0 for gamma dose. Figure 5 shows a simulated parallel-opposed irradiation (based on data in Fig. 4, but with gamma RBE equal to 0.5) demonstrating a therapeutic ratio of approximately 3 anywhere within the head phantom[3]. Minimum and maximum background dose refers to 0 and 3 ppm of ^{10}B, respectively. Note the high uniformity of the dose to normal brain. The absence of "hot-spots" enables maximum dose to be delivered to tumor.

MONTE CARLO BASED TREATMENT PLANNING DEVELOPMENT FOR NCT

We have developed a treatment planning procedure which incorporates Monte Carlo simulation and a true three-dimensional treatment planning program called NCTPLAN[4,5]. Figure 6 shows the procedure schematically. NCTPLAN first automatically specifies a customized Monte Carlo model for each individual patient, then incorporates CT or MRI into the results of the Monte Carlo simulation. Finally, it displays various forms of isodose contours superimposed on corresponding arbitrarily oriented anatomical image planes. Figure 7 shows one transverse plane through the head of a patient with an occipital glioblastoma multiforme with superimposed isodose contours representing a bilateral irradiation with the MITR-II epithermal neutron beam[5]. The thick "100%" contour is the "advantage depth" (AD) contour, where any tumor tissue inside this contour will receive higher radiation dose than the peak dose to any normal structures[4]. The isodose contours inside the AD contour show the variations in tumor dose that will occur, while the isodose contours outside the AD contour show the variations in normal structure dose. Additional treatment planning parameters can also be displayed including normal structure or tumor dose histograms, radiation type histograms, etc. A special elliptical Monte Carlo head

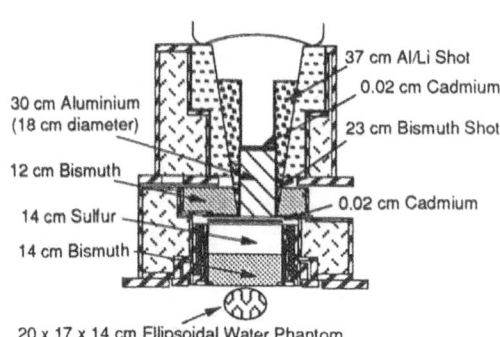

37 cm Al/Li Shot

0.02 cm Cadmium

30 cm Aluminium
(18 cm diameter)

23 cm Bismuth Shot

12 cm Bismuth

14 cm Sulfur

0.02 cm Cadmium

14 cm Bismuth

20 x 17 x 14 cm Ellipsoidal Water Phantom

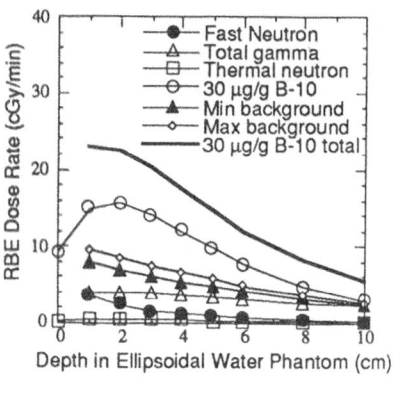

Fig. 3. Components of the epithermal neutron beam filter elements currently installed in the medical therapy beam line of the MITR-II. This beam is designated M-055.

Fig. 4. Depth/dose distribution for a unilateral irradiation of an ellipsoidal water phantom with the M-055 epithermal neutron beam. ^{10}B distribution in tumor and normal brain is 30/3 ppm.

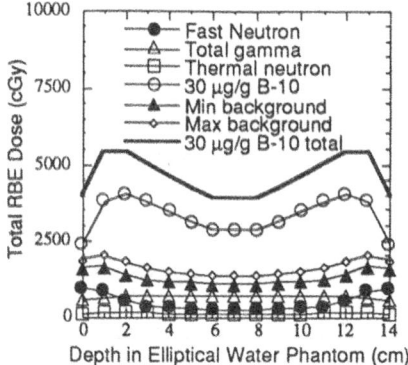

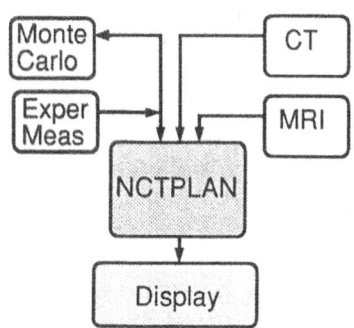

Fig. 5. Simulated fractionated bilateral irradiation using data from Fig. 4, except that gamma RBE is assumed to be 0.5

Fig. 6. Schematic representation of the information flow and functional modules for the NCT treatment planning program NCTPLAN.

model similar to the physical head model employed for experimental dosimetry permits proper experimental calibration of the neutron beam source data used by the Monte Carlo code.

HIGH RESOLUTION NEUTRON-INDUCED ALPHA-TRACK AUTORADIOGRAPHY

We have developed a technique for quantitative distribution of boron in ultra-thin histological frozen sections[6,7]. The Lexan track detector used is selectively sensitive to the high LET of the ^{10}B reaction products, while its submicron thickness together with the 1-2μ thick frozen tissue sections used ensures a high spatial resolution of 1-2μ. Moreover, the technique does not require the tissue and detector to be separated at any time so that the final product provides a superimposition of the stained tissue and the etched track detector. Computer software has been also developed to aid in the quantitative analysis of these autoradiograms. Figure 8 shows the principle of this technique. Figure 9 (left) shows an autoradiogram of a GL261 mouse glioma after the animal had been administered an oral dose of p-boronophenylalanine (BPA). The tissue microanatomy and the etched alpha particle and ^{7}Li recoil tracks are clearly seen. Using the blurred mask subtraction form of image processing, tracks are automatically identified, counted, and then mapped back into the original image, as shown in Fig. 9 (right). Such autoradiograms are used to examine

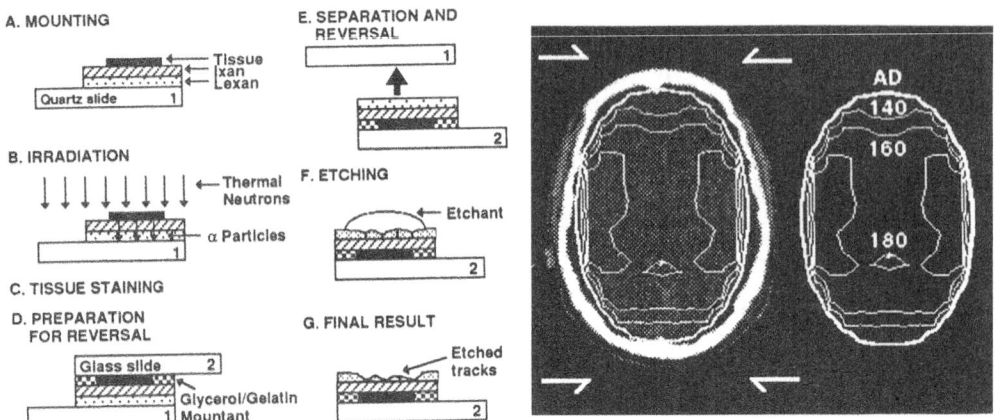

Fig. 7. Transverse plane through patient's brain with bilateral simulated irradiation with the M-055 epithermal neutron beam. The thick contour is the 100% or AD contour. Isodoses inside the AD contour give tumor dose.

Fig. 8. Schematic description of the high resolution alpha-track autoradiography technique. Theoretical modeling suggests a spatial resolution of 1-2μ.

the subcellular distribution of various boron compounds, to quantify boron concentration in microliter size blood samples, and to examine the pharmacokinetic behavior of various boron compounds.

PROMPT-GAMMA ANALYSIS OF BORON IN MACROSCOPIC LIQUID SAMPLES

We have constructed an analytical prompt-gamma boron analysis facility[8] utilizing a diffracted and sapphire filtered tangential thermal neutron beam at MITR-II. Currently, liquid samples of blood and urine of 0.5-3 cc in volume can be analyzed. Figure 10 shows the prompt-gamma spectra obtained from whole heparinized blood, with the Doppler-broadened ^{10}B peaks being clearly visible to the left of the annihilation peak from hydrogen in the sample; analysis of the latter provides an internal neutron fluence monitor. Also shown are interfering prompt gamma peaks from sodium and lithium which must be accounted for. Figure 11 is a nomogram showing the tradeoff between sensitivity, measurement time, and estimated measurement error. For instance, 3 ml blood samples with 1 ppm of ^{10}B can measured with an accuracy of ±5% in 25 minutes.

BIODISTRIBUTION AND PHARMACOKINETIC STUDIES IN MICE

We have carried out a series of biodistribution and pharmacokinetic studies of BPA compound after its oral administration to GL261 glioma bearing C7BL/6 mice. Figure 12 shows the results of a recent study[7], from which it was concluded that (i) BPA seems to attain a homogeneous subcellular distribution in tumor; (ii) tumor-to-normal brain and tumor-to-blood boron ratios of 3-3.5:1 and 11-13:1, respectively, are attained between 3 and 8 hours post BPA administration.

SURVIVAL STUDIES IN MICE

We have carried out NCT treatment survival experiments on GL261 glioma bearing C7BL/6 mice after oral administration of 95% ^{10}B enriched racemic BPA. Radiation dose levels were manipulated by varying the administered pharmacological doses and estimating

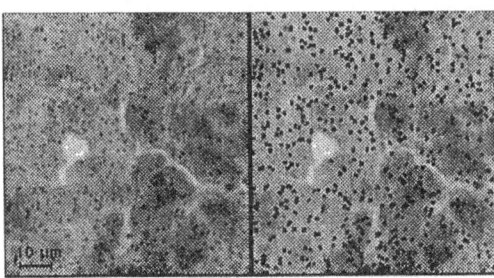

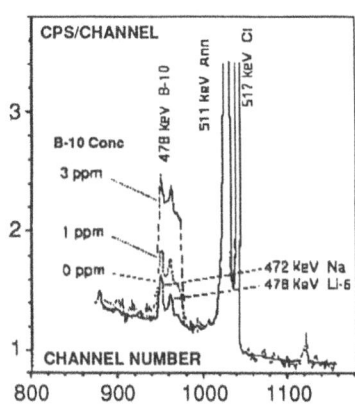

Fig. 9. High resolution autoradiogram of a GL261 mouse tumor after the animal had been administered an oral dose of BPA and killed six hours later.

Fig. 10. Prompt gamma spectrum of whole heparinized blood measured using the MITR-II prompt gamma analysis facility.

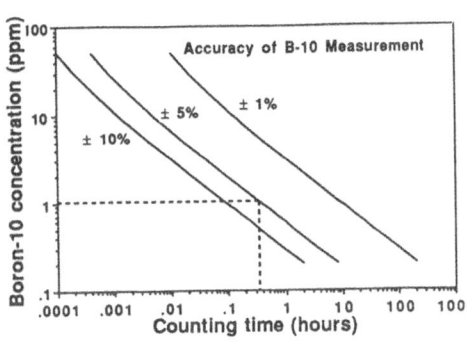

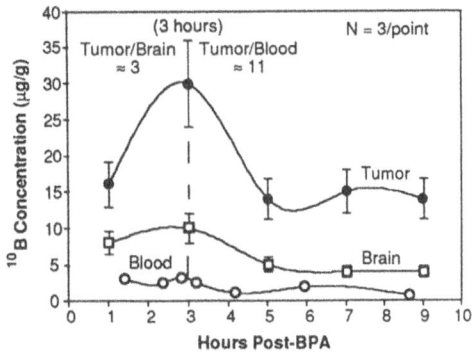

Fig. 11. Nomogram for MITR-II prompt gamma analysis facility showing tradeoff between sensitivity, measurement time, and statistical errors.

Fig. 12. Pharmacokinetic study of BPA distribution in tumor bearing mice. All ^{10}B assays were done by alpha-track autoradiography.

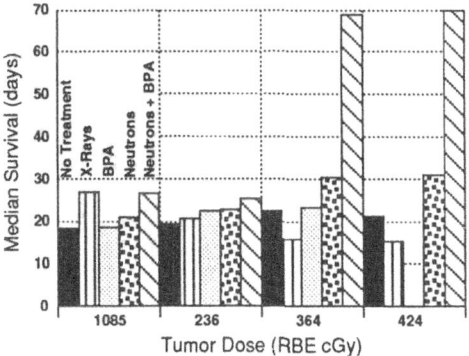

Fig. 13. Median survival for NCT treated and control mice at four specified tumor RBE dose levels. ^{10}B doses were estimated from earlier pharmacokinetic study.

the ratio of tumor boron concentration-to-administered pharmacological dose, based on the biodistribution and pharmacokinetic studies described above. Figure 13 shows the median survival of the NCT treated mice relative to control groups[7]. While the two lower dose groups show no NCT efficacy, NCT treatment at the two higher dose levels does show statistically significant increase in median survival at a level of $p \leq 0.03$.

BPA BIODISTRIBUTION, PHARMACOKINETICS, AND TOXICITY IN HUMANS

NEMC/MIT, Boston University Medical Center, Brookhaven National Laboratory, Stonybrook Medical Center, North Shore Hospital (Long Island), and Ohio State University Medical Center are collaborating in a human biodistribution study to examine the potential suitability of BPA for clinical trials of NCT. Currently, approximately 15 ocular and cutaneous melanoma and glioblastoma patients have been studied. Tumor, normal brain, and skin boron distributions have been analyzed by high resolution alpha-track autoradiography, while the blood and urine samples have been analyzed by prompt-gamma. Initial results indicate tumor/normal ^{10}B ratios slightly better than in Fig. 12, and tumor/blood ratios slightly worse.

ACKNOWLEDGMENTS

This research is supported in part by U.S. Department of Energy Grant No. DE-FGO2-87ER6060, by the Chairmen's Research Funds of the NEMC Departments of Radiation Oncology and Neurosurgery, and by a U.S. Department of Energy Reactor Sharing Grant awarded to the MIT Nuclear Reactor Laboratory.

REFERENCES

1. S. D. Clement, J. R. Choi, R. G. Zamenhof, J. C. Yanch, and O. K. Harling, "Monte Carlo Methods of Neutron Beam Design for Neutron Capture Therapy at the MIT Research Reactor (MITR-II)," In: Neutron Beam Design, Development, and Performance for Neutron Capture Therapy, Plenum Press, NY (1990).

2. J. R. Choi, S. D. Clement, O. K. Harling, and R. G. Zamenhof, "Neutron Capture Therapy Beams at the MIT Research Reactor," In: Neutron Beam Design, Development, and Performance for Neutron Capture Therapy, Plenum Press, NY (1990).

3. J. R. Choi, R. G. Zamenhof, J. C. Yanch, R. Rogus, and O. K. Harling, "Performance of the Currently Available Epithermal Neutron Beam at the Massachusetts Institute of Technology Research Reactor (MITR-II)," These proceedings.

4. R. G. Zamenhof, S. D. Clement, O. K. Harling, J. F. Brenner, D. E. Wazer, H. Madoc-Jones, and J. C. Yanch, "Monte Carlo Based Dosimetry and Treatment Planning for Neutron Capture Therapy of Brain Tumors," In: Neutron Beam Design, Development, and Performance for Neutron Capture Therapy, Plenum Press, NY (1990).

5. R. G. Zamenhof, J. Brenner, J. C. Yanch, D. E. Wazer, H.Madoc-Jones, S. Saris, and O. K. Harling, "Treatment Planning Techniques for Neutron Capture Therapy of Glioblastoma Multiforme Using an Epithermal Neutron Beam from the MITR-II Research Reactor and Monte Carlo Simulation," These proceedings.

6. R. G. Zamenhof, S. Clement, K. Lin, C. Lui, D. Ziegelmiller, and O. K. Harling, "Monte Carlo Treatment Planning and High Resolution Alpha-Track Autoradiography for Neutron Capture Therapy," Strahlentherapie und Onkologie, 165:188 (1989).

7. G. Solares, R. G. Zamenhof, S. Saris, D. Wazer, S. Kerley, M. Joyce, H. Madoc-Jones, L. Adelman, and O.K. Harling, "Biodistribution and Pharmacokinetics of p-Boronophenylalanine in C57BL/6 Mice with GL261 Intracranial Tumors, and Survival Following Neutron Capture Therapy," These proceedings.

8. R. Rogus, O. K. Harling, I. Olmez, and S. Wirdzek, "^{10}B Prompt Gamma Boron Analysis Using a Diffracted Neutron Beam," These proceedings.

NCT PROGRAM AT THE UNIVERSITY OF MISSOURI-COLUMBIA

R.M. Brugger, J.A. Shih, H.S. Wu, H.B. Liu, X.S. Luo

Nuclear Engineering Program and Research Reactor, University of Missouri-Columbia, Columbia, MO 65211, USA

At the University of Missouri-Columbia (MU), developments continue on specific parts of NCT. These are the epithermal beam design, Gd as an alternative agent to B, dose predictions and treatment planning, and accelerator based neutron sources.

EPITHERMAL NEUTRON BEAM: At the workshop on "Neutron Beam Design, Development and Performance" held in Boston in March 1989 [1], beam designs for a number of epithermal neutron beams were presented. Among this set was a design for an epithermal beam from the Missouri University Research Reactor (MURR) [2]. The Monte Carlo calculations for the neutron fluxes and gamma doses of this beam showed that, if built, this beam would be a very clean and intense epithermal neutron beam for NCT. Since that meeting, improvements have been made in the design to accommodate a beam shutter and to provide more flexibility in patient positioning. Also, capital cost and operating cost projections have been made.

The MURR operates at 10 MW, and has operated at 10 MW, 90% of the time since August 1974. In the new design, the beam is still in the thermal column of the MURR and the core of the reactor and the Be reflector are not changed. Two graphite wedges facing the thermal column hole will be replaced with Al wedges. The Pb shield will be replaced with Al plates. At the inner end of the thermal column indentation, an Al_2O_3 moderator will be assembled. The beam face and sides will be shielded with Bi or Pb. The patient irradiation position will be at the outer face of the biological shield where there will be ample room to position the patient in any orientation. This longer beam also allows space for thick shielding doors plus a tank that can be flooded. These will be effective beam controls to protect the patients and physicians during the preparation periods.

Outside the reactor biological shielding a treatment room will be assembled large enough to allow for easy patient handling and support equipment, i.e., 5 m x 3.5 m. The room will be designed and built to meet the requirements for a medical room with the proper safety systems and interlocks. In this treatment facility, the reactor will not be shut down and started up to accommodate patients but the reactor will be run continuously. Thus the source of neutrons will be available at all times and the beam to the patient will be controlled by the beam shutter and the floodable tank. Estimates of the cost of constructing and installing this beam in the MURR are less than $1 million. It is estimated that this beam

could be in service within a year after it is funded. The incremental
operating costs of this beam and the supporting facilities will be modest
since the reactor already is operating serving other functions. All
necessary support facilities, i.e. hospitals and veterinary facilities are
nearby within the University. A major advantage of the MURR location is
the participation of students; engineering, science and medical students.

Detailed calculations have been made of the neutron and gamma fluxes
and currents that will be realized with the new MURR NCT beam. These
calculations were made using the code MCNP and the central computer at the
BNL. Uncertainties were reduced to less than 10% statistical errors
(except as noted) by following many neutron histories in each calculation.
At least two ways have been suggested to describe the quality and quantity
of epithermal beams and both of these ways can be applied to the MURR beam.
First consider the calculation of the flux and dose in a small tissue
sample in air at the patient position. For the MURR beam, the Monte Carlo
calculations give the results presented in Table I.

TABLE I.   Calculated Fluxes and Doses from the New MURR Beam

Power Reactor (MW)	10
Epithermal Neutron Flux at Patient Position (n/cm^2 sec)	7.9×10^9
Neutron Induced Dose in Tissue in Air Per Epithermal Neutron at Patient Position (Rad/n/cm^2)	2.8×10^{-11}
Gamma Dose from Beam in Tissue in Air Per Epithermal Neutron at Patient Position (Rad/n/cm^2)	$0.3\ (\pm\ 0.1) \times 10^{-11}$
Current to Flux Ratio	0.78

The second way of presenting the quality and intensity of epithermal
beams is by the dose-in-phantom method proposed by Harling for the Boston
Workshop. Figure 1 shows the calculated doses for the MURR beam in a
tissue phantom at the patient position. As anticipated from the flux in
air and dose/flux calculations presented above, these doses are quite good.
The recent Monte Carlo calculations show that a very effective epithermal
neutron beam for NCT can be produced at the MURR. This beam could form the
center of a reasonably costed, conveniently located, and complete program
of NCT with graduate student participation.

The doses in a tissue phantom placed at the patient position. The symbols
signify the doses from: ▼neutrons > 10 ev, ▲ all neutrons, △ gammas,
● total background, ◆ 3 μg/g ^{10}B total, ◇ 30μg/g^{10}B, ■ 30 μg/g ^{10}B total.

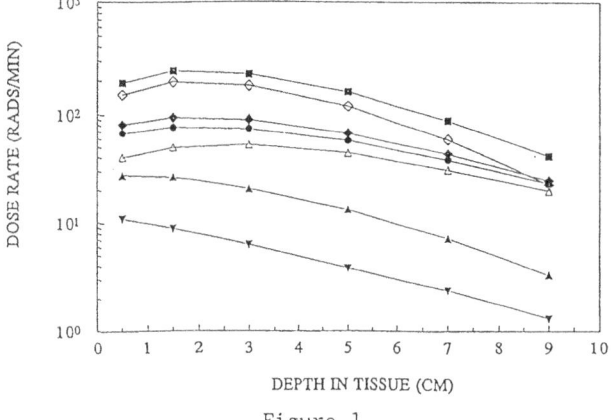

Figure 1

GADOLINIUM AS AN NCT AGENT: Studies continue of ^{157}Gd as an alternative agent of B continue at MU. Monte Carlo calculations of the dose magnitude and distribution with ^{157}Gd (GdNCT) and dose measurements in phantoms have been performed. The results show that GdNCT offers comparable dose distribution to BNCT. Auger electrons following the Gd prompt gamma emission which have been observed in the measurements should enhance the therapeutic effect of GdNCT. Solid Gd as brachytherapy seeds has also been evaluated. Monte Carlo based treatment planning indicates that more than 5,000 cGy of gamma dose from the Gd can be delivered to a volume of a few tens of cm^3. Measurements in air and phantoms verified the calculations. An image technique which displays the distribution and the concentration of ^{157}Gd has been developed. This technique allows a ^{157}Gd concentration from 20 μg/g to 500μg/g in thin samples to be quantified. The intrinsic spatial resolution of this imaging system is 70 μm. The details of these developments are presented in these proceedings.[3]

TREATMENT PLANNING: Dose distributions obtained from Monte Carlo codes are being developed to characterize the dose distributions within head models irradiated by the MURR epithermal neutron beam. Isodose curves in the head models are computed with a PC based program. Standard combinations of beam characteristics, field size, head orientation, and geometrical configuration are being designed and optimized for specific cases. Dependence of dose distributions on these factors will be evaluated and separately compared with each combination. Finally, the predicted isodose curves will be checked by calibration experiments with phantoms.

ACCELERATOR BASED NEUTRON SOURCES: Part of the MU program is focusing on several different reactions that can be supported by small accelerators to evaluate their effectiveness in producing epithermal neutrons for BNCT. For the more promising reactions, moderators will be designed using the Monte Carlo computer code to approach the best neutron yield and therapeutic neutron spectrum. Each reaction with moderators will be compared to a proposed [4] Li^7(p,n)^{7}Be reaction and moderator to see if improvements can be realized.

ACKNOWLEDGEMENTS: The authors thank the MURR for support during this research. The support from Brookhaven National Lab and specifically Ralph Fairchild, Vili Benary, and Yakov Kamen was especially significant. The accelerator based neutron source development is now supported by a grant from DOE.

REFERENCES

[1]   Neutron Beam Design, Development, and Performance for NCT, Otto Harling, et al, Plenum Press, New York, NY, 1990
[2]   R.M. Brugger and W.H. Herleth, "Intermediate Neutron Beam from the MURR", ibid, pages 153-166
[3]   R.M. Brugger, J.A. Shih, H.S. Wu, H.B. Liu, X.S. Liu, "NCT Program at the University of Missouri-Columbia", presented at the 4th International Symposium on Neutron Capture Therapy, Sydney, Australia, December 3-7, 1990
[4]   C.K. Wang, T.E. Blue, and J.W. Blue, "An Experimental Study of the Moderator Assembly for a Low-Energy Proton Accelerator Neutron Irradiation Facility", ibid, pages 271-280

GOALS OF THE EUROPEAN COLLABORATION ON
BORON NEUTRON CAPTURE THERAPY

Detlef Gabel

Department of Chemistry, University of Bremen, Germany

INTRODUCTION

Since 1989, the Commission of the European Community (CEC) funds, through their program Europe against Cancer, a Concerted Action European Collaboration on Boron Neutron Capture Therapy.

The European Collaboration has two main goals. Goal 1 is to initiate clinical trials of glioma at the High Flux Reactor Petten at the earliest possible time. Goal 2 is to create all necessary conditions to initiate clinical trials of other tumors and treatment at other facilities.

In this overview the activities of the European Collaboration towards the two goals are summarized.

TASKS NECESSARY FOR CONSIDERATION OF CLINICAL TRIALS

For Goal 1, the following tasks were identified as necessary to achieve before clinical trials can begin:

- Design, construction and installation of an epithermal neutron beam
- Physical and biological characterization of the beam
- Installation of a suitable treatment room with corollary facilities
- Pharmacokinetics and toxicity studies of boronated tumor seekers
- Establishment of a response function for healthy tissue to the treatment intended
- Development of an adequate treatment planning modality.

Beam Development

The High Flux Reactor (HFR) of the Joint Research Center (JRC) of the Commission of the European Communities has been made available to modification for boron neutron capture therapy (BNCT). The reactor is a 45 MW light water swimming pool reactor. It is used mainly for materials testing. The availability of the reactor is very high.

One horizontal beam hole of the reactor, the HB11/HB12 hole, can be used for modifications necessary for BNCT. In 1989, a program was started to design an epithermal neutron beam. MCNP (Monte Carlo neutron and photon) calculations were carried out at the AEA Harwell (P. Watkins, G. Constantine and others) and the ECN Petten (F. Stecher-Rasmussen, W. Freudenreich and others), first for the beam tube HB7. This beam tube was available for preliminary measurements and experimental validation of the correctness of the calculations. Following this, calculations have been completed for HB11. A filter consisting of Cd (1 mm), Al (150 mm), S (50 mm), Ti (10 mm) and Ar (1500 mm) was found to yield a beam beleived to have suitable properties for BNCT.

The irradiation location is around 5 m from the reactor core, and consequently the beam has little divergence at the treatment location. Table 1 lists the calculated parameters of the beam and compares them to other epithermal beams suggested or constructed for BNCT.

Table 1

Comparison of the HB11 epithermal neutron beam with other epithermal beams

	HB11[1] calc.	BMRR[2][a] meas.	PBF[3] calc.	MIT[4][a] meas.
neutron flux (n cm^{-2} s^{-1})	$1.1 \cdot 10^9$	$1.8 \cdot 10^9$	$14. \cdot 10^9$	$0.25 \cdot 10^9$
fast neutron dose per incident neutron ((Gy·cm^2)·10^{13})	7.8	4.87	1.9	20.1
gamma dose per incident $3 \cdot 10^{12}$ n cm^{-2} (Gy)	0.5	0.3	0.18	3.3
peak thermal neutron flux at depth in tissue per incident neutron [b]	≥ 2.7	1.6	2.7	1.7
fast neutron dose at surface per thermal neutron at depth ((Gy·cm^2)·10^{13})	≤ 2.9	3.0	0.7	11.8
time needed to deliver $3 \cdot 10^{12}$ n cm^{-2} (min) [c]	45	28	3.6	198

Footnotes to Table 1
[a] The neutron flux for the MIT and BMRR beams and the numbers derived from it refer to neutrons with energies above 1 eV, whereas the flux and numbers for the other beams consider neutrons of all energies.
[b] These numbers indicate the geometry of the beam, a value of 3 pertaining for a parallel beam, one of 1.5 for an isotropic beam.
[c] assuming exposure to full beam without diameter control. The actual treatment time will be longer than this, depending on the extent of beam diameter control. For the HB11 and PBF beams, the increase will be smaller than for the BMRR and MIT beams.

Treatment Facilities

The treatment of glioma is the first clinical goal of the European Collaboration. It was considered important to utilize to as high a degree as possible all the experience that has been gained with other types of radiation therapy. Therefore, the treatment room at the HB11 has been designed to permit bilateral irradiations of the head; i.e., a half circle of 2 m radius is available for patient placement. The exact positioning will be carried out with lasers defining the dose point. An observation area is to be installed, and an adequate patient rest and surveillance area has been conceived. The facility will be able to allow treatment of glioma and other patients well in excess of 1000 full treatments per year. Treatment will probably be carried out in a series of around 5-6 fractions.

PRECONDITIONS FOR THERAPY

In Europe, BNCT is planned to be tried clinically by the end of 1991 or beginning of 1992. It is planned to treat glioma patients, with $Na_2B_{12}H_{11}SH$ (BSH) as the boron compound. Before the treatment can be tried, it must be established in a suitable animal model that the risk of the treatment is low. In order to achieve this, the tolerance of healthy tissue to BNCT conditions needs to be determined in animals, and the pharmacokinetics of the boron compound in question needs to be established in both animals and patients.

Healthy tissue tolerance

Healthy tissue tolerance will be studied in dogs. The dogs will be given BSH in different amounts, and will then be exposed to different levels of neutron irradiation. From the initial studies on healthy tissue tolerance in dogs carried out in the United States, as well as from the dose-depth profiles of such beams in phantoms, the likely tissue at risk is not the skin, but tissue at a few centimeters depth (i.e. brain tissue). White matter necrosis may occur with such treatment, and this will take several months to develop.

In previous experience of the late 50's and early 60's, skin was the most radiosensitive organ. This was due to both the high boron concentration in the skin and the simultaneous use of a thermal neutron beam. With beams of moderate mean energy, and using the presently available boron compounds, skin appears to be no longer the dose limiting healthy tissue.

When this study includes different levels of boron concentration and neutron exposure, operational factors for the effectiveness of a given boron concentration and a given neutron fluence can be derived from a knowledge of the dose components at different depths. These factors then allow the necessary exposure planning.

Due to the importance of localization of boron, the maximally tolerated dose will be compound dependent. Thus, studies with one compound (e.g. BSH) will not yield much information for treatment using a different boron compound (e.g. p-dihydroxyboryl phenylalanine). Equally, studies for one target organ (e.g. brain tissue) cannot, even for the same compound, be transferred easily to other treatment areas.

Pharmacokinetics of BSH

The pharmacokinetics of the boron compound needs to be known in both the animal model and in man in order to transfer results from the animal study to patients. Therefore, the European Collaboration has placed great emphasis on a thorough pharmacokinetic study of BSH in brain tumor patients. Data on the boron concentration in different tissues and their time dependence are being collected.

A number of centers are involved in this study, especially Lausanne, Bremen, Leiden, and Lund.

For BSH, which is presently used in Japan for treating gliomas, no compound related toxicity was found.

Provided that the study on healthy tissue tolerance does not result in unacceptable damage to the tissue exposed, treatment trials for glioma will be able to start towards the middle of 1992.

DEVELOPMENT OF OTHER NEUTRON SOURCES

It must be envisaged that the construction of a nuclear reactor for BNCT in a hospital environment will meet considerable difficulties. It is therefore desirable to look into the conversion of existing reactors for BNCT, and the construction of accelerator-based neutron sources.

The possibility to use a plate of U-235 at the end of the thermal column of a reactor as an intense source of neutrons, may be an attractive alternative. Also here, a filter may provide a beam of suitable characteristics.

Spallation neutrons produced by bombarding a target with protons could be moderated down to appropriate energies and may be useful for BNCT.

The centers most involved in these aspects are Paris, Ispra, and Villigen.

DEVELOPMENT OF NEW TUMOR SEEKERS

The future perspectives of BNCT are closely linked to, and indeed dependent on, the development of new and improved tumor seekers. Within the European Collaboration, this aspect has therefore a high priority.

Work is being carried out, among others, on the synthesis of boronated analogues of porphyrins, lipid ethers, and melanoma seekers as examples for low-molecular weight tumor seekers, and on growth factors, peptide hormones and antibodies as examples for high molecular weight tumor seekers.

Synthesis will be followed by distribution studies in appropriate test systems, toxicity studies, and pharmacokinetics.

Laboratories involved include Uppsala, London, Bremen, München, Glasgow, and Pavia.

BNCT AS ADJUVANT IN FAST NEUTRON THERAPY

The moderation of fast neutrons down to thermal energies also occurs in fast neutron therapy. It has been suggested before to use the thermalized neutrons to enhance the dose to the tumor, via pre-irradiation administration of boron. It has been demonstrated that a dose enhancement can be observed in fast neutron beams used for clinical purposes. The same holds true for reactor fission neutrons.

Work on these goals is being pursued in Essen, München, and Villigen.

Participating centers and internal structure

In the European Collaboration, 46 centers from 11 countries in Europe participate. These are:

Austria	University of Graz, Graz
Belgium	Catholic University of Louvain, Brussels
France	Centre Henri Becquerel, Rouen Commissariat à l'Energie Atomique, C.E.N. Saclay, Gif-sur-Yvette University of Rouen
Federal Republic of Germany	GSF, Neuherberg Klinik Rechts der Isar, München Kernforschungsanlage Jülich

	Reaktorstation Garching
	Physikalisch-Technische-Bundesanstalt, Braunschweig
	Technical University München
	University of Bremen
	University of Essen
	University of München
	University of Göttingen
	University of Stuttgart
	University of Münster
	Zentralkrankenhaus St. Jürgen-Straße, Bremen
Greece	University of Ioannina
Ireland	University of Cork
Italy	Foundation "Clinica del Lavoro", Pavia
	Joint Research Centre, Ispra
	National Institute of Nuclear Physics of Pavia
	National Research Council, Pavia
	University of Pavia
Sweden	Studsvik AB, Nyköping
	University of Lund
	University of Uppsala
Switzerland	Centre Hospitalier Universitaire Vaudois, Lausanne
	Paul-Scherrer-Institut, Villigen
The Netherlands	Academisch Ziekenhuis, Leiden
	ECN, Petten
	Institute of Radiotherapy, Nijmegen
	Joint Research Centre, Petten
	Netherlands Cancer Institute, Amsterdam
United Kingdom	Belvidere Hospital, Glasgow
	CEGB, Berkeley Nuclear Laboratories, Berkeley
	Charing Cross Hospital, London
	AEA Harwell, Oxford
	Scottish Universities, Research and Reactor Centre, Glasgow
	The Churchill Hospital, Oxford
	The Hospitals for Nervous Diseases, London
	The Radcliffe Infirmary, Oxford
	University of Edinburgh
	University of Strathclyde, Glasgow

It is expected that each center will provide funds for its own research through their own grants. The European Collaboration can only pay for costs that are associated with the coordination of the work of the different groups. Thus, funds from the European Collaboration can be used for personnel and materials exchange, for meetings and workshops, and only limited support for salaries of personnel necessary for coordinating the work of the different groups.

Because there is no direct competition of the groups for the money of the European Collaboration, no antagonistic behavior has emerged within the European Collaboration. Indeed, the working atmosphere has been dominated by a high degree of cooperation.

Besides the formal structure of a project leader, assisted by a Project Management Group (D. Chiaraviglio, Pavia; L. Dewit, Amsterdam; H. Fankhauser, Lausanne; R. Huiskamp, Petten; B. Larsson, Villigen; R. Moss, Petten; P. Schofield, Harwell), no formalized groups have been created to deal with specific tasks. Instead, all members are invited to participate in and suggest meetings and working parties for areas of common interest.

COOPERATION WITH OTHER GROUPS

The European Collaboration is determined to maintain a policy of open and free interaction with all other groups interested in BNCT. Thus, the European Collaboration has made available all data and results on, e.g., beam design, and will continue to do so. It has adopted this policy because nothing can be gained from a restricted exchange of information and results. This is even more so because of limited availability and access to suitable neutron sources, and the impact that successful or unsuccessful therapy trials have on other programs world-wide.

The European Collaboration enters into cooperation and information distribution unconditionally. However, all other groups world-wide are challenged to do the same, so that maximum benefit can be achieved for patients everywhere.

FUTURE PERSPECTIVES OF THE EUROPEAN COLLABORATION

The primary goals of the European Collaboration, as described here, are presently being funded to the middle of 1992. However, the work, and the need for cooperation, does not stop then.

Clinical trials will then have begun. The fact that several centers will send patients, and the need for thorough follow-up from the sending institutions, will necessitate a very intense exchange of results and experiences between the centers.

The development of new compounds, and the development of other neutron sources, are tasks where the mutual stimulation of the European groups, together with their contacts world-wide, will prove beneficial for the progress towards these goals.

For both of these reasons, a follow-up or continuation of the European Collaboration seems desirable and necessary.

ACKNOWLEDGMENT

The work of the European Collaboration of Boron Neutron Capture Therapy is supported by the Commission of the European Community. Financial support of national agencies and foundations for the individual projects makes this Collaboration possible. Thanks are due to R. Alberts for skillful and competent organizational and secretarial assistance in the coordination of this project.

REFERENCES

[1] P.D.T. Watkins, "Additional Calculations Performed at Harwell for the Petten HB11 BNCT Facility"; European Collaboration on Boron Neutron Capture Therapy (1990)
[2] R.G. Fairchild, J. Kalef-Ezra, S.K. Saraf, S. Fiarman, E. Ramsay, L. Wielopolski, B. Laster, F. Wheeler, "Installation and Testing of an Optimized Epithermal Neutron Beam at the Brookhaven Medical Research Reactor (BMRR)"; in Neutron Beam Design, Development and Performance for Neutron Capture Therapy, Plenum Press, Basic Life Scienes Vol 54, 185-200 (1990)
[3] F.J. Wheeler, personal communication (1990)
[4] O.K. Harling, personal communication (1990); data for filter combination M55

CRITIQUE OF MIT WORKSHOP ON NEUTRON BEAM DESIGN, DEVELOPMENT AND PERFORMANCE FOR NEUTRON CAPTURE THERAPY

Otto K. Harling,[1] John A. Bernard,[1] and Robert G. Zamenhof[2]

[1]Nuclear Reactor Laboratory, Massachusetts Institute of Technology
Cambridge, Massachusetts 02139, USA

[2]Tufts-New England Medical Center, Boston, Massachusetts 02111, USA

INTRODUCTION

The March 29-31, 1989 workshop at MIT dealt with beam design and performance for neutron capture therapy. This paper will provide a limited critical overview of some of the subjects and issues which were discussed in the Workshop. The authors have attempted to include differing views and approaches represented by the Workshop participants where scientifically defensible.

EPITHERMAL NEUTRON BEAM DESIGN APPROACH

The goal of epithermal beam design is to produce beams which can effectively treat the entire brain through the intact skull, including its deepest parts, in a reasonable time and with low enough background contamination to assure that tumor will be destroyed while most normal tissue will survive. An integrated approach to beam design and development must include consideration of the optimum energy and angular dependence of the beam incident upon the brain tissue and the incident background components as well as those generated in the brain tissue. Epithermal neutrons in the energy range of ~ 1 eV to ~ 20 keV were shown to be useful for treating deep-seated cancers. These limits are not precise and some latitude is possible. An epithermal beam should be able to provide ~ 10^{13} n/cm^2 in a reasonable time, e.g., in six one-hour fractions; however, there is no hard limit on irradiation time per fraction.

Filters and moderators can be used to produce epithermal beams in the desired energy range with sufficiently low contamination from fast neutrons, gamma rays, and thermal neutrons. Materials such as Al_2O_3, Al, D_2O, S, AlF_3, SiO_2, Be, BeO, and Ti are all useful for moderation and/or filtration. For filters the cross section should be low for energies in the desired range and increase significantly at higher energies. Al and S are good examples of candidate filter materials. For gamma-ray shielding, Bi and Pb are useful, and it is not yet clear which is best for epithermal beams. Slow neutrons can be removed with ^{10}B, Cd and ^{6}Li. Cadmium has the most desirable cross-section shape, rising steeply near 0.5 eV, but it must be shielded from the patient position due to its intense high-energy capture gammas. Lithium-6 produces few gamma rays, but captures a significant fraction of useful epithermal neutrons. Boron-10 produces a relatively low energy gamma ray at 478 keV, which is relatively easy to shield, but also absorbs many useful epithermal neutrons due to the 1/v dependence of the (n,α) cross section.

COMPUTATIONAL METHODS OF BEAM DESIGN

Deterministic techniques for solution of the Maxwell-Boltzmann transport equation, e.g. using the DOT code from the Oak Ridge National Laboratories, can provide complete characterization of the beam through computation of the detailed fluxes as a function of energy, angle, and position in the tissue phantom. Modeling of complex geometries may require approximations and a relatively coarse mesh in space, angle, and energy may have to be accepted in the solution.

Monte Carlo codes such as MCNP, developed by Los Alamos Scientific Laboratory, are capable of modeling complex geometries. This particular code also uses the exact cross section for each neutron energy and is, therefore, particularly useful for exploring resonance neutron filters. However, the inherent efficiency of transporting source neutrons to the target tissues is 10^{-6} or less for Monte Carlo. Therefore, extreme biasing in selecting neutrons of interest, to reduce computation time, may result in large errors.

Both the deterministic and Monte Carlo techniques are useful for epithermal neutron beam design, but limitations of both approaches must be well understood and experimental verification should be an important part of the design process.

Ideal beam studies, e.g. using MCNP, have provided guidance for BNCT beam design. Such studies have shown that good beam performance can be obtained for a wide range of energies, 0.5 eV$\leq E \approx 30$ keV. The upper boundary is not subject to a sharp cutoff and some neutrons up to energies as high as 50-70 keV are acceptable in a practical beam.[1] Ideal beam studies can also provide useful guidance concerning phantom design, angular dependence, and size of beams for BNCT.[2]

EXPERIMENTAL VERIFICATION OF BEAMS

There was general agreement that experimental verification of beam designs is both useful and necessary.

Although neutron energy spectrum measurements of actual beam designs are judged to be useful, considerable effort must be expended to obtain neutron energy spectra from ~ 1 eV to the MeV region, and the accuracy of such measured spectra is generally quite limited.

Final proof of the performance of epithermal beams, short of actual patient treatments, is the measurement of all dose components in a representative head phantom. The phantom should be as anatomically similar as possible to the shape and composition of a human brain and head. For example, cylindrical polyethylene phantoms, while convenient to use and useful for comparisons of relative beam performance, provide significantly different results compared to more realistic ellipsoidal-shaped phantoms based, e.g., on the Snyder[3] brain model and containing brain equivalent material. For realistic comparisons, it is especially important to use compositions which have the correct hydrogen density. Water is a convenient material since its hydrogen density is the same as that for brain.

Measurements in phantom should include a complete three-dimensional characterization of all dose components, including thermal flux, epithermal flux, gamma dose rate, and fast neutron dose rate. The $^{14}N(n,p)$ and $^{10}B(n,\alpha)$ dose rates can be calculated. Thermal and epithermal neutron fluxes can be measured using accepted ASTM[4] procedures with small, minimally perturbing gold foils or wires. Gamma-ray and fast neutron dose rate measurements in-phantom are difficult to obtain because these dose components must be separated. One of the few satisfactory approaches to in-phantom gamma and fast neutron dosimetry is the dual chamber method of Attix.[5]

Figures of merit to assist in making objective comparisons of various BNCT beams can be derived in various ways. We recommend the figures of merit recommended and used for the MIT Workshop. These include the advantage depth (AD), which is a measure of the useful penetration of the beam; the advantage ratio (AR), which provides a measure of the ratio of tumor dose to normal tissue dose; and the advantage depth dose rate

(ADDR), which is a measure of the dose rate at the advantage depth. These figures of merit are based on doses calculated or measured in phantoms.

If complete in-phantom dose versus depth distributions cannot be measured, then measurements of, for example, fast neutron dose and epithermal flux in air can be used to compare the quality of different epithermal beams.

SOME ISSUES RAISED AT THE WORKSHOP'S RAPPORTEURS' SESSION

Dose Delivered to Sensitive Organs During BNCT

In the treatment of intracranial tumors by BNCT, a number of radiosensitive tissues need to be considered as limiting the dose that can be delivered to tumor. These include: scalp, cerebral gray and white matter, the tissues lining the larger blood vessels such as arterioles and venules, the endothelial cells of the capillaries, and other tissues which may accumulate above normal quantities of boron. The latter may include the retina, lens, pituitary, brainstem, substantia nigra, etc. The potential injuries caused to these structures during BNCT treatment will depend on their depth in the brain, their hydrogen content, and their boron uptake and microscopic boron distribution.

The microdistribution properties of different boron compounds in various tissues will influence the microscopic biologically effective boron doses that these tissues will receive, and hence their dose tolerance parameters. For example: the boron compound $Na_2B_{12}H_{11}SH$ (BSH), a "blood brain barrier" type compound, accumulates to negligible degrees in normal tissues protected by an intact blood brain barrier, while the compound p-boronophenylalanine (BPA) appears approximately to attain equal concentrations in all normal tissues with substantially lower concentrations in blood. In the case of scalp, which from irradiation by an epithermal neutron beam would receive the highest fast neutron dose of any tissue while simultaneously being in a region of relatively low thermal neutron flux, the effective boron dose may be relatively small compared to the fast neutron dose. Therefore, differences in the microdistribution of these different boron compounds in the scalp would be less influencial on their dose tolerance.

Single exposure dose tolerance experiments (with and without BSH compound) on canine brains using the epithermal neutron beam at the Brookhaven National Laboratory's BMRR have demonstrated that doses to scalp in excess of approximately 2,000 cGy may produce moderate to severe scalp necrosis. Since there was some evidence that increased levels of BSH in blood resulted in higher total dose tolerance of the scalp, a particularly important role of fast neutrons in causing such injury might be inferred. In contrast, single exposure irradiations of canine brains (with BSH) using a thermal neutron beam at MIT's MITR-II, which contains negligible fast neutron dose, have shown that 4,000 cGy total scalp dose is very easily tolerated, resulting only in mild discoloration of fur and no histologically evident injuries to the brain. This also points out inferentially the importance of minimizing the fast neutron dose to the scalp.

The type of radiation injury (i.e., whether acute or delayed, and its degree) will also be strongly dependent on the fractionation schedule employed, in that fractionation will protect against low LET injury components; 4-6 fractions will approximately halve the biological effect of low LET radiations and theoretically improve the chances for homogeneous uptake of boron by all tumor cells.

CURRENT STATUS OF NCT BEAMS

At the time of the MIT Workshop there existed two clinically usable reactor-based epithermal beams (BMRR and MITR-II) with several under development. There are a number of reactors worldwide which have the potential to provide epithermal beams for BNCT. We judge that fission reactors offer the only realistic opportunities for epithermal BNCT beams over the next several years, although relatively compact, low-energy, high-current accelerator sources are currently under development. These offer several potential attractions for neutron beam production in a hospital-based patient treatment facility. ^{252}Cf based sources have also been proposed in this context.

SUMMARY

The conclusion of the rapporteurs of the MIT Workshop is repeated below since it continues to represent a good summary of the status of neutron source and beam development for NCT:

"It is the consensus of this workshop's rapporteurs that the technology currently available for epithermal beam design, construction, and dosimetric characterization is sufficient to make the neutron irradiation component of NCT safe and potentially effective for clinical therapy. A few facilities already possess existing epithermal beams suitable for clinical applications, while other facilities are in the course of designing and/or constructing such beams."

ACKNOWLEDGEMENTS

The authors wish to acknowledge the input from the Workshop Rapporteurs and other Workshop participants and the support of the U.S. Department of Energy under Grant No. DE-FG02-87ER60600.

REFERENCES

1. S. D. Clement, J. R. Choi, R. G. Zamenhof, J. C. Yanch, and O. K. Harling, "Monte Carlo Methods of Neutron Beam Design for Neutron Capture Therapy at the MIT Research Reactor (MITR-II)," in: Basic Life Sciences, Volume 54, O. K. Harling, J. A. Bernard, and R. G. Zamenhof, eds., Plenum Press, New York (1990).

2. J. C. Yanch and O. K. Harling, "A Monte Carlo Study of Ideal Beams for Epithermal Neutron Beam Development for Boron Neutron Capture Therapy," this symposium.

3. W. S. Snyder, M. R. Ford, G. G. Warner, and H. L. Fisher, Jr., "Estimates for Absorbed Fractions for Monoenergetic Photon Sources Uniformly Distributed in Various Organs of a Heterogeneous Phantom, MIRD," J. Nucl. Med., Suppl. No. 3, Pamphlet 5, p. 47 (1969).

4. ASTM E262-77, "Standard Method for Measuring Thermal Neutron Flux by Radioactivation Techniques."

5. F. H. Attix, "Introduction to Radiological Physics and Radiation Dosimetry," John Wiley and Sons, Inc., New York, p. 479 (1986).

PROGRAMME FOR BNCT WITH ACCELERATOR-PRODUCED keV

NEUTRONS AND RELATED CHEMICAL AND BIOLOGICAL STUDIES

A. Andersson[4], J. Andersson[4], J-O. Burgman[4], J. Capala[4], J.Carlsson[4], H. Condé[4],
J. Crawford[8], S. Graffmann[7], E. Grusell[4], A. Holmberg[4], E. Johansson[4],
B. S. Larsson[5], B. Larsson[4], T. Liljefors[4], P. Lindström[1,4], J. Malmquist[1],
L. Pellettieri[2], O. Pettersson[4], J. Pontén[3], A. Roberti[5], K. Russel[4], H. Reist[8],
L. Salford[6], S. Sjöberg[1], B. Stenerlöw[4], P. Strömberg[4] and B. Westermark[3].

From the Departments of Chemistry[1], Neurosurgery[2], Pathology[3], Radiation
Sciences[4] and Toxicology[5], Uppsala University, Uppsala Sweden; he Departments
of Neurosurgery[6] and Oncology[7], University of Lund, Lund, Sweden;
and the Paul Scherrer Institute[8], CH-5232 Villigen PSI, Switzerland

INTRODUCTION

Boron neutron capture therapy (BNCT), with slow neutrons, is based on the large cross-section of the stable boron isotope, ^{10}B, for the thermal neutron capture. Upon capture of a neutron, the ^{10}B nucleus is transformed to a highly excited ^{11}B compound nucleus that promptly disintegrates into two antiparallel, highly energetic and cell-killing fragments, one $^4He^{2+}$ and one $^7Li^{3+}$ ion, with ranges of 9 and 5 micrometers, respectively. By more or less selective accumulation of ^{10}B in suitable chemical form in or in close contact with the target cells, the probability of target cell sterilization is significantly increased, after therapeutic slow-neutron irradiation.

BNCT was originally conceived in 1936[1]. Partly for lack of basic knowledge, partly for technical reasons, it took half a century to introduce the idea clinically and get it accepted on the basis of favourable treatment results[2]. BNCT using thermal neutrons from fission reactors is at present used in Japan, in cases of malignant brain tumours and skin melanoma. Also in preparation are reactor-based facilities for intermediate energy neutrons ("keV neutrons") that would permit more efficient irradiation of deep-lying targets, without the concern for damage to the skin and other intervening tissues[3]. The appropriate energy range is around 10 keV, in single or opposing field BNCT. When the aim is multidirectional irradiation, as in our programme, somewhat higher energies, say 10 - 100 keV could be used, without undue risk of damage caused by recoiling nuclei. A rotating source would also permit some tailoring of the neutron capture probability distributions within the brain or the body. Taken together with the difficulties connected with the safety of nuclear reactors in hospital environments - be it a real problem or not - the desired versatility in configuration of the keV neutron fields in BNCT calls for studies of the usefulness accelerator-produced neutrons for multidirectional intermediate energy neutron irradiation. Thus the production of the keV neutron by spallation reactions induced by accelerated protons in heavy element targets has been studied as part of a Swedish-Swiss collaboration[4]. The aim is the design of a keV neutron source that could be rotated relative to the patient. Indirectly, the successful operation of such a device could be a step towards the introduction of hospital-based BNCT.

Various target-moderator combinations have been tried using 72 MeV protons from the Philips I Injector Cyclotron I at the Paul Scherrer Institute (PSI). The experimental neutron spectra thus found have been compared to and supplemented by theoretical calculations[5]. A proposal for a prototype facility for accelerator-based BNCT with the high-current PSI Injector Cyclotron II is now in preparation[6]. In this proposal the concept of a rotating proton beam hitting a ring-shaped spallation target in the depth of a moderator structure is introduced[7]. In this paper, this idea is referred to , and the biological and clinical implications discussed.

This paper summarizes four presentations at the symposium[8-11].

A SPALLATION SOURCE FOR BNCT

When medium-energy protons are stopped in a heavy metal target, such as tungsten, the evaporation neutron spectrum shows a peak energy of less than 2 MeV. By proper choice of moderator material and configuration, it is possible to reduce the energy of the bulk of these neutrons to the energy interval suitable for BNCT with keV neutrons. The 72 MeV proton beams available at the injector cyclotrons are well suited for the design study, and for eventual biological and clinical tests with the planned prototype neutron source for BNCT. This was demonstrated in the first experiments with low-current proton beams from the Philps Injector Cyclotron I that included measurements of moderated spallation neutron spectra by time-of-flight techniques; and the mapping of neutron capture probability distributions in a perspex phantom[6]. Results of these experiments show that thermal neutron fluences suitable for BNCT in the depth of the brain could be produced by keV neutron fields emanating from a tungsten target bombarded with less than 0.2 mA of 72 MeV protons.

Here we limit ourselves to problems concerned with treatment of cerebral disorders, but the new concepts and findings may help to pave the way for the use of BNCT in cases of infiltrating neoplasms, pathological vessels, and regional metastatic disease in the abdomen or in extremities. Whether accelerator-based BNCT would be eventually useful against systemic disease, by whole-body keV neutron irradiation, is still hard to say.

This programme is closely connected with the European Collaboration on BNCT[3]. The primary goal is a useful BNCT for advanced malignant brain tumours and for inoperable vascular malformations, as a supplement to existing methods of surgery, stereotaxic radiosurgery, and radiotherapy. A basic philosophy is to consider BNCT as an adjuvant therapy, in the context of precise external photon or particle therapy. By such a combination of modalities it should be possible to further optimize radiotherapy for maximum benefit of the patient. The bulk of primary tumour, or the nidus of an arterio-venous malformation, where the density of target cells is high could the be treated with a relatively high dose, while peripheral or scattered target cells in surrounding tissues could be more selectively attacked by highly cell-killing fragments of disintegrating boron nuclei.

To meet the clinical expectations, the aim of our chemical and biological research is to develop and test a variety of principles that would be useful for directing [10]B to tumour cells, or to the endothelium of pathological vessels. In a number of basic scientific projects presented at this conference we therefore address problems of boron compound synthesis and cytoaffinity, boron pharmaco-kinetics in animal models and human subjects, as well as the radiobiology of neutron capture reactions in tumour cells, tumour models, and healthy tissues. A main theme is the design of boron-loaded biomolecules with specificity for target cells. The epidermal growth factor, EGF, conjugated with boron-loaded dextran is the latest and most promising example[9]. EGF-dextran conjugates are being tested with favourable results, in experiments on cultured human glioma cells and in tumours transplanted into immunodeficient mice and rats.

Awaiting the availability of heavily boron-loaded, cell-seeking biomolecules, such as EGF or suitable antibody fragments, the radiobiological study is based on low-molecular weight boron compounds with affinity for melanin[12]. In this way [10]B could be accumulated in melanotic melanoma cells that are useful in model experiments, in vitro as well as in vivo. The effects of neutron capture on endothelial cells are similarly studied by use of boronated dextran, at relatively high concentration, in the medium of cell cultures or in the blood of experimental animals[13].

BORONATION OF EGF VIA DEXTRAN

The aim of the project is to synthesize low molecular weight boron compounds and to conjugate these with EGF-dextran and other tumor-seeking substances. Special emphasis is placed on the principle of using epidermal growth factor, EGF, as the targeting biomolecule and dextran as the carrier of boron. Such conjugates are small (molecular weight 20 - 30 kD) in comparison with antibodies or antibody fragment conjugates.

Several tumours of squamous carcinoma, glioma or melanoma types have EGF receptor amplification with a factor of at least ten, in some cases up to hundred times, more receptors than most normal cells[14-20]. Thus, there is a large potential for tumour therapy in using boron-rich compounds that bind to the EGF receptor. The alternative approach of using antibodies and/or antibody-fragments binding to the EGF receptor will also be applied to allow comparison between antibody and growth factor guided targeting.

The chemical approach is that dextran is activated with a reagent specific for coupling with amino groups. The activated dextran is allowed to react first with the amino end in EGF, or another seeking compound, and then with low molecular weight boron compounds containing amino groups. By suitable choice of the reaction conditions a large number of boron containing molecules could be coupled via the dextran spacer.

Dextran-based conjugates

We use dextran as a link between the tumour-seeking biomolecule and the boron compound. Dextran is used as a blood substitute in medical care (Macrodex) and is in itself not toxic or immunogenic. There exists a number of well-known methods to conjugate different molecules to dextran. We have shown, in introductory experiments, that the conjugates can be coupled together by so called CDAP (1-cyano-4-dimethylamino-pyridinium-tetrafluoroborate) activation which was first applied for activation of sepharose 4B by Kohn and Wilcheck[21]. The activated dextran can be coupled to any substance that contains at least one free amino group. The low molecular compound, (S)-carboranylalanine and high molecular compounds such as EGF, antibodies and antibody fragments all fulfil this criterion. Most polypeptides and proteins have in most cases at least one free amino group. The method is therefore of general interest. An advantage is also that all ingredients can be coupled to dextran in one single step. The dextran is activated and the boron compound and the tumour-seeking polypeptides or proteins can be added in arbitrary molar proportions. The principles for the synthesis (activation and coupling) of conjugate is illustrated with a carborane-dextran-EGF conjugate (**CDE**) in Fig. 1.

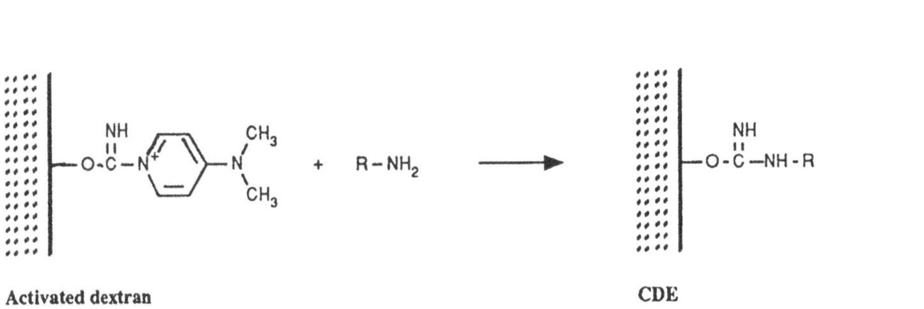

Fig. 1. Synthesis of a CDE. R-NH$_2$ represents EGF or an amino substituted carborane.

Dextran is activated with CDAP. EGF and amino substituted carboranes like (*S*)-carboranylalanine are coupled to the activated dextran via their amino groups. After coupling the conjugate is purified in two or three steps. The capacity of the conjugate to bind to the EGF-receptor is determined in an *in vitro* assay using human glioma cells in culture, U-343-MGaCl2;6 cells. These cells have a high amount of EGF receptors[22-24].

We have conjugated EGF to dextran using the amino group on the N-terminal of EGF. The N-terminus not involved in the binding site. The EGF- dextran conjugate binds to the EGF-receptors on the cultured glioma cells[25].

Radioactivity delivered to the U-343-MGaCl2;6 cells by ^{125}I-EGF-dextran or EGF-dextran-^{3}H remained cell-associated for long periods of time, more than 20h, in contrast to the radioactivity carried by free EGF which disappeared from the cells within a few hours (Fig. 2).

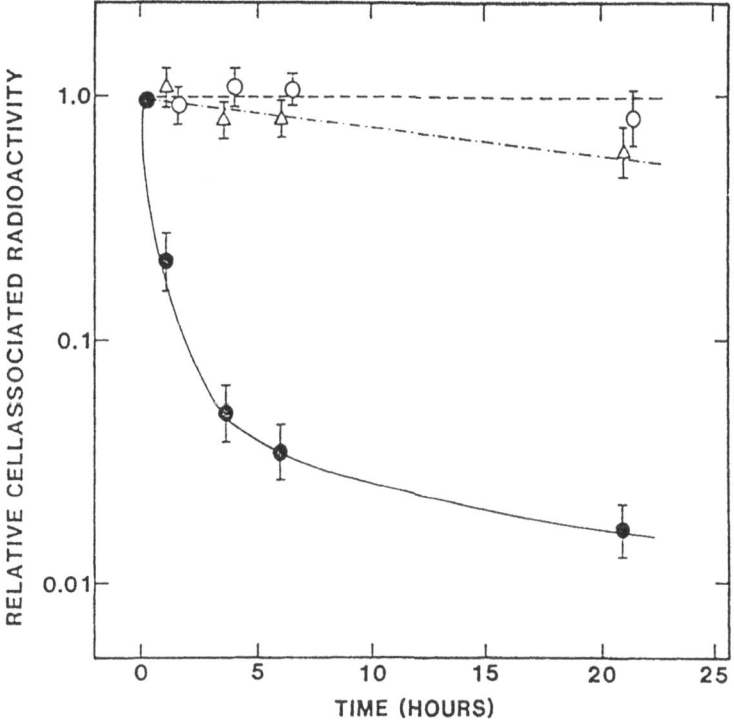

Fig. 2. Cell-associated radioactivity as a function of time after incubation at 37° C with EGF-dextran- [3]H (○), ^{125}I-EGF-dextran (△)and ^{125}I-EGF (●). The cells were washed after the incubations and thereafter grown in normal culture medium for varying times. The cell-associated radioactivity, directly after incubation, was normalized to unity. The values for the background samples incubated with dextran-^{3}H were in the range 0.01 - 0.03. Triple samples were analysed for each point and mean values and maximum variations are shown[25].

It seemed, in pilot experiments, possible to accumulate radioactivity in the cells through repeated exposure to the conjugate. The cells synthesized new EGF-receptors between the exposures.

We have in preliminary experiments tried to conjugate the boron containing amino acid (S)-carboranylalanine and EGF to dextran, CDE-1. The conjugates seemed to bind to the EGF-receptors (Fig. 3). However the amount of boron in the conjugates has not yet been determined.

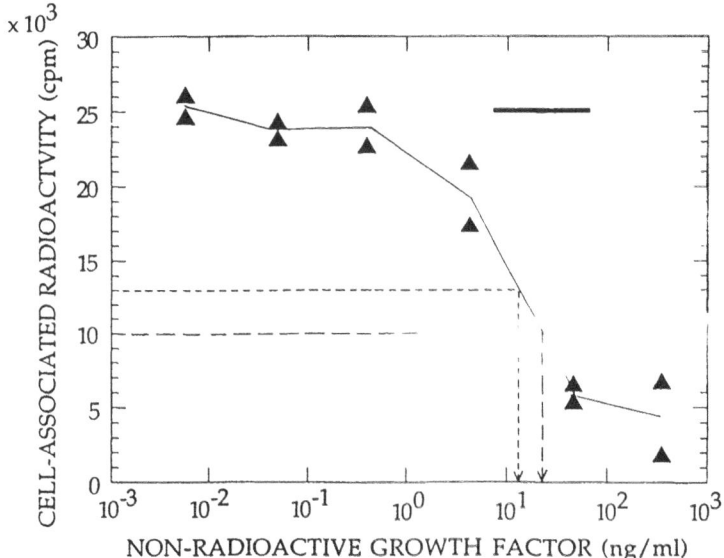

Fig. 3. The figure shows, with filled triangles, how increased concentrations of non-radioactive EGF inhibit binding of ^{125}I-EGF to the EGF-receptor of human glioma U-343-MGaCl2;6 cells. (S)-Carboranylalanine-dextran-EGF (CDE-1) was added in two relative concentrations; 1.0 and 0.33 as indicated with the long and short dashed lines respectively. The inhibition of ^{125}I-EGF binding by CDE-1 and the corresponding "effective EGF concentrations" are shown with these dashed lines. The thick bar at the upper right part of the figure shows the binding level of ^{125}I-EGF in control cultures.

The probably most important property of the EGF-dextran conjugates is the ability of the conjugate bound radioactivity to remain cell-associated for a long time. This must be valuable for use in BNCT for getting enough boron into tumour cells and prevent degradation in the lysosomes[25].

SYNTHESIS OF CARBORANES CONTAINING AMINO GROUPS

Our synthetic efforts are directed toward the preparation of boron compounds containing a primary amino function such as amino acids and primary amines. The boron compounds will be carboranes and carborane anions, mainly 1,2-dicarba-*closo*-dodecaborane(12)derivatives and their 7,8-dicarba-*nido*-dodecahydro-undecaborate (-1) anion analogues. Here we report methods for synthesis of optically active carboranylamino acids and aminoalkylcarboranes .

We have in our initial studies chosen to work with conjugates containing the enantiomeric forms of carboranylalanine.

Asymmetric synthesis of (R)- and (S)-carboranylalanine

In 1976 the first synthesis of optically active o-carboranylalanine (II) was reported. In a nine-step synthesis, starting with diethyl N-acetamidomalonate and involving an enzymatic resolution of N-acetylpropargylglycine, (S)-II was obtained in an overall yield of 1.9%[26] In a later report the same research group[27] described a modified nine-step version with an overall yield of 4.5%.We have performed three successful syntheses of (S)-carboranylalanine according to this route. However the low yield and the very lengthy procedure prompted us to find an alternative.

We have performed a three-step synthesis of the enantiomeric o-carborany-alanines[28], starting with the commercially available enantiomers of 2-*t*-butyl-1-*t*-butyloxycarbonyl-3-methyl-4-imidazolidinone (I) introduced by Fitzi and Seebach[29]. The synthesis of (R)-carboranylalanine is illustrated in Fig. 4. The overall yield was 20 % starting from (R)-I.

We are presently working on the asymmetric synthesis of other amino acids containing carboranyl groups and their corresponding *nido*anions.

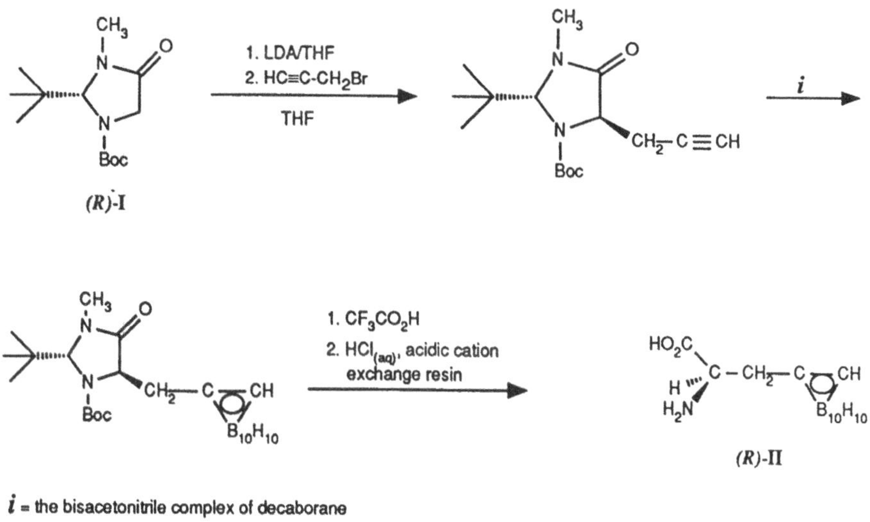

i = the bisacetonitrile complex of decaborane

Fig. 4. Asymmetric synthesis of (R)-carboranylalanine , (R)-II.

Synthesis of aminoalkylcarboranes

We are using the alternative Gabriel reagent, di-*t*-butyl imidodikarbonat[30], for preparation of aminoalkylcarboranes starting with haloalkylsubstituted acetylenes or carboranes. In a recent dissertation from Professor Hawthornes research group[31] a similar approach was used for the preparation of 1,2 bis-(3-amino-propyl)-1,2-dicarbadodecaborane.

We have found that di-*t*-butyl imidodikarbonat can be alkylated as an ion pair in ca 90% yield under the general conditions for alkylation of weak acids described by Brändström[32].

The method is exemplified by the synthesis of the hydrochloride of aminomethylcarborane with an over all yield of 25%. In this case one of the *t*-butyloxycarbonyl groups was lost during the formation of the carborane.

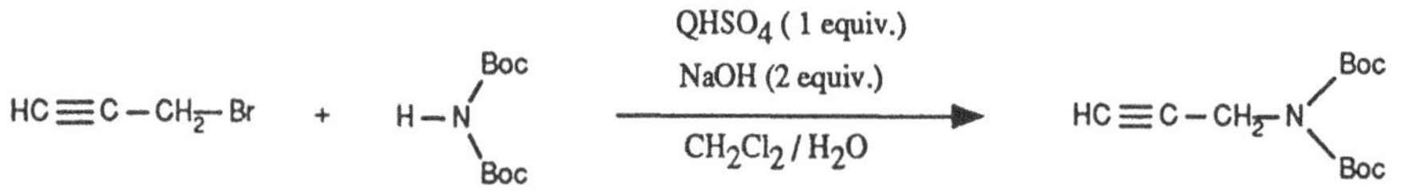

QHSO$_4$ = tetrabutylammonium hydrogen sulphate

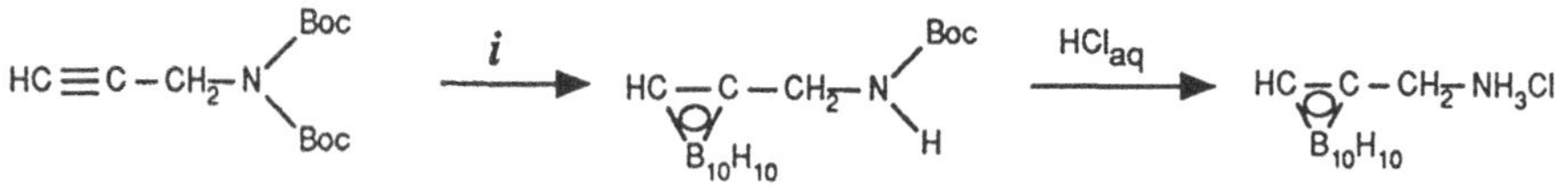

i = the bisacetonitrile complex of decaborane

Fig. 5. Synthesis of the hydrochloride of aminomethylcarborane.

ANALYSIS OF BORON COMPOUNDS WITH ICP-MS

Accurate methods for the quantitative determination of boron in biological and synthetic material are essential for research in BNCT.

Inductively coupled plasma mass spectrometry (ICP-MS) is a sensitive and selective method for the analysis of the total concentration of most elements and nuclides, viz. ^{10}B and ^{11}B.

The aim of this study is to examine if ICP-MS can be used for fast, accurate and sensitive determination of boron in biological tissues and synthetic compounds of boron.

Accurate estimations of the isotope ratio is a prerequisite for the use of isotopic dilution technique for determining boron concentration. By comparing different modes (survey scan using conditional Saha factors[34], peak jumping and isotope ratio) we have studied the sensitivity of ICP-MS for the estimation of boron and the boron isotope ratio in BSH ($Na_2B_{12}H_{11}SH$), 1-(bromomethyl)-carborane and boric acids with different isotopic ratios. The measurements were performed on a VG PQ1 ICP-MS using soft ware version 3.1 A. The results are presented in Tables 1-3.

TABLE 1 ESTIMATION OF BORON BY SAHA-CORRECTION

Sample	Expected conc. ng/ml	Found conc. ng/ml	Rel.error, %
Boric acid, BDH*	50	53	5.7
Boric acid, BDH*	100	100	-
BSH**	88.7	92 (n=2)	3.6
SRM 952***	94.2	94.2 (n=2)	-
SRM 1643b****	94	100 (n=2)	6.0

*) BDH Spectrosol
**) $Na_2B_{12}H_{11}SH$
***) Enriched boric acid (94.949 % ^{10}B), SRM 952 (NBS)
****) Trace elements in water, 1643b (NBS)

In the different compounds, the error in the estimation of boron was less than 10 %. By using Saha-correction, it was possible to get quantitative information within a short time. In the same run, it is possible to detect the amount of contaminant elements in synthetic compounds.

TABLE 2 ESTIMATION OF BORON USING ^{115}In AND ^9Be

Sample	INTERNAL STANDARD ^{115}In			INTERNAL STANDARD ^9Be		
	Expected conc. ng/ml	Found conc. ng/ml	Rel.error, %	Expected conc. ng/ml	Found conc. ng/ml	Rel.error, %
Boric acid, BDH	10	10	-	50	46	8.0
BSH	88.7	90	1.4	88.7	87 (n=2)	1.9
SRM 1643b	94	101	6.9	94	91 (n=3)	3.2

Different internal standards ^{115}In and ^9Be were used to compare the ability to compensate for changes in plasma etc. For ICP-MS, the element ^{115}In is generally used for the mass range 4 - 245. We thought that ^9Be would be an alternative for elements of lower mass. The detection limit of boron estimated as 3s of the blank yielded 1 ng/ml which is in accord with earlier observations[35].

Because of its accuracy and speed of analysis, the Saha corrected estimation of boron may be a routine method for analysis of boron in synthetic compounds and biological tissues. Boron analysis by ICP-MS is precise and accurate within a detection limit of 1 ppb and a relative error of $\pm 10\%$.

Isotope ratio analysis of boron compounds is a precise method and will be used in future work for analysis of boron concentrations by the isotope dilution method.

TABLE 3 ISOTOPE RATIO OF $^{11}B/^{10}B$

Sample	Conc., ng/ml	Found ratio	Stand.dev.
Boric acid, BDH	10	4.55 (n=2)	0.12
Boric acid, BDH	50	4.60 (n=4)	0.07
Boric acid, BDH	100	4.49	0.05
BSH	88.7	4.23 (n=2)	0.04
SRM 952	94.2	0.052	0.002
BrMeCar*	120	4.54	0.04
SRM 1643b	94	4.11	0.05

*) 1-(bromomethyl)-carborane

ACKNOWLEDGEMENTS

The experimental work has been financially supported by the Swedish Cancer Society, the Swedish Medical Research Council, the Swedish Natural Science Research Council, and the Swedish Board of Technical Development.

REFERENCES

1, G. L. Locher, Biological effects and therapeutic possibilities of neutrons, *Am. J. Roentgenol. and Radium Ther*. 36: 1 (1936).

2. H. Hatanaka, S. Kamano, K. Amano, S. Hojo, K. Kano, S. Egawa, and H. Yasukochi: Clinical experience of boron-neutron capture therapy for gliomas - a comparison with conventional chemo-immuno-radiotherapy, in: "Boron Neutron Capture Therapy for Tumours," H. Hatanaka, ed., Nishimura Co. Ltd, Niigata, Japan (1986), pp 349-378.

3. D. Gabel, Goals and achievements of the European Collaboration on boron neutron capture therapy, in: these proceedings.

4. H. Condé, E. Grusell, B. Larsson,, E. Ramström, T. Rönnqvist, O. Sornsuntisook, S. Villa, J. Crawford, H. Reist, B. Dahl, N. G. Sjöstrand, and G. Russel, Status report on the development of a spallation source for neutron capture therapy, in: "Clinical Aspects on Neutron Capture Therapy," R. G. Fairchild et al., eds., Plenum Publ. Corp., New York (1989), pp. 319-323.

5. P. Strömberg, Pers. comm. 1990.

6. J. F. Crawford, H. Condé, K. Elmgren, E. Grusell, B. Larsson, B. Nilsson, O. Pettersson, H. Reist, T. Rönnqvist, and G. Russel, Neutron beams for capture therapy produced by 72 MeV protons, in: these proceedings.

7. A. Andersson, J. Burgman, J. Capala, J.Carlsson, H. Condé, J. Crawford, S. Graffmann, E. Grusell, A. Holmberg, E. Johansson, O. Jonsson, B. S. Larsson, B. Larsson, P. Lindström, L. Pellettieri, O. Pettersson, J. Pontén, M. Pråhl, A. Roberti, K. Russel, H. Reist, L. Salford, S.Sjöberg, B. Stenerlöw, P. Strömberg, and B.Westermark, Programme for accelarator-based neutron capture therapy, in: Proceedings from the European Particle Accelerator Conference, Nice, France (June 1990).

8.. A. Andersson, J. Andersson, J-O. Burgman, J. Capala, J.Carlsson, H. Condé,J. Crawford, S. Graffmann, E. Grusell, A. Holmberg, E. Johansson, B.S. Larsson, B.Larsson, T. Liljefors, P. Lindström, L. Pellettieri, O. Pettersson, J. Pontén, A. Roberti, K. Russel, H. Reist, L. Salford, S.Sjöberg, B. Stenerlöw, P. Strömberg, and B.Westermark, Programme for BNCT with accelerator produced keV neutrons and related chemical and biological studies, in: Abstracts from this symposium p. 47.

9. A. Andersson, J.Carlsson, J. Capala, B.Larsson, P Lindström, O. Pettersson, and S. Sjöberg, Boronation of EGF via dextran, in: ibid. p 34.

10. S. Sjöberg, P. Lindström, A. Andersson, J.Carlsson, A. Holmberg, B.Larsson, and O. Pettersson, Asymmetric synthesis of carboranyl amino acids for for boronation of EGF-dextran and other macromolecules of therapeutical interest, ibid. p. 68.

11. A. Andersson, J.Carlsson, E. Johannson, B. Larsson, T. Liljefors, P. Lindström, and S. Sjöberg, Analysis of boron compounds with ICP-MS, ibid, p87..

12. B. S. Larsson, B. Larsson, and A. Roberto, Boron neutron capture therapy for malignant melanoma: An experimental approach, *Pigm. Cell. Res.* 2, 356 (1989).

13. B. Larsson, J. Carlsson, H. Börner, J. Forsberg, A. Fourcy, and M. Thellier, Biological studies with cold neutrons: An experimental approach to the LET problem in radiotherapy, in : "Progress in Radio-Oncology II," K. H. Kärcher et al. eds., Raven Press, New York (1982), pp. 151-157.

14. T. A. Libermann, N. Razon, A. D. Bartal, Y. Tarden, J. Schlessinger, and H. Soreq, expression of epidermal growth factor in human brain tumors, *Cancer Res.* 44:753-760 (1984).

15. J. Filmus, M. N. Pollak, R. Cailleau, and R. Buick, MDA-468, a human breast cancer cell line with a high number of epidermal growth factor (EGF) receptors, has an amplified EGF receptor gene and is growth inhibited by EGF, *Biochem. Biophys.* 128:898-905 (1985).

16. T. A. Libermann, H. R. Nusbaum, N. Razon, R. Kriz, I. Lax, H. Soreq, N. Whittle, M. D. Waterfield, and J. Schleissinger, Amplification, enhanced expression and possible rearrangement of receptor gene in primary human brain tumors of glial origin, *Nature* 313:144-147 (1985).

17. G. Carpenter, Receptors for epidermal growth factor and other polypeptide miogens, *Ann. Rev. Biochem.* 56:881-914 (1987).

18. S. H. Bigner, P. C. Burger, A. J. Wong, M. H. Werner, S. R. Hamilton, L. H. Muhkbaier, B. Vogelstein, and D. D. Bigner, Gene amplification in malignant human gliomas: clinical and histopathologic aspects, *J. Neuropathol. Exp. Neurol.* 47:191-205 (1988).

19. S. Ozawa, M Ueda, N. Ando, O. Abe, S. Minoshima, and N. Shimzu, Selective killing of squamous carcinoma cells by an immunotoxin that recognizes the EGF receptor, *Int. J. Cancer* 47:191 (1989).

20. I. D. Campbell, R. M. Cooke, M. Baron, T. S. Harvey, and M. J. Tappin, The solution structures of epidermal growth factor and transforming growth factor alfa, *Progress in Growth Factor Research* 1: 13 -22 (1989).

21. J. Kohn, and M. Wilchek. 1-Cyano-4-dimethylamino pyridinium tetrafluoroborate as a cyanylating agent for the covalent attachment of ligand to polysaccharide resins, *FEBS Letters*, 154:209-210 (1983.).

22. B. Westermark, A. Magnusson, and C. H. Heldin, Effect of epidermal growth factor on membrane motility and cell locomotion in cultures of human glioma cells, *J. Neuroscience research* 8:491-507 (1982).

23. M. Nister, B. Wedell, C. Betsholtz, M. Bywater, M. Petterson, B. Westermark, and J. Mark, Evidence for progressional changes in the human malignant glioma line U-343MGa: analysis of karyotype and expression of genes encoding the subunit chains of platelet-derived growth factor, *Cancer Research*, 47:4953-4960 (1987).

24. M. H. Werner, P. A. Humphrey, D. D. Bigner, and S. H. Bigner, Growth effects of epidermal growth factor (EGF) and a monoclonal antibody against the EGF receptor on four glioma cell lines, *Acta neuropathol.* 77:196-201 (1988).

25. A. Andersson, A. Holmberg, J.Carlsson, J.Carlsson, J. Pontén, and B. Westermark, Binding of epidermal growth factor-dextran conjugates to cultured glioma cells, *Int. J. Cancer* in press (1991).

26. O.Leukart, M. Caviezel, A. Eberle, E. Escher, A. Tun-Kyi, and R. Schwyzer, L-o-Carboranylalanine a boron analogue of phenylalanine, *Helv. Chim. Acta* 59: 2184 (1976).

27. J-L Fauchére, O. Leukart, A. Eberle, and R. Schwyzer, The synthesis of (4--Carboranylalanine, 5-Leucine)-enkephalin, *Helv. Chim. Acta*, 62:1385-1395 (1979).

28. P.L Lindström, and S. Sjöberg, Manuscript in preparation.

29. R. Fitzi, and D. Seebach, Resolution and use in amino acid synthesis of imidazolidinone glycine derivatives, Tetrahedron 44, 5277 (1988).

30. L. A. Carpino, New methods of introducing the carbo-*t*-butoxy amino-protecting group; Preparation and use if *t*-butyl cyanoformate and *t*-butyl iminodicarboxylate, *J. Org: Chem.* 29:2820 (1964).

31. J. L. Maurer, The synthesis of glycosyl carboranes and carboranyl diacids and diamines as precursors to reagents for boron neutron capture therapy, Dissertation, University of California, Los Angeles, USA (1989).

32. A. Brändström "Preparative Ion Pair Extraction,"Apotekarsocieteten/Hässle Läkemedel, Stockholm, Sweden (1974).

33. J. Malmquist, and S. Sjöberg, Unpublished observations.

34. T. D. B. Lyon, G. S. Fell, R. C. Hutton, and A. N. Eaton, Evaluation of inductively coupled plasma mass spectrometry (ICP-MS) for simultaneous multi-element trace analysis in clinical chemistry, *JAAS* 3:265-271 (1988).

35. A. L. Gray, and A.R. Date, Inductively coupled plasma source mass spectrometry using continuum flow ion extraction, *Analyst* 108:1033-1050 (1983).

PERFORMANCE OF THE CURRENTLY AVAILABLE EPITHERMAL NEUTRON BEAM AT THE

MASSACHUSETTS INSTITUTE OF TECHNOLOGY RESEARCH REACTOR (MITR-II)

J.R. Choi[1], R.G. Zamenhof[2], J.C. Yanch[1], R. Rogus[1], and O.K. Harling[1]

[1] Nuclear Reactor Laboratory, Massachusetts Institute of Technology
138 Albany Street, Cambridge, MA 02139, USA.

[2] Department of Radiation Oncology, Tufts New England Medical Center
750 Washington Street, Boston, MA 02111, USA.

ABSTRACT

This paper describes the performance of the currently available epithermal neutron beam at MITR-II. This beam is one of the few clinically useful epithermal neutron beams available for BNCT in the world. The MITR-II epithermal neutron beam has a peak thermal neutron flux of greater than 4×10^8 n/cm^2 s at 2 cm depth in tissue. Assuming a B-10 concentration of 30 μg/g in tumor and an effective 10 to 1 ratio of B-10 in tumor to healthy tissue, the most important figures of merit for the beam are as follows. The advantage depth (useful therapeutic penetration) is in excess of 7 cm. The dose rate to tumor at the advantage depth is 9.6 RBE cGy/min. The integral ratio of dose to tumor vs. dose to healthy tissue is greater than 3 when measured along the centerline of an ellipsoidal water phantom. When used in bilateral irradiation of tumors, this beam can treat the entire brain with therapeutic advantage ratio of greater than 2.9. In addition, plans for improving the current epithermal beam through straightforward modifications are presented. This improved beam is expected to have peak thermal neutron flux in excess of 10^9 n/cm^2 s with proportionally greater therapeutic dose rate and higher advantage ratio than the current epithermal neutron beam.

INTRODUCTION

Significant modifications have been made to the MITR-II epithermal neutron beam facility since the beam design workshop held at Massachusetts Institute of Technology.[1] Figure 1 illustrates the current

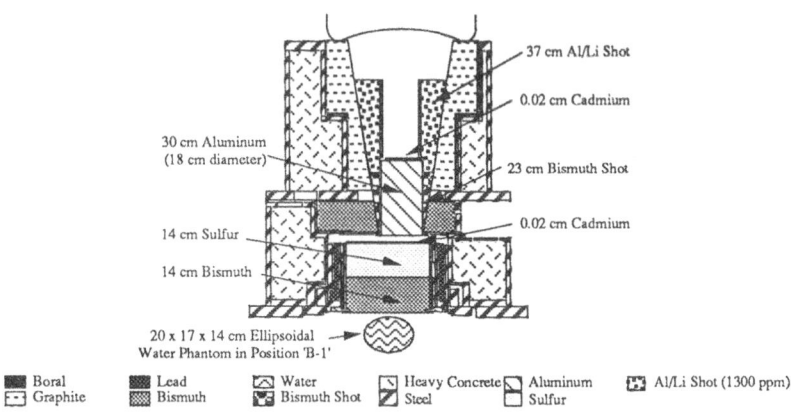

Figure 1. Cross section of the current M-055 epithermal neutron beam filter at MITR-II

configuration of the MITR-II epithermal neutron beam. The central region of the filter materials have been moved down near the beam collimator to approximate a moderator configuration. The filter is composed of 30 cm of aluminum, 14 cm of sulfur, and 14 cm of bismuth. The aluminum and the sulfur sections are topped by 0.02 cm of cadmium. The outer cone region in the graphite collimator is filled with 37 cm of aluminum shot doped with 1300 ppm of lithium placed above 23 cm of bismuth shot. The effective diameter of this epithermal beam is the same as the width of the final bismuth collimator which is approximately 30 cm. As with previous epithermal filter arrangements, this beam can be changed back to a thermal beam in a few hours.

PERFORMANCE CHARACTERIZATION

Measurements to characterize this beam were made in two different phantoms. One was a cylindrical acrylic phantom 18 cm in diameter and 23 cm in height filled with water. The other was an ellipsoidal phantom made out of acrylic that closely approximated the standard human brain according to Snyder et al,[2] dimension of 20 cm by 17 cm by 14 cm, also filled with water. Calculations based on densities and hydrogen atom percentages show that water accurately approximates the hydrogen density, the most important element for BNCT phantoms, of average human brain (6.69×10^{22} atoms/cc for water, 6.68×10^{22} atoms/cc for brain).

Table 1.   Measured performance of the M-055 epithermal neutron beam at MITR-II in a 18×20 cm cylindrical water phantom and a $20 \times 17 \times 14$ cm ellipsoidal water phantom. The beam is incident upon the flat end of the cylindrical phantom and parallel to the 14 cm elliptical axis of the ellipsoidal phantom. Values are normalized to 5 MW_t reactor power.

Phantom	Inc. Φ_{epi} flux	Peak Φ_{th} flux	Gold Cd ratio*
Cylindrical water	2.6×10^8 n/cm^2 s	4.4×10^8 n/cm^2 s @ 2 cm	2.7
Ellipsoidal water	3.0×10^8 n/cm^2 s	4.3×10^8 n/cm^2 s @ 2 cm	2.7

*   Gold Cd ratio obtained for gold foil thickness of 40 mg/cm^2.

The principal performance characteristics of the current epithermal neutron beam (M-055) are listed in Table 1. The peak thermal neutron flux is greater than 4×10^8 n/cm^2 s at 2 cm depth in both phantoms. At 7 cm depth, along the beam axis at the midline of the brain, the beam provides nearly one-third of this peak neutron flux. The cadmium ratio measured on top of the phantoms is 2.7 and the effective calculated epithermal neutron current, assuming a 1/E distribution in the epithermal energy region (0.4 eV to 10 keV), is $2.6 \sim 3.0 \times 10^8$ n/cm^2 s.[3]

Table 2 lists the measured performance characteristics of the M-055 beam in the ellipsoidal water filled phantom using the terminology and RBEs used for the MIT workshop.[4] The table lists two sets of results, one assuming boron-10 concentration of 30 μg/g in tumor and an effective boron-10 dose ratio of 10

Table 2.   Advantage depth (AD), advantage depth dose rate (ADDR), advantage ratio (AR), and percentage of low LET, high LET, and $^{10}B(n,\alpha)^7Li$ reaction dose that results from the M-055 epithermal neutron beam at MITR-II incident on the $20 \times 17 \times 14$ cm ellipsoidal water phantom based on measured depth dose distribution and assumed boron distribution at 5 MW_t reactor power.*

	30 ppm ^{10}B in tumor with tumor/brain ratio of 10 to 1	50 ppm ^{10}B in tumor with tumor/brain ratio of 4 to 1
RBE Advantage depth (max/min)	8.0/7.1 cm	9.6/6.8 cm
RBE Advantage depth dose rate	9.6 cGy/min	14 cGy/min
RBE Advantage ratio (maximum)	3.1	4.5
% low LET RBE dose**	21	15
% high LET RBE dose**	13	9
% $^{10}B(n,\alpha)^7Li$ RBE dose**	65	76

*   RBE factors of 2.3 for (n,α) reactions, 1.6 for high LET proton recoil and $^{14}N(n,p)^{14}C$ reactions, and 1.0 for low LET reactions were used in all dose calculations; the figures of merit AD, ADDR, and AR and the source of the RBEs are defined in Ref [1].

**   Doses are integral RBE doses measured from the surface to the maximum advantage depth.

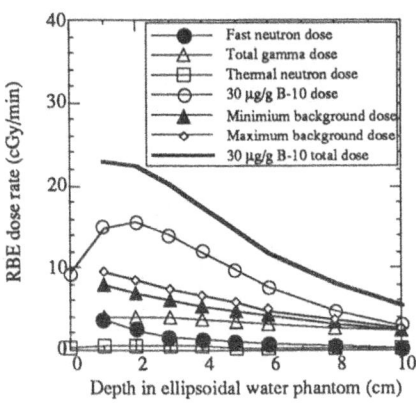

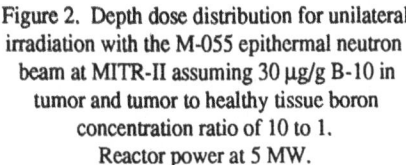

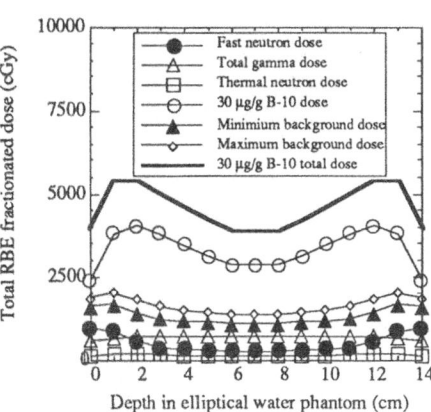

Figure 2. Depth dose distribution for unilateral irradiation with the M-055 epithermal neutron beam at MITR-II assuming 30 μg/g B-10 in tumor and tumor to healthy tissue boron concentration ratio of 10 to 1. Reactor power at 5 MW.

Figure 3. Depth dose distribution for bilateral irradiation with the M-055 epithermal neutron beam at MITR-II assuming 30 μg/g B-10 in tumor and tumor to healthy tissue boron concentration ratio of 10 to 1. (Figure derived from figure 2)

to 1 for concentration in tumor versus healthy tissue (which correspond to biodistribution characteristics of boron sulfhydril (BSH) compound including a 1/3 capillary factor); and the other assuming boron-10 concentration of 50 μg/g in tumor and tumor-to-tissue ratio of 4 to 1 (corresponding to biodistribution characteristics of boron phenylalanine (BPA) compound). Figure 2 shows the corresponding dose depth rate distribution for the former boron-10 distribution and a unilateral irradiation of the ellipsoidal phantom. In either case, the majority of the dose delivered to the tumor from this neutron beam is due to the $^{10}B(n,\alpha)^7Li$ reaction.

Figure 3 shows the depth dose distribution, derived from measurements along the central beam axis (see figure 2), for bilateral irradiation using the M-055 epithermal neutron beam on an ellipsoidal water phantom. For this figure, tumor concentration of boron-10 was assumed to be 30 μg/g and tumor to healthy tissue boron concentration was assumed to equal 10. It is assumed that the dose will be delivered in 4 - 6 fractions with an effective RBE of 0.5 for gamma rays.[5] The RBE for fast neutrons or $^{14}N(n,p)^{14}C$ and for $^{10}B(n,\alpha)^7Li$ reactions are 1.6 and 2.3 respectively. What is remarkable from this figure is that the background dose to the healthy brain remains relatively constant at all depths. This is especially desirable for clinical trials, because it places no part of the brain at greatly increased risk and thus allows the maximum therapeutic dose to be delivered to the tumor region, wherever it may be located. For example, with a local maximum dose of 2000 RBE cGy to the healthy brain, one can deliver 3900 ~ 5400 RBE cGy to the tumor region throughout the entire depth in brain. This corresponds to an advantage ratio of 2.9.

PLANS FOR FUTURE WORK

Work is under way to further significantly improve the current epithermal neutron beam at MITR-II. The proposed stage I changes illustrated in figure 4 are based on results from dozens of different filter configurations previously installed and characterized. The inner aluminum filter will be replaced by a larger sulfur filter 25 cm in diameter and 50 cm in height. Simple experiments conducted at MITR-II using large aluminum and sulfur plates indicated that sulfur is significantly better as a filter material than aluminum. Increasing the filter diameter to 25 cm from 18 cm should result in proportionally greater neutron flux. Preliminary analysis indicates that this new filter arrangement will increase the peak epithermal neutron flux by about a factor of two. Likewise, the ADDR is expected to increase significantly. The fast neutron contribution to the dose is expected to decrease, resulting in improved AR.

If the steps outlined above result in the improvements of the beam as expected, we have plans to further increase the intensity and the quality of the epithermal neutron beam. The sulfur filter would be made much larger by removing portions of the graphite collimator. This filter design shown in figure 5 is expected to give much higher epithermal neutron current, some of which could be traded for better fast neutron and incident gamma ray attenuation. This stage II epithermal neutron filter design incorporates a large sulfur filter

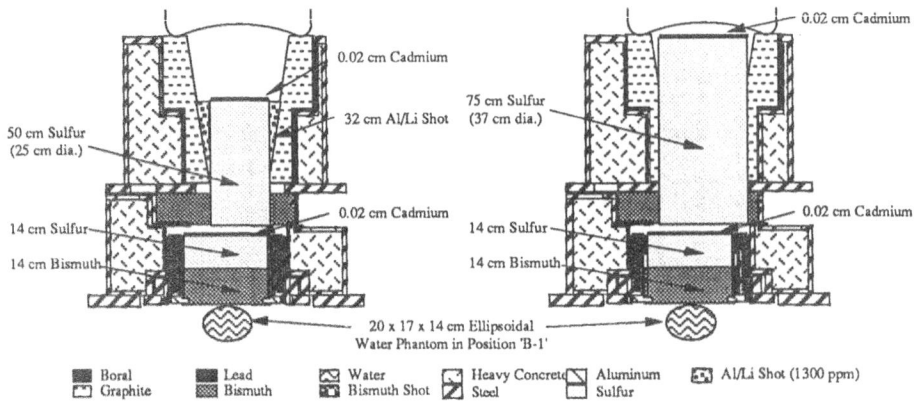

Figure 4. Cross section of the proposed stage I epithermal neutron beam filter at MITR-II.

Figure 5. Cross section of the proposed stage II epithermal neutron beam filter at MITR-II.

37 cm in diameter and 75 cm in height and eliminates the need for aluminum shot that is used to fill the outer cone region in the present filter designs. This with the increased sulfur thickness is expected to give 30 to 50% improvement in the fast neutron attenuation over the stage I configuration. Initial estimates show that a minimum global advantage ratio of over 4 can be obtained with ADDR over 20 cGy/min. Such a beam would, for example, be able to deliver over 4000 RBE cGy to the tumor region while limiting the healthy brain dose to less than 1000 RBE cGy. In either stage I or stage II configurations, the ability to switch to a thermal neutron beam within a few hours will be retained.

CONCLUSIONS

The modifications made to the medical beam of the MITR-II Research Reactor have produced one of the few currently available and clinically useful epithermal neutron beams in the world. The current epithermal neutron beam has the capability to treat tumors located anywhere in the brain with good therapeutic advantage. The rather straight forward modifications planned for the future should further improve the capabilities of this epithermal neutron beam.

ACKNOWLEDGMENTS

The authors wish to thank Dr. John Bernard and the rest of the MITR-II operations group for their support and assistance in all aspects of this work. This research was funded by the U.S. Department of Energy, Office of Health and Human Assessments, under the Grant No. DE-FG02-87ER-6060.

REFERENCES

1. Harling, O.K. et al. eds., Neutron Beam Design, Development, and Performance for Neutron Capture Therapy, Basic Life Science, Vol. 54, Plenum Press, New York (1990)

2. Snyder, W.S. et al. , "Estimates for Absorbed Fractions for Monoenergetic Photon Sources Uniformly Distributed in Various Organs of a Heterogeneous Phantom," MIRD, J. Nucl. Med., Suppl. No. 3, Pamphlet 5, p. 47 (1969)

3. ASTM E262-77, Standard Method for Measuring Thermal Neutron Flux by Radioactivation Techniques.

4. Choi, J.R. et al. , "Neutron Capture Therapy Beams at the MIT Research Reactor," Neutron Beam Design, Development, and Performance for Neutron Capture Therapy, Harling, O.K. et al. eds., Basic Life Science, Vol. 54, Plenum Press, New York, p. 201 - 218 (1990)

5. Hall, E.J. , Radiobiology for the Radiologist, 3rd Ed., J. B. Lippincott Co., Philadelphia, p 165 (1988)

A COMPACT TRIGA REACTOR FOR

BORON NEUTRON CAPTURE THERAPY

William L. Whittemore

General Atomics

San Diego, California

INTRODUCTION

Hatanaka[1] has reviewed the many clinical results for the treatment of glioblastoma using Boron Neutron Capture Therapy (BNCT) carried out at the Musashi TRIGA 100 kW reactor facility. Mishima[2] has reviewed the successful application of BNCT to the treatment of malignant melanoma at the same facility. Aizawa[3] has reported details of the Musashi TRIGA reactor for the thermal neutron treatment of more than 100 patients and outlined improvements for this small reactor. During the last years, the perception has been growing that epithermal neutrons ($\bar{E}$ <8.5 keV) are much more suitable for a variety of reasons than thermal neutrons for the treatment of deep seated malignancies.

Extensive efforts in Europe, Japan, Australia and the United States have been directed to the development of BNCT beam parameters suitable as a goal for the modification of existing, higher power reactors or for new reactors dedicated for BNCT. It appears that a need will continue for higher flux thermal neutron sources (possibly with larger than the presently used treatment cross sectional area) for malignant melanoma cases near the surface of the skin. In addition, there is a need for appropriately high flux sources of epithermal neutrons for the deeper seated malignancies. The general consensus is that a full therapy epithermal neutron treatment should take less than one hour. This will require an epithermal neutron fluence at the patient of about 3 to 5×10^{12} n/cm^2 (E $\leq$8.5 keV). Fractionation (perhaps up to 5) may be used. Typically a reactor with a leakage flux at core edge of $>10^{13}$ n/cm^2.s (thermal) and $\sim 10^{14}$ n/cm^2.s (>10 keV) will easily satisfy the above requirements.

In supplying the needs for BNCT, it will be of utmost important that the reactor meet the strictest safety standards. Not only must the background radiation in the beam be carefully controlled, but the reactor itself even in unusual or abnormal operation must pose no threat to the patient or the public. A new reactor to be constructed for BNCT should have such recognized safety features that it can be safely sited in a hospital or hospital complex. Several TRIGA reactors have already been sited in hospital complexes (Heidelberg Cancer Research Center; Hanover Medical College; Omaha Veterans Hospital) and in university buildings on campus (University of California at Irvine; University of Arizona).

Progress in Neutron Capture Therapy for Cancer
Edited by B.J. Allen *et al.*, Plenum Press, New York, 1992

GENERAL REACTOR REQUIREMENTS FOR BNCT

Except for the Brookhaven Medical Research Reactor (BMRR) and the BNCT medical facility constructed below the MIT research reactor, all other facilities for BNCT have been using, or plan to use, existing research or test reactors with modified thermal columns, beam ports, or both. Since these latter reactors are usually general purpose research facilities they frequently incorporate geometries or embedded components that are less than suitable for BNCT.

The BMRR facility has undergone extensive calibration efforts to characterize a suitable epithermal neutron source for BNCT. These efforts have been carried out jointly by the staffs at Brookhaven National Laboratory and the Idaho National Engineering Laboratory (INEL).[4,5,6] For the BMRR facility a full therapeutic dose of 25 Gy can be delivered in about 50 min with a total patient fluence of 5.6×10^{12} n/cm^2. The accompanying gamma ray dose is 0.62 Gy.

An important design consideration for either a thermal or epithermal neutron source for BNCT is the area at the source end of the beam forming system. A collimator that is large at the reactor end and tapers to the small aperture required at the patient end is ideal, taking full advantage of the available reactor leakage flux. A typical radial beam port with parallel walls uses only a portion of the available leakage flux. As examples, the thermal column modified into essentially a tapered port enabled the 100 kW Musashi TRIGA reactor to perform effective BNCT treatment.[3] On the other hand, the parallel walled, radial beam port HB11 at the Petten reactor requires a 45 MW reactor power level to produce a flux at the patient comparable with that obtained with the 3 MW BMRR facility which uses a large, tapered port.

To tailor the fast neutron leakage flux to the desired epithermal flux (E $\leq$ 8.5 keV), one can use filters, spectrum shifters, or special moderators.[4,5,6] The distinction often blurs in the large number of approaches that have been considered. In any case, it will be important to remove excess hydrogen and graphite from the beam path. In the following, the specific beam tailoring system for a TRIGA reactor will not be considered in detail because it is evident from the many studies that have been reported that the important features of a suitable reactor source will be the area of the fast neutron leakage surface and the magnitude of the fast neutron leakage flux ($>$10keV).

TRIGA REACTORS FOR BNCT

Reactors with TRIGA $U-ZrH_x$ fuel elements are known worldwide for their high degree of safety and their flexibility in satisfying widely differing customer needs. The $U-ZrH_x$ fuel is capable of supplying a large flux-per-Watt so that, in general, less steady state power is needed to supply the desired neutron fluxes.

Safety Features

The special features of $U-ZrH_x$ fueled reactors that provide the large safety for TRIGA reactors are threefold:

- large, prompt, negative coefficient of reactivity[7],

- high fuel temperature capability with safety limit of 1150°C[8] and,

- large fission product retention even at high temperatures[8].

The large, prompt, negative temperature coefficient of reactivity ($\sim 10^{-4}$ $\Delta k/k^\circ C$) derives from the hardened thermal neutron spectrum as the fuel temperatures of the $U-ZrH_x$ matrix rises.[7] The high temperature capability is due to the large chemical stability and the special metallurgical features of $U-ZrH_x$.[8] The large fission product retention is due to the trapping of fission products within the ZrH_x matrix and the slow diffusion of these products even at temperatures as high as $1000^\circ C$.[8] The fission product retention has been experimentally determined for all types of TRIGA fuel including the more recent LEU fuel.

It should be noted that an additional safety feature of the TRIGA LEU fuel is the long core life[9] (several thousands of MWD) before fuel handling is required for fuel shuffling or fuel replacement. This results in far less fuel handling than for other types of reactor fuel and thus considerably reduced chance for mishandling of the fuel.

Operational Safety

The above safety features of the TRIGA fuel combine to provide an exceptional degree of operational safety both in routine and abnormal circumstances. The negative feedback coefficient of reactivity assures that large amounts of reactivity can be added without danger to the reactor. The smaller TRIGA reactors (≤ 3 MW) can be pulsed routinely with 2% to 3% $\Delta k/k$ with no damage to the core. While the larger TRIGA reactors (≥ 5 MW) are not intended for pulsing operation, their fuel has all the safety characteristics described above and can safely sustain prompt reactivity insertions of the same magnitude as above, even though the gap resistance and resulting fuel temperatures may be altered for continued operation. A TRIGA fueled reactor can tolerate without damage a control rod ramp accident during startup that could destroy reactors with plate-type fuel. The resulting TRIGA fuel temperatures for this event are well within safe operating limits.

A loss-of-coolant flow event in a $U-ZrH_x$ core can be tolerated without any additional, auxiliary cooling, relying entirely on natural convective cooling. A 3-MW forced cooled TRIGA responds to loss of coolant flow[10] with a rising fuel and core water temperature that forces the power automatically to a lower, safe power level without a reactor scram. A loss-of-coolant flow test was performed on the 14 MW Romanian TRIGA reactor during the startup commissioning program.[11] With loss of flow, the reactor scrammed but no other action was required; the fuel temperatures fell monotonically from the operating values using only natural convective cooling.

The rapid startup (few seconds duration) capability of any TRIGA reactor may be valuable for BNCT applications. Because of the safety features described above, a controlled reactivity insertion can be safely used to increase the power from a few Watts to full power (e.g., 3 MW, or 10 MW) with no overshoot in a few seconds. This may be a convenience in starting the irradiation for a patient.

It may be useful to note that the TRIGA fuel has an excellent record of containment. Of the over 10,000 fuel rods fabricated, only a dozen stainless steel clad fuel rods have developed leaks of fission products. It is interesting to note that the high retention of fission products in the fuel matrix makes it very difficult to locate a leaking fuel element. The result of this large retention of fission products is that no TRIGA reactor requires a containment building, not even the 14-MW Romanian TRIGA reactor. A normal confinement reactor hall is sufficient to protect the public.

Table 1 presents a comparison of the thermal neutron fluxes available at core edge for TRIGA reactors ranging from the 100 kW Musashi reactor to a 10 MW reactor using a newly proposed fuel cluster with a 19-rod hexagonal array. Table 1 also presents a similar comparison for fast neutron fluxes ($\geq$10 keV) at core edge. This table also includes parameters for certain other reactors of interest; namely, BMRR, Petten, INEL TRIGA core, and HIFAR (Australia). The fast flux values for the Petten,[12] INEL TRIGA core,[13] and HIFAR[14] reactors were calculated from the published flux-per-unit lethargy spectra. The value for BMRR was estimated from the IAEA published core average fast flux.

TRIGA REACTOR PROPOSED FOR BNCT

To illustrate how a relatively simple, standard TRIGA reactor can be constructed specifically for BNCT, Figure 1 presents a sketch of a modified 3-MW Mark II TRIGA reactor. For thermal neutron BNCT, Table 1 shows that the proposed facility would provide a flux increased 28 times above that for the Musashi 100 kW TRIGA reactor. For epithermal neutron BNCT, Table 1 suggests that the performance of a 3 MW TRIGA reactor core is comparable to that for the 3 MW BMRR facility. Note that the leakage flux from a 3 MW TRIGA reactor can be enhanced by installing a weak neutron poison centrally in the core to flatten the core flux distribution. Neuman has already proposed this idea for the 10 MW INEL extended TRIGA core.[13] With this enhancement the 3 MW TRIGA core and the BMRR reactor appear to have similar capabilities as a source for epithermal BNCT.

The variation in reflector around the core in Figure 1 is chosen to satisfy a number of requirements. A portion uses graphite to optimize thermal neutron leakage for a suitably modified thermal column (tapered collimator). The epithermal BNCT treatment port (tapered collimator) is supplied with a leakage flux having a minimum of water reflector and no graphite. Also shown in Figure 1 are two radial beam ports that could be used for cell studies in a BNCT program.

For a substantial improvement in epithermal neutron performance compared to that available with a 3 MW reactor, a 10 MW TRIGA reactor using standard 1.37 cm fuel rods in either a 16-rod or 19-rod cluster would provide more than a factor of 5 improvement. Neuman has already reported a specialized version of a 10-MW reactor using TRIGA U-ZrH$_x$ fuel.[13] This design uses an extended core with a low average power density. The compact TRIGA cores for 10 MW have higher power densities, and hence larger fluxes and, at the same time, have all the safety characteristics already discussed earlier in this paper.

SUMMARY

TRIGA U-ZrH$_x$ fuel in either the standard Mark II format ($\leq$3 MW) or in larger power reactors (e.g., 10 MW) can provide very efficient and cost effective sources of thermal and epithermal neutrons for BNCT. The 3 MW power level can provide a full epithermal BNCT treatment in less than one hour and a full thermal BNCT treatment in much less than one hour.

Of all the types of research reactor fuel, the TRIGA U-ZrH$_x$ fuel is recognized by licensing authorities as providing the safest reactor operation. Reactivity accidents that would seriously damage or destroy

Figure 1. A 3 MW TRIGA Mark II Reactor for BNCT Using
Thermal and Epithermal Neutrons

REACTOR	POWER LEVEL (MW)	$\odot$ (th)	$\odot$(epi) (> 10 keV)
MUSASHI TRIGA MK II	0.10	1.1×10^{12}	--
TRIGA MK II	0.25	2.5×10^{12}	5.3×10^{12}
TRIGA MK II WATER REFLECTED NATURAL CONVECTION	1.0	1.3×10^{13} $(0.7 \times 10^{13})[1]$	0.6×10^{13}
NATURAL CONVECTION	2.0	2.1×10^{13} $(1.1 \times 10^{13})[1]$	0.9×10^{13}
FORCED COOLING	3.0	3.1×10^{13} $(1.6 \times 10^{13})[1]$	1.35×10^{13}
INEL-TRIGA FUEL EXTENDED CORE	10.0	$7 \times 10^{12}[2]$	7.6×10^{13}
COMPACT TRIGA CORE (16-ROD) SQUARE ARRAY-WATER REFLECTED	10.0	9×10^{13}	8×10^{13}
COMPACT TRIGA CORE (19-ROD) HEX ARRAY WATER REFLECTED	10.0	1.4×10^{14}	1.3×10^{14}
PETTEN HB11	45	--	6.6×10^{13}
HIFAR 10H	10	--	$5 \times 10^{12}[3]$
BMRR	3	--	$\sim 2.5 \times 10^{13}[4]$

(1) GRAPHITE RELECTED
(2) INCLUDES BISMUTH FILTER
(3) WITH 9 cm OF D_2O BETWEEN CORE AND BEAMPORT
(4) ESTIMATED FROM CORE AVERAGE PUBLISHED AS 1.5×10^{13} n/cm^2.s AT 1 MW

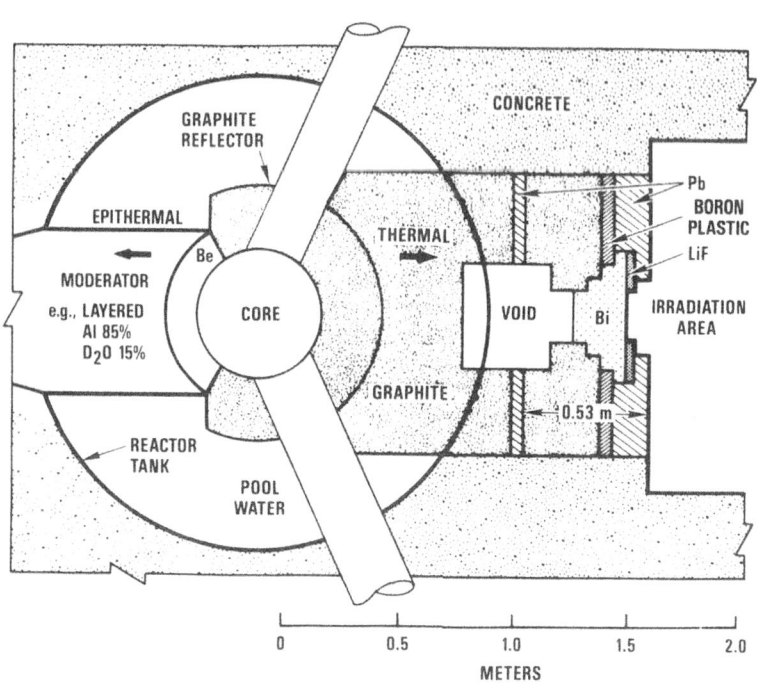

Table 1. Comparison of Neutron Fluxes at Core Edge for BNCT Application (Various Reactors)

other types of reactors are simply unusual occurrences for a reactor with TRIGA fuel, with no damage to the reactor or risk to the patient or public. Because of the widely recognized safety of the TRIGA reactor based on more than 65 worldwide installations, a TRIGA reactor would be a suitable choice for a BNCT installation in or near a hospital complex.

REFERENCES

1. H. Hatanaka, Clinical Results of Boron Neutron Capture Therapy, in: "Neutron Beam Design, Development, and Performance of Neutron Capture Therapy," O. K. Harling, et al., ed., Plenum Press, New York (1990).
2. Y. Mishima et.al., New Thermal Neutron Capture Therapy for Malignant Melanoma: Melanogenesis-Seeking ^{10}B Molecule-Melanoma Cell Interaction from InVitro to First Clinical Trial, in "Pigment Cell Research," Vol 2, No. 4, Alan R. Liss, Inc., New York (1989).
3. O. Aizawa, Research on Neutron Beam Design for BNCT at the Musashi Reactor, in: "Neutron Beam Design, Development, and Performance for Neutron Capture Therapy," O. K. Harling, et al., ed., Plenum Press, New York (1990).
4. F. J. Wheeler, et al., Physics Design for the Brookhaven Medical Research Reactor Epithermal Neutron Source, Ibid
5. G. K. Becker, et al., Neutron Spectrum Measurements in the Aluminum Oxide Filtered Beam Facility at the Brookhaven Medical Research Reactor, Ibid.
6. R. G. Fairchild, et al., Installation and Testing of an Optimized Epithermal Neutron Beam at the Brookhaven Medical Research Reactor (BNRR), Ibid.
7. G. B. West, et.al., Kinetic Behavior of TRIGA Reactors, in General Atomics document GA-7882, March 1967.
8. M. T. Simnad, The U-ZrH$_x$ Alloy: Its Properties and Use in TRIGA Fuel, in General Atomics document E-117-833, February 1980.
9. 10 MW TRIGA LEU Fuel and Reactor Design Description, in General Atomics document: UZR-14 (Rev.), October 1979.
10. R. Chesworth and G. West, Update on World-Wide Use of TRIGA-LEU Fuel Including Loss of Flow Tests, to be included in Proc. Int. RERTR Mtg, Newport, Rhode Island, September 23-27, 1990.
11. W. L. Whittemore, Startup Testing of Romania Dual-Core Test Reactor, in General Atomics document, TOC-13, September 1980.
12. R. L. Moss, Progress Towards Boron Neutron Capture Therapy at the High Flux Reactor Petten, in: "Neutron Beam Design, Development, and Performance for Neutron Capture Therapy," O. J, Harling et al., ed., Plenum Press, New York (1990).
13. W. A. Neuman, Neutron Beam Studies for a Medical Therapy Reactor, Ibid.
14. B. V. Harrington, A Calculational Study of Tangential and Radial Beams in HIFAR for Neutron Capture Therapy," Ibid.

DESIGN, CONSTRUCTION AND INSTALLATION OF AN EPITHERMAL NEUTRON BEAM FOR

BNCT AT THE HIGH FLUX REACTOR PETTEN

R.L.Moss[1], F.Stecher-Rasmussen[2], K.Ravensberg[2],
G.Constantine[1][3] and P.Watkins[1][3]

[1]Commission of the European Communities, Joint Research
Centre (JRC), Petten, The Netherlands
[2]Netherlands Energy Research Foundation (ECN), Petten
The Netherlands
[3](Formerly) AEA Technology, Harwell, United Kingdom

INTRODUCTION

Following the formation in 1987, of both the European Collaboration group on Boron Neutron Capture Therapy (BNCT) and the Petten BNCT group, steps were taken to design and implement an epithermal neutron beam for BNCT applications at the High Flux Reactor (HFR) at Petten. The installation would serve as a European facility, which once the modality of BNCT is proven would be the pathfinder for implementation of BNCT at other European nuclear sites.

Due to its favourable nuclear and geometric characteristics, the beam tube HB11 was chosen as the candidate beam tube for BNCT applications. To reconfigure the beam tube to produce the required epithermal neutrons, it was first necessary to remove the existing mirror system and then to install the appropiate filter materials. Due to the fixed operating schedule of the HFR, with only one long shut-down period per year during the summer weeks for maintenance and upgrading actions, installation of the new facility was planned for the summer stop period in 1990. To take full advantage of the period leading up to this (18 months), experience was gained in designing and carrying out nuclear measurements on a smaller beam tube, HB7.[1] This gave valuable guidance towards the design at the larger beam tube, HB11. Extensive nuclear calculations to design the facility have been performed (see Watkins, this symposium), the final design was chosen at the beginning of 1990. Manufacture of the required filter components, plus newly designed main and emergency beam shutters was completed in time for installation during this summer's (1990) shut-down period.

HFR PETTEN AND BEAM TUBE HB11

The HFR at Petten is a multi-purpose nuclear materials testing reactor, operating at 45MW(th), cooled and moderated by light water.[2] The reactor is primarily used for in-core nuclear materials irradiation experiments. Radiating outwards on 3 sides of the reactor vessel are 12 horizontal beam tubes. At the north side of the reactor, the beam tube HB11 is a specially designed high flux facility which was installed during the reactor vessel replacement exercise in 1984 when the old thermal column was replaced. The beam tube faces one whole side of the reactor vessel. At the exit end, the tube has a 35 x 35 cm square cross-section. The potential to create a high flux, large cross-section (greater than head size) beam tube is apparent.

DESIGN OF THE EPITHERMAL NEUTRON BEAM AT HB11

The following requirements of the neutron beam at the therapy position were stipulated :

- neutron flux $> 1.0 \times 10^9$ neutrons / cm^2 s

- average neutron dose $< 8.0 \times 10^{-11}$ rads cm^2 / neutron, (or mean neutron energy < 8.0 keV),

and - gamma dose rate < 50 cGy / hr

The requirements were chosen to enable a treatment to be completed in a reasonable time (< 1 hour), probably in 6 fractions (≈ 10 min). The average neutron dose can be re-interpreted using the ICRU neutron dose function (ie. 10^{-11} rads cm^2/neutron ≈ 1 keV) to produce a mean energy in keV's. This is considered a good indication of the quality of the beam and reflects the fast neutron contamination in the beam. The incident gamma dose rate must be sufficiently small as not to dominate the total (incident + induced) gamma dose rate at the tumour site.

The beam diameter should be at least head size to enable, if felt necessary whole head irradiations. In addition, there must be the available space in the irradiation room to enable the head to be exposed from two laterally opposing directions. Furthermore, the radiotherapists stipulated that the beam should be able to be closed within 15 seconds to allow in case of emergency medical staff to enter the treatment room in a sufficient time.

For the design calculations, the coupled neutron/photon transport code MCNP,[3] version 3A, was used. Of the hundreds of combinations of filter materials, core configurations and spectrum shifters that were analysed, the chosen HB11 set-up consists of the standard reactor core (ie. no change in any of the periphery reflector elements), no spectrum shifter (ie. no solid material at the reactor end of the beam tube) and a filter material combination of: Al, S, Ti, Cd and liquid Ar.

The Al+S+Ti filter combination is a well tried principle from designs performed elsewhere[4]. The liquid argon is an excellent gamma attenuator and was shown to perform better than other candidate materials such as Bi and ^{10}B. The filter lay-out and dimensions are shown schematically in fig.1.

CONSTRUCTION AND INSTALLATION OF THE HB11 BEAM COMPONENTS

The following engineering constraints on the design had to be addressed : removal of the existing highly active material (mirror system); a circular beam is required from a rectangular tube; the argon must remain liquid; the argon system must have sufficient control to fill and evacuate the cryostat chamber when necessary, be able to control, check and regulate within seconds any loss or gain in temperature and pressure of the argon, and to have all critical components duplicated for back-up purposes; a main beam shutter should close the beam within 15 seconds; and an emergency shutter must be installed to replace

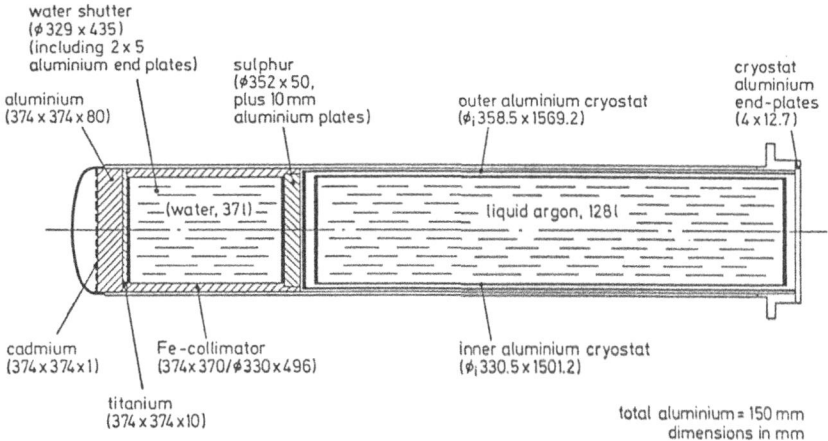

Fig 1 . Filter arrangement, including emergency water shutter

any eventual failure of the main beam shutter or evacuation of the argon cyrostat.

The removal of the activated mirror system was performed without any undue exposure to personnel. The solid filter components, Cd, Al and Ti, required no special manufacturing constraints. The sulphur component was prepared by casting molten sulphur into a circular aluminium casing. The sulphur block was interlaced with aluminium sheeting to enhance internal cooling. The circular components, including the emergency water shutter, were placed into iron shoulders to fit into the square beam tube. The liquid argon cryostat is a double-contained, vacuum insulated chamber. The control and feed system consist of two pump-cooler-compressor units, cryogenic vacuum insulated piping, cryogenic valves and an array of pipework for gas (N_2 and Ar) supply and extraction.

The main beam shutter, positioned behind the filter components, consists of an outer casing (96x140x75cm), with an inner drum 92cm diameter. The drum rotates about an horizontal axis and contains a 30cm diameter beam hole. The structure is made of alternating layers of lead and borated polyethylene plates, which are stepped in the mid-position to avoid possible neutron streaming.

ACKNOWLEDGEMENTS

The installation was completed as scheduled in August 1990.

REFERENCES

1. G.Constantine et al, "Progress in neutron beam development at the HFR Petten (Feasibility study for a BNCT facility)", Proc. 7th ASTM-EURATOM Symposium on Reactor Dosimetry, 27-31 August 1990, Strasbourg, France.

2. H.Röttger et al.,"High Flux Materials Testing Reactor Petten, Characteristics of the Facilities and Standard Irradiation Devices", EUR 5700 EN, 1986/87.

3. J.F.Breimeister (Ed),"MCNP - A General Monte Carlo Code for Neutron and Photon Transport", LA-7596-M, Rev.2.

4. G.Constantine et al, "Harwell research on beams for neutron capture therapy", Proc. of the Third Int. Symp. on Neutron Capture Therapy, (Bremen, May/June 1988), J. Strahlentherapie und Onkologie, Vol 165, No.2/3, 1989.

MODELLING AN EPITHERMAL NEUTRON BEAM FOR A DIDO TYPE REACTOR

USING MCNP - A MONTE CARLO CODE

D.Ross[1], G.Constantine[2] and D.R.Weaver[1]

[1] School of Physics and Space Research, The University of Birmingham, Birmingham B15 2TT, England.
[2] Currently at ANSTO, Lucas Heights, Australia

INTRODUCTION

Epithermal neutron beams are currently being developed for use in BNCT. They have the advantage over thermal beams in that they can achieve better penetration and can therefore treat deeper tumours. It has been shown that the optimum energy range for epithermal neutrons is approximately from 0.5 eV to 10 keV[1]; energies above this range give significant damage due to proton recoil.

The original aim of this project was to design an epithermal neutron beam for Harwell's DIDO reactor 10H beam tube, but the reactor was closed down in March, 1990. DIDO was a 25MW(th) research reactor, cooled and moderated by D_2O. To model the reactor the Monte Carlo code MCNP[2] was used. Initially, calculations were made to model an experimental set-up that was used in 1987 to carry out cell irradiations with an Al/S/Ar filtered beam[3]. Using this experience a study was begun to design an optimum epithermal beam for the 10H beam tube, a 10 inch diameter horizontal tube which penetrates the shield and radial reflector to within 9 cm of the core.

THE 1987 EXPERIMENTAL Al/S/Ar BEAM

The DIDO reactor core contains 25 fuel elements, each consisting of four concentric, 75% enriched uranium/aluminium alloy tubes surrounded by an outer aluminium tube. A closed-ended aluminium tube or thimble was placed within one of these fuel elements, as shown in Figure 1, and neutrons were scattered up this to form a beam. The beam was then filtered by a combination of 48.3cm of aluminium, 30cm of sulphur, 42cm of liquid argon, 0.1cm of titanium and $0.0456 gcm^{-2}$ of boron-10. The neutron measurements were taken from a position above the dose point and adjusted to the lower height by assuming an inverse square law with distance from the graphite scatterer at the core centre level. Calculations showed that this assumption was not completely accurate and the results had to be increased by 9% compared with previously published results[3].

Calculations were made on a quarter core model, using mirror planes to simulate the remainder. Both the vertical experiment and the 10H beam tube were included. The neutron source for the calculation was specified as a fixed source with a Watt fission spectrum emitting $\nu = 2.45$ neutrons per fission event. The spatial distribution of the source was determined by three independent parameters according to measured data: (1) a discrete distribution specifying the proportion of the source within each fuel element, (2) an axial power distribution and (3) a radial distribution specifying the proportion of the source within each of the four concentric fuel tubes. Due to unsatisfactory Argon data in the MCNP files, more recent data[4] have been used to provide energy dependent attenuation factors. A point detector was used for tallying. The computer used was a Mistral Computer Systems Hitech-10 workstation.

A comparison of the experimental results and calculations for the vertical beam tube is shown in Table 1; the neutron results show good agreement. However the calculated photon dose is less than half the measured dose. 55% of the calculated photon dose originates from neutron capture by the aluminium thimble, the rest mainly from aluminium present in the fuel element alloy, and from polythene and steel surrounding the dose point. The prompt and delayed photons from fission and the gammas from the decay of ^{28}Al, were found to produce little dose. The reason for the discrepancy is uncertain. However there are several photon contributions which are not modelled yet due to lack of data including gamma production in the argon filter and from thermal neutron capture by the fission products.

THE 10H THERAPY FACILITY

An extensive series of calculations has been performed on a quarter core model, see Figure 2, similar to the previous section, with the fuel element previously thimbled now modelled normally and the dose point now just outside the biological shield. The first series tried filter combinations of boron-10, cadmium, aluminium, sulphur and argon; using the filter transmission option to include various filter combinations in one run. Each run took approximately 400 minutes, to achieve an accuracy of less than 5%. The results showed: (a) cadmium and boron are both effective thermal neutron filters, and (b) 1cm of titanium reduced the neutron dose per unit flux (N_D) by up to a factor of two, though at the expense of reducing the neutron flux by a similar factor. The best combinations had a total neutron flux of 1×10^9 ncm^{-2}s^{-1}, a total neutron dose rate per unit flux (N_D) of around 3.5×10^{-11} cGycm^2 and a photon dose rate per unit neutron flux (P_D) of around 2.5×10^{-11} cGycm^2.

Next the effect of using spectrum shifters was calculated. Initial calculations took over 2000 minutes but it was found that this could be reduced to 800 minutes by performing two separate runs. The first run provided fast and epithermal neutron results, with an importance distribution biased to particles heading towards the 10H beam tube, and the second run was unbiased and provided thermal neutron and photon results.

Transferring aluminium from the filter to the wet spectrum shifter (within the D$_2$O) resulted in N_D increasing, due to the displacement of the D$_2$O, a marked increase in flux, and a small drop in P_D. However any advantage in using a wet spectrum shifter is outweighed by

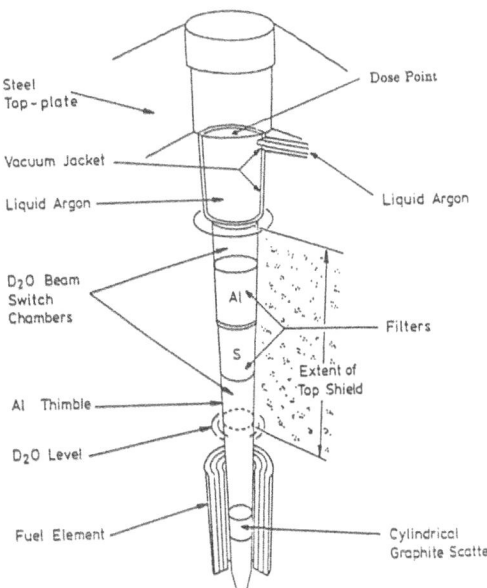

Fig 1. The Experimental Beam Facility

Table 1. Comparison of Results

	Experimental Results	Calculated Results
Neutron Flux (ncm^{-2}s^{-1})	(1.80 ± 0.15) $\times 10^7$	(1.93 ± 0.04) $\times 10^7$
Neutron Dose in Water (mGy hr^{-1})	(70 ± 4)	(84 ± 3)
Photon Dose in Water (mGy hr^{-1})	(60 ± 10)	(25.0 ± 1.0)

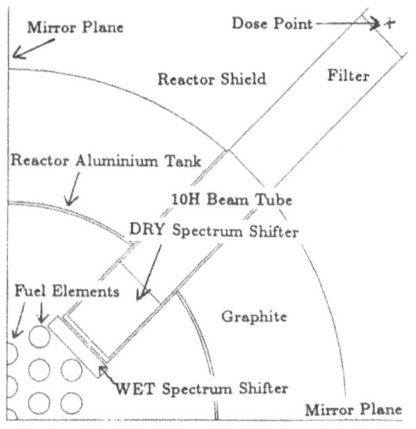

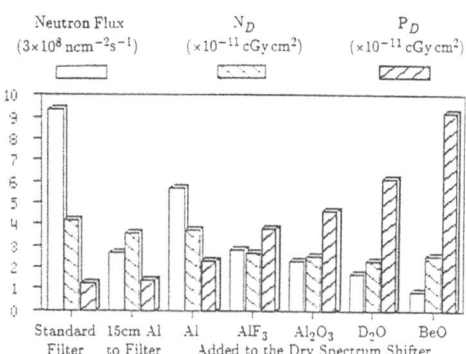

Fig2. Model of the DIDO Reactor.　　　Fig3. Effects of Adding to a Standard Filter

engineering difficulties and possible loss in reactivity. Next, aluminium was moved from the filter to the core end of the beam tube - known as a dry spectrum shifter. In comparison with the optimum filter combinations there was no improvement in N_D, with the neutron flux and P_D increasing by similar ratios. Figure 3 shows the effect of adding 15cm of Al to a standard filter. Trials with titanium in the dry spectrum shifter resulted in higher values of N_D than by using it as a filter. To increase the moderation in the dry spectrum shifter region, Al_2O_3, AlF_3, BeO, D_2O were tried. Figure 3 shows the effect of adding 15cm of these to a standard filter configuration. On performing a series of calculations with various lengths of these spectrum shifters no obvious preferred choice was found. They decreased N_D compared to the aluminium spectrum shifter but at the expense of lower neutron fluxes and higher P_D. The optimum spectrum shifter seems to be a combination of Al and one of these spectrum shifters.

Several modifications were made to the model to see their effect. The cadmium/europium control arms were modelled to see if they would increase the photon dose but there was no noticeable change because the arms were not in the line-of-sight of the dose point. A full core representation was modelled, however there was no noticeable change in the results. Future calculations will track the particles through the filter region, observe the effects of various lengths of titanium, and model mixed combinations of dry spectrum shifters.

In conclusion, DIDO reactors can provide an epithermal beam for BNCT with a low neutron dose per unit flux. A compromise will have to be made between filters which provide low values of P_D and dry spectrum shifters which can provide lower N_D, and judgments will need to be made in comparing the relative merits of high neutron flux, low N_D and low P_D.

ACKNOWLEDGEMENTS

The authors wish to thank the Science and Engineering Research Council and the UK Department of Health for their support and Dr D. J. Picton and Dr P. R. D. Watkins for their general assistance.

REFERENCES

1. R. G. Fairchild et al, Neutron capture therapy at Brookhaven National Laboratory, in: 'Proc. Wkshop. on NCT, BNL.' R. G. Fairchild and V. Bond eds. (1986).
2. J. F. Briemeister(ed), 'MCNP - A general Monte Carlo code for neutron and photon transport, Version 3A.' Los Alamos Laboratory, LA-7396-M, Rev.2 (1986).
3. C. A. Perks, G. A. Constantine and R. Birch, The design and dosimetry of an Al/S/Ar filtered neutron beam. Rad. Prot. Dosim., 23:329 (1988).
4. V. McLean, C. L. Dunford, P. F. Rose, 'Neutron cross sections, Vol.2 - neutron cross-section curves', Academic Press (1986).

MCNP CALCULATIONS FOR THE DESIGN AND CHARACTERISATION OF THE PETTEN BNCT EPITHERMAL NEUTRON BEAM

P. Watkins[1,3], G. Constantine[1,3], F. Stecher-Rasmussen[2],
W. Freudenreich[2], R.L. Moss[3] and R. Ricchena[4]

[1]AEA Technology, Harwell, United Kingdom.
[2]Netherlands Energy Research Foundation ECN, Petten, Holland
[3]Commission of the European Communities, JRC, Petten, Holland
[4]Commission of the European Communities, JRC, Ispra, Italy

INTRODUCTION

The filter assembly which has recently been installed in the HB11 beam tube of the High Flux Reactor (HFR) at Petten has been the culmination of two years of intensive activity. This has included a lengthy series of calculations to optimise the facility for BNCT. Previous work[1] had shown the effectiveness of a combination of "spectrum shifter" and filter in producing an epithermal neutron beam of the required characteristics. Here a "spectrum shifter" is a device, placed close to the source, which moderates unwanted high energy neutrons to lower energies within the beam. In contrast a "filter" is positioned some distance from the source and simply removes unwanted neutrons from the beam.

The calculations sought to establish the best choice of spectrum shifter and filter for the HB11 facility. The target beam characteristics were;

Neutron intensity	$> 1.0 \times 10^9$ neutrons $cm^{-2}s^{-1}$
Average beam energy	< 8 keV
Photon dose	< 0.5 Gy per 3.0×10^{12} neutrons

CHOICE OF CALCULATIONAL METHOD.

The beam tube geometry of HB11 (see **Moss**, this symposium) combined with a therapy position 5 metres from the core dictated a transport theory solution. The complex geometry of the facility presented severe modelling problems for deterministic methods so the Monte Carlo code MCNP[2], version 3A, was chosen instead. MCNP could model the geometry exactly, has an extensive library of continuous energy cross-section data and has a coupled neutron-photon mode. Other features of the code permitted the rapid surveying of many filter/spectrum shifter combinations. All of the calculations were performed on a dedicated workstation thus avoiding the excessive cost usually associated with lengthy Monte Carlo simulations.

The MCNP models employed a detailed whole, or half, core representation of the reactor with the beam tube modelled out to the therapy position.

Point detector tallies were used to record neutron and photon data at this position. In general coupled neutron-photon calculations were performed.

Two features of MCNP were used extensively. First, the multiplication of any tally by an energy dependent function. Thus dose responses could be folded into the tallies. Secondly the inclusion of energy dependent attenuations allowed a tally to be modified to simulate intervening material which simply attenuated particles. Many sets of such attenuators may be defined for each tally. Representing the filter components as such attenuators allowed many potential filters to be surveyed at once. Strictly this approach is only valid for thin regions of material since no account is taken of multiple scattering. However the geometry of HB11 produces a very forward peaked flux so this effect is negligible.

The neutron data for argon supplied with MCNP (ENDF/B-IV) were known to be poor. Instead a recent tabulation of the total cross-section was converted into an attenuation function which was input into MCNP as a tally modifier. A completely validated set of argon data is still awaited.

The "average energy" of the beam was defined via the neutron dose

$$\text{average dose} = \frac{\int (\text{dose function}).(\text{flux}) \, dE}{\int (\text{flux}) \, dE}$$

this may be converted back to an equivalent average energy by inverting the dose function.

OPTIMISATION OF SPECTRUM SHIFTER AND FILTER CONFIGURATIONS

Spectrum shifters of aluminium, alumina, D_2O and graphite were examined. These were combined with many possible filter materials, namely argon, aluminium, sulphur, titanium and cadmium. Unfortunately the spectrum shifters gave only small improvements which were judged insufficient to overcome the installation problems. Subsequent calculations concentrated on optimising the arrangement of materials in the filter.

Argon was included in the filter to reduce the photon component of the beam with only a small effect on the neutrons. A thin layer of cadmium at the core side of the filter removes thermal neutrons and reduces activation of the filter. The aluminium "window" at about 24 keV produces a neutron spectrum emerging from the aluminium with a peak at this energy, effectively reducing the average energy of the beam. The other materials, sulphur and titanium, preferentially remove neutrons at higher energies thereby softening the beam further.

Several hundred combinations and thicknesses of filter materials were considered. Some 200000 neutron histories or more were simulated for each filter configuration to obtain acceptable statistical accuracy on the results. The final filter arrangement and corresponding beam parameters were as follows;

15 cm Al; 5 cm S; 1 cm Ti; 0.1 cm Cd; and 150 cm liquid Ar

Neutron intensity   = 1.1 x 10^9 neutrons $cm^{-2}s^{-1}$
Photon dose   = 0.5 Gy per 3.0 x 10^{12} neutrons
Average beam energy   = 7.8 keV
(Fast Neutron Dose / Epithermal neutron $\approx$ 7.9 x 10^{-11} cGy/neutron/cm^2)

PHOTON CALCULATIONS

Initially coupled neutron-photon calculations used a half core model without the cadmium control absorbers. For the neutron tallies this was adequate since uncollided core neutrons gave a negligible contribution. However the photon tallies were dominated by uncollided particles and so the photon source had to be defined accurately. Moving to a whole core model complete with cadmium control absorbers had only a small effect on the neutron parameters but raised the photon dose by about 40%.

The coupled neutron-photon calculations accounted for photon production in those materials which were modelled explicitly and for which data was available. This did **not** include photon production in the argon. Prompt photons from fission were modelled but not the delayed contribution from the fission products. Their effect was estimated with a separate series of photon-only calculations. The spatial distribution of these fission product photons was assumed identical as the neutron source in the coupled neutron-photon calculations. However the time dependence of the photon spectrum from the fission products was given as summations of exponentials[3]. These calculations established that only a small fraction of the total photon dose, about 10%, came from the fission products.

EVALUATION OF OTHER QUANTITIES

Apart from optimising the filter and evaluating the beam parameters MCNP simulations were used for many other purposes. Sufficient histories were simulated for neutron spectra to be estimated with acceptable levels of accuracy at various positions along the beam and within the core. The effect of changes to the reactor core were also investigated. In particular the power distribution was shown to have a marked effect on the neutron intensity. However changes to the beryllium reflector elements between the core and the beam tube influenced the results at the therapy position only slightly.

MCNP simulations also supported several series of measurements of the HB11 beam (see **Stecher-Rasmussen**, this symposium). These measurements used Bonner spheres and proton recoil counters to record the neutron spectra. Boron plates of various thicknesses in front of the Bonner spheres modified the response. Calculations estimated the spectra with the boron plates modelled as tally attenuators. The response functions of the Bonner spheres were included as tally multipliers. The resultant MCNP spectra were used as first estimates in a spectrum adjustment process. These measurements provided some validation of the MCNP calculations.

MCNP simulations were also performed for the HB12 beam tube both for validation purposes and also with the objective of establishing the feasibility of this beam tube as a second, smaller, BNCT facility.

REFERENCES

1. **Constantine, G.**; Neutron Capture Therapy Beam Design at Harwell, p 71, Basic Life Sciences, Vol 54, Neutron Beam Design, Development and Performance for Neutron Capture Therapy. Plenum Press. 1990
2. **Briesmeister, J.F.(ed)**; MCNP - A General Monte Carlo Code for Neutron and Photon Transport. LA-7396-M, Revision 2
3. **LaBauvre, R.J., England, T.R. and George, D.C.**; FITPULS, A Code for Obtaining Analytic Fits to Aggregate Fission-Product Decay-Energy Spectra, LA-8277-MS, 1980.

MONTE-CARLO CALCULATION RESULTS FOR THE EPITHERMAL NEUTRON BEAM AT THE BROOKHAVEN MEDICAL REACTOR

J. Gajewski[1], E. B. Ramsay[1], L. E. Reinstein[1], S. Saraf[2], R. Fairchild[2]

[1]State University of New York at Stony Brook, New York 11794, U.S.A.
[2]Brookhaven National Laboratory, Upton, New York 11973, U.S.A.

INTRODUCTION

As a first step towards developing a treatment planning system for BNCT, the Brookhaven Medical Research Reactor (BMRR) and its epithermal neutron filter have been modeled in detail using the Monte-Carlo code MCNP[1]. The geometry of the reactor as defined in MCNP is shown to scale in Figure 1, where the various components of the Al-Al$_2$0$_3$ filter are indicated, the thick black lines being Al. The thicknesses of materials in the filter along their centers are 45.72cm of Al$_2$0$_3$, 19.65cm Al, 0.75cm, Cd and 11.5cm Bi. The geometry as modeled takes advantage of the symmetry of the reactor and a reflecting plane passes through the core center. The geometry in 3 dimensions is built up from a total of 90 basic cells (cylinders, slabs etc.) with 19 different materials representing 26 nuclides. The distance from the core center to port face is 170.9 cm which requires that variance reduction techniques be used in order to obtain good statistics at the port face with a reasonable CPU effort. The 90 geometric cells are further subdivided into 240 spaces where the importances are varied such that particles heading towards the port are made more significant than those heading away.

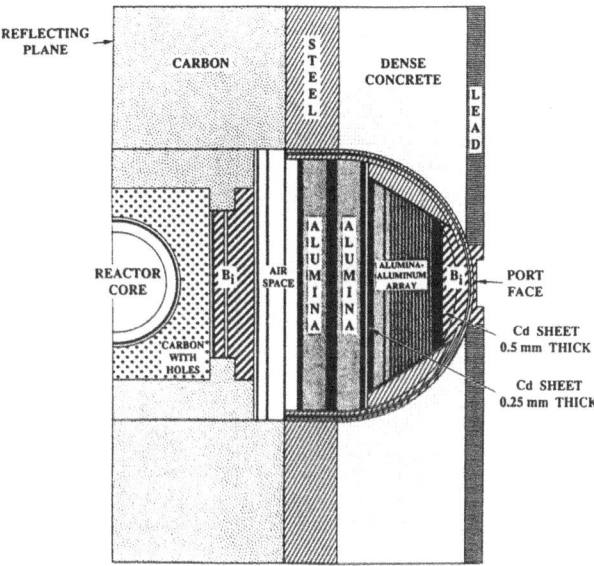

Figure 1. MCNP Model of the Brookhaven Medical Research Reactor

The reactor core was taken to be homogeneous in density, has a Watt fission energy spectrum and a position distribution determined from the power distribution for uranium consumption. The results given by MCNP are per neutron released in the reactor core and require a multiplication factor in order to get absolute numbers. The factor used in this work is equal to the theoretical estimate of the number of neutrons released for a reactor power of 1 MW and is equal to 7.6×10^{16} n/s. All calculations were performed either on a DEC Microvax II or an IBM 3090. Calculation times on the IBM were typically 500 minutes and two to three days on the Microvax. All future calculations will be carried out on an IBM RISC 6000/320 Work-station for which a complete treatment planning system will be developed.

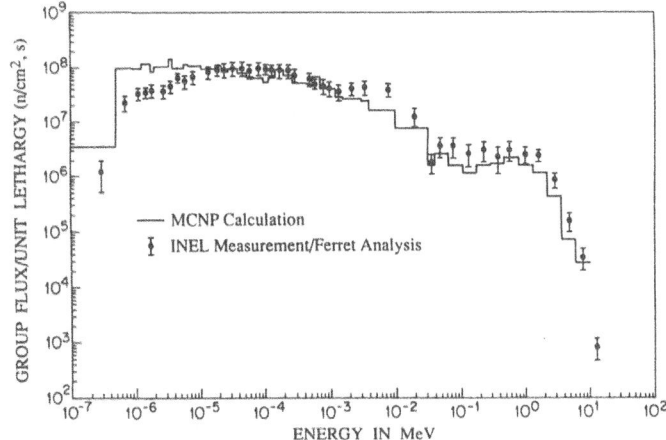

Figure 2. BMRR Neutron Spectrum (Power = 1MW)

Table 1. Summary of Measured and Calculated Beam Parameters

Power = 1 MW	Measured	Calculated 15 cm Bi	Calculated 11.4 cm Bi
Fast neutron flux density in n/cm^2.s (E > 10 KeV)	3.4×10^7	1.7×10^7	2.14×10^7
Epithermal neutron flux density in n/cm^2.s (0.4ev < E < 10kev)	6.0×10^8	7.3×10^8	8.3×10^8
Thermal neutron flux density in n/cm^2.s (E < 0.4 eV)	2.4×10^7	1.4×10^7 (2.5×10^7)	1.58×10^7 (2.9×10^7)
Absorbed dose from fast neutrons for soft tissue free in air in rads/min	1.75	0.9	1.1
Absorbed dose from gammas for soft tissue free in air in rads/min	0.4	0.15	0.47
Thermal-neutron flux density in n/cm^2.s (for peak flux at ~ 2cm depth in phantom)	9.3×10^8 no filtration 6.3×10^8 (1 mm ^{6}Li)	1.05×10^9 no filtration 5.5×10^8 (1 mm ^{6}Li)	1.18×10^9 no filtration 6.06×10^8 (1 mm ^{6}Li)

RESULTS

Figure 2 shows the calculated neutron spectrum as compared to a spectrum measurement made by the Idaho National Engineering Laboratory (INEL) using activation foils having energy responses[2] over the indicated range. In Table 1, the values for various measured parameters are compared with calculations. The original design goal for the epithermal filter called for 15cm of Bi at the port but in the final as-built configuration only 11.4cm was used as a result of space limitations. The table shows calculations for the design intent of 15cm Bi and the as-built configuration of 11.4cm. The agreement is generally good except in the epithermal region where the calculations suggest a 38% higher epithermal flux than measured. In the thermal region, the calculated data in brackets is what one obtains if the thermal flux is defined up to 0.5eV. Figure 3 shows the experimental and theoretical thermal flux depth distributions in a 16.6cm diameter cylindrical phantom filled with tissue equivalent fluid and placed against the port face first with and then without a 1mm ^{6}Li filter between the port and the phantom. The agreement between the calculations and experiments is excellent for the Lithium filtered case but off by approximately 15% at the depth of the peak flux for the case of no filtration. Effective dose distributions in a cylindrical tissue equivalent phantom are shown in figure 4 for a reactor power of 3 MW and with 1mm ^{6}Li sandwiched between the port face and the phantom. RBE's of 1.6 are used for the nitrogen and fast-neutron dose, and 2.3 for the ^{10}B dose. The gamma dose calculated is smaller than that measured by a factor of 2 and the reason for the discrepancy is not clear at this time.

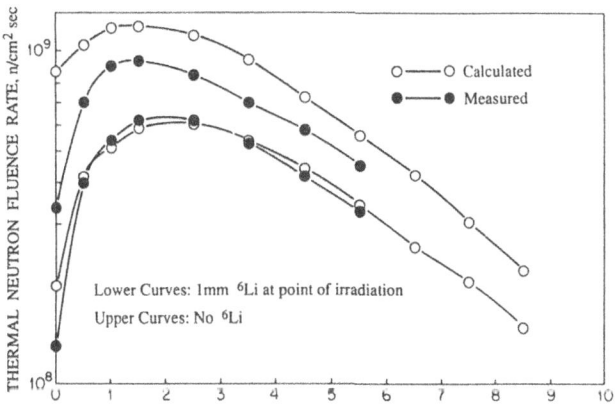

Figure 3. Thermal-neutron Flux Densities in a Tissue Equivalent Head Phantom (Power = 1MW)

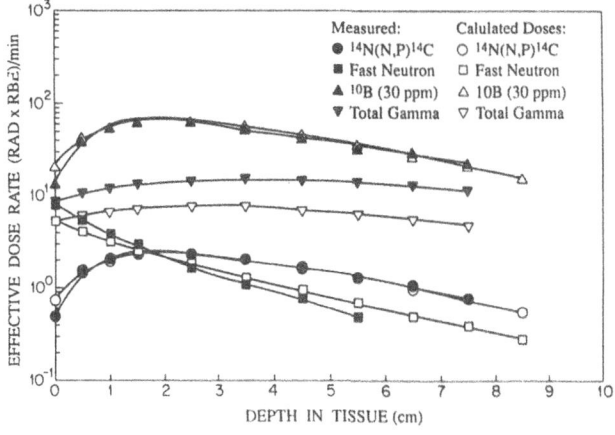

Figure 4. Dose Distributions in Phantom Head (Power = 3MW)

REFERENCES

1) "MCNP - A General Monte Carlo Code for Neutron and Photon Transport, Version 3A", J.F. Briemeister, ed, Los Alamos National Laboratory, LA-7396-M, Rev 2 (1986)

2) G.K Becker, Y.D. Harker, L.G. Miller, R.A. Anderl, F.J. Wheeler, "Neutron Spectrum Measurements in The Aluminum Oxide Filtered Beam Facility at the Brookhaven Medical Research Reactor" in Neutron Beam Design, Development, and Performance for Neutron Capture Therapy, O.K. Harling, J.A. Bernard and R.G. Zamenhof, eds, Plenum Press, N.Y., 235 (1990)

DESIGN CONSIDERATIONS FOR THE PROPOSED HIFAR THERMAL AND

EPITHERMAL NEUTRON CAPTURE THERAPY FACILITIES

G.J.Storr[1], B.J. Allen[1], B.V. Harrington[1], L.R. Davis[2], M.M. Elcombe[1] and H. Meriaty[1]

[1] Australian Nuclear Science and Technology Organisation PMB 1,
Menai NSW 2234, Australia.
[2] Australian Institute of Nuclear Science and Engineering,
Lucas Heights NSW 2234, Australia.

At the Australian Nuclear Science and Technology Organisation (Ansto) the 100kW reactor Moata has been used successfully for Boron Neutron Capture Therapy (BNCT) of murine melanoma xenografts. [1] Envisaged large animal and human irradiations would require a beam from the High Flux Australian Reactor (HIFAR). Attaining a therapeutic beam for BNCT at HIFAR presents a challenge in physical design and engineering, as there is restricted access to core neutrons. Major modifications to the HIFAR shielding are precluded as this action would require a long shutdown and a significant and costly safety analysis. The only feasible existing beam tube that may provide a BNCT beam is the 28 cm diameter 10H re-entrant hole, located at the core mid-plane. The 10H end-plate is located approximately 9 cm from two outer core fuel elements, separated from them by D_2O. The 10H facility is currently used for neutron diffraction studies, and has a collimator installed which reduces the beam to a 5 cm square hole. Figure 1 shows a vertical section of the reactor and the relative position of the 10H facility.

A description of the 10H beam hole is contained in a calculational optimisation study [2] of an epithermal beam for HIFAR. A major component of the study was a comparison of different filter combinations located at the core end of 10H to maximise therapeutic gain at depth in a one-dimensional phantom model. Dose rates in the phantom were shown to lie close to the lower limit of acceptability for BNCT.

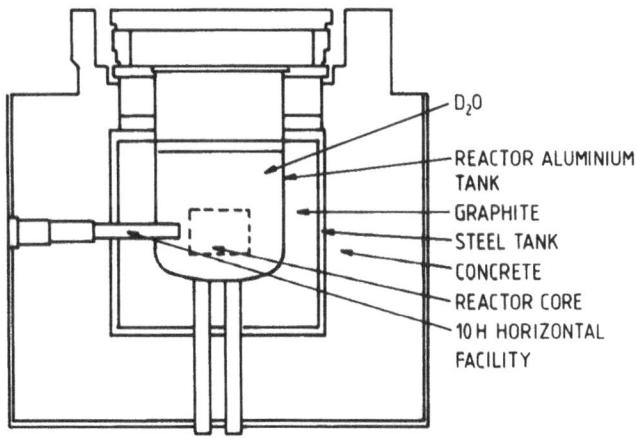

Figure 1. Vertical section of HIFAR and 10H facility

Table 1. HIFAR 10H BEAM CHARACTERISTICS (at 10MW)

Parameter	Previous measurement	Measured value	Calculation
Gamma dose rate ($Gy\ h^{-1}$)		88.1	66.0
Thermal neutron flux, ϕ_o ($10^9\ n\ cm^{-2}\ s^{-1}$)	0.78 (1972) 1.17 (1970) 1.10 (1966)	0.91 (Au) 0.94 (Mn) 0.82 (Cu)	1.31
Flux per unit lethargy/Thermal flux, ($\phi(u)/\phi_o$)	0.049 (1966, 5eV)	0.058 (Au, 5 eV) 0.059 (Mn) 0.056 (Cu)	0.056
Flux per unit lethargy, $\phi(u)$ ($10^9\ n\ cm^{-2}\ s^{-1}$)		0.47	0.80

For example, the results from calculation of a filter combination of 0.05 cm of ^{6}LiF, 5.0 cm Pb and 12.0 cm AlF_3 gives an RBE dose rate at a depth of 5 cm of approximately 16 cGy/min, which leads to an irradiation exposure time of about 2 hours for a target dose of 2000 cGy.

Additional calculations are now proceeding on a new beam design using the discrete ordinates transport code DORT [3] and the Monte Carlo code MCNP [4], that will, for example, allow us to study the effects of varying filter position and filter materials. A further improvement to the earlier work is the development of a two-dimensional phantom model for dose calculations. However, a full characterisation of the beam requires measurements of neutron and photon fluxes for comparison with calculational models and to determine absolute values for existing beam parameters.

Initial measurements have been carried out this year during periods when the facility has become available, and measurements made in previous years have been re-analyzed. Neutron beam parameters have been determined from activation measurements of gold, manganese and natural copper foils. The technique [5] requires careful cadmium ratio measurements combined with calculated parameters to determine the epithermal index of the beam and hence an effective cross-section [6] for the target foil, so a thermal flux and epithermal flux (assuming a 1/E slowing down spectrum) can be determined. Gamma dose rate has been measured with two types of EXRADIN ionisation chambers of tissue equivalent and Mg materials. The chambers were calibrated against standard sources located at Ansto. Access to the beam is restricted by the spectrometer shielding, presenting difficulties for other measurement techniques in the 10H facility. Measurements were made 360 cm from the 10H end-plate, and the results in Table 1 are adjusted to the estimated patient position (320 cm) by considering the beam hole as a long narrow cylindrical duct. [7]

Table 1 also gives a historical compilation of corrected 10H beam parameters. Harrington's calculated results for a 10H beam model are included in the table. The AUS [11] 3-D diffusion module POW3D [12] was used to calculate the scalar flux on the core side of the 10H end plate, which was then used to normalize subsequent transport calculations. A uniform core loading of 110 grams of U235 per fuel element and coarse control arm (CCA) angle of 22 degrees was assumed in the reactor calculation. The transport code DORT [3] was used to calculate the directional flux along 10H. The results were adjusted to the estimated patient position by the same attenuation factor as for the experimental results.

There is a discrepancy between the calculated and the measured thermal flux, and gamma dose rates. There appears to have been a significant drop (possibly due to collimator corrosion) in the measured 10H thermal flux between 1970 and 1972 that could go some way to resolving the measured and calculated difference in ϕ_o. The rest of the difference can be accounted for by errors in the measurements of $\approx 10\%$, and the calculational assumptions of a homogenous distribution of fuel elements in the core and a fixed CCA angle. The difference between the measured and calculated gamma dose rates is significant, though it is not unexpected due to assumptions made in the calculational models. [2] The calculated gamma dose is essentially the gamma dose from the reactor core. Induced gammas from structural reactor components and rigs have not be included, and could partly account for the discrepancy between measured and calculated gamma doses. The calculated and measured (at 5 eV) neutron flux spectrum results are in good agreement, even considering the errors associated with the activation technique. Errors on the gamma dose rate measurement are of similar order. Measurements for Cu and Mn foils give a similar ratio of $\phi(u)/\phi_o$ but it is recognised for these foils that the 1/v contribution to the reaction rate, gives an integral result for $\phi(u)$ between the Cd cutoff and the resonance energies.

The use of a resonance self-shielding technique will be employed for future measurements in this energy range. Calculations over the resonance energy range of 5 - 580 eV suggest a 1/E slowing down spectrum is an adequate assumption for 10H, with the values for $\phi(u)$ determined by assuming a 1/E spectrum between 1 eV and 10 keV. Measurements to determine neutron and photon parameters from beams at low power are currently being planned and the MCNP code will be used to model the experimental arrangements in order to validate later designs for the 10H beam.

A therapeutic epithermal beam requires filters to take advantage of the tissue kerma minimum between $\approx$ 1 eV and 10 keV and thus maximise dose at depth and reduce dose to the skin. The filter combinations studied previously at Ansto [13] suggest areas where improvements in design can be achieved and these are now being considered. Information from our calculations and other researchers [2,8,9,10] have provided us with a basis to estimate the reduction in epithermal flux in 10H by a factor of 20 for a conceptual filter of about 30 cm Al or S, 100 cm of liquid Ar and an appropriate thermal neutron shield. Attaining a therapeutic epithermal beam from the 10H facility therefore requires augmentation to compensate for the decrease in beam intensity due to beam filters and shields. This would be partially achieved by increasing the beam diameter to 25 cm, and fully achieved by also increasing the operating power to the current safety case limit of 15 MW. Hence it is reasonable to expect a therapeutic epithermal beam of $0.5\times10^9\,\mathrm{n\,cm^{-2}\,s^{-1}}$ can be achieved, and that total exposure time required would be 165 minutes, or 5 fractions of 30 minutes each.

The option of installing a thermal neutron beam from 10H is also being considered. Single crystal silicon cooled to liquid nitrogen temperatures (or lower) has been demonstrated to filter epithermal and fast neutrons and gamma-rays [14], while transmitting $\approx$ 50% of thermal neutrons for every 50 cm of silicon crystal. Silicon has a fast neutron window in its cross-section at 144 keV, that would require filtering with a material like sulphur which has a resonance near 144 keV. The transmitted thermal beam intensity of $\approx$ $10^9\,\mathrm{n\,cm^{-2}\,s^{-1}}$ would be utilised at the shield face. Alternatively neutron guides [15] could provide thermal beams remote from HIFAR with the advantages of beam sharing and low patient background environment if superior guides could be manufactured. Nickel coated glass guides totally internally reflect neutrons at glancing angles to the guide walls less than 0.1° per angstrom wavelength of neutron, implying a transmission of neutrons of wavelength 4 angstroms proportional to $(2\times0.4)^2$. The much larger solid angle transmittance for thermal wavelengths through single crystal silicon and the reported attenuation indicates that current guide materials would provide thermal fluxes an order of magnitude less than a single crystal silicon filter. Improved guide materials of supermirror and multilayer coatings may provide a competitive thermal beam option in the near future.

Our design considerations to date indicate that a therapeutic epithermal beam from the HIFAR 10H facility is feasible, however further calculations and experiments are now underway to confirm this position.

REFERENCES

1. B.J. Allen, S. Corderoy-Buck, D.E. Moore, Y. Mishima, M. Ichihashi, Local control of murine melanoma xenografts in nude mice by neutron capture therapy, in these Proceedings.
2. B.V. Harrington, Optimisation of an Epithermal Beam in HIFAR for Boron Neutron Capture Therapy. ANSTO/E662. (1987).
3. W.A. Rhoades, R.L. Childs, The DORT Two-Dimensional Discrete Ordinates Transport Code, Nuclear Science and Engineering, Vol. 99, 88-89. (1988).
4. J.F. Briesmeister, ed. MCNP - A General Monte Carlo Code for Neutron and Photon Transport, Version 3A. LA-7396-M, Rev 2 (1986).
5. J.W. Connolly, A. Rose, T. Wall, Integral reaction rates and neutron energy spectra in a well moderated reactor. AAEC/TM 191. (1963).
6. C.H. Westcott, The Specification of Neutron Flux and Nuclear Cross-sections in Reactor Calculations. J. Nuclear Energy, Vol 2, 55-76. (1955).
7. B.R. Bergelson, V.P. Mashkovich, Attenuation of neutrons, in Engineering Compendium on Radiation Shielding. Vol. 1. R.G. Jaegar, E.P. Blizard, A.B. Chilton, M. Grotenhuis, A. Honig, Th. A. Jaegar and H.H Eisenlohr, eds. Springer-Verlag, New York, 497-508. (1968).

8. J.R. Choi, S.D. Clement, O.K. Harling, R.G. Zamenhof, Neutron Capture Therapy beams at the MIT Research Reactor in Neutron Beam Design, Development and Performance for Neutron Capture Therapy, eds., O.K. Harling, J.R. Bernard, R.G. Zamenhof, Basic Life Science Series, Vol. 54, Plenum NY, (1990).

9. F.J. Wheeler, The Power Burst Reactor Facility as an Epithermal Neutron Source for Brain Cancer Therapy, in Workshop on Neutron Capture Therapy, eds., R.G. Fairchild, V.P. Bond, BNL 51994 (1986).

10. European Collaboration. Boron Neutron Capture Therapy of Tumours. Newsletter 3. (1990).

11. G.S. Robinson, A Guide to the AUS Modular Neutronics Code System. AAEC/E645. (1987).

12. J.M. Barry, B.V. Harrington, J.P. Pollard, Aus Module POW3D - A General Purpose 0,1,2 and 3D Multigroup Diffusion Code Including Feedback-Free Kinetics. To be published.

13. B.V. Harrington, A Calculational Study of Tangential and Radial Beams in HIFAR for Neutron Capture Therapy, in Neutron Beam Design, Development and Performance for Neutron Capture Therapy, eds., O.K. Harling, J.R. Bernard, R.G. Zamenhof, Basic Life Science Series, Vol. 54, Plenum NY, (1990).

14. R.M. Brugger, A Single Crystal Silicon Thermal Neutron Filter. Nucl. Inst. Methods. 135, 289-291, (1976).

15. B. Jacrot, Utilization of Neutron Guide Tubes for Neutron Inelastic Scattering, in Instrumentation for Neutron Inelastic Scattering Research. IAEA, Vienna. (1970).

NEUTRON BEAM PARAMETERS ON LVR-15 REACTOR FOR NEUTRON CAPTURE THERAPY

J.Burian, M.Marek, J.Rataj

Nuclear Research Institute, Rez, Czechoslovakia

INTRODUCTION

Some years ago, a research group was formed in Prague, Czechoslovakia, to study Boron Neutron Capture Therapy (BNCT). The important task for physicists was to design a suitable neutron source. First we concentrated on the design of a thermal beam and experimental verification of the beam parameters. Then the modeling and measurements for an epithermal beam were performed. Some difficulties arose when the reactor VVR-S was being reconstructed as the multi-purpose experimental reactor LVR-15. For this reason, physical tests had to be repeated under the new conditions /1/.

THERMAL NEUTRON BEAM

The configuration of moderating and shielding materials was designed by using multigroup transport codes. It was composed of layers of graphite, heavy water, lead and a bismuth block of high purity (99.999%). Activation and gamma sources in lead were lowered by using a thin boron carbide layer. The detailed design is shown in Fig. 1.

Calculational and experimental methods

To calculate the neutron and gamma space-energy distribution in moderating and shielding layers the two-dimensional code DOT and the coupled neutron-gamma data library DLC-36/CLAW were used.

The thermal and epithermal flux densities were measured by foil activation. The neutron spectrum over a wide energy range was determined with a Bonner moderation spectrometer. The gamma background in a human head phantom was mapped using a scintillation spectrometer with pulse shape discrimination.

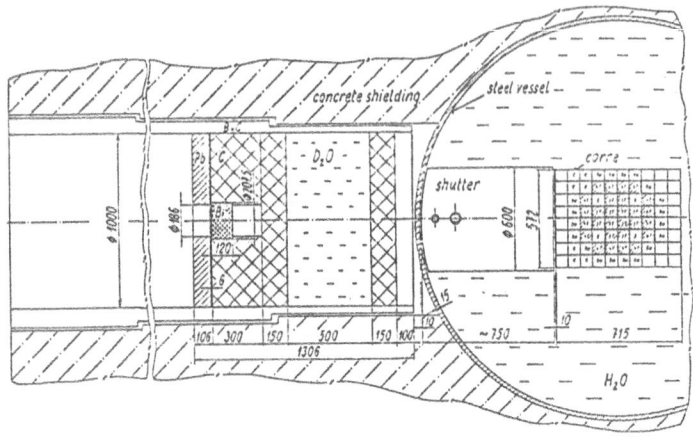

Fig.1 The LVR-15 thermal beam configuration, map view

A small semiconductor detector was used to map the thermal neutron flux in the head phantom. The important dosimetric characteristics were obtained from thermoluminescent detectors.

Results

Results of the calculation were published in the proceedings of the MIT Workshop /2/.

The parameters of the thermal neutron beam were measured in a beam free in air, in a cylindrical polyethylene phantom and in a human head phantom (a human skull and water).

The main parameters of a free beam for reactor power 1 MW:

		calculated	measured
Thermal flux	$1/cm^2s$	1.38×10^9	1.04×10^9
Epithermal flux	$1/cm^2s$	1.70×10^6	5.00×10^6
Neutron dose	cGy/min	1.16	1.90
Gamma dose	cGy/min	7.68	2.90
30 µgB10/g dose	cGy/min	22.30	–

EPITHERMAL NEUTRON BEAM

The transport calculations for the modeling of the epithermal beam facility were carried out. Some results for filter blocks with Al_2O_3 (50 cm), Al (60 cm), C + Al (15 + 60 cm) layers are shown in Fig. 2. For C + Al geometry one and two-dimensional results are normalized to the same integral flux.

The first epithermal beam filter configuration considered was C + Al. The block is composed of layers of lead, graphite of nuclear purity, aluminium, lead with a boron carbide cover and a 0.5 mm cadmium sheet. The detailed design is in Fig. 3.

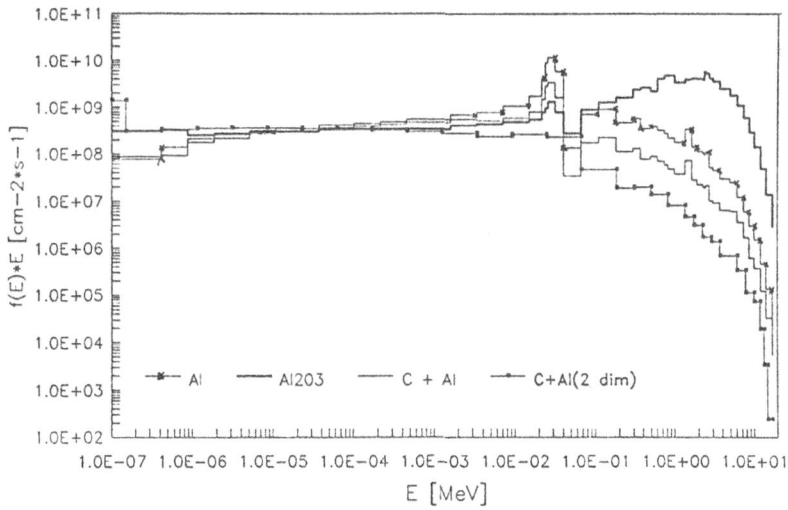

Fig.2 Neutron spectra for different filter materials

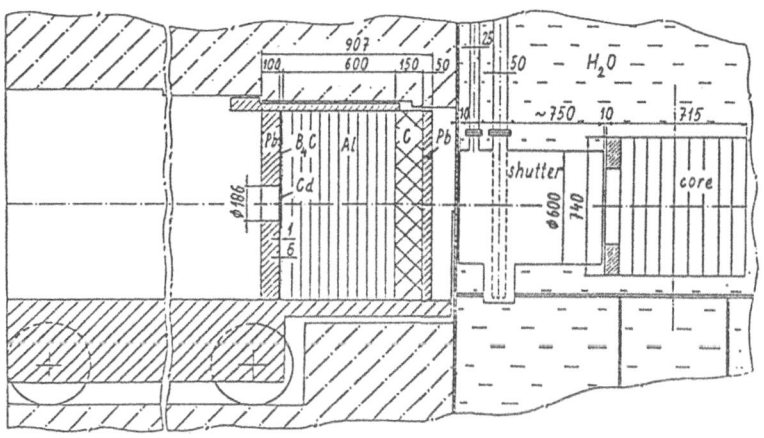

Fig.3 The LVR-15 epithermal beam configuration,
elevation view

Results

The investigated design is preliminary and in many aspects will be gradually improved. The measurements verifying the epithermal beam parameters were realized on the LVR-15 reactor recently; therefore only some results are incorporated in this paper.

The epithermal energy range was assumed to be 0.414eV – 9keV and the fast neutron range above this. The level of gamma dose is very high, but when a Bi filter was used the neutron fluxes decreased by only a factor of two and gamma dose by more then a factor of three.

The main parameters of the free beam for reactor power 1 MW:

		calculated	measured
Epithermal flux	1/cm^{2}s	2.97x10^9	1.35x10^9
Fast flux	1/cm^{2}s	1.40x10^8	-
Neutron dose	cGy/min	14.30	-
Gamma dose	cGy/min	51.00	40.00
30 μgB10/g dose	cGy/min	48.70	-

Measured thermal neutron flux distributions in the human head phantom are shown in Fig. 4 for thermal and epithermal beams.

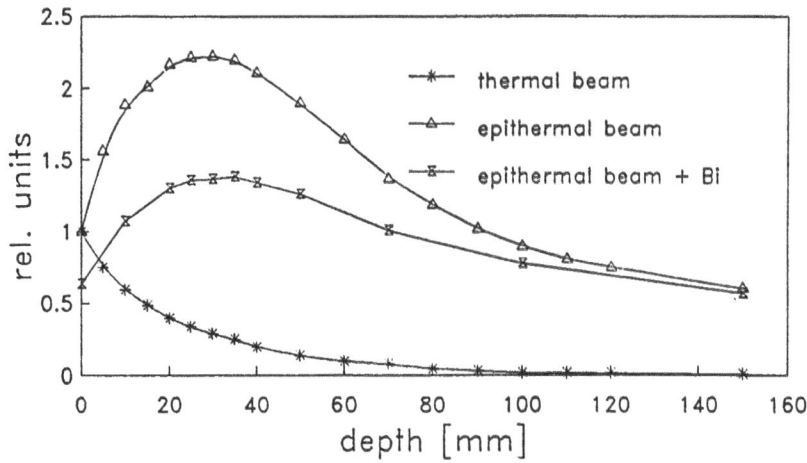

Fig. 4 Thermal neutron flux distribution in the phantom

CONCLUSIONS

International experience and contacts would be desirable in the next stage of our studies in order to improve the parameters of the epithermal beam mainly by reducing the fast neutron and gamma background.

REFERENCES

1. J. Burian, "The Physical Tests for Realization of Neutron Capture Therapy in Czechoslovakia", <u>Strahlenther. Onkol.</u> <u>165 (2/3),12, 1989.</u>

2. J. Burian, J. Rataj, "Neutron Beam Design and Performance for BNCT in Czechoslovakia", in Neutron Beam Design. Development and Performance for Neutron Capture Therapy, Ed. O. K. Harling, J. A. Bernard, R. G. Zamenhof, Plenum Press, NY, P. 229 (1990).

STUDY ON THE BEST DESIGN OF NEUTRON

IRRADIATION FACILITY FOR BNCT

Otohiko Aizawa and Hiroshi Yamada

Atomic Energy Research Laboratory
Musashi Institute of Technology
Ozenji 971, Asao-ku, Kawasaki, Japan

INTRODUCTION

We have two principles for design studies; the first one is the "best design" which has no restrictions in the case of a design of a newly built reactor, and the second one is an "optimum design" which has some restrictions in the case of remodeling for some existing reactors. The first modification of the Musashi reactor was a so-called "optimum design" work[1]. We have already performed the neutron beam design work[2][3] for an enhancement of the thermal and epithermal flux. The present study aims at the "best design" for BNCT, starting from an "optimum design". The design criteria are as follows: (1) $\Phi_{th} \geq 3 \times 10^9 (n/cm^2 sec)$ for thermal beams, (2) $\Phi_{epi} \geq 1.5 \times 10^9 (n/cm^2 sec)$ for epithermal beams, on condition of $\Phi_f \leq 3 \times 10^6 (n/cm^2 sec)$ and $\gamma \leq 150 (R/h)$ at the reactor power of 500 kW. If we want to get the flux values for 1 MW reactor, we can easily get them by multiplying the 500 kW values by a factor of 2.

ARRANGEMENT OF DESIGN CALCULATIONS

Library Used and Definition of Epithermal Total Flux

A two dimensional discrete ordinate transport code[4] DOT3.5 was employed for the design calculations by adopting the S_{12} and P_3 approximations. The group constants used are the neutron and gamma coupled cross sections based on the BUGLE Library[5]. Here we define the epithermal total flux as the integrated flux from 0.1 eV to 3,350 eV, and if we assume an 1/E spectrum in this energy region, we get the equation:

$$\Phi_{epi} = \int_{0.1}^{3.350} \Phi(E) \cdot dE = \int_{0.1}^{3.350} \frac{\lambda}{E} dE = 10.4 \times \lambda \qquad (1)$$

As we have measured λ at the "old" irradiation port of the Musashi reactor by using a cadmium-covered gold foil as 1.55 x $10^6 (n/cm^2 sec)$, Φ_{epi} can be obtained from eq. (1) as $\Phi_{epi} = 10.4 \times 1.55 \times 10^6 = 1.6 \times 10^7 (n/cm^2 sec)$.

Source Intensity Normalization and Assumption for Design Calculations

The design calculation was initiated for the "old" configuration at the Musashi reactor by using a shell source at the core side as shown in Fig. 1.

Progress in Neutron Capture Therapy for Cancer
Edited by B.J. Allen *et al.*, Plenum Press, New York, 1992

The size of the mesh used for the calculations was 24 x 80 and 24 x 48 in R-Z geometry for 2.5 cm and 5.0 cm mesh-intervals in Z-direction, respectively. The mesh-interval in R-direction was kept constant at 2.5 cm. As the calculated results usually depend on the mesh-interval of calculations, we have determined the source normalization factors as 1.33 and 0.71 for 2.5 cm and 5.0 cm mesh-interval calculations, respectively. The results are tabulated in Table 1.

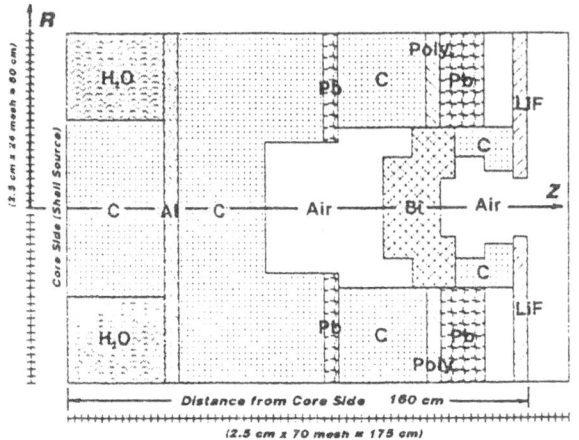

Fig. 1 "Old" configuration
at the Musashi reactor

As the present study aims at the "best design" for BNCT at the reactor power of 500 kW, we assume that we can use, in the following calculations, a source intensity 5 times higher than what we are available. To make the explanation more convenient, we define the words, "spectrum shifter", "neutron filter", "gamma filter" and "neutron collimator" as shown in Fig. 2. The irradiation port was assumed to be located at about 2 meters from the core side.

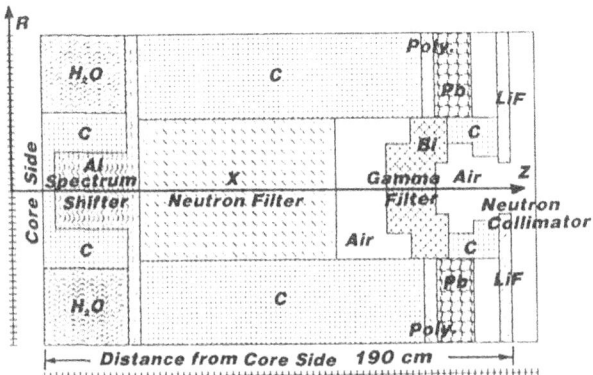

Fig. 2 Geometrical model of calculations
for the "best design"

Table 1. Neutron Flux and Gamma-Dose
of the Musashi Reactor

(TRIGA–II, 100 kW)

'Old" Irradiation Port at The Musashi Reactor		Neutron Flux (n/cm²sec)			Gamma Dose rate
		Thermal	Epithermal ★	Fast ★★	(R/h)
Exp.		1.3×10^9	1.6×10^7	1.0×10^8	25–30
Cal.	2.5 cm mesh cal.	1.0×10^9	1.6×10^7	1.8×10^8	40
	5.0 cm mesh cal.	0.6×10^9	1.6×10^7	1.1×10^8	23

★ defined by equation (1). Normalized with this flux.
★★ Integrated flux from 821 keV to 17.3 MeV.

Table 2. Results of Design Calculations

Distance from Core Side   190 cm
Spectrum Shifter: Aluminum 30 cm fixed   (500 kW Reactor)

Neutron Filter	Thickness (cm)	Thermal (n/cm²sec)	Epithermal (n/cm²sec)	Fast (n/cm²sec)	Gamma (R/h)
Al	55	3.3×10^9	1.9×10^9	4.5×10^8	151
	60	2.8×10^9	1.7×10^9	2.9×10^8	130
	65	2.4×10^9	1.5×10^9	1.9×10^8	111
C	40	3.8×10^9	4.4×10^7	3.0×10^8	148
	45	3.3×10^9	2.2×10^7	1.8×10^8	125
	50	2.7×10^9	1.1×10^7	1.1×10^8	104
Si	75	4.0×10^9	9.1×10^8	3.4×10^8	164
	80	3.6×10^9	8.0×10^8	2.5×10^8	147
	85	3.2×10^9	7.0×10^8	1.8×10^8	131

Choice of Materials for Spectrum Shifter and Neutron Filter

As a result of the investigation for various combinations of spectrum shifters and neutron filters by using the materials of aluminum, alumina, single-crystal silicon, zirconium-deuteride and carbon, it was found that aluminum is the best spectrum shifter and also the best neutron filter for epithermal beams.

As for the thermal beams, the materials of single-crystal silicon, aluminum, carbon, alumina and zirconium-deuteride were investigated as spectrum shifters. The results showed that the ratios of thermal and fast neutron fluxes were almost the same, and that the intensities of thermal neutron fluxes were higher in the order of silicon, aluminum and carbon. We decided to use aluminum as a spectrum shifter for thermal beams, because it was also the best spectrum shifter for epithermal beams.

Final Adjustment by Fine Mesh Calculations

By using the configuration shown in Fig. 2, the neutron filter was changed as aluminum, carbon and single-crystal silicon. The results are shown in Table 2 as a function of the thickness of the neutron filter. From this table we can see that "*Al 60*" and "*Al 65*" satisfy the design criteria for epithermal beams, and "*C 40*", "*C 45*", "*Si 80*" and "*Si 85*" satisfy the design criteria for thermal beams.

REFERENCES

1. O. Aizawa, K. Kanda, T. Nozaki and T. Matsumoto, "Remodeling and Dosimetry on the Neutron Irradiation Facility of the Musashi Institute of Technology Research Reactor for Boron Neutron Capture Therapy," Nucl. Technol., 48; 150 (1980)

2. O. Aizawa, "Research on Neutron Beam Design for BNCT at the Musashi Reactor," Neutron Beam Design, Development, and Performance for Neutron Capture Therapy, pp. 109-124 (1990)

3. O. Aizawa, "Neutron Beam Design for Enhancement of Thermal and Epithermal Flux at the Musashi Reactor," Proc. Int. Conference on the Physics of Reactors: Operation, Design and Computation, Vol. 4, pp. 133-142 (1990)

4. W. A. Rhoades and F. R. Mynatt, "The DOT III Two-Dimensional Discrete Ordinate Transport Code," Oak Ridge National Laboratory, ORNL-TM-4280 (1973)

5. R. W. Roussin, "DCL-75/BUGLE-80 Coupled 47-Neutron, 20-Gamma-ray, P_3 Cross-Section Library for LWR Shielding Calculations," Oak Ridge National Laboratory (1980)

STUDSVIK THERMAL NEUTRON FACILITY

Orn-Anong Pettersson[1], Per Svensson[2], Börje Larsson[1] and Erik Grusell[1]

[1] Department of Radiation Sciences, Uppsala University
Box 535, S-75121 Uppsala, Sweden
[2] Studsvik AB, S-61182 Nyköping, Sweden

INTRODUCTION

The Studsvik thermal neutron facility at the R2-0 reactor originally designed for neutron capture radiography has been modified to permit irradiation of living cells and animals. A hole was drilled in the concrete shielding to provide a cylindrical channel with diameter of 25.3 cm. A shielding water tank serves as an entry holder for cells and animals. The advantage of this modification is that cells and animals can be irradiated at a constant thermal neutron fluence rate of approximately 10^9 n cm^{-2}s^{-1} (at 100 kW) without stopping and restarting the reactor. Topographic analysis of boron done by neutron capture autoradiograghy (NCR) can be irradiated under the same conditions as previously.

THERMAL FACILITY DESIGN AND OPERATION

A thermal neutron facility has been constructed for biological and analytical purposes at the R2-0 reactor in Studsvik. The reactor is of the swimming pool type with a maximum power of 1 MW. The reactor core is made up of MTR- type fuel elements with Al-clad uranium aluminium alloy plates containing 90% ^{235}U. The fluence rate at the centre of the core at maximum power is 10^{13} n cm^{-2}s^{-1}.

As in a previous report,[1] a tank of heavy water is used as moderating material. A lead sheet 75 mm thick was placed between the moderator and the water pool to attenuate gamma radiation from the reactor core. The NCR specimens position indicated as autoradiography position in fig.1 has the effective size of 30 x 30 cm^2. A concrete block behind the NCR position serves as a radiation shield. For safety reasons, the concrete block has to be in place before starting the reactor.

Before operation, the reactor core is moved to the side wall close to the heavy water moderator. The reactor takes about 40 minutes to reach the required power. Before modification, the specimens could not be removed till the induced activity had gone down to an acceptable level. This took 30 minutes or more and was unacceptable for living animals or cells. The facility was therefore modified by drilling a cylindrical channel - diameter 25.3 cm in the concrete block so that specimens could be changed without removing the concrete block. A natural water tank 100x 90 x 68 cm^3 is placed behind the concrete block for shielding and as an entry for an animal cage (fig.1). The temperature of the water in the tank can be controlled to any specific temperature from 20 to70 degrees.

The specimen is loaded into a plexiglass cylinder which is guided into the irradiation position when the reactor has reached the required power and taken out when the irradiation is finished. The cylinder is 58.0 cm long,the inner diameter 22.8 cm and is sealed at one end. It was constructed so that when required it could be flushed with air or other gas with adjustable flow rate. The animal or cell culture holder can be varied in shape and size.

MATERIALS AND METHOD

The measurement of the neutron fluence at the neutron capture autoradiography position was done by a cadmium covered indium foil and by bare and cadmium covered gold foils. To determine

Progress in Neutron Capture Therapy for Cancer
Edited by B.J. Allen *et al.*, Plenum Press, New York, 1992

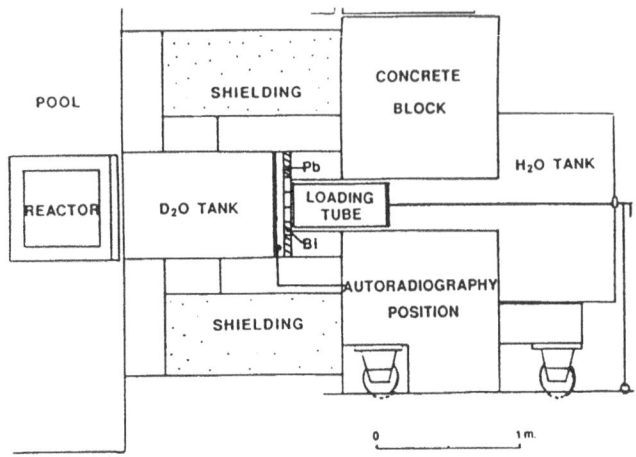

Fig. 1. Layout of the facility.

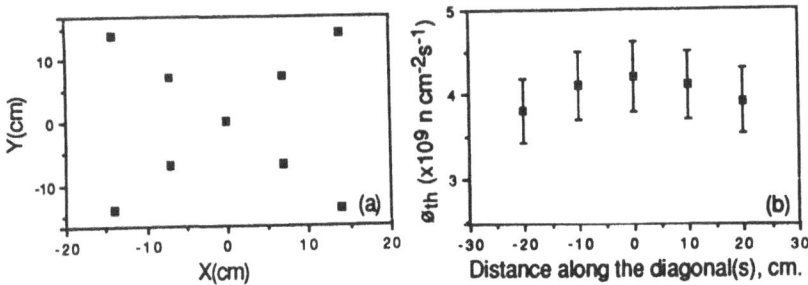

Fig. 2 (a) Position of foils placed along the diagonal of the plexiglass support
(b) Thermal neutron fluence rate at the NCR position

the distribution of the thermal neutrons over the surface of the specimens, 9 gold foils — distance 10 cm between each foil — were placed along the diagonal of the plexiglass plate (Fig.2a) used to support NCR specimens.The foils were irradiated at a power of 100kW. Zirconium foils were irradiated at the power of 200 kW to measure the ratio of the epithermal to thermal neutron fluence.

Five gold foils (average thickness of 18 mg cm^{-2}) and five thermoluminescence dosimeters (TLD-700 of low ^{6}Li content) were placed along the diameter of the plexiglass cylinder in the position nearest to the heavy water moderator. Four more sets were put along its axis. During irradiation, the TLDs were covered with a lithium polyethylene sheet and the gold foils were covered by thin aluminium foil.The experiments were done at a power of 20 kW so that the presence of thermal neutron fluence during the TLD measurement is not too high. The activity of the foils was measured by a Ge(Li) detector.

RESULTS

At the neutron capture autoradiography position, the ratio of epithermal to thermal neutron fluence from Zirconium measurement was of the order of 10^{-4} while the activity of ^{115m}In from the Cd covered indium could not be observed. These results agree with those of the previous report.[1] Figure 2 shows the measured results of gold foils along the diagonal line of the plexiglass plate. The variation of the fluence was found to be within 10 % - an acceptable homogeneity. The fluence along the diameter and the axis of the plexiglass cylinder is shown in figures 3a and 3c. The corresponding gamma dose measured by TLD 700 is presented in figures 3b and 3d.

DISCUSSION

The gamma dose rate at the NCR position was not measured since the gamma radiation level is not critical for this purpose. The ratio of the high energy neutron fluence to the thermal neutron

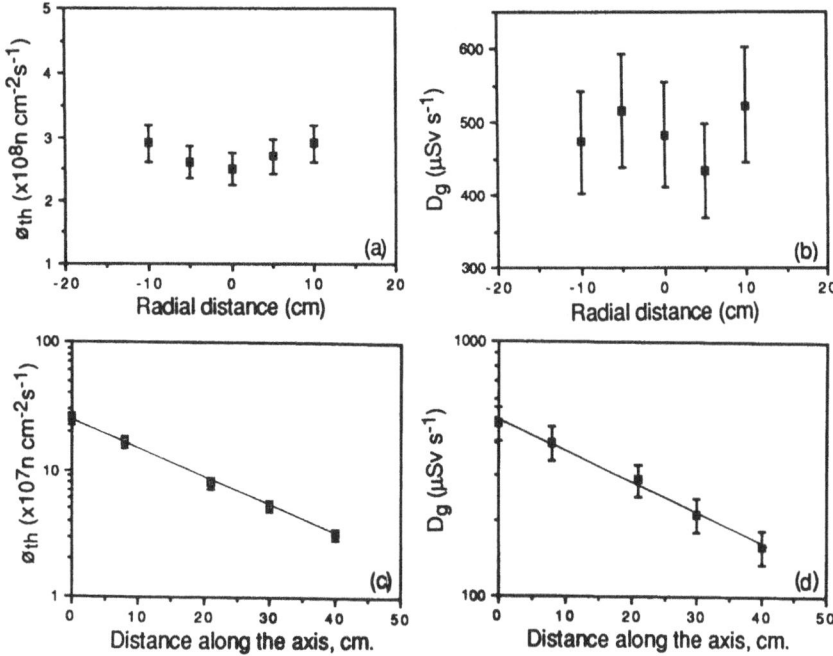

Fig. 3. Thermal neutron fluence rate and gamma dose rate: (a) & (b) along the diameter, (c) & (d) along the axis of the plexiglass cylinder.

fluence is different from the calculation presented previously[1] since some details have been changed.

Results show that: (a) The contribution from epithermal neutron compared to thermal neutron fluence was low. (b) The gamma dose rate at the living specimens position was 2 mSv s^{-1} at the thermal neutron fluence rate 1×10^9 n cm^{-2}s^{-1}. This is about 10 times the dose rate from nitrogen capture in the specimen.[2] The gammas mainly come from capture of neutrons by hydrogen in the water tank. Further, if necessary, extra gamma shielding can be designed. (c) The fluence rate tends to be higher at the edge of the plexiglass cylinder due possibly to the back scattering from the water around it. Since animals are put in the shielding cage and the part irradiated will not be close to the cylinder's wall, this will not cause a great variation of the fluence at the site of interest.

In concludsion, the Studsvik thermal neutron facility provides a high intensity broad beam of thermal neutrons with a very low contribution of fast neutrons. This is very useful for NCR and studying the effect of boron neutron capture reactions in cell cultures and small experimental animals. For cell cultures serveral samples can be irradiated at the same time.

ACKNOWLEDGEMENTS

The authors wish to thank the Studsvik staff for their efficient assistance. The work was supported by the Swedish National Research Council, the Studsvik AB and the International Sciences Program, Uppsala University.

REFERENCES

1. B.Larsson, et al, Neutron Microradiography for Cell-seeking Boron Compounds, in: "Neutron Radiography," proceeding of the Second World Conference, Paris, June 16-20,(1986).
2. D. Gabel, et al, The Relative Biological Effectiveness in V79 Chinese Hamster Cells of the Neutron Capture Reactions in Boron and Nitrogen, Rad. Res.98:307 (1984)

EFFECTIVE THERMAL NEUTRON COLLIMATION FOR NEUTRON CAPTURE THERAPY

USING NEUTRON ABSORPTION AND SCATTERING REACTIONS

Tooru Kobayashi, Shusuke Fujihara* and Keiji Kanda

Research Reactor Institute, Kyoto University
Kumatori-cho, Sennan-gun, Osaka 590-04, Japan

INTRODUCTION

The thermal neutron field available at the Heavy Water Facility of Kyoto University Reactor (KUR) is usually isotropic and the field size is larger than the target. For this reason, collimation of thermal neutrons is needed for clinical irradiations[1,2]. The collimator materials chosen to minimize the secondary gamma rays, are lithium-6 used as a thermal neutron absorber, and graphite used as a thermal neutron scatterer. However a collimator, a few cm in diameter using neutron absorbing materials significantly reduces the neutron flux and increases the clinical irradiation time. The shorter irradiation time nevertheless is desirable for patients. In order to reduce irradiation times for patient treatment, we have manufactured a cone shaped thermal neutron collimator using polyethylene which has a high scattering cross section. The characteristics of cone shaped collimators were determined by experiments and calculations. It is noted that the technique of thermal neutron irradiation for neutron capture therapy should be changed according to the characteristics of thermal neutron beam components and also the depth of the tumor.

EXPERIMENTS

Figure 1 shows the vertical section of the Heavy Water Facility of the KUR. The size of the irradiation room is 2.4 x 2.4 x 2.4 m. The inner wall surface is covered by boron neutron shielding material. The center line of the irradiation field is 90 cm above floor level. Thermal neutrons are obtained from the bismuth surface which is 60 cm in diameter. The irradiation equipment on a rail can be used to hold and/or handle test samples whith maximum diameter of 8 cm and length of 20 cm during the KUR operation at the power of 5 MW.

Figure 2 shows the cone shaped collimators and a polyethylene phantom . Polyethylene has a high hydrogen density and good manufacturing characteristics and is therefore a

---

* Present address: Kansai Electric Power Co., Inc.
3-3-22, Nakanoshima, Kita-ku, Osaka 530, Japan

Progress in Neutron Capture Therapy for Cancer
Edited by B.J. Allen *et al.*, Plenum Press, New York, 1992

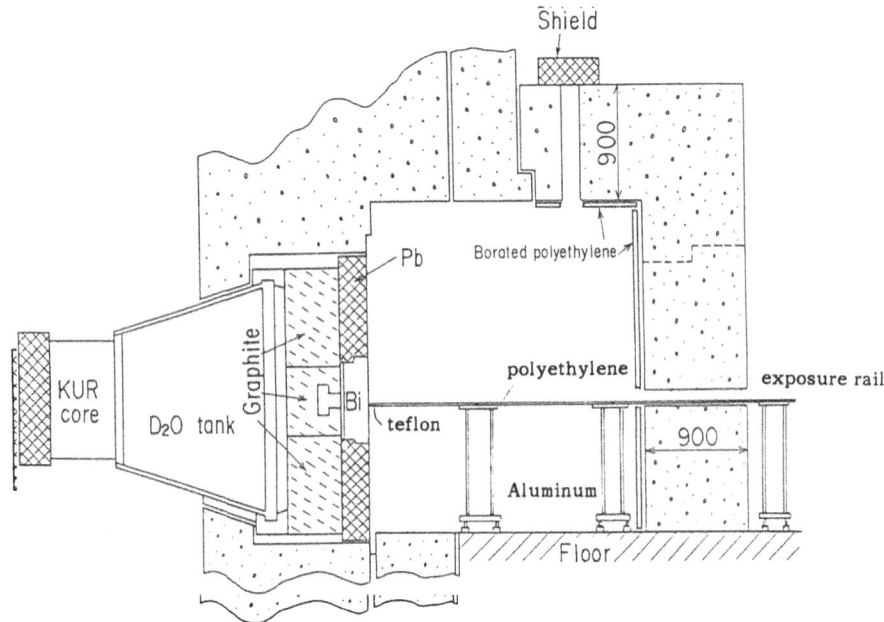

Figure 1. Vertical cross section of Heavy Water Facility of the KUR
and its exposure equipment

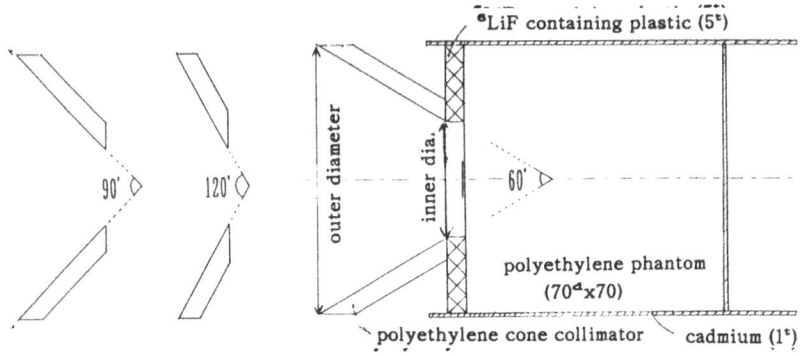

Figure 2. A polyethylene cone collimator and a phantom for experiments

suitable material for the cone shaped collimator. We manufactured the cone shaped collimators with different cone angles (60°,90°,120°), and cone sizes (inner diameter: 20, 30, 40 mm, outer diameter: 40, 50, 60, 70 mm). The wall thickness of 5 mm for the cone shaped collimator was determined by experiments for thermal neutron reflection characteristics. A polyethylene phantom 7 cm in diameter and 7 cm in thickness was used for the experiments. To shield against thermal neutrons when measuring the depth dose distribution in the phantom, the phantom surface except for the irradiated area, was covered by cadmium (1 mm in thickness) and plastic containing 30 % ^{6}LiF (5 mm in thickness). Experiments were systematically performed for several cone collimators of constant wall thickness of 5 mm. Thermal neutron flux was measured by irradiating gold wire 0.25 mm in diameter.

CALCULATIONS

We aimed to calculate the characteristics of the thermal neutron beam at the bismuth surface of the Heavy Water Facility of the KUR. The two dimensional transport code DOT-3.5 was used to calculate thermal neutron flux distributions in the KUR core to bismuth layer. The one dimensional transport code ANISN was used for the angular dependence of thermal neutrons at the bismuth surface. The thermal neutron energy spectrum was assumed to be the 60 ° C Maxwellian distribution. Because of the complicated geometry between the bismuth surface and cone shaped collimators with phantom, a Monte Carlo code MCNP-V3 was used.

RESULTS AND DISCUSSION

Firstly, we checked the reflection characteristics in order to choose a scattering material for the collimator. Table 1 shows the thermal neutron flux measured on the surface facing the core for several materials which were put at 5 cm from the center of the bismuth surface. The intensity of the thermal neutron flux depends on the neutron absorption and scattering of each material. The differences between the measured neutron fluxes of the materials are caused by neutron reflection from each material. Hydrogenous material is effective as a scattering material even though its thickness is small. The optimum wall thickness of the cone shaped collimators was determined by these experiments using polyethylene thicknesses of 2, 4, 6, 8 and 10 mm.

Figure 4 shows the measured and calculated thermal neutron flux at the center of the phantom surface used to check the optimum cone angle. In these cases, the distances from the bismuth surface to phantom were 30 cm, 90 cm and the cone shaped collimators were both 6 cm in outer diameter, 3 cm in inner diameter and 5 mm wall thickness . We also checked two other cases with distances of 10 cm and 60 cm. These data showed that the optimum cone angle depends on the distance of the phantom from the bismuth surface. It depends mainly on the combination of isotropic and parallel beam components. We also examined the relationship of cone size and the optimum cone angle. The relationship between them is not strong.

Figure 5 shows the calculated depth dose distribution when the distance of the phantom from the bismuth surface is changed from 0 to 90 cm. It reflects the change of the ratio of parallel to isotropic beam components. The thermal neutron field having a large parallel beam component produces a flux peak inside a phantom. The relaxation constants deeper than 10 mm in the phantom are almost the same. The thermal neutron distribution up to a depth of 10 mm in phantom can be affected by the distance from the bismuth surface. Namely, by changing the parallel beam component versus the isotropic one, the depth dose distribution in tissue can be controlled. When the distance between the bismuth surface and

Table 1. Characteristics of thermal neutron reflection

Materials	(thickness x diameter)	thermal neutron flux (x10⁹ n/cm².s)
Cadmium	1.4 x 65 mm	2.5
Borated Polyethylene	10 x 65	3.2
Aluminum	10 x 65	3.1
Bismuth	10 x 65	3.4
Teflon	10 x 65	3.6
Polyethylene	10 x 65	4.7

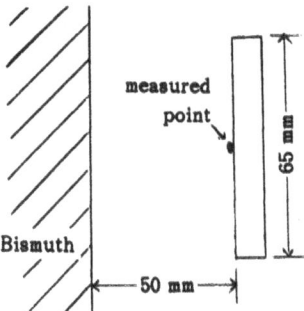

Figure 3 The geometry for the
experiments of Table 1

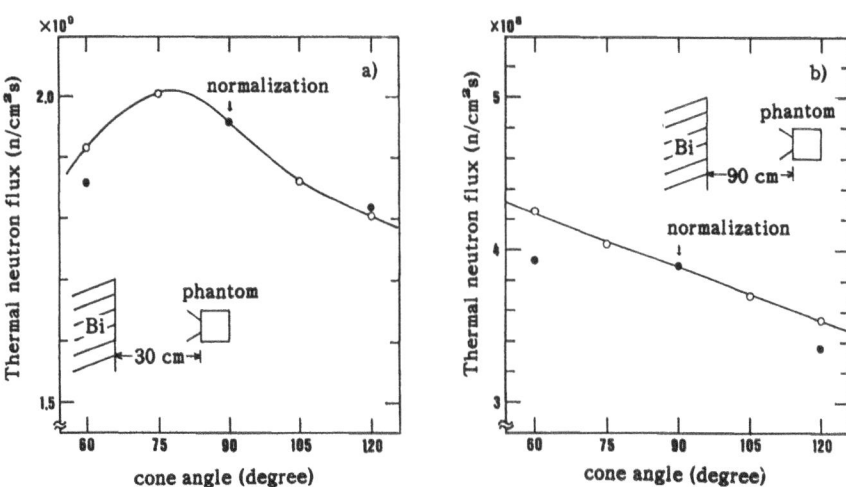

Figure 4. The optimum cone angle for thermal neutron flux at the phantom surface
depended on distance from bismuth surfase, a) = 30 cm and b) = 90 cm.
○ : calculation   ● : experiment

the phantom becomes large, the thermal neutron flux of the phantom surface decreases. In the case of the KUR at the power of 5 MW, thermal neutron fluxes at 10 cm, 30 cm, 60 cm and 90 cm distance from the bismuth surface were 3.7×10^9, 1.9×10^9, 7.8×10^8 and 3.9×10^8 n/cm^{2}s, respectively. So, in actual clinical irradiation, we have to take care of decreasing intensity when the combination of isotropic and parallel beam components are controlled.

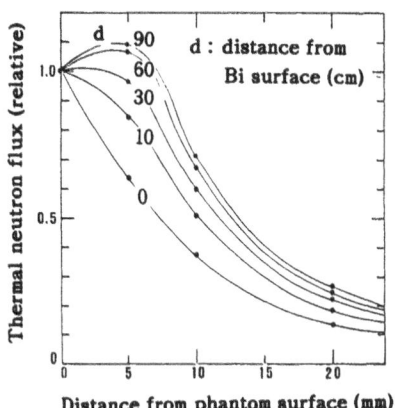

Figure 5. Calculated thermal neutron flux distribution in a polyethylene phantom. Parametric survey calculations for characteristics of beam direction components.

CONCLUSIONS

(1) The isotropic thermal neutron field is effective for the cutaneous tumor such as skin cancer. By using a cone shaped collimator, increase of available thermal neutron fluence rate of about 20 % is easily obtained at the surface of the tissue.

(2) On the other hand, the parallel thermal neutron beam is more effective for the treatment of deep seated tumors.

(3) It is useful and beneficial in neutron capture therapy to use the two components of thermal neutron irradiation fields, that is, the parallel beam component and the isotropic beam component.

REFERENCES

1. T. Kobayashi, K. Kanda, Y. Ujeno and M. R. Ishida, "Biomedical Irradiation System for Boron Neutron Capture Therapy at the Kyoto University Reactor," in Neutron Beam Design Development and Performance for Neutron Capture Therapy, O. K. Harling, et al. ed., Plenum Press, New York, USA, p.321 (1990).

2. K. Kanda, T. Kobayashi, K. Ono, T. Sato, T. Shibata, Y. Ujeno, Y. Mishima, H. Hatanaka, and Y. Nishiwaki, "Elimination of Gamma Rays from a Thermal Neutron Field for Medical and Biomedical Irradiation Purposes," IAEA-SM-193/68, IAEA, Vienna, Austria, March 10-14, 1975, Biomedical Dosimetry, p. 205.

REEVALUATION OF THERMAL NEUTRON FIELD OF THE KUR
HEAVY WATER FACILITY FOR BIOMEDICAL USES
(OPTIMIZATION OF BISMUTH, HEAVY WATER AND GRAPHITE LAYERS)

Yoshinori Sakurai, Shusuke Fujihara[*], Tooru Kobayashi and Keiji Kanda

Research Reactor Institute, Kyoto University
Kumatori-cho, Sennan-gun, Osaka 590-04, Japan

INTRODUCTION

The object of this study is to optimize the Heavy Water Facility of the Kyoto University Reactor (KUR) through experiment and calculation with a view to modifying the facility. The heavy water facility thermalizes fast neutrons from the reactor core with the heavy water layer and shields against gamma-rays with the bismuth layer. It produces a thermal neutron field of high quality for neutron capture therapy (NCT). At present, the thicknesses of heavy water, graphite and bismuth layers are 140, 48 and 15 cm, respectively.

The following three conditions need to be satisfied for the facility to be used for NCT;

   1) obtain a sufficient intensity of thermal neutrons,
   2) minimize the contamination of fast and epithermal neutrons; and,
   3) eliminate gamma-rays as much as possible.

These conditions do not need to be changed and have already been partly realized in the present facility[1]. We have tried to review the thickness of the heavy water, bismuth, graphite and lead layers, paying particular attention to the heavy water and bismuth layers in order to optimize the design of the facility.

The role of heavy water is to thermalize fast neutrons from the nuclear reactor core. Heavy water also yields fast neutrons by $D(\gamma,n)H$ reactions. Therefore, by increasing the thickness of the heavy water layer, the ratio of fast neutron to thermal neutron dose rate decreases until at a certain thickness an equilibrium value is reached[2].

On the other hand, the role of the bismuth layer is to shield against primary gamma-rays from the reactor core and other sources. But bismuth itself yields secondary gamma-rays by (n,γ) reactions. And so, by increasing the thickness of the bismuth layer, the ratio of thermal neutron flux to gamma-ray dose rate reaches an equilibrium value[3].

In calculations to optimize the thickness of heavy water and bismuth layers we used newly evaluated data for bismuth[4].

---

* Present address : Kansai Electric Power Co., Inc.
               3-3-22, Nakanoshima, Kita-ku, Osaka 530, Japan

Progress in Neutron Capture Therapy for Cancer
Edited by B.J. Allen *et al.*, Plenum Press, New York, 1992

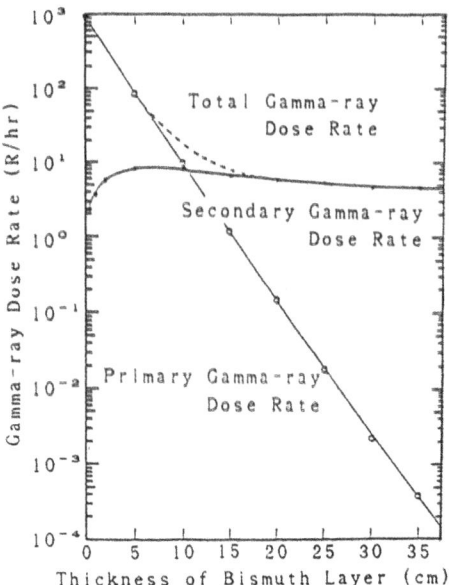

Figure 1   Components of gamma dose at
the mid point of the bismuth
for varying thickness of the
bismuth layer.

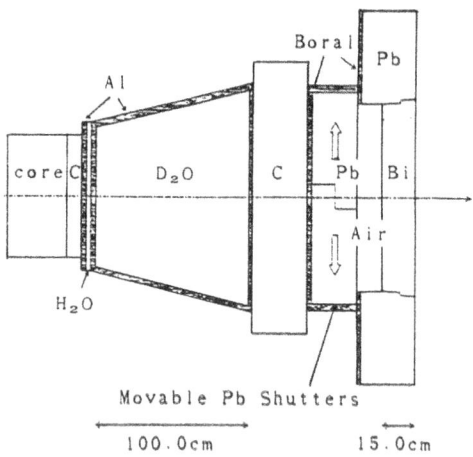

Figure 2   Aspect of the future
KUR Heavy Water Facility

CALCULATIONS

Nuclear data for bismuth had not been included in any cross section library. We requested the Nuclear Data Center of Japan Atomic Energy Research Institute and the Sigma Committee of Japan to prepare the evaluated cross sections for bismuth. A new set of cross sections based on JENDL-3 was prepared for biomedical design purposes[4].

For optimization calculations, a one dimensional transport code named ANISN in the SRAC code system[5,6] was adopted. The heavy water thickness was varied from 60 to 130 cm in 10 cm steps and the bismuth layer thickness from 0 to 27 cm in 3 cm steps. The order of the Pn and Sn approximations was set to be 3 and 8, respectively. In the finite plane calculation, every region was assumed to be the same size in X and Y directions. The number of energy groups for neutrons and gamma rays was 21 and 9, respectively.

Additionally, a two dimensional transport calculation was performed for the purpose of comparison with experiments. Here, we used the DOT 3.5[7,8] code and the order of Pn and Sn approximations was set to be 3 and 8, respectively.

EXPERIMENTS

The calculated results for varying thickness of the bismuth layer, were compared with experiments. In addition to the fixed bismuth layer of 15 cm thickness and 60 cm diameter, a part of the graphite layer 30 $\times$ 30 cm^2 and 0-15 cm thickness was replaced by bismuth blocks to obtain 15, 20, 25 and 30 cm total bismuth thickness. The thermal neutron flux was measured by gold foils of 0.05 mm thickness and 3 mm diameter. The gamma ray dose was measured by TLDs : BeO dosemeters (UD-170L) 0.8 mm in diameter and 10 mm in length manufactured by the Matsushita Co. Ltd., encased in ^{6}LiF cylinders of 2 mm thickness.

RESULTS AND DISCUSSION

As the heavy water thickness increases, the thermal neutron flux decreases , but the ratio of fast to thermal neutrons reaches an equilibrium value at the heavy water thickness of about 100 cm. We decided upon this value as the optimized thickness of the heavy water layer.

As the thickness of the bismuth layer increases, the thermal neutron flux decreases, but the ratio of gamma-ray dose rate to thermal neutron flux does not decrease to less than a certain value which is the equilibrium value. We decided that the optimized thickness of the bismuth layer is in the range of 15 to 20 cm for the KUR heavy water thermal neutron facility. Figure 1 shows the calculated primary and secondary gamma ray dose components. From figure 1, it is easy to see the optimized bismuth thickness which mainly depends on the primary gamma ray intensity.

Overall, the thickness of the moderator filter facility can be reduced by about 40 cm and the thermal neutron flux can be increased more than 10 times over the present value without changing the beam quality. Moreover, because of flexibility in the thickness of the graphite layer, we can make room for increasing the thickness of the lead layer and for adding the movable boral-lead shutters, which reduce the neutron and gamma-ray contamination during reactor operation (Figure 2).

Additionally, according to the results of experiments and two dimensional calculations, aluminum used as a structural material in the facility affects the γ/n ratio significantly. We need to take careful account of materials and structure in optimizing the design of a facility.

CONCLUSIONS

A 2-dimensional transport calculation shows that 15 cm of bismuth is optimum for gamma-ray shielding. The graphite layer thickness does not

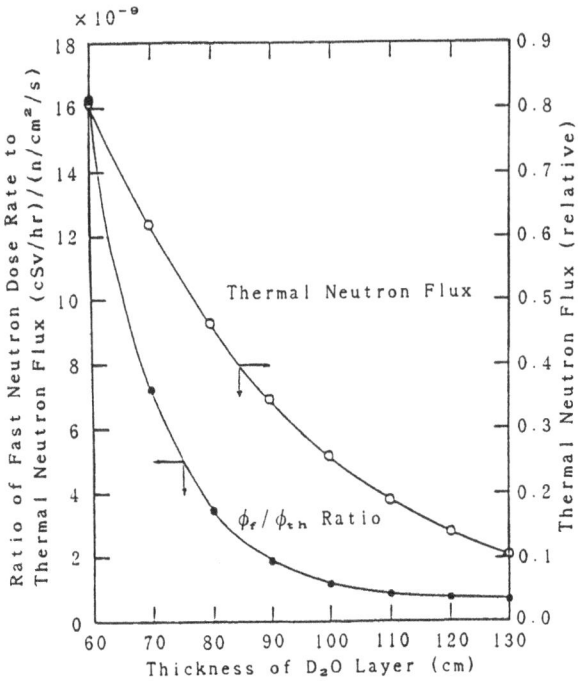

Figure 3 Thermal neutron flux and the ratio of
fast neutron dose rate to thermal
neutron flux at the bismuth surface
for varying heavy water thickness.

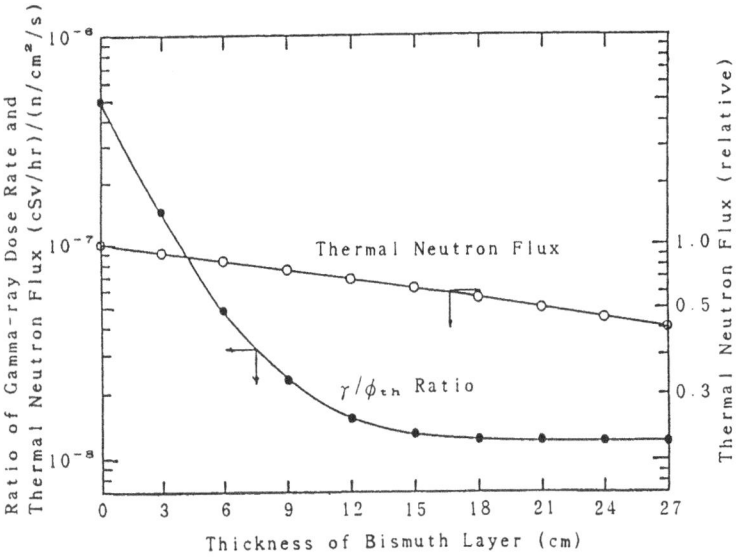

Figure 4 Thermal neutron and the ratio of gamma-ray dose rate
to thermal neutron flux at the bismuth surface for
varying bismuth thickness.

greatly affect the beam quality and thickness in the range of 0-50 cm can be selected in order to accommodate other experimental conditions. Conclusions are the following;

(1) the optimum thickness of the heavy water layer is around 100 cm (Figure 3),
(2) the optimum thickness of the bismuth layer is around 15 cm (Figure 4); and,
(3) the thickness of the graphite layer is selected freely.

ACKNOWLEDGEMENTS

The authors wish to acknowledge Dr. Seiji Shiroya, Mr. Hironobu Unesaki and Mr. Chihiro Ichihara of Kyoto University Research Reactor Institute for their helpful suggestions and discussions of the calculation method. The authors thank the Nuclear Data Center of Japan Atomic Energy Research Institute and the Sigma Committee of Japan for preparing the evaluated cross sections for bismuth. The authors thank the core design group of Mitsubishi Atomic Power Industry for preparing the data sets for bismuth.

REFERENCES

1) K.Kanda, T.Kobayashi, K.Ono, T.Shibata, Y.Ujeno, Y.Mishima, H.Hatanaka and Y.Nishiwaki, Biomedical Dosimetry, IAEA, (1975) 205-223.
2) K.Aoki and K.Kanda, J. Nucl. Sci. Technol., 20[10] (1983) 812-821.
3) T.Kobayashi, Thesis of doctor degree, (1983) 59-60.
4) "JSSTDL-295/J3", A.Hasegawa, private communication (1989).
5) K.Tsuchihashi, Y.Ishiguro, K.Kaneko and M.Ido, JAERI-1302 (1986).
6) K.Koyama, K.Minami, Y.Taji and S.Miyasaka, JAERI-M 7155 (1977).
7) F.R.Mynatt, et al., ORNL-TM-4280, (1973).
8) F.R.Mynatt, et al., CCC-276, (1975).

DESIGN OF AN ACCELERATOR-BASED EPITHERMAL

NEUTRON BEAM FOR BORON NEUTRON CAPTURE THERAPY

J.C. Yanch[1], X-L. Zhou[1], R.E. Shefer[2], R.E. Klinkowstein[2], and G.L. Brownell[1]

[1]Department of Nuclear Engineering and Whitaker College of Health Sciences and Technology, Massachusetts Institute of Technology, Cambridge, MA, USA

[2]Science Research Laboratory, Somerville, MA, USA

INTRODUCTION:

Recent interest in the production of epithermal neutrons for use in boron neutron capture therapy (BNCT) has prompted an investigation into the feasibility of generating such neutrons with a tandem cascade accelerator[1,2]. Accelerator-produced neutrons in the range of roughly 200-800 keV are generated in a lithium compound target via the $^7Li(p,n)^7Be$ nuclear reaction in a tandem cascade accelerator currently under development by Science Research Laboratory, Somerville, MA. Details of the design of the proton accelerator and operating characteristics will be presented elsewhere in these proceedings[3]. Recognizing that the accelerator-produced neutrons will be too energetic for use in neutron capture therapy, a detailed dosimetric study was undertaken to determine the energy, or range of energies most suitable for NCT. This study was carried out using three-dimensional Monte Carlo transport calculations; results are discussed briefly here. Once the most suitable range of energies for BNCT was determined, it was then possible to design an appropriate moderator assembly to shift the energy of the neutrons down to the therapeutically useful levels. Such an assembly has been designed with the aid of computer simulation; calculations of treatment parameters indicate that the accelerator neutron beam can provide dose rates and advantage depths comparable to currently available reactor beams for neutron capture therapy.

I. IDEAL BEAM STUDIES:

The computer simulation code MCNP[4] was used to examine the dosimetric effects of neutron beams of varying energies on brain tissue (and hence to determine an optimal energy range for BNCT in the brain). Two phantoms composed of brain-equivalent material were modelled (see Figure 1). The first phantom was cylindrical in shape (16.0 cm in diameter x 16.0 cm height). A monoenergetic plane wave of neutrons was directed onto the flat surface of the cylinder. The disc-shaped source was centered on the axis of the cylinder and its diameter was varied to examine the effect of beam size on depth- and radial-dose distribution in the phantom. The geometry of the second phantom was based on a Monte Carlo brain and skull model reported by Deutsch and Murray[5].

To estimate the contribution of individual dose components as a function of depth and of radial distance from the longitudinal axis, the phantom models were divided into several 1 cm thick disks and into eight concentric cylinders. The following flux components were assessed as a function of depth: thermal neutrons (cut-off energy: 0.36 eV), fast neutrons, and (n,γ) photons. The neutron (including the $^{14}N(n,p)$ reaction) and photon fluxes were modified by

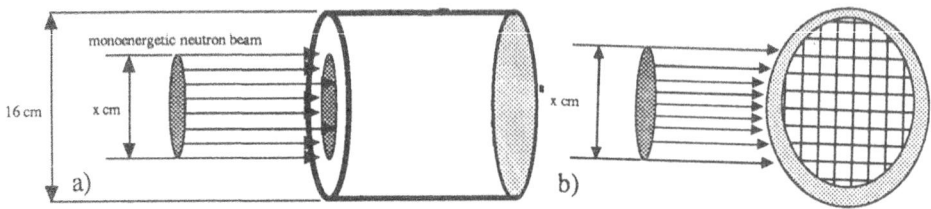

Figure 1. Phantoms modelled in ideal beam study. a) 16.0 cm diameter x 16.0 length cylinder, b) ellipsoidal head phantom (after Deutsch and Murray[4]).

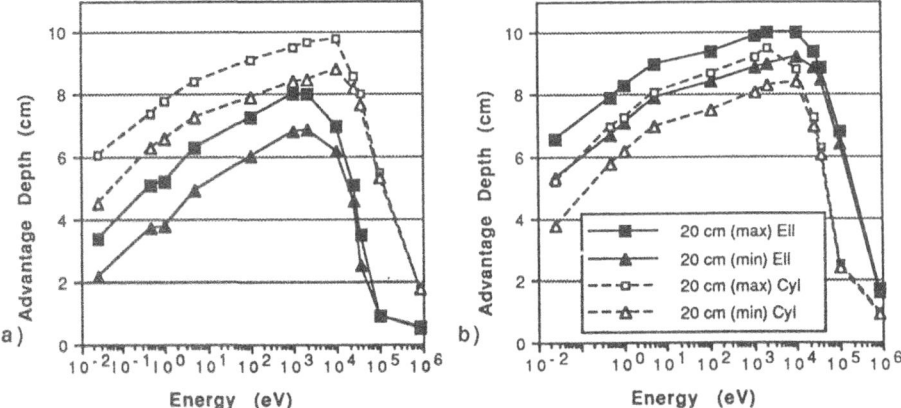

Figure 2. Maximum and Minimum advantage depths versus neutron energy based on ^{10}B tumour/healthy tissue ratios of 30:0 and 30:3, respectively. a) beam size = 0.0 cm, b) beam size = 20.0 cm.

the KERMA-dose conversion factors of Caswell et. al.[6], and Zamenhof et. al.[7] respectively. To estimate the ^{10}B(n,α)^{7}Li contribution to dose, the thermal neutron flux was multiplied by either a factor of 3 (to represent 3 μg/g ^{10}B in healthy tissue) or a factor of 30 (to represent 30 μg/g ^{10}B in tumour) and then modified by ^{10}B fluence-to-KERMA conversion factors, also listed by Zamenhof et. al.[7].

Two figures of merit were used to evaluate the performance of the various neutron beams: the advantage depth (AD) and the advantage ratio (AR). Both have been used extensively by many authors[8]. Advantage depth represents the depth in tissue at which the dose to tumour will equal the maximum dose to the healthy tissue. The advantage ratio is equal to the integral of the total tumour dose, divided by the integral of the total background dose (assuming no ^{10}B in healthy tissue) over the entire effective treatment depth (i.e. from 0.0 cm to the maximum advantage depth).

Also calculated is the percent contribution of the various dose components to the integrated treatment depth. The dose components were grouped into high LET (fast neutrons and the ^{14}N(n,p) reaction), low LET (induced gammas) and the ^{10}B reaction products.

AD, AR and percent dose components were calculated for each of several monoenergetic neutron beams with energies ranging from 0.025 eV (thermal) to 800 keV (the maximum neutron energy of the accelerator-produced neutrons). For each neutron energy tested, the beam diameter was varied in order to examine the effect of beam size on the figures of merit.

Results of the Ideal Beam Study:

Figures 2a and 2b show maximum and minimum advantage depths as function of neutron energy, for two different beam sizes impinging on both the cylindrical (dashed curves) and the elliptical (solid curves) phantoms. Dose components are measured within a 2 cm diameter axial cylinder through the center of the phantom. It is seen that, for a given beam size, advantage depth increases with increasing energy; a peak is reached at some energy (dependent on beam size) between 1.0 keV and 10 to 20 keV at which point it decreases rapidly with further increases in energy. Also, as beam size increases, the energy at which the AD peaks (both AD_{max} and AD_{min}) also increases.

The maximum AD obtained with a very narrow beam is produced by an energy of 1.0 keV, however for a large beam, this energy rises to 10 keV. The "optimal" beam energy thus *appears* to be a function of beam size. However, this is simply an artifact of measuring dose components in a 2 cm diameter cylinder in the phantom (i.e. a situation roughly simulating the experimental condition of measuring dose components with gold foils or small ion chambers placed along the central axis of the phantom). When the entire phantom width is used in dose measurements, the maximum AD occurs at 10 keV for all beam sizes. This is discussed in more detail elsewhere[9]. Similar trends are seen in either phantom however some differences are apparent, especially at smaller beam sizes.

Calculated advantage ratios are plotted as function of neutron energy in Figures 3a and 3b, for two beam sizes and for the two phantom shapes. Again, measurements are made within a 2 cm diameter central cylinder. For any given beam size, the advantage ratio is always a maximum at thermal energies and decreases as the energy is increased, reaching a value of 1.0 at high energies where the tumour dose becomes entirely swamped by the background dose component (primarily the fast neutron dose). This decrease in AR illustrates the increasing effect that higher-energy neutrons have in healthy tissues, primarily at the surface. A smaller AR is an inevitable consequence of the improved penetration offered by neutrons with greater than thermal energies. Again, some differences exist between the two phantom shapes, especially at low energies[9].

From Figures 2 and 3 the optimal range of ideal energies for BNCT of brain tumours can be determined. Used as the criterion is the ability of a neutron beam to treat, with large advantage ratio, to the midline of the brain (7.0 cm). To be conservative the minimum advantage depth with its assumption of 3 µg/g ^{10}B in healthy tissue is used. Examine the curve representing AD_{min} (triangles) on Figure 2b. It is seen that all energies in the range of roughly 4 eV to 40 keV will successfully treat to the midline of the brain. The optimal energy, 10 keV, lies within that range and will treat, in the brain, to a depth of 9.0 - 10 cm.

A fairly wide range of energies (4 eV - 40 keV) is thus seen to be useful for neutron capture therapy. At energies below 4 eV it is no longer possible to treat to the midline (i.e. AD < 7.0 cm); however, the AD falls off only slowly with a decrease in beam energy suggesting a lower energy beam may in fact be useable. Neutron energies higher than 40 keV, on the other hand, will not be useful. The advantage depth falls off rapidly at $E_n > 40$ keV indicating that higher energy beams will contribute only fast-neutron dose to the healthy tissues at the brain surface and will provide no net benefit to tumour treatment.

Figure 4 plots the percentage RBE-weighted dose composition as a function of energy for a 16 cm beam impinging on the cylindrical phantom. It is apparent that all neutron energies up to roughly 40 - 50 keV will ensure that 75 - 85 % of the dose to a tumour within the the advantage depth will be due to ^{10}B reaction products. Increasing the energy above 40 - 50 keV will mean

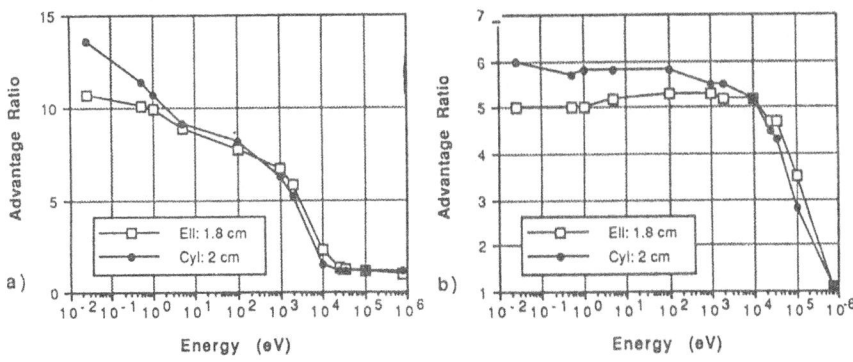

Figure 3. Advantage ratio versus neutron energy in elliptical and cylindrical phantoms, a) beam size = 0.0 cm, b) beam size = 20.0 cm.

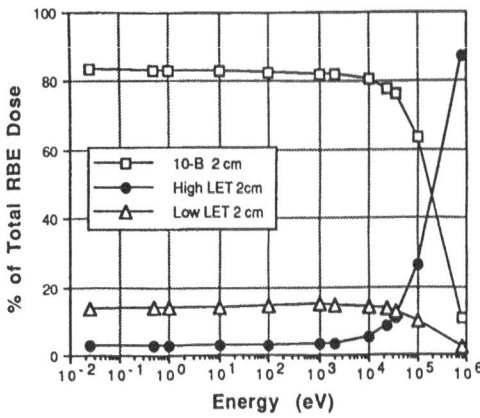

Figure 4. Percent dose contribution at maximum advantage depth versus energy.
Dose components are as described in text.

that more of the dose in that volume of tissue will be due to fast neutrons than to ^{10}B. The lower limit of 4 eV is seen to be less critical. There is even a slight increase in the relative importance of ^{10}B to the tumour dose as the neutron energy falls below 4 eV.

The range of neutron energies found here to be therapeutically useful in brain-equivalent material, 4 eV to 40 keV, is roughly similar to that found by Clement et. al.[7] in a polyethylene phantom. It is much higher, however, and also more extensive than the range deemed suitable by Wang et. al. (1.0 eV - 1.0 keV)[10].

II. MODERATOR ASSEMBLY DESIGNS

Conclusions from the ideal beam study indicate that neutrons emerging from the accelerator target, while much lower in energy than those from a reactor, are too energetic for patient therapy (E_{max} = 800 keV for a 2.5 MeV proton beam)[3]. MCNP has again been used to perform a systematic study of a wide range of moderating, filtering and reflecting materials, and to develop a design that will be useful for shifting the energy of the neutrons down to the therapeutically useful levels (4 ev to 40 keV). Due to a low neutron yield from the lithium target itself (relative to a reactor source), it was important to avoid designing any component in such a way as to unnecessarily reduce neutron flux at the patient position. Thus, for example, materials with low absorption cross-sections were chosen and an attempt was made to limit the distance between the accelerator target and the patient to avoid excessive spreading out of the beam. The major conclusions of these simulations are summarized below.

Moderator Material

A moderator material with a large scattering cross-section is essential; a small absorption cross-section will minimize neutron loss. Also, in order to maintain a large neutron flux at the patient end of the moderator assembly, it is critical that neutron moderation be accomplished in the shortest possible distance. Thus the moderator should be of low mass number so that the average energy loss per interaction is high. Also, a light nucleus is desirable for maintaining the angular directivity of the neutrons as they emerge from the lithium target. Another consideration is the degree of gamma production. Because of the need to limit the extent of materials between the accelerator and the patient, the addition of gamma shielding would be undesirable. Light hydrogen, therefore, is not a useful candidate. Finally, an ideal moderator would have a larger interaction cross-section for fast neutrons than for lower-energy neutrons. This would limit fast-neutron contamination of the therapy beam and would prevent the output spectrum becoming saddle-shaped.

A large number of candidate moderating materials were evaluated with respect to moderating efficiency, directivity of the scattered neutron beam and low secondary gamma production. The materials D_2, BeO, Al_2O_3 and TiO_2 were then selected for more detailed evaluation.

Simulations showed that D_2O (followed by BeO) is superior in terms of both moderating efficiency (fraction of neutrons scattered into the 4 eV - 40 keV bin) and total surviving fraction. All subsequent simulations used D_2O as the moderating material.

Moderator Thickness

D_2O moderator thickness in the range t = 3 - 30 cm were simulated. The surviving neutron fraction in the 4 eV - 40 keV energy bin rises rapidly to a peak at t = 9 cm and declines thereafter. This rise in therapeutic fraction is coupled with a sharp decline in the fast to therapeutic neutron ratio. However, subsequent simulations of dose distributions in a phantom showed that even larger moderator thicknesses (15 - 27 cm) are required to reduce the fast neutron component sufficiently to treat tumours near the midline of the brain.

Filter

Unwanted components of the moderated neutron spectrum can be further reduced by filtering. Two aspects were considered: filtering of the high energy component and filtering of the thermal component. Thermal neutrons may be effectively removed from the beam with ^6Li which has a high thermal neutron capture cross-section and low gamma production cross-section. Simulations with different lithium thickness interposed between the moderator and phantom indicate that a small thickness (~ 0.01 cm) of ^6Li significantly increases the advantage depth. However, thicknesses larger than approximately 0.1 cm begin to cause a significant reduction in tumour dose rate by affecting the low energy (4 - 100 eV) end of the therapeutic neutron component. It was therefore concluded that a ^6Li thickness of 0.02 - 0.1 cm is optimal.

Filtering the high energy neutron component (above 40 keV) while maintaining a high therapeutic neutron flux is more difficult. Four materials, Al, S, Fe and Si have transmission windows in the 4 eV - 40 keV range. Of these Al was found to be superior to S and Si for this application. However, the small beneficial effect of the Al filter on the spectral shape was partially offset by the reduced surviving therapeutic fraction and the concomitant increase in gamma flux. A larger ratio of epithermal/fast neutrons could be obtained by simply increasing the thickness of D_2O than by incorporating Al into the design, in any configuration. Al was therefore not used.

Reflector

Reflection of neutrons emerging from the moderator in directions not compatible with patient treatment is essential for maximization of therapeutic neutron flux. Four materials were evaluated for use as neutron reflectors: graphite, lead, bismuth and Al_2O_3. Of these, lead was found to have superior properties in terms of overall reflectivity, low gamma production and low degree of moderation of the neutron spectrum. The overall reflectivity was found to saturate at a thickness of 18 cm for normal neutron incidence.

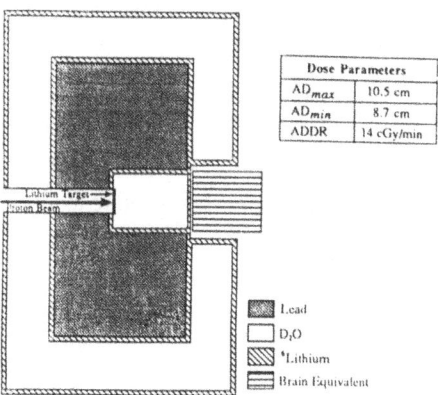

Figure 5. Design of moderator-reflector-shielding assembly. Dose parameters calculated in a cylindrical phantom of brain-equivalent material are also included.

Shielding

Some neutrons will penetrate the reflector and will contribute an undesirable radiation dose to the rest of the patient and may cause neutron activation in components of the therapy room. Shielding of these neutrons can best be carried out by moderating (with D_2O) to slow the neutrons down to thermal energies, and then absorbing the thermal neutrons with a substantial thickness of ^6Li. Alternative (and less costly) shielding strategies will also be considered.

Final Design

A final configuration is shown in Figure 5. Irradiation parameters (advantage depth (AD), advantage ratio (AR) and advantage depth dose rate (ADDR)[8]) were measured in a cylindrical phantom composed of brain-equivalent material. With a D_2O moderator thickness of 23 cm, followed by .02 cm ^6Li, maximum and minimum advantage depths of 10.5 cm and 8.7 cm were obtained. The advantage ratio is 4.6 and a tumour at the advantage depth would receive a dose rate of 14 rads/min. We believe that these parameters are comparable to currently available reactor beams for neutron capture therapy. As a result, physical construction of the moderator/reflector/ shielding design described above is currently underway.

ACKNOWLEDGMENT

The MCNP version used in this study, version 3b, is installed on SUN SPARC workstations in the Whitaker College Biomedical Imaging and Computation Laboratory at MIT. This investigation was supported by Grant No. DE-FG01-89ER60874 from the US Department of Energy.

REFERENCES

1. G.L. Brownell, J.E. Kirsch and J. Kehayias, Accelerator production of epithermal neutrons for neutron capture therapy, in: *Neutron Capture Therapy*, H. Hatanaka, Ed., Nishimura Co., Ltd., Nigita, Japan (1986).
2. R.E. Shefer, R.E. Klinkowstein, J.C. Yanch and G.L. Brownell, A versatile new accelerator design for epithermal neutron production for neutron capture therapy, in: *Neutron Beam Design, Development and Performance for Neutron Capture Therapy*, O.K. Harling, J.A. Bernard and R.G. Zamenhof, eds., Plenum Press, New York (1990).
3. R.E. Shefer, R.E. Klinkowstein, J.C. Yanch and G.L. Brownell, Production of epithermal neutrons for BNCT with a tandem cascade accelerator, these proceedings.
4. J. F. Briesmeister, MCNP - A general Monte Carlo code for neutron and photon transport. *Los Alamos National Laboratory, LA 7396-M Rev. 2* (1986).
5. O.L. Deutsch and B.W. Murray, Monte Carlo dosimetry calculation for boron neutron capture therapy in the treatment of brain tumors, *Nucl. Tech.*, 25:320-339 (1975).
6. R.S. Caswell, J.J. Coyne and M.L. Randolph, Kerma factors of elements and compounds for neutron energies below 30 MeV, *Int. J. Appl. Radiat. Isot.*, 33:1227-1262 (1982).
7. R.G. Zamenhof, B.W. Murray, G.L. Brownell, G.R. Wellum and E.I. Tolpin, Boron neutron capture therapy for the treatment of cerebral gliomas. 1: Theoretical evaluation of the efficacy of various neutron beams, *Med. Phys.*, 2:47-60 (1975).
8. S.D. Clement, J.R. Choi, R.G. Zamenhof, J.C. Yanch and O.K. Harling, Monte Carlo methods of neutron beam design for neutron capture therapy at the MIT Research Reactor (MITR-II), in: *Neutron Beam Design, Development and Performance for Neutron Capture Therapy*, O.K. Harling, J.A. Bernard and R.G. Zamenhof, eds., Plenum Press, New York (1990).
9. J.C. Yanch, X.L. Zhou, G.L. Brownell, A Monte Carlo investigation of the dosimetric properties of monoenergetic neutron beams for neutron capture therapy, to appear in *Rad. Res.* (March 1990).
10. C. Wang, T.E. Blue and R. Gahbauer, A neutronic study of an accelerator-based neutron irradiation facility for boron neutron capture therapy, *Nucl. Tech*, 84:93-107 (1989).

AN INTEGRATED NEUTRONIC AND THERMAL-HYDRAULIC DESIGN

STUDY FOR AN ACCELERATOR NEUTRON IRRADIATION FACILITY

Thomas E. Blue
T-X Bruce Qu
Richard N. Christensen
Peng Guo
James W. Blue*

The Ohio State University, Columbus, OH 43210, USA
*Cleveland Cinic, Cleveland, OH 44135, USA

INTRODUCTION

The major components of an Accelerator Neutron Irradiation Facility (ANIF) for BNCT are a radio-frequency quadrupole (RFQ) proton accelerator, a ^{7}Li target, and a moderator assembly. Neutrons generated by bombarding the ^{7}Li target with 2.5 MeV protons are too energetic to be used for BNCT, and are moderated as they traverse the moderator assembly to the patient. For treating glioblastoma multiforme, the neutrons should have epithermal energies (in the range of 1 eV to approximately 10 keV) as they exit the moderator assembly.

BACKGROUND/PREVIOUS STUDIES

Moderator Assembly Figures of Merit for a 5 cm Diameter Target

For an Accelerator Epithermal Neutron Irradiation Facility (AENIF), the neutronic properties which a good moderator material should possess are (1) large Σ_s, the neutron scattering cross section; (2) moderate ξ, the average increase in the lethargy of a neutron per collision; and (3) small $\Sigma_a(n,\gamma)$, the neutron cross section for radiative capture. For the AENIF, a good reflector material should have large Σ_s, small ξ, and small $\Sigma_a(n,\gamma)$.

In order to assess the suitability of the AENIF neutron field, we have identified two figures of merit: (1) the useful (i.e. E > 1 eV) neutron flux (Φ_u) at the irradiation point in air (a point on the centerline of the moderator assembly 3 cm from the exit window) and (2) the ratio of the neutron kerma to the useful fluence ($<k_n>$) for a differential volume of tissue at the irradiation point. The optimization of the design figures of merit for a 5 cm diameter target for the AENIF resulted in the moderator assembly that is shown in Fig.1. It consists of a cylinder of BeO, which is 25 cm in diameter and 22.5 cm in height, surrounded by a 30 cm thick alumina reflector. Also, 0.01 g/cm^2 of ^{6}Li is placed at the moderator assembly exit window to reduce thermal neutron contamination at the irradiation point. For the AENIF moderator assembly with a 30 mA proton beam Φ_u equals $(9.0 \pm 0.3) \times 10^8$ neutrons/cm^2·sec. Also, $<k_n>$ is $(4.4 \pm 0.5) \times 10^{-11}$ cGy·cm^2, which is equivalent to the kerma factor for 5 keV neutrons.[1]

METHODS

Our analysis models two distinct physical processes: (1) neutron generation in the ^{7}Li target and (2) neutron transport in the moderator assembly. Neutron generation in the ^{7}Li target was calculated by simulating the production of neutrons as protons slow down in the target, using the doubly differential cross section for the ^{7}Li(p,n)^{7}Be reaction [2] and the stopping power for protons in lithium.[3] Neutron transport in the moderator assembly was modeled using the MORSE [4] and MCNP [5] Monte Carlo neutron transport codes.

INTEGRATED NEUTRONIC AND THERMAL-HYDRAULIC DESIGN OF THE TARGET ASSEMBLY PLUS MODERATOR ASSEMBLY

To this point, we have decoupled the neutronic design of the moderator assembly from the thermal-hydraulic design of the target. The AENIF moderator assembly design which is presented above represents the first step in an iterative neutronic and thermal-hydraulic design process. The design is based on a 5 cm diameter target. Since the beam heat flux decreases

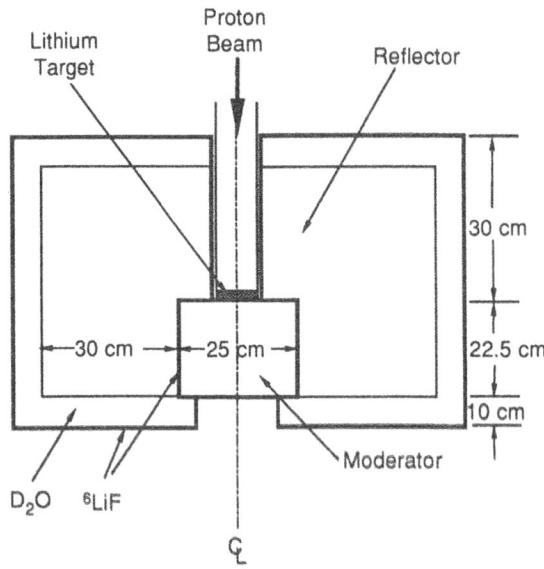

Fig. 1 Configuration of AENIF Moderator Assembly with a 5 cm Diameter Circular Target

inversely with increasing target area, and since the target thermal-hydraulic design criteria are more easily achieved for smaller beam heat flux, we have considered the effect of increasing target area on the neutronic performance of the AENIF moderator assembly.

Neutronic Effect of Increasing Target Diameter

We have calculated the design figures of merit for the AENIF moderator assembly with 5, 15, and 25 cm diameter circular targets, in order to assess the effect of increases in circular target diameter on the neutronic performance of this assembly. The figures of merit Φ_u and $<k_n>$ are presented in Table 1. One can see from the table that Φ_u decreases with increasing

Table 1. Design Figures of Merit (FOM) for an AENIF Moderator Assembly with 5, 15, and 25 cm Diameter Circular Targets

FOM	Diameter		
	5 cm	15 cm	25 cm
Φ_u(n/cm$^2\cdot$sec/10mA)	$(3.0 \pm 0.1) \times 10^8$	$(2.9 \pm 0.1) \times 10^8$	$(2.2 \pm 0.1) \times 10^8$
$<k_n>$ (cGy/cm^2)	$(4.5 \pm 0.8) \times 10^{-11}$	$(4.6 \pm 0.7) \times 10^{-11}$	$(3.5 \pm 0.5) \times 10^{-11}$

target diameter: Φu for the 25 cm diameter target is $(73 \pm 4)\%$ of Φu for the 5 cm diameter target. In contrast $<k_n>$ is better for the 25 cm diameter target than it is for the 5 cm diameter target: $<k_n>$ for the 25 cm diameter target is (78 ± 18) % of $<k_n>$ for the 5 cm diameter target.

Thermal-Hydraulic Effect of Increasing Target Diameter

Our first step (described above) in achieving an integrated neutronic and thermal-hydraulic target assembly plus moderator assembly design was to find a neutronically acceptable AENIF moderator assembly design based on a 5 cm diameter target. As a second step (described above), we determined how the neutronic performance of the AENIF moderator assembly is affected by increasing the target's diameter. To proceed further (described below) in integrating the neutronic and thermal-hydraulic target assembly plus moderator assembly designs, we specified an initial thermal-hydraulic target design. With this initial thermal-hydraulic target design, we continued our iterative design process by determining what target diameters are acceptable from a thermal-hydraulic viewpoint.

Our initial target is 0.25 mm thick solid lithium on a 5 mm thick Cu backing. The Cu backing is cooled by flowing heavy water. A Cu backing has been chosen because of copper's high thermal conductivity. Flowing heavy water has been chosen, because neutrons can lose too much energy in single collisions with protons for light water to be an acceptable component of an AENIF target assembly. The range of 2.5 MeV protons in solid lithium is ~250 μm . The lithium thickness of the target is approximately equal to the protons' range. However, only the first 90 μm contribute to neutron production, since the threshold for the ^{7}Li(n,p)^{7}Be reaction is 1.88 MeV.[2]

The thermal-hydraulic design criteria for the target are: 1) the lithium targets' temperature shall at no point exceed the lithium melting temperature of 180°C, and 2) the maximum heat flux (q"$_{max}$) at the target/water interface shall not exceed the critical heat flux (q"$_{chf}$). For forced convective cooling, there is a trade-off with system pressure (P) between the two target design criteria: $T_{max} < 180°C$ and q"$_{max}$ <q"$_{chf}$. As P increases, 180°C - T_{max} decreases [6], but q"$_{chf}$- q"$_{max}$ increases [7]. To establish an acceptable system pressure we have calculated 180°C - T_{max} and q"$_{chf}$- q"$_{max}$, as a function of system pressure, for targets which are 15 and 25 cm in diameter. For forced convective saturated nucleate boiling, q"$_{chf}$ and T_{max} are rather insensitive to changes in the effective hydraulic diameter (D_e) of the coolant channel, for reasonably large D_e. For our case, the coolant channel is rectangular with a width which greatly exceeds its thickness (t), and D_e ~2t. Assuming t = 1 cm, and a coolant flow velocity of 3 m/s, both of the target thermal-hydraulic design criteria can be fulfilled for a target diameter of 25 cm with P ~ 0.7 bar.

INTEGRATED TARGET ASSEMBLY PLUS MODERATOR ASSEMBLY NEUTRONIC PERFORMANCE

We have established that a 25 cm diameter target is large enough that both thermal-hydraulic design criteria can be achieved. Also, from a neutronic point of view, a 25 cm diameter target is acceptable for the AENIF moderator assembly. We neglect the small effect of the 1 cm thick layer of D_2O in the target assembly upon the neutronic performance of the integrated target plus moderator assemblies. Then the values for the figures of merit which characterize the neutronic performance of the integrated target plus moderator assemblies are simply the entries in Table 1 for the 25 cm diameter target.

The magnitude of Φ_u for the AENIF moderator assembly with a 30 mA proton beam, is comparable with the magnitude of Φ_u for reactor neutron beams of similar spectra, which are extracted with special beam filters from nuclear reactors which are in the mega-watt power range. As an example, Φ_u for the Brookhaven National Laboratory Medical Research Reactor (BMRR) beam is 6.2×10^8 neutrons/cm²•sec for the BMRR operating at 1.0 MW. In order to compare in more detail the BMRR beam and the AENIF neutron field, the calculated neutron flux spectra for the BMRR BNCT beam [8] is plotted in Fig. 2 along with the calculated neutron flux spectra for the integrated AENIF moderator and target assemblies. The units of the neutron flux for the BMRR beam are neutrons per cm²•sec per unit lethargy per MW of

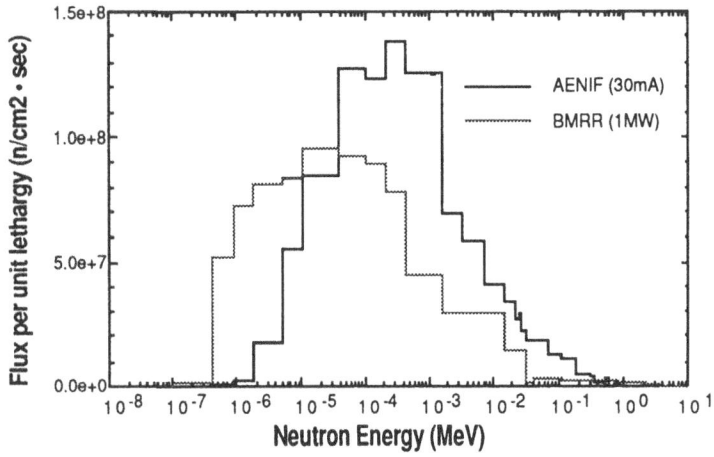

Fig. 2 The Neutron Flux Spectra for the AENIF and the BMRR

reactor thermal power. As can be seen from Fig. 2, the neutron flux in the epithermal region (i.e. from 1 eV to 10 keV) is comparable for the AENIF operating at 30 mA and for the BMRR operating at 1.0 MW. For neutron energies from 0.4 eV to 40 eV, the neutron flux for the BMRR operating at 1 MW is greater than the neutron flux for the AENIF operating at 30 mA. For neutron energies from 40 eV to 400 keV, the neutron flux for the BMRR operating at 1 MW is less than the neutron flux for the AENIF operating at 30 mA. However, for neutron energies from 400 keV to several MeV, the neutron flux spectrum for the BMRR exceeds the neutron flux spectrum for the AENIF, because the $^7Li(p,n)^7Be$ reaction does not produce neutrons with energies greater than 790 keV for a proton kinetic energy of 2.5 MeV. As a consequence of the differences in the spectra, the average kerma factors for a differential volume of tissue irradiated in the two beams is less for the AENIF than for the BMRR. For the BMRR BNCT beam, $<k_n>$ is 4.5×10^{-11} cGy•cm² [8], while as stated above, for the AENIF $<k_n>$ is $(3.5 \pm 0.5) \times 10^{-11}$ cGy-cm².

CONCLUSION

A 0.25 mm thick lithium target on a 5 mm thick Cu backing, with the Cu backing cooled by flowing heavy water, can be maintained as a solid with a 30 mA 2.5 MeV proton beam bombarding the target, if the beam is uniformly distributed over a 25 cm diameter circular target area. We calculate that with a 25 cm diameter circular target our AENIF moderator assembly produces a useful neutron flux (Φ_u) equal to (2.2 $\pm$ 0.1) x 10^8 neutrons/cm^2 •sec/10mA. The ratio of the neutron kerma to the useful fluence ($<k_n>$) equals (3.5 $\pm$ 0.5)x10^{-11} cGy-cm^2.

ACKNOWLEDGMENT

This work was supported in part by the National Cancer Institute under Grant 1 RO1 CA 47298-01 and by the U.S. Department of Energy under contract DE-AC02-76CH00016.

REFERENCES

1. C.K. Wang, T. E. Blue, and R. A. Gahbauer, "A Neutronic Study of an Accelerator-Based Neutron Irradiation Facility for Boron Neutron Capture Therapy," Nucl. Tech. 84: 93-107(1989).

2. H. Liskien and A. Paulsen, "Neutron Production Cross Sections and Energies for Reactions ^{7}Li(p,n)^{7}Be and ^{7}Li(p,n)^{7}Be*," Atomic Data and Nuclear Data Tables 15: 57-84 (1975).

3. H.H. Anderson and J. F. Zeigler, "Hydrogen Stopping Powers and Ranges in All Elements", (Pergamon Press Ltd., 1977), Vol. 3, p. 16.

4. M.B. Emmett, "The MORSE Monte Carlo Radiation Transport Code System," ORNL-4972, Oak Ridge National Laboratory (1975).

5. J. F. Briesmeister, ed., "MCNP - A General Monte Carlo Code for Neutron and Photon Transport, Version 3B," LA-7396-M, Los Alamos National Laboratory, (1989).

6. R. Bjorge, G. Hall, and W. Rohsenow, "Correlation for Forced Convection Boiling Heat Transfer Data," Int. J. Heat Mass Transfer 25: 753, (1982).

7. J. G. Collier, "Convective Boiling and Condensation," 2nd Edition, McGraw-Hill, pp. 293-294, (1981).

8. F. J. Wheeler, D. K. Parsons, B. L. Rushton, and D. W. Nigg, "Epithermal Neutron Beam Design for Neutron Capture Therapy at the Power Burst Facility and the Brookhaven Medical Research Reactor," Nucl. Tech. 92:106-117 (1990).

AN EPITHERMAL NEUTRON SOURCE FOR BNCT USING A TANDEM

CASCADE ACCELERATOR

R. E. Shefer[1], R. E. Klinkowstein[1], J. C. Yanch[2] and G. L. Brownell[2]

[1]Science Research Laboratory, Inc., Somerville, MA, USA

[2]Department of Nuclear Engineering, MIT, Cambridge, MA, USA.

I. Introduction

The development of boron neutron capture therapy into a viable modality for the treatment of tumors will depend, in part, on the availability of neutron sources with the required dose and spectral characteristics which are compatible with installation and operation in a clinical setting. This paper describes the design of a neutron irradiation facility based on neutrons produced via the $^{7}Li(p,n)^{7}Be$ nuclear reaction.[1] A lithium target is bombarded by a multimilliampere proton beam from a new electrostatic accelerator developed at Science Research Laboratory (SRL). The salient features of the tandem cascade accelerator (TCA) are compactness, low power consumption, and the ability to deliver high proton currents to a target at energies of up to several million electron volts.

II. Production of Neutrons via the $^{7}Li(p,n)^{7}Be$ Nuclear Reaction

The neutron yields, energy spectra and angular distributions for the $^{7}Li(p,n)^{7}Be$ nuclear reaction were calculated analytically from published cross-section data[1] and stopping powers for protons in lithium for bombarding energies of 2.5 MeV down to the reaction threshold $E_T = 1.88$ MeV. Since the mean proton scattering angle relative to its initial direction is less than 2° over a path which is one mean range in length, scattering of the protons in the target material was assumed to be negligible.

Figure 1 shows the total neutron yield as a function of proton energy for a 1 mA proton beam on a lithium metal target. The figure illustrates the very rapid rise in yield as the proton energy is increased above threshold. For a 2.5 MeV beam, a total yield of 8.96×10^{11} neutrons/second per milliampere is obtained. The neutron yield and energy spectrum are strong functions of both angle and proton bombarding energy. Figure 2 shows the calculated neutron energy spectrum in ±5° bins at five angles relative to the proton beam direction for a 2.5 MeV protons incident on a thick lithium target. The neutron flux from the target is forward directed with a maximum neutron energy at 0° of 800 keV.

The neutron energy spectrum may also be varied by changing the bombarding proton energy. The kinematics of the Li(p,n) reaction dictate an approximately linear increase in maximum neutron energy with proton energy.[2] As the proton energy is decreased below 2.5 MeV, the spectrum at a given angle will be truncated at the maximum neutron energy corresponding to the proton bombarding energy but will otherwise retain the same characteristic shape illustrated in Figure 2. For example, for a proton energy of 2.2 MeV, the maximum neutron energy at 0° is 490 keV. In this respect, it is clearly advantageous to reduce the proton energy; however, the decrease in maximum neutron energy is accompanied by a decrease in yield. The decrease in moderated neutron yield

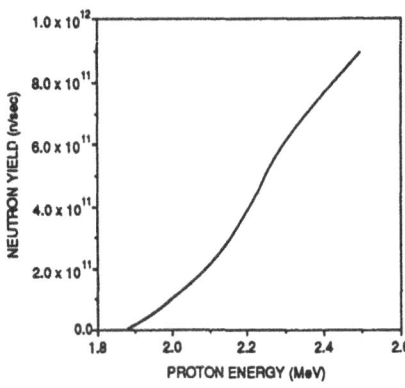
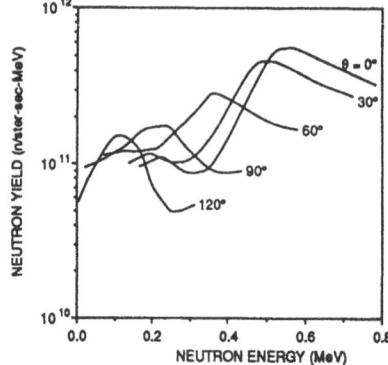

Figure 1. Neutron yield versus proton energy for 1 mA beam on Li target.

Figure 2. Neutron energy spectrum at five angles for 2.5 MeV, 1 mA proton beam on Li target.

will be slower than linear with proton energy since less moderation will be required for the spectra with lower maximum neutron energies. Additionally, the minimum neutron energy generated may be varied by reducing the lithium target thickness below one proton range. In this way, the neutron flux may be made more highly monochromatic, again with a corresponding decrease in yield.

Monte-Carlo simulations[2] of neutron and photon transport in a tissue equivalent phantom show that the neutron energies produced by the Li(p,n) reaction are too high to be used directly for therapy due to the unacceptably large proton recoil dose to surface tissue. The neutron beam must be moderated to energies in the 4 eV - 40 keV range in order to treat tumors at depth with therapeutic advantage. The design of a D_2O moderator and collimator assembly suitable for the irradiation of tumors at the midline of the brain is presented elsewhere in these proceedings.[3] MNCP simulations of the dose-depth distributions of the moderated neutrons in a brian equivalent phantom predict that an accelerator source utilizing a 2.5 MeV, 4 mA proton beam can deliver a total tumor dose of 2000 RBE-cGy to the midline of the brain in less than 3 hours. The moderated accelerator produced beam is comparable with reactor-produced epithermal beams with respect to dose rate and dose composition.[3] Thus, the lower maximum neutron energy and low gamma contamination of the Li(p,n) beam compensate for the lower available unmodered neutron yield when compared with a reactor source.

III. Production of Intense Proton Beams with a Tandem Cascade Accelerator

As discussed above, accelerator production of a sufficient neutron flux for BNCT requires a high current (4 mA), low energy (2.0-2.5 MeV) proton beam. A high current electrostatic accelerator, the TCA, is under development at Science Research Laboratory. This accelerator utilizes a recently developed high current negative ion source[3] in conjunction with a high current solid state power supply to provide a compact, low cost proton accelerator well suited for neutron production. The TCA is a tandem electrostatic accelerator which utilizes a symmetrical, series-feed cascade multiplier to supply a dc accelerating potential to the high voltage terminal. A negative ion beam (H^-) is continuously injected at low energy into the accelerating column of the TCA. A carbon stripping foil, located in the terminal, converts H^- to H^+ with high efficiency. The positive ion beam is then accelerated to ground potential where it attains a final energy corresponding to twice the terminal potential. The operating parameters of the TCA under development for BNCT are listed in Table 1. Fabrication of a prototype accelerator with these specifications is currently underway.

The linear geometry of the TCA allows very high beam extraction efficiency to be achieved which results in reduced maintenance and shielding requirements. The high gradient cascade rectifier power supply is power efficient, and the tandem design means that both the ion source and target are at ground potential during operation and are both easily accessible. A high degree of compactness is achieved by a patented SRL design which matches the power supply gradient to the accelerating column gradient. This allows the power supply to be mounted directly onto the accelerating column and eliminates the requirement for external power supply chassis. The TCA requires no

Table 1. Tandem Cascade Accelerator Specifications

Accelerator Type	Tandem Electrostatic
Terminal Voltage	1.0 - 1.25 MV
Beam Energy	2.0 - 2.5 MeV
Proton Beam Current	5 mA
Input Power	25 kW
Total Overall Length	2.6m
Outer Diameter	83 cm
Weight (excl. shielding)	1800 lb

RF or magnetic fields which greatly reduces the system weight, power dissipation and heat load on auxiliary systems when compared with cyclotron or RFQ accelerators. A possible layout for a TCA-based epithermal neutron irradiation facility is illustrated in Figure 3. The dimensions of the moderator/collimator assembly are described in detail in an accompanying paper in these proceedings.[3]

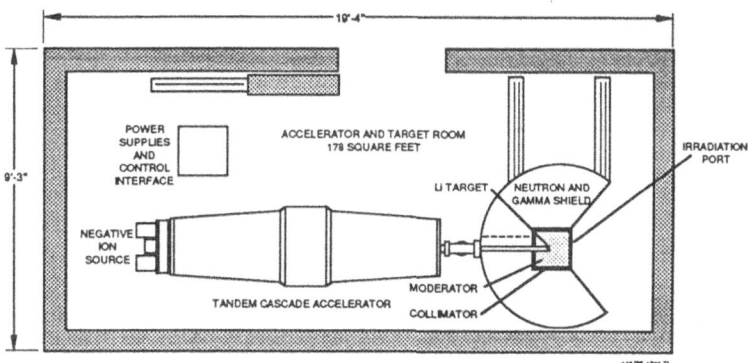

Figure 3. Layout of epithermal neutron source

Several lithium target materials and configurations have been considered for the TCA neutron source. The total 10 kW power load from the 4 mA, 2.5 MeV beam may be spread over a large surface area by operating the target at oblique incidence. The nominal proton beam diameter at the exit aperture of the accelerator is 2 cm. By inclining the target at 18° relative to the beam direction, the areal power loading is reduced to 1 kW/cm^2. Since the ^{7}Li(p,n)^{7}Be reaction has a threshold energy of 1.88 MeV, it is not necessary to slow the protons below this energy in the lithium layer. Utilizing a thin lithium target layer facilitates heat removal from the lithium and allows a large fraction of the beam energy to be deposited directly in a cooled copper heat sink which serves as a substrate for the lithium layer. For the angle of incidence given above, a lithium thickness of 28 μm will reduce the proton beam energy to the reaction threshold. Under these conditions, the maximum temperature in the lithium layer will be within 1°C of the temperature of the lithium-copper interface. It should therefore be possible to maintain a lithium metal layer at a temperature well below its melting point (T_m = 181°C) during bombardment. A lithium metal target in this configuration is currently being tested using a prototype TCA at Science Research Laboratory.

References

(1) R.E. Shefer, R.E. Klinkowstein, J.C. Yanch and G.L. Brownell, in Neutron Beam Design, Development and Performance for Neutron Capture Therapy, O.K. Harling, J.A. Bernard and R.G. Zamenhof, eds., Plenum Press, NY (1990) 259.

(2) H. Liskien and A. Paulsen, Atomic Data and Nuclear Data Tables, 15 (1975) 57-84.

(3) J.C. Yanch, X.L. Zhou, R.E. Shefer, R.E. Klinkowstein and G.L. Brownell, these proceedings.

(4) K.R. Kendall, M. McDonald, D.R. Mosscrop, P.W. Schmor, D. Yuan, Rev. Sci. Instrum 57 (1986) 7.

ACCELERATOR BASED NEUTRON SOURCES FOR NEUTRON CAPTURE THERAPY

Erik Grusell

Department of Radiation Sciences, Uppsala University, Uppsala, Sweden

INTRODUCTION

Accelerator based neutron sources are an attractive alternative to nuclear fission reactors for several reasons; size, cost and safety being the most obvious. Although the first clinical trials with keV neutrons for neutron capture therapy (NCT) will be made with reactor produced neutrons, a second generation hospital based clinical unit might well be equipped with an accelerator for the production of neutrons. Such an accelerator could also be used for other purposes, such as radionuclide production.

MATERIAL AND METHODS

In this work three methods of producing neutrons by bombarding a target with energetic charged particles will be considered, viz.: spallation in tungsten by 72 MeV protons[1,2,3], 2,5 MeV protons on a ^{7}Li target[4,5,6], and deuterium of 20 MeV on a beryllium target[7].
Monte Carlo transport calculations have been made for all three alternatives, equipped with different moderator assemblies as described below. Comparisons have been made regarding the following aspects:
1. Boron-10 capture dose distributions in a spherical 20 cm diameter water phantom.
2. Boron-10 capture dose at the dose maximum (i.e. 2 cm depth in all cases) normalised to unit energy deposited in the target.
3. The maximum boron-10 dose divided by the maximum fast neutron dose (which is attained at the surface).
The dose in 1 has been calculated by multiplying the low energy neutron fluence by the appropriate kerma factors[8] for ^{10}B capture at a ^{10}B concentration of 30 ppm. The transport calculations were made without ^{10}B in the water, i.e. the result after multiplying with the kerma factors represents the dose a small volume containing 30 ppm of ^{10}B would receive if surrounded by water with no ^{10}B in it. For the Monte Carlo calculations the transport code MCNP[11] was used.
The moderator configuration in the spallation and d-Be calculations is shown in fig 1, taken from ref 3. For the p-^{7}Li source the moderator geometry is shown in fig 2, taken from ref 5, where it is described as optimized. In the calculations, the water phantom was placed close to the BeO moderator, and only the heavy water shielding closest to the phantom was included.

SPECTRA FROM THE TARGETS

The neutron spectrum from a heavy target bombarded by 72 MeV protons consists of two parts, an isotropic evaporation spectrum with a maximum intensity at a few MeV, and a forward peaked component extending all the way up to the full proton energy. This latter part is only a few percent and has been neglected in the calculations[3].
2,5 MeV protons on lithium-7 give a forward peaked spectrum with maximum neutron energy of 0,8 MeV, allowing a much smaller moderator[4,5]. In the calculations the data given in figs 2 to 5 of ref 6 were used to model the spectrum.

Progress in Neutron Capture Therapy for Cancer
Edited by B.J. Allen *et al.*, Plenum Press, New York, 1992

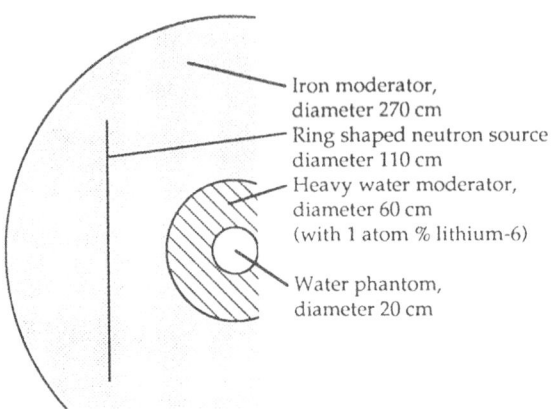

Iron moderator,
diameter 270 cm

Ring shaped neutron source
diameter 110 cm

Heavy water moderator,
diameter 60 cm
(with 1 atom % lithium-6)

Water phantom,
diameter 20 cm

Fig 1. Geometry of iron/heavy water moderator
used with the spallation and d-Be sources.
(From ref 9, Larsson et al.)

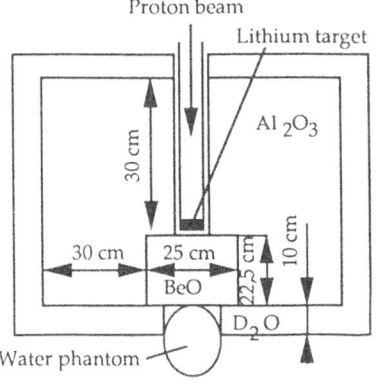

Fig 2. Geometry of BeO moderator and alumina
reflector used with the p-Li source.
(From ref 5, Wang et al.)

Table 1. Neutron yield per unit energy deposited in the target for
different neutron production methods.

neutron production method	total number of neutrons produced per unit energy (n/Ws)
72 MeV protons on W	$1,7 \times 10^{10}$
2,5 MeV protons on Li	$2,8 \times 10^{8}$
20 MeV deuterons on Be	$8,5 \times 10^{8}$

124

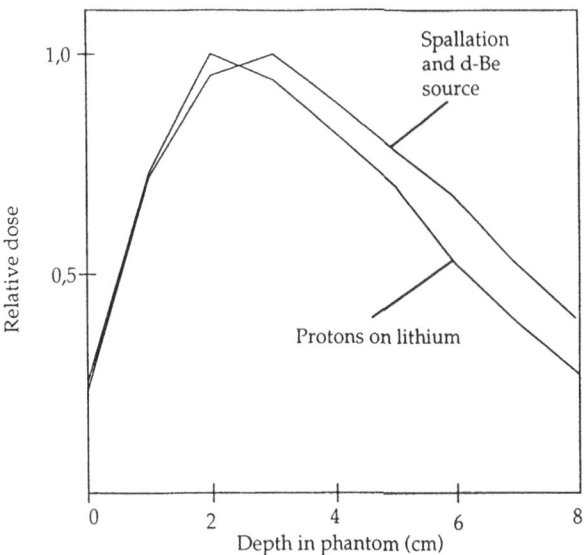

Fig 3. Relative 30 ppm boron-10
dose along central axis.

Table 2. Absorbed dose from the neutron capture reaction in boron-10
in a small volume with 30 ppm of boron-10 at 2 cm depth ,
per unit energy deposited in the target.

neutron production method	absorbed dose per unit energy (Gy/Ws)
72 MeV protons on W	$4{,}2 \times 10^{-7}$
2,5 MeV protons on Li	$8{,}8 \times 10^{-8}$
20 MeV deuterons on Be	$1{,}9 \times 10^{-8}$

Table 3. Maximum boron capture dose per unit fast neutron dose

neutron production method	maximum boron capture dose per unit fast neutron dose at surface
72 MeV protons on W	8,5
2,5 MeV protons on Li	8,5
20 MeV deuterons on Be	8
reactor	8,5

The 20 MeV deuterium on beryllium source gives a forward peaked spectrum with a maximum intensity at a neutron energy of 8 MeV, and an isotropic component similar to the evaporation spectrum above. This latter component is 20 percent of the total number of neutrons[7].

INTENSITY OF THE DIFFERENT SOURCES

The yield expressed as number of neutrons per unit energy deposited in the target is given in table 1.

Because of the different sizes of the moderators the neutron fluence at the phantom surface is not proportional to the number of neutrons produced. In table 2 the maximum absorbed dose at 2 cm depth from the capture reaction in boron 10 in a concentration of 30 ppm is given.

DOSE DISTRIBUTIONS

The relative dose distributions from the capture reaction in a small volume with 30 ppm of ^{10}B along the central axis in a water phantom of diameter 20 cm is shown in fig 3. The maximum dose is reached at a depth of approximately 2 cm in all cases. It is seen that the spallation and d-Be sources give a somewhat better penetration. The filtered reactor boron-10 depth dose curve reported in ref 10 resembles the protons on lithium curve.

FAST NEUTRON CONTAMINATION

The fast neutron depth dose curves also resemble the corresponding curves reported for reactors with approximately a 25% level at 2 cm depth. The maximum fast neutron dose relative to the maximum thermal fluence is shown in table 3, where the maximum ^{10}B dose (at 30 ppm and 2cm depth) divided by the maximum fast neutron dose is given. Reactor data are also included for comparison[10].

DISCUSSION

When using the moderator configurations described above, the thermal neutron fluence distributions are somewhat better for the spallation and d-Be sources, in terms of penetration.The corresponding curve for thefiltered reactor beam resembles the one for protons on lithium[10]. The fast neutron contamination is equivalent for all three configurations.

The photon dose has not been taken into consideration as for all cases the photon dose from hydrogen capture in the phantom itself can be made dominating by appropriate shielding without disturbing the neutron fluence.

When it comes to heat liberation in the target, the spallation source gives the highest boron-10 dose per unit energy deposited in the target, as is apparent form table 2.

Acknowledgement. This work has been supported by the Swedish National Board for Technical Development.

References

1.   J. F. Crawford, and B. Larsson, Proc. First Int. Symp. on Neutron Capture Therapy, BNL, Upton, New York, USA (1983)

2.   H. Condé,E. Grusell, B. Larsson, C.-B. Pettersson, L. Thuresson, J. Crawford, H. Reist, B. Dahl, and N. G. Sjöstrand, "Time of Flight Measurements of the Energy Spectrum of Neutrons Emitted from a Spallation Source and Moderated in Water", Nucl. Instr. and Meth. in Phys. Res., A261:587-590 (1987)

3.   E. Grusell, H. Condé, B. Larsson,T. Rönnqvist, O. Sornsuntisook, J. Crawford,H. Reist, B. Dahl, N. G. Sjöstrand, and G. Russel, "The Possible Use of a Spallation Neutron Source for Neutron Capture Therapy with Epithermal Neutrons", Basic Life Sciences Vol. 54, Neutron Beam Design, Development, and Performance for Neutron Capture Therapy, O. K. Harling et al. eds., Plenum Press, New York, (1990), p249-258

4.   G. L. Brownell, J. E. Kirsch, and J. Kehayaias, Proc. Second Int. Symp. on Neutron Capture Therapy,Hatanaka, H. ed., (Nishimura, Niigata, Japan 1986)

5. C. K. Wang, T. E. Blue, and J. W. Blue, "An Experimental Study of the Moderator Assembly for a Low-Energy Proton Accelerator Neutron Irradiation Facility for BNCT", Basic Life Sciences Vol. 54, Neutron Beam Design, Development, and Performance for Neutron Capture Therapy, O. K. Harling et al. eds., Plenum Press, New York, (1990), p271-280

6. R. E. Shefer, R. E. Klinkowstein, J. C. Yanch, and G. L. Brownell, "A Versatile, New Accelerator Design for Boron Neutron Capture Therapy: Accelerator Design and Neutron Energy Considerations", Basic Life Sciences Vol. 54, Neutron Beam Design, Development, and Performance for Neutron Capture Therapy, O. K. Harling et al. eds., Plenum Press, New York, (1990), p259-270

7. S. Cierjacks, ed. Neutron Sources for Basic Physics and Applications, Pergamon Press, Oxford, England (1983)

8. Neutron Dosimetry for Biology and Medicine, ICRU report 26, (Washington, USA 1977)

9. A. Andersson et al., "Programme for Accelerator-Based Neutron Capture Therapy", in Proc. of the 2nd European Particle Accelerator Conference, P. Marin and P. Mandrillon, eds., p S79-S81, Editions Frontières, Paris (1990)

10. R. G. Fairchild, J. Kalef-Ezra, S. K Saraf, S. Fiarman, E. Ramsay, L. Wielopolski, B. H. Laster, and F. J. Wheeler, Basic Life Sciences Vol. 54, Neutron Beam Design, Development, and Performance for Neutron Capture Therapy, O. K. Harling et al. eds., Plenum Press, New York, (1990), p185-199

11. J. F. Briesmeister, ed., "MCNP - A General Monte Carlo Code for Neutron and Photon Transport, Version 3A", Los Alamos National Laboratory, LA-7396-M, Rev.2, 1986

NEUTRONS FOR CAPTURE THERAPY PRODUCED BY 72 MEV PROTONS

J. F. Crawford and H. Reist
Paul Scherrer Institute, CH-5232 Villigen, Switzerland

H. Conde, K. Elmgren and T. Rönnqvist
Department of Neutron Research, University of Uppsala
PO Box 535, S-75221 Uppsala, Sweden

E. Grusell, B. Nilsson, O. Pettersson and P. Stromberg
Department of Radiation Sciences, University of Uppsala
PO Box 535, S-75221 Uppsala, Sweden

B. Larsson
Strahlenbiologisches Institut, August-Forel-Strasse 7, CH-8029 Zürich

Introduction Neutrons (and protons) move in nuclear matter with an energy which is roughly the same in all nuclei, and which can be thought of as a temperature (of about 10^{11} K). Neutrons from the fission process therefore emerge with an energy corresponding to this temperature; so do most but not all neutrons from the 'spallation' process, in which fast protons strike nuclei and liberate neutrons. The use of a proton beam or a reactor for the production of neutrons for capture therapy (NCT) thus present basically similar problems: to reduce the energy of the neutrons from the MeV level at which they emerge to the few keV required for NCT. There are however significant differences: the total intensity of a spallation source is much lower – some four orders of magnitude between the layout planned at the Paul Scherrer Institute (PSI) and the Petten reactor, for example. On the other hand, the source is much smaller: of the order of a cubic centimetre as against the cubic metre of a typical reactor. This means that it can be made mobile, as in the PSI layout, and in practice one can work closer to it. Again, less γ radiation is produced by a spallation source.

Simple Moderators In order to develop some understanding of our materials and options, and also to economize on computer time, we started with very simple, spherical layouts. Studies were made of Fe, Al, Ti, V, Pb, Sn, U, W, Si, SiO_2, Be, D_2O, H_2O, O_2 and CD_4, some with H or D doping, as possible moderators/filters/shifters, using the program MCNP[1].

Figure 1 shows the neutron fluence spectra from two simple layouts: Al and Fe spheres of radius 0.6m. It can be seen that the spectra have maxima at about 24 keV, because the materials have cross-section minima there. Since the other, higher energy, minima in Al and Fe do not overlap in quite this way, and since NCT requires keV neutrons, we decided to examine the properties of mixtures of these two elements. As one might expect from Figure 1, the relative proportion has a considerable effect on the spectrum, and in particular on the two parameters of most interest: average energy and fluence. Further studies led to the data in Figure 2, which show clearly that the average energy has a minimum at an Al/Fe ratio of about 1:1 by atom, and the fluence is not much below its maximum. While the fluence at this ratio is adequate (see below), the mean energy is still too high. To reduce it, the effects of layers of carbon and heavy water were tested. It was found that 10-20 cm of either material reduced the mean energy to the levels appropriate for NCT, and that considerably higher neutron fluences were obtained with heavy water than with carbon.

At PSI, the injector cyclotrons can deliver a few hundred μA of 72 MeV protons. Since a heavy target such as tungsten will yield about 1 neutron for every 5 incident protons of this energy [2,3,4], a beam of 80μA will liberate about 10^{14} neutrons s^{-1}. The required flux of 10^9 cm^{-2}s^{-1} therefore implies a neutron fluence per initial neutron of 10^{-5} cm^{-2}. Such a proton beam will also dump about 6 kW of heat in the target, for which cooling arrangements must be made.

Backgrounds In NCT, γ dose is considered critical. As mentioned above, spallation sources produce fewer γs than a reactor. In a special MCNP run, even 50 MeV γs, created at the centre of a 1:1 Al/Fe sphere 0.6m in radius, yielded a dose at the surface of only 3×10^{-19} Gy per initial γ. By extrapolating the very low rate of such γs from measurements at 52 MeV [6], it follows that this presents no significant problem, even with a generous allowance

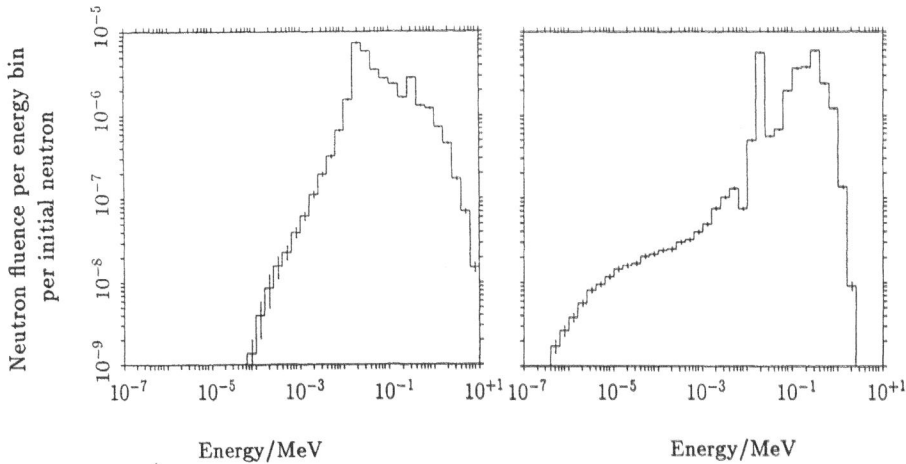

Figure 1. The surface neutron fluence spectra per initial neutron, for *Al* (left) and *Fe* (right) spheres of radius 0.6m. The central neutron source had an evaporation spectrum with parameter 1.2895 MeV.

for build-up, much of which would be absorbed in the heavy water or carbon layer.

The main concern is therefore with γs produced in the moderator. In early calculations for this paper, one γ, of mean energy about 2 MeV, was delivered to the patient position for every 9-10 neutrons. Since most neutrons delivered to the phantom are in fact captured by hydrogen in the phantom with the emission of a 2.2 MeV γ, the γ dose is dominated by these neutron capture γs; hence the total γ dose can be reduced by only a limited amount. On the other hand, the quoted γ rate from the moderator converts to a dose about three times the design goal accepted by the European Community Concerted Action (CA) of 1 Gy per 3×10^{12} cm^{-2} [5]. In consequence, we decided to investigate the possibilities of reducing the γ rate by a factor of three. It was found that this could be done by the use of a 25 mm layer of lead between the Al/Fe and heavy water layers. This reduced the neutron fluence at the surface of the heavy water by only 5%.

As this paper was being prepared, cross-section data for fast neutrons up to 100 MeV had only just become available, for only a few elements. An MCNP calculation for a 0.6m sphere of 1:1 Al/Fe by atom, with 72 MeV neutrons created in a needle beam at the centre, shows that the fluence emerging from the sphere at near 90° to the initial neutron direction contains

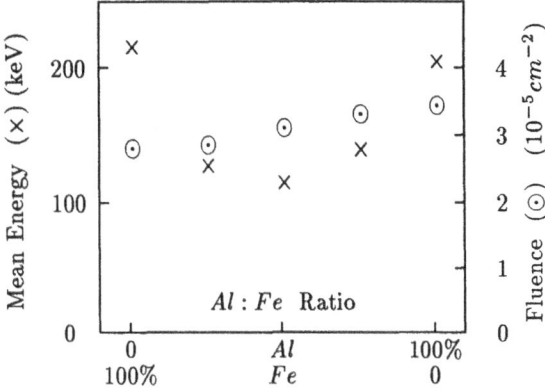

Figure 2. The effect of varying the $Al : Fe$ atom ratio on mean energy (LH scale) and fluence (RH scale). Statistical errors from MCNP, which are not shown, are only a few percent.

< 1% of neutrons above 10 MeV. Since neutrons of above a few MeV are present in the initial spallation spectrum at only the percent level[7,8], it can be concluded that fast neutrons are not significant in the present context, although a calculation for the complete layout cannot yet be carried out because some cross-section data are missing.

A Conceptual Spallation Neutron Facility A possible facility for brain tumour treatment based on these ideas is shown in Figure 3. The proton beam is delivered to a magnetic field on the axis, where it is deflected to hit the ring-shaped neutron production target. In normal operation, the magnetic field is rotated about the axis about once per minute, so that the point from which neutrons are emitted orbits the patient's head. This is done largely to distribute the skin dose and improve the neutronics inside the phantom, but also to facilitate cooling the production target. A preliminary design for the magnet, including the current and cooling water supplies, has been worked out at PSI [9].

The neutron fluences from the layouts so far described still contain about 20% below 1 eV. To reduce this, the heavy water layer was loaded with 1% ^6Li by atom. (This was for simplicity of computation; whether Lithium would in practice be added in this form or as a thin foil is a matter of convenience.) The result was a fifty-fold reduction in the flux at thermal energies; above 1keV, the effect was about 10%.

The results of a preliminary dose calculation are shown in Figure 4, for a representative layout of the type sketched in Figure 3. The phantom was a 20 cm diameter sphere of brain-like material: H 10.6%, C 14.0%, N 1.84%, O 72.6% by weight. It was surrounded by a $D_2O + Li$ layer 20 cm thick, which in turn was surrounded by a 90 cm layer of Al/Fe, 50:50 by atom. The moderator materials extended as far as a plane tangential to the downstream side of the phantom. The ring neutron source had a radius of 47.9 cm, and was centred 47.9 cm from the centre of the phantom; it was an evaporation source[1], i.e. it had an energy spectrum $E/E_o^2 \exp(-E/E_o)$, with $E_o = 1.2895$ MeV. There was no lead γ shield.

Conclusion It can be seen from Figure 4 that the advantage depth is about 10 cm, an improvement on previous calculations of similar layouts[4]. This rather high value is attributed to neutrons entering the phantom through so much of its surface, rather in the manner of opposed neutron beams. Further, since 10^{17} initial neutrons can be produced in 1000 seconds by an 80 μA beam (see above), a dose of 30 Gy could be delivered to a deep-seated tumour in a total of about two hours, fractionated as required. We may conclude that such a facility is comparable, in terms of advantage depth and dose rate, with reactor facilities.

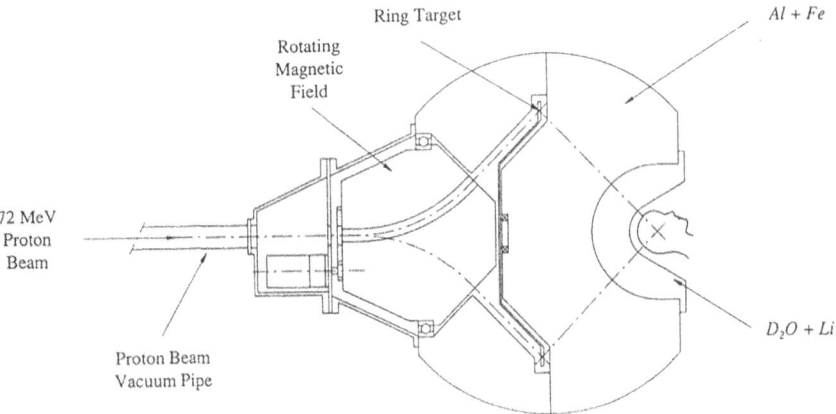

Figure 3. Conceptual spallation neutron facility for brain tumour treatment.

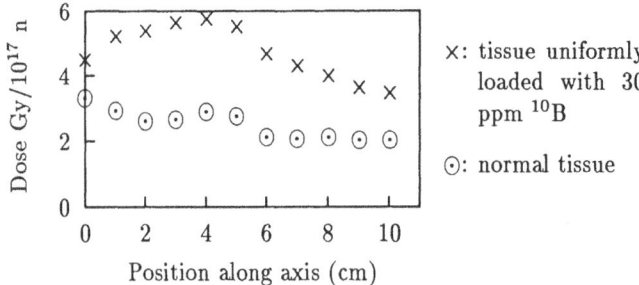

Figure 4. Dose for brain treatment in a representative layout of the type shown in Figure 3, and described in the text. Dose in Gy per 10^{17} source neutrons is plotted against distance along the phantom axis; the origin is where the axis enters the phantom. Statistical errors range up to 0.2 Gy per 10^{17} neutrons.

REFERENCES

[1] J. F. Briesmeister (Ed), 'MCNP - A General Monte Carlo Code for Neutron and Photon Transport, Version 3A' Los Alamos National Laboratory, LA-7396-M, Rev. 2 (1986).

[2] H. Condé, E. Grusell, B. Larsson, C.-B. Pettersson, L. Thuresson, J. F. Crawford, H. Reist, B. Dahl and N. G. Sjöstrand, Nuclear Instruments and Methods in Physics Research A261, 587-590 (1987).

[3] H. Condé, J. F. Crawford, B. Dahl, E. Grusell, B. Larsson, C.-B. Pettersson, H. Reist, N. G. Sjöstrand, O. Sornsuntisook, and L. Thuresson, Strahlentherapie und Onkologie 165, 2/3, 340-342 (1989).

[4] E. Grusell, H. Condé, B. Larsson, T. Rönnqvist, O. Sornsuntisook, J. F. Crawford, H. Reist, B. Dahl, N. G. Sjöstrand, and G. Russell, 'The Possible Use of a Spallation Neutron Source for Neutron Capture with Epithermal Neutrons', pp249-258 in 'Neutron Beam Design, Development and Performance for Neutron Capture Therapy', Eds O. K. Harling, J. A. Bernard and R. G. Zamenhof, Plenum Press, New York (1990).

[5] D. Gabel, private communication.

[6] T. Nakamura, M. Yoshida and K. Shin, NIM 151, 493-503 (1978).

[7] T. Nakamura, M. Fujii and K. Shin, Nucl. Sci. and Engineering 83, 444-458 (1983).

[8] T. A. Broome, D. R. Perry and G. B. Stapleton, Health Physics 44, 487-499 (1983).

[9] D. George and V. Vrankovic, PSI Magnet Group, private communication.

A MONTE CARLO STUDY OF IDEAL BEAMS FOR EPITHERMAL NEUTRON

BEAM DEVELOPMENT FOR BORON NEUTRON CAPTURE THERAPY

J.C. Yanch and O.K. Harling

Nuclear Reactor Laboratory, Massachusetts Institute of Technology
Cambridge, MA   02139   USA

A series of "ideal neutron beam" studies has been carried out using Monte Carlo simulation with the goal of providing guidance for epithermal neutron beam design for boron neutron capture therapy (BNCT). An "ideal beam" is defined as a monoenergetic, photon-free source of neutrons with user-specified size, shape and angular dependence of neutron current. Although discrete-energy, uncontaminated neutron sources are currently largely unobtainable, there are a number of computational techniques that allow simulation of such sources, thereby permitting an otherwise difficult or impossible investigation. For example, the Monte Carlo code MCNP[1] has been used extensively in studies of beam design and dosimetry in neutron capture therapy; MCNP installed on SUN SPARC workstations in the Whitaker College Biomedical Imaging and Computation Laboratory at MIT was also used in the current study.

METHOD

This study examines the effect of beam diameter and angle of neutron emission on an elliptical phantom composed of brain-equivalent material. The geometry of this phantom is that of the Deutsch and Murray[2] adaptation of the Snyder elliptical brain model[3]; dimensions of the phantom are 13.5 cm (beam direction) x 19.5 cm x 16.6 cm. The ellipse was divided into several concentric cylinders and 0.9 cm thick disks. Individual dose components were measured in each compartment as described in reference[4], and variously combined to provide a number of dosimetric parameters including Advantage Depth (AD), Advantage Ratio (AR), and advantage depth dose rate (ADDR)[5]. ^{10}B concentration in the tumour was assumed to be 30 µg/g; maximum and minimum advantage depths were determined by assuming either zero or 3 µg/g ^{10}B in healthy tissue, respectively.

Neutron beam energy was varied from 0.025 eV to 800 keV. The shape of the ideal neutron source was kept circular, however the source size and the maximum angle (θ_{max}) into which neutrons were allowed to emerge from the source were varied. Fixing the neutron angle at 0° simulates the situation of a well-collimated therapy beam, that is, either there is no scattering material placed low in the beam near the patient or the patient is positioned at some distance away from the beam port. On the other hand, increasing the value of θ to 90° mimics the situation in which a scattering material (e.g. Bismuth) is placed low in the beam line and/or the patient is located very close to the beam port.

Four beam diameters were considered (6.0, 12.0, 16.5 and 33 cm) and the maximum emission angle was varied between 0° (a plane wave of neutrons) and 90° (representing an isotropic beam). Emission angle was obtained by uniformly sampling from cos 0° to cos θ_{max}; azimuthal angle was uniformly sampled from 0° to 360° . The source-to-phantom distance was fixed at 0.1 cm.

RESULTS

Results indicate that for any source configuration examined (i.e. for any source size or emission angle), a large range of ideal energies is capable of producing ADs greater than 7 cm and is thus able to treat at least to the midline of the brain. The exact range, however, is a function of both beam size and neutron emission angle, and ^{10}B concentration in tumour and normal tissue.

Progress in Neutron Capture Therapy for Cancer
Edited by B.J. Allen *et al.*, Plenum Press, New York, 1992

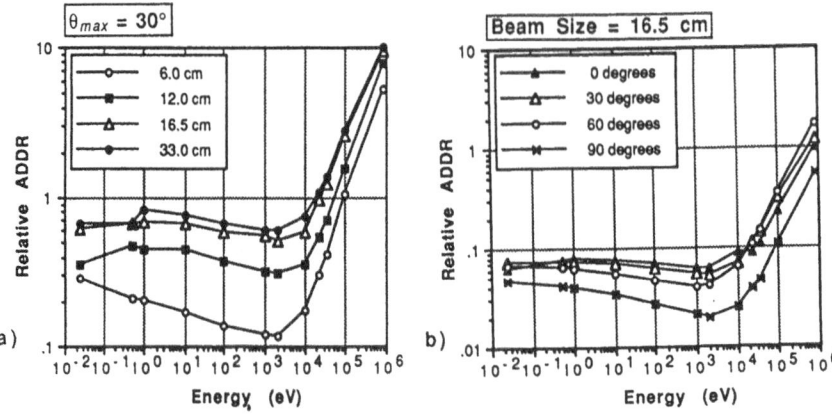

Figure 1. Relative ADDR vs. Energy. a) Effect of beam size on dose rate; θ_{max} is fixed at 30°.
b) Effect of θ_{max} on dose rate; beam size is fixed at 16.5 cm.

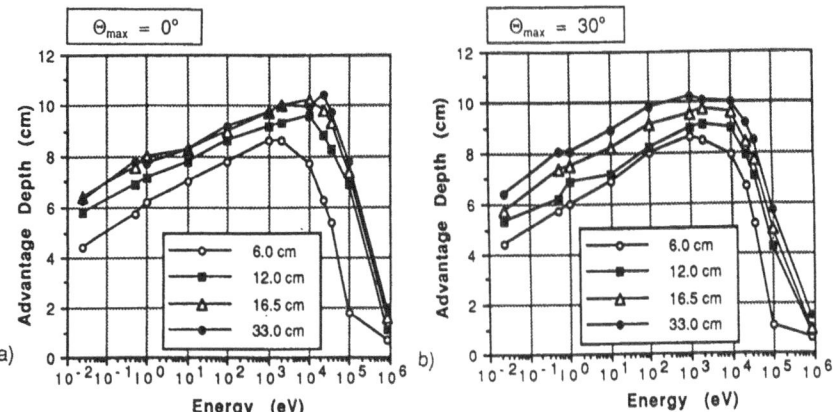

Figure 2. Maximum AD vs. Energy. a) Effect of beam size on AD; θ_{max} = 0°. b) θ_{max} fixed at 30°.

1. Effect of Beam Size and θ_{max} on ADDR

To examine the effect of beam size on dose rate the neutron flux was kept constant for all beam diameters. A plot of relative ADDR vs energy shows a wavelike shape (see Figures 1a and 1b). That is, ADDR tends to be maximized at roughly 1 eV and minimized at 2 keV before becoming very large at high energies due to the effect of fast neutrons and the reduction in AD at these energies. The extent of the dose rate difference between 2 keV and 1 eV varies between approximately 50 % and 100 % (depending on the beam size and the value of θ_{max}).

As shown in Figure 1a, for a given value of θ_{max}, ADDR tends to increase as beam size is increased. Figure 1b illustrates the effect of altering the maximum neutron emission angle on ADDR. As the beam becomes more isotropic, the dose rate at the AD in the phantom decreases.

2. Effect of Beam Size and θ_{max} on AD

The effect of increasing beam size (while keeping θ_{max} fixed) is to increase the advantage depth at all energies (see Figures 2a and 2b). When θ_{max} is zero (Figure 2a), the limit of increase in AD occurs when beam size reaches the size of the phantom itself. However, as θ_{max} is increased, and neutrons are allowed to enter the phantom at increasing angles, the AD continues to rise with beam size even when the beam becomes larger than the phantom (Figure 2b). This implies that for beams larger than the patient's head and that are not mono-directional, increasing beam size or placing a scattering object close to the patient's head will improve AD. It should be noted that as θ_{max} increases the dose rate will drop, implying a trade-off between AD and the irradiation time. Comparing Figures 2a and 2b indicates that for a small beam, neutron energies in the range of 10 eV - 20 keV will be capable of treating to the midline of the brain. As beam size increases, the range of suitable energies also increases. With a 12.0 cm beam, neutrons in the range 1 eV to 40 keV will be therapeutically useful; for even larger beams, the range is extended even further.

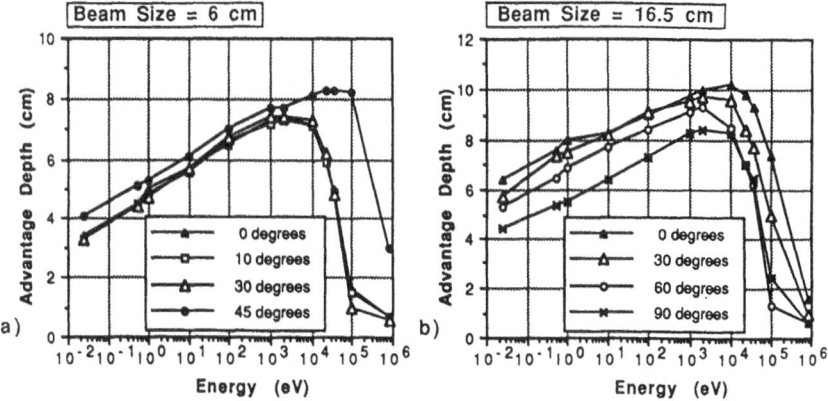

Figure 3. Maximum AD vs Energy. a) Effect of θ_{max} on AD; beam size = 6.0 cm.
b) Effect of θ_{max} on AD; beam size = 16.5 cm

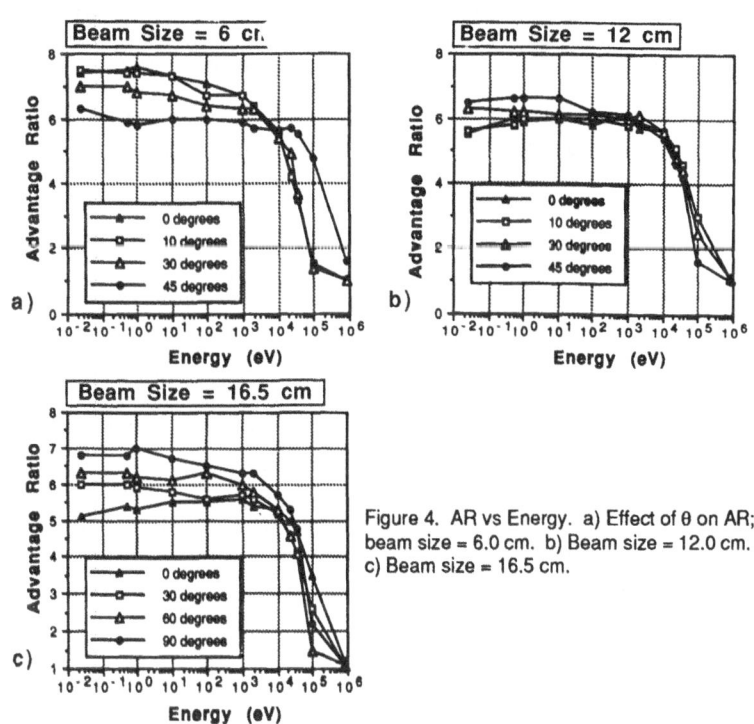

Figure 4. AR vs Energy. a) Effect of θ on AR; beam size = 6.0 cm. b) Beam size = 12.0 cm. c) Beam size = 16.5 cm.

With a small beam (see Figure 3a), the effect of increasing θ_{max} is minimal until θ_{max} becomes large. When θ_{max} = 45°, AD is increased at all energies and the curve is seen to peak at a higher neutron energy than is the case when θ_{max} < 45°. For larger beams, the effect of an increasing θ_{max} is to decrease AD at all energies, as illustrated in Figure 3b, and again, to push the peak of maximum AD to higher neutron energies.

3. Effect of Beam Size and θ_{max} on AR

When beam size is small, increasing the value of θ_{max} causes a reduction in AR, except at high energies (see Figure 4a). However, this trend quickly reverses as beam size is increased. With a 12.0 cm beam (Figure 4b), θ_{max} appears to affect AR very little until θ_{max} reaches 45°. At larger beam sizes, AR increases ᴀᴤ the beam becomes more isotropic (Figure 4c).

SUMMARY

Results of ideal beam studies are able to provide information that cannot be obtained experi-mentally. This information can offer guidance to those designing epithermal neutron beams for BNCT. An extensive ideal beam study has been carried out and some results have been discussed here; other results will be presented elsewhere. The following is a summary of the pertinent results discussed in this paper:

1. The advantage depth dose rate increases rapidly with beam size until the beam approaches the size of the phantom. The ADDR shows approximately a factor of two variation with energy and is highest at 1 - 10 eV.

2. The ADDR for beams of the size of the phantom, or larger, is maximized for neutrons which have an angular divergence of less than about 30°.

3. Beam energies in the range 1 eV to 40 keV are generally able to treat at least to the midline of the brain, for most beam sizes and neutron emission angles. However, when the beam is very small, this range shrinks to 1 eV - 20 keV for emission angles of 0° - 30°.

4. For beam sizes larger than 6 cm, the effect of θ_{max} is to increase AD and to push the maximum to higher energies; also, increasing θ_{max} will increase the AR of the beam.

REFERENCES

1. Briesmeíster, J.F., MCNP - A general Monte Carlo code for neutron and photon transport. *Los Alamos National Laboratory, LA 7396-M Rev. 2*, 1986.
2. Deutsch, O.L., and B.W. Murray, Monte Carlo dosimetry calculation for boron neutron capture therapy in the treatment of brain tumours, *Nuclear Technology*, **26**:320-339, 1975.
3. Snyder, W.S., M.R. Ford, G.G. Warner and H.L. Fisher, Estimates of absorbed fractions for monoenergetic photon sources uniformly distributed in various organs of a heterogeneous phantom, MIRD, *J. Nucl. Med. Suppl.*, 3 pamphlet 5, 1969.
4. Yanch, J.C., X.L. Zhou and G.L. Brownell, A Monte Carlo investigation of the dosimetric properties of monoenergetic neutron beams for neutron capture therapy, *Rad. Res.*, **126**:1-20, 1991.
5. Clement, S.D., J.R. Choi, R.G. Zamenhof, J.C. Yanch and O.K. Harling, Monte Carlo methods for neutron beam design for neutron capture therapy at the MIT Research Reactor (MITR-II), in *Neutron Beam Design, Development and Performance for Neutron Capture Therapy* (O.K. Harling, J.A. Bernard and R.G. Zamenhof, Eds.), Plenum Press, New York, 1990.

ANALYTICAL DOSIMETRY FOR SPONTANEOUS TUMOR DOGS

RECEIVING BORON NEUTRON CAPTURE THERAPY

Floyd J. Wheeler, Carol A. Atkinson,[1] and Patrick R. Gavin[2]

[1]PBF/BNCT Research Programs, Idaho National Engineering Laboratory, Idaho Falls, ID   83415-3519
[2]College of Veterinary Medicine and Surgery, Washington State University, Pullman, WA   99164-6610

INTRODUCTION

The dog irradiation project of the Power Burst Facility/Boron Neutron Capture Therapy (PBF/BNCT) Program is administered by Washington State University (WSU) with analytical and physical dosimetry provided by the Idaho National Engineering Laboratory (INEL).   One subtask of this project includes BNCT safety studies for dogs with spontaneously-occurring brain tumors.   The boron compound ($Na_2B_{12}H_{11}SH$ or BSH) was administered and single irradiations performed using the epithermal-neutron beam at the Brookhaven Medical Research Reactor (BMRR).   The main goal of the study was not to provide therapy, but to determine tumorcidal effect while administering a subtolerance dose to healthy tissue.   Irradiation times were based on delivery of 19 Gy peak physical dose to the blood.

METHODS

The reactor and beam design calculations were performed using a two-dimensional model and the DOT 4.3[1] computer code.   The neutron and gamma intensities and directions from the DOT output are used as input to a three-dimensional Monte Carlo model of the irradiation subject. Validation measurements of the Monte Carlo model were made using a lucite phantom representing the head of a Labrador dog prepared by researchers at WSU (Figure 1).   Lucite, for neutron effects, is neutronically similar to tissue.   Neutron and gamma measuring devices were placed into holes drilled into this head phantom and irradiated in the BMRR beam.   These measurements provided assurance that the analytical calculations for dose predictions in the live dogs were correct.

Unbiased calculations compare well with measured results, confirming the analytical models and methods.[2]   A simulation of several hundred neutron tracks, as produced by the Monte Carlo model, into a dog head (depicted by a sagittal magnetic resonance image) is shown in Figure 2. Typically, neutrons scatter hundreds of times before leaking out or being captured in tissue.   The delivered dose is a strong function of target-tissue size and position; therefore, simple approximations cannot be used for irradiation planning.

After the Monte Carlo calculation has simulated many (several hundred thousand or millions) neutron and gamma histories, isoflux or isodose contours can be generated.   The peak dose forms 2-3 centimeters into tissue.   It is this peak that usually determines healthy tissue tolerance and, therefore, irradiation time.   For neutron beams with significant fast-neutron component, however, the skin reaction can be limiting.   Isoflux contours developed in the dog head are shown in Figure 3.

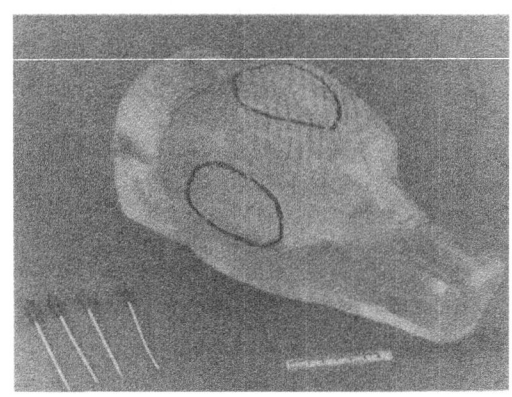

Figure 1. Lucite dog-head phantom.

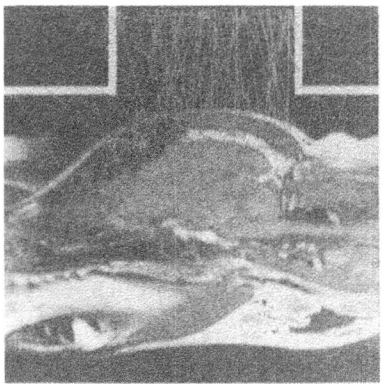

Figure 2. Monte Carlo simulation
of several hundred neutron tracks
into a dog head.

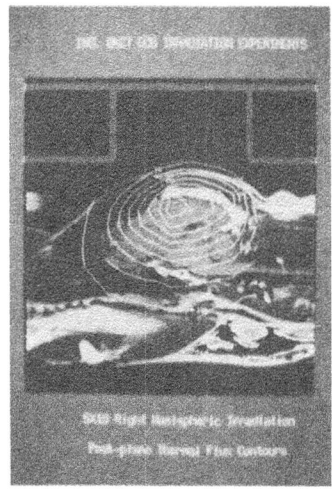

Figure 3. Isoflux contours developed in the dog head.

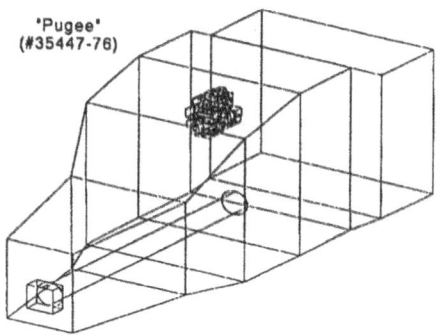

Figure 4. Wire-frame rendition of
a simple, geometric model of the
first spontaneous-tumor animal.

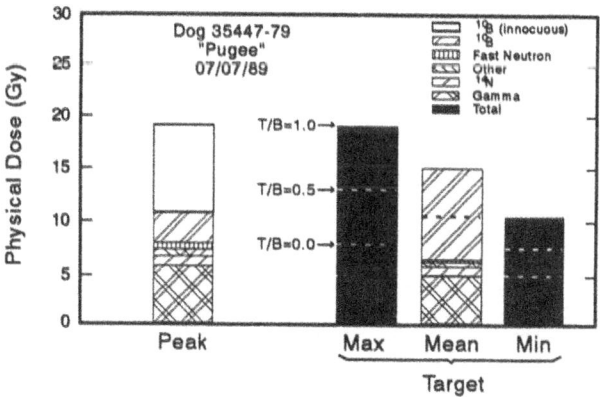

Figure 5. Dose components at the target
for the wire-frame rendition shown in
Figure 4.

The irradiations of spontaneous-tumor dogs required a unique dose-prediction model for nearly every dog since the dose rate, relative components, and dose distributions are a strong function of dog size and geometry. The preliminary models used thus far employ three-dimensional, regular-geometry primitives developed from medical image information. Final calculations are to be performed based on three-dimensional, B-spline reconstruction of the images. Figure 4 shows a wire-frame rendition of a simple, geometric model of the head, tumor, and peritumor edema present in the first spontaneous-tumor animal irradiated in the epithermal-neutron beam at BMRR. Calculations were made to determine a safe irradiation time so tumorcidal studies could be made without causing serious radiation effects in the dog. The 11-year old dog died one-year postirradiation from urinary-tract complications. Examination showed dramatic tumorcidal effect.

Figure 5 shows dose components at the target, defined here as tumor plus peritumor edema, and the peak healthy tissue location for the dog represented in the wire frame sketch shown in Figure 4. This dog was irradiated for 233 MW·min in the epithermal-neutron beam. A 9.7-cm^2 beam delimiter was used to reduce collateral dose. The peak dose in healthy tissue is actually the KERMA to the intraluminal space and a large portion of the boron dose is innocuous because of geometric sparing of the blood vessel walls.

CONCLUSIONS

1. Results of the computational model, unnormalized to experiments, show good agreement with measurement in a phantom having irregular geometry.

2. Comparisons of calculated dose and observed effect verify endothelium sparing with the BSH compound.

3. Dose rates vary substantially from animal to animal and the computational system is required to assure delivery of proper dosage.

REFERENCES

1. Rhodes, W. A. and R. L. Childs, "Updated Version of the DOT4 One- and Two-Dimensional Neutron and Photon Transport Code," ORNL-5051 (1982).

2. Wheeler, F. J., M. L. Griebenow, D. E. Wessol, D. W. Nigg, Y. D. Harker, and P. D. Randolph, "Analytical Radiation and Tissue Interaction Modeling for BNCT Dose Distribution Predictions," Fourth Japan/Australia Workshop on Neutron Capture Therapy for Malignant Melanoma, Kobe, Japan, February 13-16, 1990.

COPYRIGHT

SOME PHYSICAL FACTORS INFLUENCING THE DISTRIBUTIONS

OF THERMAL NEUTRONS AND GAMMA-RAYS IN A PHANTOM

Tetsuo Matsumoto

Atomic Energy Research Laboratory
Musashi Institute of Technology
Ozenji 971, Asao-ku, Kawasaki-shi, 215 Japan

INTRODUCTION

In boron neutron capture therapy (BNCT), the distributions of thermal neutron fluence and capture γ-ray dose rates in the brain depend on various physical factors such as the spectrum of incident neutrons, the size of the neutron irradiation aperture, the geometry and dimension of the patient's head and the ^{10}B concentration in normal and tumor tissues. For successful BNCT, it is a prerequisite to provide distributions of both thermal neutrons and capture γ-ray dose rate which take into account the preceding physical factors. The present study evaluates the effect of these factors on the depth–dose distributions. The use of heavy water by partially deuterating the tissue is being considered for the BNCT of some deep-seated tumors. The effect on the distribution of various levels of deuteration was examined.

METHODS

We reported the distributions of thermal neutron fluence and capture γ-ray dose rates in a polyethylene phantom for various neutron energy beams.[1] Results of calculations based on the two-dimensional neutron and coupled γ-ray transport code (DOT3.5) were in good agreement with experimental data. In this study, this transport code was also employed for calculations of distributions in a phantom (20 cm in diameter and 20 cm in thickness) of various compositions (polyethylene, water, tissue and brain).[2] The incident neutron spectrum measured with time of flight method was composed of a Maxwellian and a 1/E distribution for thermal and epi-thermal neutrons, respectively.

RESULTS AND DISCUSSION

1) Spectrum of incident neutrons

Figure 1a shows the measured and calculated neutron spectra incident on the tissue phantom. The spectrum can be represented by the simple form,

$$E/E_0^2 \exp (- E/E_0) + \lambda/E$$

The E_0 and λ values of the measured spectrum were determined to be 0.028 (eV) and 6.4×10^{-3}, respectively.

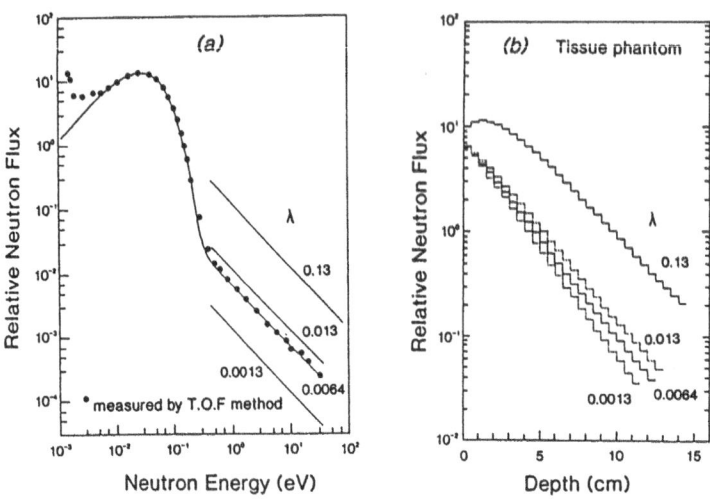

Fig.1 Measured and calculated incident neutron spectra (a) and distributions of thermal neutron fluence rate in the phantom(b)

The epi-thermal neutron content in the spectrum increases with the λ value. Figure 1b shows the calculated thermal neutron distributions in the phantom corresponding to the incident neutron spectra. The thermal neutron fluence rate at greater depths increased with the increase in epi-thermal neutron content of the incident neutron spectrum.

2) Neutron irradiation aperture (collimator)

Half- and one-tenth-value depths for thermal neutron fluence and capture γ-ray dose rates in the tissue phantom were obtained with collimator apertures of 5, 10 and 16 cm diameters (Table 1). Improved thermal neutron penetration and increased capture γ-ray dose rate were associated with a large collimator.

Table 1. Half- and one-tenth value depths for thermal neutron fluence and capture γ-ray dose rates in the tissue phantom at various aperture sizes.

	Thermal neutrons		Capture γ		
Collimator aperture (cm)	Half–value depth (cm)	One-tenth-value depth (cm)	Half-value depth (cm)	One-tenth-value depth (cm)	Dose* rate (Gyh^{-1})
5	1.5	4.25	2.5	8.0	1.22
10	2.0	5.75	3.5	10.5	1.95
16	2.5	6.75	4.5	12.5	2.40

* Associated with an incidental thermal neutron fluence rate $1.5 \times 10^9 cm^{-2}s^{-1}$

3) Phantom sizes

Two collimator aperture sizes, 5 and 10 cm in diameter and two phantoms, one 20 cm in diameter and 20 cm long, the other, 10 cm in diameter and 10 cm long were modeled. The calculated thermal neutron fluence and capture γ-ray dose rates at depth were higher for the large phantom while radiation leakage was lower.

4) ^{10}B concentration in normal and tumor tissues

The ^{10}B concentration, uniformly distributed in a water phantom, was varied. The calculated thermal neutron fluence rate at a depth of 5 cm decreased by about 2 % for 3 ppm and 20 % for 10 ppm ^{10}B concentrations.

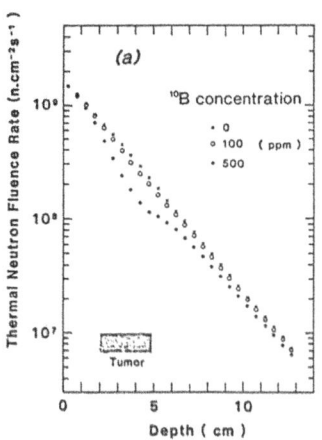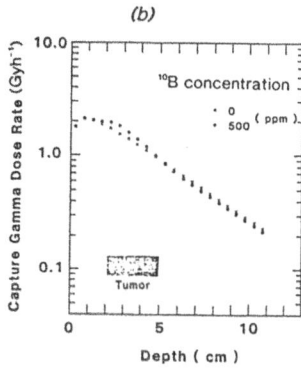

Fig.2 Distributions of (a) thermal neutron fluence and (b) capture γ ray dose rates in the water phantom with a 3 cm diameter tumor.

A tumor, 3 cm thick, at a depth of 3.5 cm in the phantom and containing ^{10}B was simulated (Fig. 2(a,b)). At the ^{10}B concentration of 30 ppm, distributions of thermal neutron fluence and capture γ-ray dose rates were only slightly affected. However, at 500 ppm, a notable reduction in thermal neutrons was observed across the ^{10}B concentration mass. These results suggest that the relationship between the concentration in the tumor and the tumor dose is not linear for concentrations greater than 100 ppm.

5) Brain water deuteration

Half- and one-tenth-value depths of thermal neutron fluence and capture γ-ray dose rates were calculated in a phantom containing D_2O at concentrations of 0 - 75 % (Table 2). A higher deuteration improved the transmission of thermal neutrons while reducing the capture γ-ray dose rate. Deuteration of the brain water appears promising for the BNCT of deep-seated brain tumors.

Table 2. Half- and one-tenth-value depths for thermal neutron fluence and capture γ-ray dose rates in the tissue phantom at various D_2O concentrations.

| D_2O (%) | Hydrogen atom. ($\times 10^{24} cm^3$) | Thermal neutrons | | Capture γ |
		Half-value depth (cm)	One-tenth-value depth (cm)	Dose rate* (max) (Gyh^{-1})
0	0.06686	2.0	5.75	2.10
25	0.05014	2.25	6.50	1.70
50	0.03343	2.50	7.50	1.20
75	0.01672	2.75	8.75	0.62

* Associated with an incidental thermal neutron fluence rate $1.5 \times 10^9 cm^2 s^{-1}$.

REFERENCES

1) T Matsumoto and O Aizawa Head phantom experiment and calculation for NCT using various neutron beams. Stralenther. Onkol. 165:98(1989)
2) T Matsumoto Transport calculations of the influence of physical factors on depth-dose distributions in boron neutron capture therapy. Phys. Med. Biol. 35:971(1990)

CHARACTERIZATION OF THE BMRR AND PBF EPITHERMAL-NEUTRON

BEAMS IN PHANTOM USING THREE-DIMENSIONAL DETERMINISTIC

RADIATION TRANSPORT THEORY

D. W. Nigg, F. J. Wheeler, and P. D. Randolph

PBF/BNCT Research Programs, Idaho National Engineering
Laboratory, Idaho Falls, ID   83415-3519

INTRODUCTION

Calculation of physically-realistic radiation dose distributions for Boron Neutron Capture Therapy (BNCT) is a complex, three-dimensional problem. The Monte Carlo stochastic simulation technique has traditionally been the primary method for performing such calculations. A three-dimensional deterministic approach to the problem would offer some complementary advantages. Recently-completed work at the Idaho National Engineering Laboratory (INEL) has established that the three-dimensional discrete-ordinates (S_n) formulation offers such an approach. The method has been validated in detail against measurements taken in a canine-head phantom irradiated in the epithermal-neutron beam at the Brookhaven Medical Research Reactor (BMRR) located at Brookhaven National Laboratory (BNL) in Upton, NY. In addition, three-dimensional deterministic calculations of all relevant BNCT dose components have been completed for the three-dimensional phantom in the proposed INEL Power Burst Facility (PBF) epithermal-neutron beam.

ANALYTICAL METHOD

The basic numerical approach in the discrete-ordinates method is well known. A version of the TORT[1] three-dimensional discrete-ordinates code, developed at Oak Ridge National Laboratory, is currently employed to perform the discrete-ordinates analysis discussed here. This code was adapted at INEL for operation on an Apollo DN-10000 engineering workstation computer.

EXPERIMENTAL VALIDATION

A canine brain irradiation program for research into various biological effects is being conducted by INEL. This experimental campaign is directed by INEL PBF/BNCT Program participants at Washington State University, Pullman, WA. An epithermal-neutron beam, designed at INEL and recently installed at the BMRR in cooperation with BNL BNCT researchers, is currently employed as the neutron source for the canine studies. Figure 1 shows the BMRR reactor with the epithermal-neutron beam installed.

Prior to use of the BMRR beam with live subjects, the neutron-flux levels that are produced by this beam were experimentally characterized using a lucite canine-head phantom (Figure 2). This phantom has a large number of regularly-spaced holes drilled into it as shown. Copper-gold alloy wires were inserted into catheters placed into these holes to measure neutron activation (and, therefore, neutron flux) as a function of

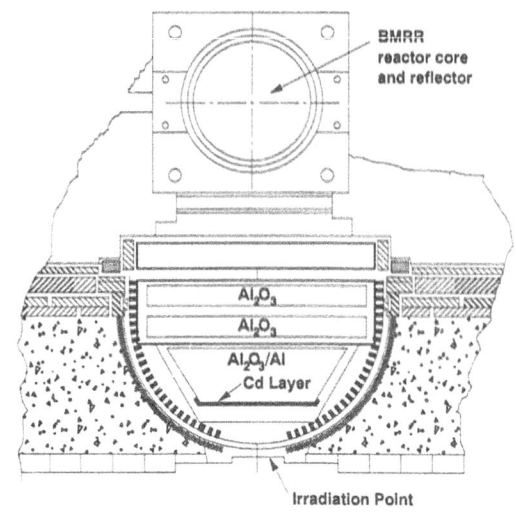

Figure 1. BMRR with epithermal-neutron beam installed.

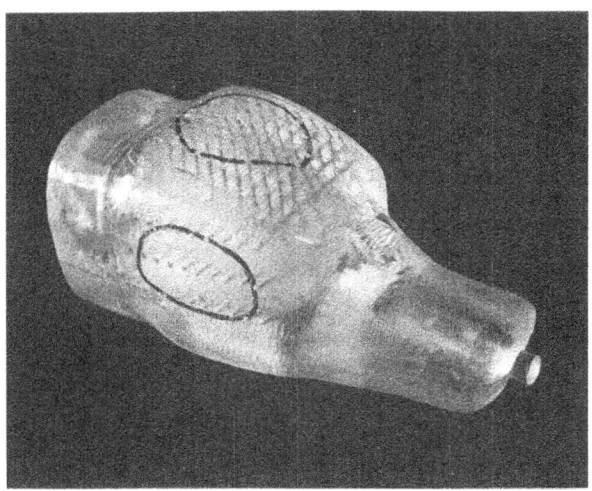

Figure 2. Lucite canine-head phantom.

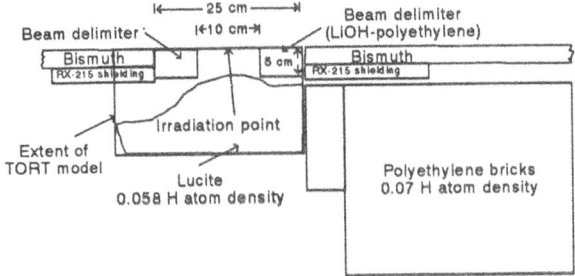

Figure 3. Canine phantom and beam delimiter positioning at BMRR beam output port.

146

Table I. Clinical BNCT Irradiation Parameters

Parameter*	Tumor at 2 cm		Tumor at 4 cm		Tumor at 6 cm	
	BMRR (3 MW)	PBF (20 MW)	BMRR (3 MW)	PBF (20 MW)	BMRR (3 MW)	PBF (20 MW)
Total dose rate at tumor location (cGy/min)	43.2	607.0	33.4	501.5	19.7	309.0
Boron (n,α)dose rate at tumor location (cGy/min)	31.2	434.8	23.5	348.6	13.1	201.4
Time required for 1000 cGy total dose at tumor location (min)	23.1	1.6	29.9	2.0	50.8	3.2
Surface tissue dose from fast neutrons for 1000 cGy total dose at tumor location (cGy)	53.1	21.1	68.8	26.4	116.8	42.2
Surface tissue dose from all components for 1000 cGy total dose at tumor location (cGy)	439.4	349.3	568.7	436.6	966.2	698.5

* 30 ppm uniform ¹⁰B assumed. No RBE applied. All data from discrete-ordinates calculation at beam centerline for lucite dog-head phantom assuming 10x10-cm epithermal-neutron beam for both PBF and BMRR

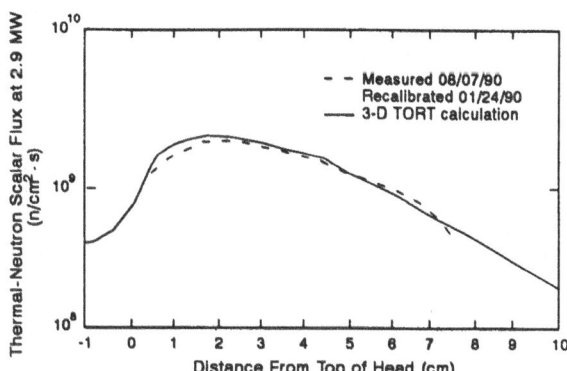

Figure 4. Typical comparison of calculation and measurement for flux along beam centerline.

depth below the top of the head in several locations. The use of these two materials allows the thermal-neutron flux (which is proportional to the boron dose) to be measured separately from the total flux. The lucite phantom was positioned in the beam near the irradiation point (Figure 3). A lithiated polyethylene beam delimiter was used to control the size of the beam aperture (approximately 10 x 10 cm). Additional polyethylene bricks were used to simulate the body of an actual dog. The region that includes the head phantom and delimiter was modeled as shown. A fixed angular flux boundary condition at the top of the geometry was used to represent the incoming beam. A 47 neutron, 20 gamma group cross-section library with a third-order Legendre polynomial scattering expansion was used. The calculation required 670 minutes on the Apollo DN-10000.

Measured scalar thermal fluxes were obtained for several flux-wire positions.[2] A typical comparison of calculation and measurement is shown in Figure 4 for the flux along the beam centerline. The irradiation was carried out at an indicated BMRR power of 2.9 MW, yielding a peak measured thermal-neutron flux along the beam centerline of 1.91×10^9 neutrons/cm$^2 \cdot$ sec. This is in very good agreement with the calculated scalar thermal-flux value of 2.02×10^9 neutrons/cm$^2 \cdot$ sec, especially considering the fact that all calculations, both those discussed here for the phantom and the associated discrete ordinates calculations employed to characterize the incoming BMRR beam[3] are based entirely on first principles, with normalization only to the reactor power. There are no empirical correction factors or source renormalizations of any type.

APPLICATION

Once the analytical methods were validated against experiment, hypothetical BNCT dose distributions in the lucite phantom were calculated for the BMRR epithermal-neutron beam and for the proposed PBF epithermal-neutron beam.[3] The PBF reactor has characteristics that make it an almost ideal source of epithermal neutrons for BNCT. The proposed filter is composed of aluminum and heavy water and will provide an intense, well-collimated, epithermal-neutron beam with a minimal level of undesirable contaminants (i.e., fast neutrons).

Three-dimensional distributions of all significant BNCT physical dose components were obtained by convoluting the calculated energy-dependent three-dimensional scalar fluxes in the phantom for each beam with appropriate energy-dependent KERMA factors for each dose-contributing interaction and summing over all interactions.[2] Some calculated results for selected positions along the beam centerline are shown in Table I. The PBF beam will produce a significantly smaller healthy tissue dose for a given tumor dose at a particular depth. For example, if one takes the healthy surface tissue dose to be limiting (because of the high relative biological effectiveness (RBE) fast-neutron component), the PBF beam is estimated to deliver approximately 40% more dose at a depth of 6 cm than is the case with the BMRR beam. This may correspond to a difference in cell survivor fraction of as much as two orders of magnitude.

At shallower depths, the performance of the BMRR beam begins to approach that of the PBF beam. It can be seen, however, from the table below that at a depth of only 2 cm the difference in achievable dose rate is still about 25%. It may also be noted that if postulated RBE factors were to be included, the difference in performance between the two beams would be greater than shown here. In particular, the PBF beam has a significantly smaller fast-neutron component.

In summary, full three-dimensional BNCT dose distribution calculations using the discrete-ordinates method, with particle scattering completely and explicitly taken into account have been completed for both the PBF and BMRR epithermal-neutron beams. This is the first known application of a three-dimensional deterministic analysis method to the problem of calculating radiation dose distributions for BNCT. The technique has been shown to be a practical and useful tool for this application.

REFERENCES

1. Rhodes, W. A. and R. L. Childs, "The TORT Three-Dimensional Discrete Ordinates Neutron/Photon Transport Code," ORNL-6268 (November 1987).

2. Nigg, D. W., et al., A Demonstration of Three-Dimensional Deterministic Radiation Transport Theory Dose Distribution Analysis for Boron Neutron Capture Therapy," (accepted for publication) <u>J. Med. Phys. 18:</u> (1) (1991).

3. Wheeler, F. J., et al., "Epithermal Neutron Beam Design for Neutron Capture Therapy at the Power Burst Facility and The Brookhaven Medical Research Reactor," <u>Nucl. Tech. 92:</u> 106-114 (October 1990).

COPYRIGHT

BEYOND THE EPITHERMAL-NEUTRON BEAM:

THE ANALYTICAL PHYSICIST'S ROLE

Floyd J. Wheeler, David W. Nigg, and Daniel E. Wessol

Idaho National Engineering Laboratory, EG&G Idaho, Inc.
Idaho Falls, ID 83415-3519

INTRODUCTION

Just four years ago, the epithermal-neutron beam, even a beam of marginal intensity and purity, was just a hope. Today, epithermal-neutron research beams of varying characteristics exist at the Joint Research Center (JRC) near Petten, The Netherlands (Europe), Brookhaven National Laboratory (BNL) (Upton, NY), and Massachusetts Institute of Technology (MIT) (Cambridge, MA). Concepts for modification of existing facilities, or construction of new facilities, exist at several sites worldwide. The challenge for the physicist, at least in the case of reactors, is no longer in providing the neutron source. The challenge now is to support the clinician, the biologist, and the chemist in effective implementation of Neutron Capture Therapy (NCT).

Radiation-transport models now exist that can be used to predict, from first principle, peak thermal-neutron flux in anthropomorphic phantom to within 10% of measurement.[1] This is the case for both Monte Carlo methods and three-dimensional deterministic methods. Improvements in capabilities and methods must be made so we can predict dose *in-vivo* to within 5% of actual administration and effectively communicate all the complicated, detailed results to the therapist and researcher.

Correlations of dose with biological response are presently primitive in the case of NCT. Dose and dose-equivalent are not adequate to describe NCT effect. Some work has been done to improve this situation by developing microdosimetric models, but much remains. Once the macroscopic and microscopic models have been proven to be reliable, they will be essential ingredients for: (1) providing true comparisons of alternate treatment protocols, (2) evaluating the efficacy of new chemical compounds, and (3) developing tumor-recurrence models.

As part of the Power Burst Facility/Boron Neutron Capture Therapy (PBF/BNCT) Program, we have been developing new particle transport software and an interactive patient treatment planning system for BNCT. The particle transport software has undergone validation and is being used to correlate large animal biological response following borocaptate sodium administration and epithermal-neutron irradiations.

DEVELOPMENTS IN PARTICLE TRANSPORT

Monte Carlo: We are constructing new Monte Carlo modules (rtt_MC), specifically tailored to BNCT that we feel offer improvements in the following principal areas:

1. Problem Solution Time. By tailoring the module to BNCT, efficiencies in algorithms can be gained.

2. Tracking in Irregular Geometry. The rtt_MC module has two basic geometries. First, particle tracking can be performed in geometry described as combinations of regular solid geometry primitives. Second, the option of constructing all or a part of the patient geometry directly from medical images is also being incorporated. For this option, the geometry will be described by nonuniform, rational, B-spline (NURB) surface representations.[2]

3. User Interface. The goal for the patient treatment planning system is to enable the therapist, or technician, to simulate irradiations, examine calculated results, and thus determine the therapy regime. This can be accomplished most effectively by using expertise built into the computer software and predetermined files, with a minimum of additional user input for a particular case.

4. Flux and Reaction-Rate Tallies. A problem, inherent to all Monte Carlo codes, arises when detailed space-dependent fluxes and reaction rates are desired. The rtt_MC module provides this desired detail by imposing an invisible subelement mesh over the regions of interest. During tracking, contributions to flux and reaction rate are accumulated into all appropriate subelements via a clipping algorithm (similar to those used in computer graphics). This subelement information is stored for later edits and interactive displays.

5. Gamma Coupling. The user will have the option of sampling from neutron interactions during the neutron tracing mode, as commonly done in transport codes. This sampling scheme, however, tends toward high variance because of the stochastic nature of neutron-interaction events. That is, the variance in gamma flux is exacerbated by the added burden of source variance. An optional mode in rtt_MC is to accumulate the gamma production distributions during neutron mode and store these into a file. A continuation gamma run then selects from this converged source (and from the direct beam source). An output file from the continuation run contains combined output from both the neutron and gamma runs.

Deterministic Methods: Details of the discrete-ordinates, or Sn, method for solution of the Boltzmann equation for radiation transport are well known and will only be briefly summarized here. The basic numerical approach involves partitioning the spatial geometry into mesh elements and treating the angular integrals that appear in the transport equation as weighted sums over a set of prespecified discrete angular directions. Given a description of the particle source, a solution for the resulting particle flux is iteratively calculated for each of these discrete directions and for each mesh element. The energy variable is ordinarily handled using the standard multigroup method. The recently-released TORT, three-dimensional discrete-ordinates code[3] has been successfully applied to complex-geometry phantom dosimetry. Although the TORT code is limited to orthogonal geometries, it is well written, clearly documented, and easily adaptable to a wide variety of computing hardware. In addition, it produces calculated results for the applications described here that are numerically very well-behaved and accurate.[1]

Charged-Particle Transport: The Monte Carlo technique is also employed for charged-particle transport for microdosimetry. Thus, applicable options discussed in the Monte Carlo section would also be available for charged-particle transport simulations.

The Northcliff and Schilling[4] range energy relationships have been used extensively in charged-particle studies. The Northcliff and Schilling formulisms, however, do not account for transient electron binding. Transient electron binding reduces the effective charge of the ion and is an important effect at energies below a few MeV. Ziegler, et al.,[5] incorporated this effect via the concept of expected charge and the Ziegler data are also in agreement with ICRU.[6] Thus, the Ziegler data are used in all charged-particle simulations.

Tumor Recurrence Models: The ultimate challenge for the analytical physicist lies in the ability to quantify tumor control and minimize tumor recurrence. The largest uncertainties blocking this ability are knowledge

152

of ^{10}B microdistributions and the *in-vivo* tumor response. Many theoretical models for tumor growth exist. Observation of tumor doubling time and recurrence after therapy could allow one to develop tumor recurrence models based firstly on simple assumptions, followed by refinement as the data becomes available. Information about the ^{10}B microdistributions for new compounds could, when combined with microdosimetric analysis, provide estimates of therapeutic advantage.

For such models, Alvord and Shaw[7] have introduced the concept of "the number of generations left behind." This concept is more intuitively pleasing than the use of fractional survival when describing tumor control. Figure 1 illustrates tumor growth and treatment using the concept of tumor generations, where a generation represents a doubling of tumor volume. The number of generations left behind can be estimated, given all required information, with a three-dimensional integration for all dose components over target volume with microdosimetric considerations included.

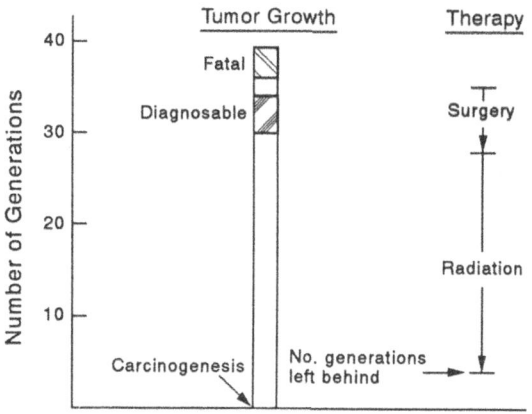

Figure 1. Number of generations left behind.

REFERENCES

1. Nigg, D. W., P. D. Randolph, and F. J. Wheeler, "A Demonstration of Three-Dimensional Deterministic Radiation Transport Theory Dose Distribution Analysis for Boron Neutron Capture Therapy," accepted for publication by J. Med. Physics in November 1990.

2. Wessol, D. E., J. Cobb, F. J. Wheeler, E. Cohen, B. Cobb, and D. Barber, "Interactive Generation of Three-Dimensional, B-Spline Objects from Planar Image Data for Multidimensional Analysis," Society of Exploration Geophysicists Sixtieth Annual International Meeting and Exposition, San Francisco, CA (September 1990).

3. Rhodes, W. A. and R. L. Childs, "The TORT Three-Dimensional Discrete Ordinates Neutron/Photon Transport Code," ORNL-6268, Oak Ridge National Laboratory, Oak Ridge, TN (November 1987).

4. Northcliff, L. C. and R. F. Schilling, "Range and Stopping Power Tables for Heavy Ions," in Nuclear Data Tables A7, 233-463 (1970).

5. Ziegler, J., J. Biersack, and U. Liltmark, The Stopping and Range of Ions in Solids, Pergamon Press, New York (1985).

6. ICRU Microsimetry Report 36, International Commission on Radiation Units and Measurements, Washington D.C. (1983).

7. Alvord, E. C., Jr. and C. Shaw, in Pathology of the Aging Human Nervous System, Chapter 11 (to be published).

COPYRIGHT

MEASUREMENTS OF LINEAL ENERGY SPECTRA FOR NEUTRON CAPTURE THERAPY USING A BORON DOPED LET CHAMBER

H.I. Amols[1], C.S. Wuu[1], S. Saraf[2], P. Kliauga[1], and L.E. Reinstein[3]

[1]Dept. Radiation Oncology, Columbia Univ., N.Y., N.Y. 10032
[2]Brookhaven National Laboratory, Upton, N.Y. 11973
[3]Dept. Radiation Oncology, SUNY at Stony Brook, N.Y. 11794

INTRODUCTION

Preclinical studies for boron neutron capture therapy (BNCT) using epi-thermal neutrons are ongoing at several laboratories. The absorbed dose in tumor cells depends on the boron concentration, thermal neutron flux at depth, size of the cell, plus fast neutron and gamma contamination in the epithermal beam. Monte Carlo computer simulations can estimate the various dose components, but dosimetry and treatment planning for BNCT present unique difficulties. Dosimetry is complicated by the admixture of thermal, epithermal, and fast neutrons, plus gamma rays; and the array of secondary high linear energy transfer (LET) particles produced within the patient from neutron interactions. Absorbed dose and radiation quality will be difficult to determine, and microdosimetry may be a viable technique for determining these quantities. Only one set of microdosimetric data for BNCT has previously been reported[1]. Spectra were measured in air for an epithermal beam, using a tissue equivalent (TE) proportional counter to assess the effects of beam filter designs. We report here the first set of in phantom microdosimetric measurements using paired TE and TE+boron chambers on an epithermal beam. Such measurements permit assessment of the dose enhancement factor, and lineal energy distributions of the boron capture reaction.

EXPERIMENTAL DESIGN

A 2.5 cm diameter TE-Rossi type[2] gas proportional counter has been built, with 50 parts per million (ppm) boron-10 incorporated into the 3mm thick walls by premixing boron nitride powder with conventional TE powder. This mixture was melted, heat molded, and machined into shape (The authors thank Mr. G. Johnson, Columbia Univ. for chamber design and fabrication). Stainless steel wire (0.05 mm) is used for the anode and helix but all other electrical pins are made of aluminum in order to reduce the total cross section for capture reactions not normally occurring in vivo. The mounting base for the detector, and all vacuum system connections are made of non-metalic materials with negligible capture cross sections. Over 99% of the capture events in the chamber (excluding reactions from hydrogen and nitrogen which occur naturally) are from boron rather than non-tissue materials necessitated by chamber design. Also 'non-tissue like' materials (steel, aluminum, and brass) only produce gamma rays after neutron capture, not high LET particles. The counting gas was a standard TE mixture of 55% propane, 40% carbon dioxide, and 5% nitrogen with the addition of boron triflouride in an amount equivalent to 50 ppm boron-10.

Progress in Neutron Capture Therapy for Cancer
Edited by B.J. Allen *et al.*, Plenum Press, New York, 1992

A second counter without boron, filled with non-boron gas was used for comparative measurements. Measurements with each detector were made using standard microdosimetry equipment[3], including a low pressure gas flow system, low noise charge sensitive preamplifier, linear amplifier, multi-channel analyzer, and Americium-241 alpha calibration source. All measurements were made at the treatment port of the Brookhaven Medical Research Reactor (BMRR), for an aluminum oxide filtered epithermal (0.5ev-30keV) neutron beam described previously[4]. Detectors were positioned in a 10 x 10 x 5 cm thick Lucite/rice phantom, centered in the uncollimated beam. The effective depth of the gas collecting volume was 2.0 cm, corresponding to the depth of maximum thermal neutron flux (via thermalization of epithermals). The reactor was run at 0.1 to 5.0 kW power to avoid detector avalanche and pulse pile up. Lineal energy spectra were measured for simulated cell diameters of 2 and 6 microns in 4-6 overlapping segments normalized to total reactor kilowatt-minutes of counting time, as determined via independent meters in the reactor control room.

RESULTS AND DISCUSSION

Lineal energy (y) spectra are plotted in Figure 1, for a 2 um cavity size (with and without boron), and for a 6 um cavity size (with boron). The y*d(y) spectra are normalized to unit dose and plotted against log(y), so that the area under the curve between any two values of 'y' is proportional to the dose fraction in that interval. Both boron spectra are dominated by

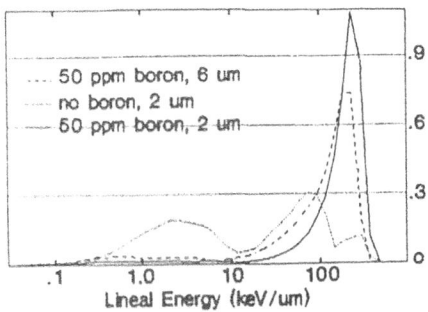

Fig. 1: Measured lineal energy spectra, y*d(y) vs. log(y) normalized to unit dose.

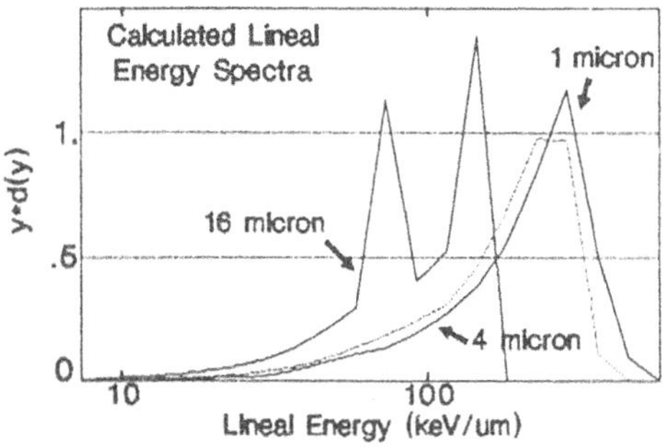

Fig. 2: Calculated lineal energy spectra y*d(y) vs. log(y) for 1, 4, and 16 μm site size.

a peak at y = 2-300 keV/μm corresponding to the LET of alpha and lithium recoils from boron capture. This peak is almost completely absent in the non-boron chamber. Some dose is observed however as TE plastic contains trace amounts of boron (0.4-0.8 ppm boron-10)[5]. The 'non-boron' spectrum is dominated by peaks at 2-3, 80, and 320 keV/μm corresponding to gammas and fast protons, Bragg peak protons, and heavy recoils respectively. The latter two peaks overlap each other, and are both due to fast neutrons. The boron spectra also show these peaks but by normalizing to unit dose, only the alpha-lithium peak is readily apparent.

As required kinematical data for boron capture are well known, the 'y' spectra for the boron chamber can be accurately predicted using algorithms presented by Caswell[6]. Typical results are shown in Fig. 2, where we plot calculated 'y' spectra for different site diameters. Calculations include only the boron-10 and nitrogen-14 reactions, and all spectra have been normalized to unit dose.

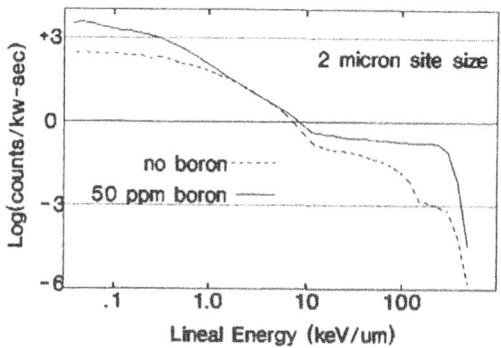

Fig. 3: Counts per kW-sec of reactor beam verses 'y' for the standard TE and boron doped chambers, for a 2 micron site diameter.

In Fig. 3 we plot detector count rates with and without boron in a 2 um site diameter normalized to kilowatt seconds of reactor beam . This shows the magnitude of the boron dose enhancement. For y>10 keV/μm, and especially for y>100 there is a significant increase in count rate. The boron spectrum also shows increased count rate for y<1 keV/μm due to the 480 keV gammas emitted after boron capture. When normalized to reactor kw-sec the difference in count rates between the two spectra yields the dose enhancement factor of boron capture. This analysis yields a 'relative dose' = 0.5 + 0.2*ppm (where ppm = parts per million boron-10). Thus, if in vivo boron concentrations were (hypothetically) 30 ppm in tumor, and 3 ppm in normal tissue, the dose enhancement factor would be 6.0 (independ-ent of RBE corrections), a value consistent with calculations.[4]

CONCLUSIONS

BNCT presents unique dosimetry problems. The reactor beam is a mix-ture of thermal, epithermal, and fast neutrons, plus gamma rays; which makes the determination of absorbed dose difficult. We have demonstrated the viability of microdosimetry for determination of absorbed dose (using a single detector), the dose enhancement factor, and the lineal energy spectra of the BNCT beam. Microdosimetry is thus a viable techniques for verifying the accuracy of dose and quality factor calculations for BNCT.

REFERENCES

1. Kliauga, P., Musolino, S. Microdosimetry of an epithermal neutron beam
   for radiotherapy. 36th Rad. Res. Soc. Mtg., Philadelphia, (1988).
2. Rossi, H.H., and Rosenzweig, W. A device for the measurement of dose as
   a function of specific ionization. Radiol. 64:404 (1955).
3. Amols, H.I., Dicello, J.F., and Lane, T.F. Microdosimetry of negative
   pions. Proc. 5th sym. microdosimetry. EUR5452 d-e-f. pp:911-928 (1975).
4. Fairchild, R.G., Kalef-Ezra, J., Saraf, S.K., et. al. Installation and
   testing of an optimized epithermal neutron beam at the BMRR. In Neutron
   beam design, development, and performance for NCT. Ed. Harling, O.K.,
   Bernard, J.A., and Zamenhof, R.G. Plenum Press, NY. pp: 185-99 (1990).
5. Smathers, J.B., Otte, V.A., Smith, A.R., et. al. Composition of A-150
   tissue equivalent plastic. Med. Phys. 4:74-77 (1977).
6. Caswell, R.S. Deposition of energy by neutrons in spherical cavities.
   Rad. Res. 27:92-107 (1966).

DOSE MEASUREMENTS AND CALCULATIONS IN THE EPITHERMAL NEUTRON
BEAM AT THE BROOKHAVEN MEDICAL RESEARCH REACTOR (BMRR)

V.Benary[1,2], R.G. Fairchild[1], J. Kalef-Ezra[1,3], D. Greenberg[1],Y. Kamen[1], S. Fiarman[1], and L. Wielopolski[1,4]

[1]Medical Dept., Brookhaven National Laboratory, Upton, NY, USA
[2]Tel Aviv University, Tel-Aviv, Israel
[3]University of Ioannina, Ioannina, Greece
[4]Radiation Oncology Dept., SUNY-SB, Stony Brook, NY, USA

INTRODUCTION

The characteristics of the epithermal neutron beam at BMRR were measured, calculated, and reported by R. G. Fairchild (1). This beam has already been used for animal irradiations. We anticipate that it will be used for clinical trials. Thermal and epithermal neutron flux densities distributions, and dose rate distributions, as a function of depth were measured in a lucite dog-head phantom. Monte Carlo calculations were performed and compared with the measured values.

MEASUREMENTS AND CALCULATIONS

Dog-Head phantom. A lucite dog-head phantom similar in size and shape to that of a Labrador retriever (Fig. 1) was constructed in our laboratory. The central part was cored to a rectangular well 4½" in depth, 3½" in length, and 3¼" in width. This was filled with different sets of horizontal lucite plates. Each set of plates had precisely machined grooves, to accommodate either foils, cadmium capsules with foils, TLD's, or silicon diodes (Fig. 2). This arrangement allowed for measurements at precise depths on the central axis. The composition and the density of lucite is, for our purposes, very similar to tissue. The phantom was irradiated with its central axis (center of the plates) aligned with the central axis of the port. A series of irradiations were conducted with the phantom touching the bare 10" x 10" port. Another series had the phantom placed against a 2"-thick LiOH collimator, with an aperture of about 4" x 4", inserted in the port. The experiments were designed:
- To check the dosimetry in an asymmetric geometrical configuration;
- To obtain dosimetric data for animal irradiations;
- To assess the influence of beam delimiters (collimators);
- To compare the measured values with the Monte Carlo calculations.

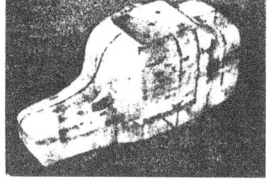

Fig. 1

Calculations. The Monte Carlo computer program MCNP was used to generate neutron fluence rates and dose rates in a dog phantom. The neutron source used in the calculations had a pancake geometry of 10" x 10" and was situated directly in front of the phantom or the collimator, when one was used. The energy spectrum of the source was the calculated spectrum reported by Wheeler et al.(2). The calculated values were compared to the measured results. The main discrepancy was observed in the calculations of the γ dose.

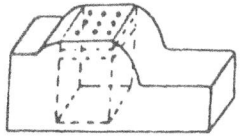

Fig. 2

Thermal and epithermal neutron fluence rates. Bare and cadmium-encapsulated gold foils were used to measure the thermal and epithermal neutron flux. The epithermal neutron fluence rate was calculated by the cadmium ratio method. The measured values of the neutron fluence rates with and without a collimator are shown in Fig. 3, and the calculated (MCNP) values are given in Fig. 4. When we compared the ratio: thermal neutron fluence rate (bare port)/thermal neutron fluence rate (collimator) at the peak and at the surface of the phantom, a skin-sparing effect was suggested when a collimator was used. The magnitude of this effect will be influenced by the combined geometry of the collimator and the phantom. The measured and the calculated values are in good agreement; however, the calculated epithermal neutron fluence rate drops faster with depth in phantom.

Effective Dose Rate. The effective dose rates for phantom irradiations on the bare port and with a collimator are given in Figs. 5 and 6 at a power of 1 MW. For the $^{14}N(n,p)^{14}C$ reaction, a N content of 1.84% by weight and an RBE of 1.6 were used. The same RBE was used for the fast neutron effective dose. The RBE used for the $^{10}B(n,\alpha)^7Li$ reaction was 2.3. The shape of the curves in Fig. 6 was influenced by the irregular shape of the phantom.

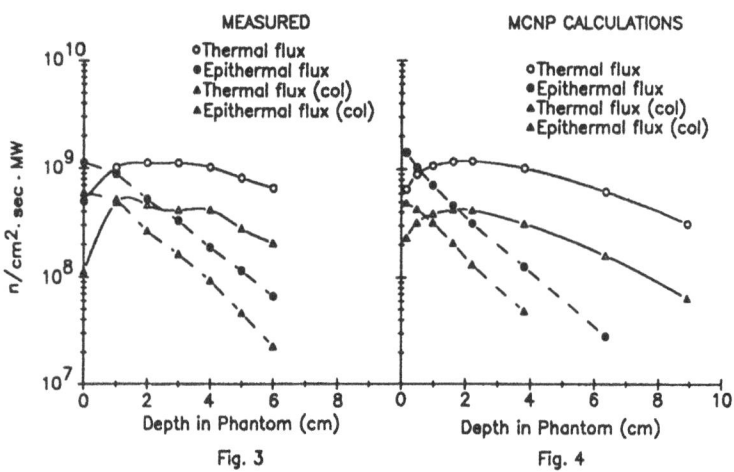

Fig. 3   Fig. 4

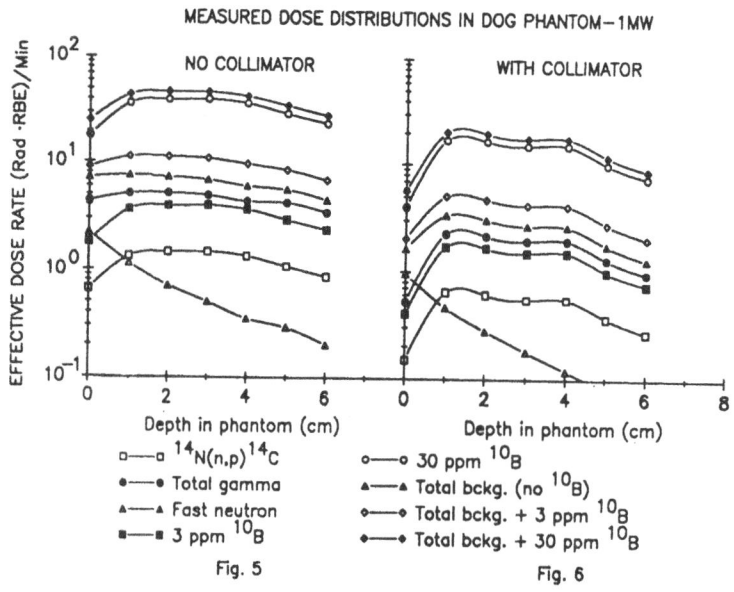

Fig. 5   Fig. 6

The calculated (MCNP) dose distributions were in good agreement with the measured values with the exception of the calculated γ doses. As can be seen in Table 1, the γ doses were much lower, probably due mainly to the cross sections used.

Table 1. Beam Parameters in Dog Phantom.

	Measured		MCNP	
	Bare	Coll	Bare	Coll
Fast neutron dose rate at 0 depth rad·rbe/MW·min	2.2	0.95	2.03	0.85
Peak total γ dose rate rad·rbe/MW·min	5.19	2.25	2.79	0.84
Fast neutron dose/th. neutron at peak rad·rbe/n·cm	$3.2 \cdot 10^{-11}$	$3.2 \cdot 10^{-11}$	$3 \cdot 10^{-11}$	$3.3 \cdot 10^{-11}$
Peak γ dose/th. neutron at peak rad·rbe/n·cm	$7.7 \cdot 10^{-11}$	$7.7 \cdot 10^{-11}$	--	--
Peak bckgr (no ^{10}B) dose rate rad·rbe/MW·min	7.53	3.35	--	--
Peak bckgr 3 ppm ^{10}B dose rate rad·rbe/MW·min	11.34	5.05	--	--
Peak bckgr 30 ppm ^{10}B dose rate rad·rbe/MW·min	47.16	20.35	--	--

INTERCALIBRATION OF EPITHERMAL NEUTRON BEAMS

Measurements and/or calculations of beam parameters in air are not enough to characterize a neutron beam. Dose components must be measured and calculated in a phantom. The compositions, shapes, and sizes of the phantoms, as well as the geometry of the beam, make it difficult to compare the performance of the different neutron beams. We suggest standardizing the phantom and the reported measured or calculated parameters in a manner similar to that which follows.

Phantom. A simple, inexpensive, and easily machined lucite right circular cylinder, 16.5 cm in diameter, 25 cm high, was built. A thin lucite tube was inserted along its central axis. Lucite rods were inserted in the tube. Each set of rods had indentations to allow the insertion of detectors (foils, TLDs, or solid state silicon diodes) at well-defined depths in the phantom. A provision is made for the insertion of a lucite tube off axis, in which measurements can be made for calculation benchmarking.

Beam Parameters in Air. It is our opinion that the parameters, measured and/or calculated at the irradiation port face, which must be reported in order to characterize the epithermal beam are:
- Neutron spectrum;
- Epithermal neutron flux density;
- Absorbed dose rate from gammas and fast neutrons free in air;
- Gamma dose and fast neutron dose per epithermal neutron.

Beam Parameters in Standard Phantom. Graphic representations of the thermal neutron flux density and dose rate distributions as a function of depth in phantom must be reported.

A beam aperture of 10 by 10 cm is suggested. In any case, the irradiation geometry must be well defined. The advantage depth and the therapeutic gain will complete the data necessary for an effective intercalibration of epithermal neutron beams.

REFERENCES

1. R.G. Fairchild et al. Installation and testing of an optimized neutron beam at the BMRR. Neutron Beam Design, Development and Performance for Neutron Capture Therapy. O.K. Harling, J.A. Bernard and R.G. Zamenhof, Eds. Basic Life. Sciences, Vol. 54, 185, Plenum Press, New York (1990).
2. F.J. Wheeler et al. Physics design for the BMRR epithermal neutron source. Neutron Beam Design, Development and Performance for Neutron Capture Therapy. O.K. Harling, J.A. Bernard and R.G. Zamenhof, eds. Basic Life Science, Vol. 54, 83, Plenum Press, New York (1990).

(Research supported by US DOE contract DE-AC02-76CH00016)

REVIEW OF TECHNIQUES DEVELOPED AT HARWELL LABORATORY FOR NEUTRON AND
GAMMA-RAY CHARACTERISATION OF FILTERED NEUTRON BEAMS FOR BORON NEUTRON
CAPTURE THERAPY

C A Perks[1], G Constantine[2] and H J Delafield[1]

[1]Radiation Dosimetry Department, AEA Environment and Energy, Harwell
Laboratory, Oxfordshire, OX11 0RA, UK
[2]Currently at: ANSTO Lucas Heights Research Laboratories, New Illawarra Road,
Lucas Heights, New South Wales, Australia

INTRODUCTION

This paper reviews techniques, developed at Harwell Laboratory over the last few years, for
determining the neutron and gamma-ray characteristics of intermediate energy neutron beams
developed for Boron Neutron Capture Therapy (BNCT) experiments.   They have been used for the
characterisation of several such beams: the iron/aluminium/sulphur[1,2] and aluminium/sulphur/
liquid argon[3] beams developed at Harwell, the Petten High Flux Reactor (HFR) HB7 developmental
beam[4] and, most recently, the HFR HB11 beam[5].   The techniques discussed include those for
neutron spectrometry, beam profiling and gamma-ray dosimetry.

NEUTRON SPECTROMETRY

A number of techniques exist for the measurement of the neutron energy spectra and intensity of
BNCT beams.   Most of the BNCT beams measured have a broad spectrum ranging from about 1 eV
up to about 30 keV, with a small fraction of neutrons transmitted through windows in the cross-
sections of the filter components being responsible for a significant fraction of the dose.   A number of
different techniques have been employed to cover the full energy range (from thermal to > 1 MeV),
with some overlap.   For various reasons these techniques can only be used at low reactor powers.
Further developments involving the multisphere spectrometry system should enable it to be used
both at low power and full power.

Proton Recoil Counter Spectrometry

High resolution proton recoil spectrometry can be used to determine neutron energy spectra in
the region from about 10 keV to 1.5 MeV.   To cover this range, three counters (type SP2, diameter
40 mm) filled with hydrogen at nominal pressures of 1, 3 and 10 atmospheres (100, 300 and
1000 kPa) are used.   Full details of the spectrometer, its calibration and the method of unfolding the
measured pulse-height distributions to give the neutron energy spectrum are described in references
6 and 7.

Spectrum Modification Spectrometry

In this technique[8], absorbers or scatterers (eg. discs of ^{10}B of various thicknesses and titanium) are interposed in the beam. The effect of increasing the thickness of the ^{10}B absorber is to attenuate the low and then progressively higher energy neutrons, while the titanium strongly scatters neutrons penetrating the window in the cross-section of aluminium at about 25 keV. The response of various detectors (eg.: a cadmium covered BF_3 counter and vanadyl sulphate bath for the Harwell Al/S/Ar beam; a cadmium covered BF_3 counter and the 38.1 mm radius multisphere for the Petten HB7 measurements; and the 38.1, 51.0 and 63.5 mm radii multispheres in the Petten HB11 measurements) is measured for a range of absorbers. The changes in the response functions of the detectors are calculated using a Monte Carlo neutron transport program (MCNP). The responses of the detectors, together with their response functions as modified with the interposed absorbers, are then used as input to an unfolding program (SENSAK[9]) to adjust a calculated neutron energy spectrum.

Multisphere Spectrometry

The multisphere spectrometer[10] consists of eight polyethylene spheres with radii ranging from 38.1 to 127.0 mm. During a measurement the spheres are irradiated sequentially. Incident neutrons are moderated by the polyethylene sphere and detected using a ^3He detector located at the centre of each sphere in turn. Each multisphere has a different neutron energy response and so the neutron energy spectrum can be derived from the observed count-rates using an unfolding program. Because of the small diameter of the beams, it has not been possible to use this type of spectrometer, except in the HB11 Petten beam. In this beam, three multispheres were used in conjuction with the spectrum modification method described above, to compensate for their restricted energy range. In this way a good overlap with the proton recoil spectrometer was achieved.

The use of this spectrometer is restricted to large diameter beams and, also, low power measurements to avoid unduly large dead time corrections to the observed count-rates. However, development of the multisphere spectrometer, replacing the ^3He counter by a suitable activation detector, is under consideration. This would allow the multisphere spectrometer to be used at both low power and full power.

GAMMA-RAY DOSIMETRY

^7LiF thermoluminescent dosemeters (TLDs) are generally used for determining the gamma-ray dose in BNCT beams. The results obtained from the TLDs were corrected for their response to thermal neutrons, which depends critically on the contamination of ^6LiF in the TLDs[11].

BEAM PROFILING

For the small diameter beams, passive methods for determining the beam profiles were needed. For the neutron fluence profiles arrays of gold foil detectors, covered with cadmium were used and for gamma-ray measurements arrays of ^7LiF TLDs have been used. Corrections were made for the neutron response of the TLDs. However, for the HB11 beam at Petten, it was possible to use a small (12.5 mm diameter and 63 mm long) BF_3 detector, covered with a 1 mm cadmium sheath, end-on to determine the neutron fluence profile. This detector was scanned across the beam using a two dimensional cross-slide mechanism adapted from a drawing board.

CONCLUSIONS

This paper has outlined techniques developed for the neutron and gamma-ray characterisation of filtered neutron beams for BNCT research. Most of the techniques are well established. However, some development, particularly to set up the multisphere spectrometer with activation detectors, will be very advantageous to future BNCT development. Attention must then be given to establishing techniques and instrumentation for routine monitoring of the neutron and gamma-ray dose, and beam quality, in BNCT beams, particularly as the first clinical trials approach.

ACKNOWLEDGEMENTS

This work is being supported by the UK Department of Health.

REFERENCES

1. C. A. Perks, K. G. Harrison, R. Birch and H. J. Delafield, The characteristics of a high intensity 24 keV, iron-filtered neutron beam, Radiat. Prot. Dosim. 15:31 (1986).
2. C. A. Perks, A. J. Mill, G. Constantine, K. G. Harrison and J. A. B. Gibson, A review of boron neutron capture therapy (BNCT) and the design and dosimetry of a high-intensity, 24 keV, neutron beam for BNCT research, The British Journal of Radiology, 61:1115, (1988)
3. C. A. Perks, G. Constantine and R. Birch, The design and dosimetry of an Al/S/Ar filtered neutron beam, in: Proc. 6th Int. Symp. on Neutron Dosimetry, Neuherberg, 12 - 16 October 1987, Radiat. Prot. Dosim., 23:329 (1988).
4. G. Constantine, P. R. D. Watkins, C. A. Perks, H. J. Delafield, D. Ross W. P. Voorbraak, A Paardekooper, W. E. Freudenreich, F. Stecher-Rasmussen and R. L. Moss, Progress in neutron beam development at the HFR Petten (feasibility study for a BNCT facility), in: Proc. 7th ASTM-EURATOM Symp. on Reactor Dosimetry, Strasbourg, 27 - 31 August 1990, to be published.
5. F Stecher-Rasmussen, G. Constantine, W. Freudenreich, W. P. Voorbraak, K. Ravensberg, C. A. Perks, H. J. Delafield, R. Moss and D. Ross, Characterisation of intermediate energy neutron beams for BNCT at the HFR in Petten, Paper to be presented at this Conference.
6. R. Birch, L. H. J. Peaple and H. J. Delafield, Measurement of neutron spectra with hydrogen proportional counters. Part 1, Spectrometry system and calibration. Report, AERE R-11397 (1984).
7. R. Birch, L. H. J. Peaple and H. J. Delafield, Measurement of neutron spectra with hydrogen proportional counters. Part 2, Analysis of proton recoil distributions, Report, AERE R-11398 (1984).
8. G. Constantine, A. Brenen, P. G. F. Moore, and C. A. Perks, Spectrum measurements on filtered neutron beams for medical applications, in: Reactor Dosimetry: Methods Applications and Standardisation, ASTM STP 1001, Harry Farrar IV and E. P. Lippincott, Eds., American Society for Testing and Materials, Philadelphia, pp 699 - 709 (1989).
9. A. K. McCracken and A. Packwood, The spectrum unfolding program SENSAK, AEEW ANSWERS (SENSAK) (1984).
10. P. M. Thomas, K. G. Harrison, and M. C. Scott, A multisphere spectrometer using a central ^{3}He detector, Nucl. Instrum. Meth., 224:225 (1984).
11. S. Croft and C. A. Perks, Corrections to the gamma-ray dosimetry measurements made in Harwell's two high intensity filtered neutron beams owing to their neutron sensitivity. in: Proc. 9th Int. Conf. on Solid State Dosimetry, Vienna, November 6 - 10 1989, Radiat. Prot. Dosim., 33:351 (1990)

RELATION BETWEEN TOLERANCE DOSE OF SKIN AND BORON-10 CONCENTRATION IN NEUTRON CAPTURE THERAPY FOR CUTANEOUS MELANOMA

Tooru Kobayashi[1], Keiji Kanda[1], Yowri Ujeno[1], Hiroshi Fukuda[2], Koichi Ando[2], Yutaka Mishima[3], Masamitsu Ichihashi[3] and Jun-ichi Hiratsuka[4]

1. Research Reactor Institute, Kyoto University,
   Kumatori-cho, Sennan-gun, Osaka 590-04, Japan
2. National Institute Radiological Sciences, Chiba 260, Japan
3. Kobe University School of Medicine, Chuo-ku, Kobe 650, Japan
4. Kawasaki Medical University, Matsushima, Kurashiki, Okayama 701-01, Japan

INTRODUCTION

In boron neutron capture therapy of cutaneous melanoma[1], damage to scalp, facial skin and eyes must be strictly avoided. Two basic irradiation conditions follow:

(1) Dose to normal skin and eyes except tumor parts must be less than the maximum tolerance dose.
(2) All of the tumor must be irradiated with more than the curative dose.

Since the absorbed dose depends on both neutron fluence and boron concentration[2,3], the upper and lower limits of irradiation dose are determined by the boron concentrations in normal tissue and tumor. In this report we describe these relationships through our clinical experiences in recently treated patients.

DOSE ESTIMATION

In boron neutron capture therapy using thermal neutrons, we have to estimate the absorbed dose in a mixed field of gamma rays and thermal neutrons. In the living body the $^{10}B(n,\alpha)^7Li$, $^{14}N(n,p)^{14}C$, $^{17}O(n,\alpha)^{14}C$, etc thermal neutron reactions yield heavy charged particles. The RBE value of gamma rays is different from that of the heavy charged particles. So for dose estimation in mixed fields RBE doses should be used. From the irradiation conditions above, the following inequalities are derived for the RBE dose for (1) normal and (2) tumor tissue. In this analysis we include the $^{10}B(n,\alpha)^7Li$ and $^{14}N(n,p)^{14}C$ reactions. Other reactions such as $^{17}O(n,\alpha)^{14}C$ are ignored because of their small contributions to total absorbed dose.

$$D_S(r) \geq G_S(r) + \{C_N \cdot R_N \cdot N_S + C_B \cdot R_B \cdot B_S(r)\} \, \Phi_S(r) \tag{1}$$
$$D_T(r) \leq G_T(r) + \{C_N \cdot R_N \cdot N_T + C_B \cdot R_B \cdot B_T(r)\} \, \Phi_T(r) \tag{2}$$

The symbols are defined as follows and (r) shows dependence on position:

$D_S(r)$	-	tolerance RBE dose for normal tissue (RBE $\cdot$ Gy)
$D_T(r)$	-	curative RBE dose for tumor tissue (RBE $\cdot$ Gy)
$G_S(r)$	-	absorbed dose of gamma rays for normal tissue (Gy)
$G_T(r)$	-	absorbed dose of gamma rays for tumor tissue (Gy)
N_S	-	^{14}N concentration for normal tissue (%)
N_T	-	^{14}N concentration for tumor tissue (%)
$B_S(r)$	-	^{10}B concentration for normal tissue (µg/g)
$B_T(r)$	-	^{10}B concentration for tumor tissue (µg/g)
$\Phi_S(r)$	-	thermal neutron fluence for normal tissue (n/cm^2)

$\Phi_T(r)$ - thermal neutron fluence for tumor tissue (n/cm^2)
R_N - the RBE of the $^{14}N(n,p)^{14}C$ reaction
R_B - the RBE of the $^{10}B(n,\alpha)^7Li$ reaction
C_B - dose conversion factor for ^{10}B {$Gy/(\mu g/g)/(n/cm^2)$}
C_N - dose conversion factor for ^{14}N {$Gy/\%/(n/cm^2)$}

Generally N_S, N_T, R_N and R_B are also dependent on position.

In clinical irradiations, the distributions of thermal neutron fluence, $\Phi_C(r)$ and of absorbed gamma dose, $G_C(r)$, for both normal and tumor tissue regions can be roughly estimated before irradiation. From the inequalities above, the maximum thermal neutron fluence for normal tissue, $\Phi_{SO}(r)$, and the minimum thermal neutron fluence for tumor, $\Phi_{TO}(r)$, are calculated as follows:

$$\Phi_{SO}(r) = \{D_S(r) - G_S(r)\} / \{C_N \cdot R_N \cdot N_S + C_B \cdot R_B \cdot B_S(r)\} \tag{3}$$
$$\Phi_{TO}(r) = \{D_T(r) - G_T(r)\} / \{C_N \cdot R_N \cdot N_T + C_B \cdot R_B \cdot B_T(r)\} \tag{4}$$

Figure 1 shows the relationships between $D_S(r)$, $D_T(r)$, $B_S(r)$, $B_T(r)$, $G_C(r)$, $\Phi_C(r)$, $\Phi_{SO}(r)$ and $\Phi_{TO}(r)$, which satisfy (3) and (4). $\Phi_{SO}(r)$ depends mainly upon $D_S(r)$ and $B_S(r)$ and $\Phi_{TO}(r)$ depends upon $D_T(r)$ and $B_T(r)$. From this figure the thermal neutron fluence, $\Phi_C(r)$, for clinical irradiations can be determined since it must lie between $\Phi_{SO}(r)$ and $\Phi_{TO}(r)$.

In the present study, we assume that tumor and normal tissue are located in the same position. The depth dose distribution is not taken into account. So these values are applicable only for the superficially located layer. Hereafter, we will use these symbols without (r). Accordingly, $\Phi_{SO}(r)$ and $\Phi_{TO}(r)$ are rewritten as Φ upper and Φ lower, respectively. To satisfy these clinical irradiation conditions, B_S and B_T, Φ upper and Φ lower must satisfy the following:

$$B_T \geq D_T \cdot B_S/D_S + \{(D_T/D_S-1)K + (D_T \cdot N_S/D_S - N_T)C_N \cdot R_N\}/(C_B \cdot R_B) \tag{5}$$
$$\Phi \text{ upper} = D_S/(K + C_N \cdot R_N \cdot N_S + C_B \cdot R_B \cdot B_S) \tag{6}$$
$$\Phi \text{ lower} = D_T/(K + C_N \cdot R_N \cdot N_T + C_B \cdot R_B \cdot B_T) \tag{7}$$

Here, K {$Gy/(n/cm^2)$} is the ratio of the total gamma ray dose to thermal neutron fluence during clinical irradiation.

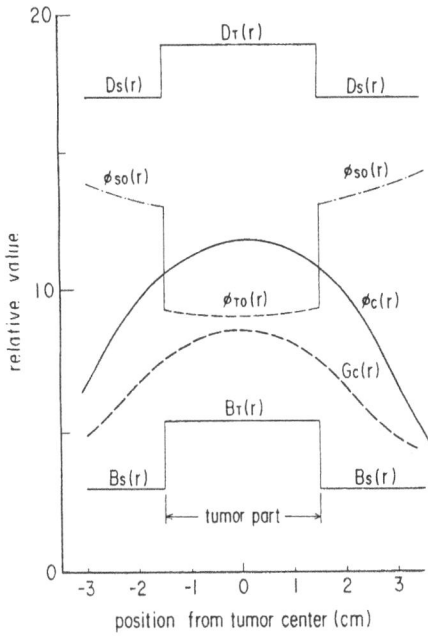

Figure 1.   Relationships among the $D_S(r)$, $D_T(r)$, $B_S(r)$, $B_T(r)$, $G_C(r)$, $\Phi_C(r)$, $\Phi_{SO}(r)$ and $\Phi_{TO}(r)$
The thermal neutron fluence for clinical irradiations $\Phi_C(r)$ is determined as lying between $\Phi_{SO}(r)$ and $\Phi_{TO}(r)$.

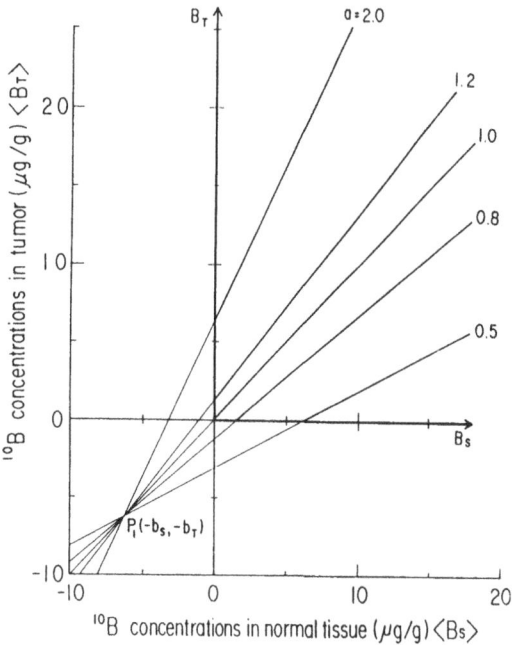

Figure 2.   The minimum ^{10}B concentration for a curative dose, B_T as a function of B_s in accordance with inequality (5.1), for D_T/D_s varying from 0.5 to 2.0, and K = 50 x 10^{-14}.

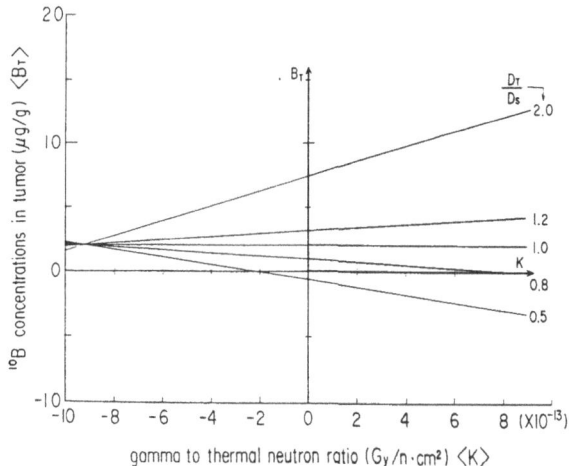

Figure 3.   The minimum ^{10}B concentration for a curative dose, B_T as a function of K in accordance with inequality (5.2), for D_T/D_s varying from 0.5 to 2.0 and B_s = 2 µg/g.

The parameter D_T/D_S was varied in inequality (5) which can be rewritten as follows:

$$B_T \geq D_T/D_S \{B_S + (N_S \cdot C_N \cdot R_N + K)/(C_B \cdot R_B)\} - (N_T \cdot C_N \cdot R_N + K)/(C_B \cdot R_B)$$
$$= a(B_S + b_S) - b_T \tag{5.1}$$
$$B_T \geq (D_T/D_S - 1)(K + N_S \cdot C_N \cdot R_N + B_S \cdot C_B \cdot R_B)/(C_B \cdot R_B)$$
$$+ B_S + C_N \cdot R_N \cdot (N_S - N_T)/(C_B \cdot R_B) \tag{5.2}$$

Except where otherwise stated, the values of parameters used in this study are as follow:
$D_S = 18$, $D_T = 25$, $K = 50 \times 10^{-14}$, $N_S = N_T = 3.48$, $R_N = R_B = 2.5$, $C_N = 6.782 \times 10^{-14}$ and $C_B = 6.933 \times 10^{-14}$. The thermal neutron energy spectrum is assumed to be the 40°C Maxwellian distribution in tissue. So we should use 85.35 b ($\times 10^{-24}$ cm^2) for the average activation cross section of gold foil or wire for thermal neutron monitors. For the specific case of cutaneous skin cancer, we examined the numerical response of both parameters, D_T and D_S, to B_T and B_S. D_T/D_S is very sensitive to the selectivity of the treatment (Figure 2). In the extreme case, where D_T/D_S is smaller than unity, ^{10}B administration is not needed. The lower limit of B_T, namely, the minimum ^{10}B concentration for a curative dose, is affected by the K value (Figure 3). In the KUR, the K values change from $2 \sim 6 \times 10^{-13}$ Gy/n/cm^2. The effect of K on B_T is only a few µg/g, at most.

From Figure 4, we can easily decide the feasibility of treatment, and also estimate the maximum and minimum thermal neutron fluences. For example the point $A(B_S, B_T)$ in Figure 4 lies above line (1), hence treatment is feasible for a patient with skin and tumor ^{10}B concentrations of B_S and B_T respectively. Of course, B_T and B_S must be estimated before irradiation.

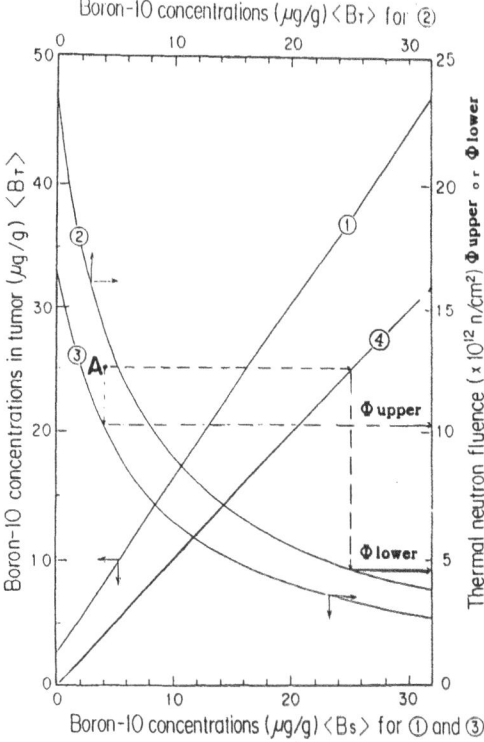

Figure 4.   An inequality for judging the feasibility of BNCT treatment and relationships
for Φ upper and Φ lower   (1) $B_T \geq 1.39B_S + 2.45$ (2) Φ lower=$1.44 \times 10^{14}/(B_T + 6.29)$
(3) Φ upper=$1.04 \times 10^{14}/(B_s + 6.29)$ (4) $B_T = B_S$

We treated two patients with malignant melanoma using KUR in 1990. Boron-10 concentrations for these cases were measured before clinical irradiation with prompt gamma ray spectroscopy[4,5] using the KUR neutron guide tube. The values for B_T and B_S were 5-10 and 2-4 µg/g respectively, with errors of several tens % derived from the assumptions in the estimation[6]. Boron-10 concentrations of these cases were not large but we finally judged that they narrowly satisfied the conditions for BNCT defined in this paper. We aimed to irradiate with thermal neutron fluences of 1.0×10^{13} and 1.35×10^{13} n/cm^2, respectively. The difference in fluence for the two cases was due to medical conditions such as tumor thickness and pre-irradiated dose.

CONCLUSION

For cutaneous melanoma, irradiation conditions can be examined numerically using tolerance and curative doses. Although the measured ^{10}B concentration or the estimated one from other data contains some inaccuracy, we can determine the intensity of thermal neutron fluence needed for the treatment.

REFERENCES

1. Mishima Y., C. Honda, M. Ichihashi, H. Obara, J Hiratsuka, H. Fukuda, H. Karashima, T. Kobayashi, K. Kanda and K. Yoshino, THE LANCET, August 12 (1989) 388-389.
2. Kobayashi T. and K. Kanda, Radiat. Res., 91 (1982) 77-94.
3. Kobayashi T. and K. Kanda, Boron-Neutron Capture Therpay for Tumors, (Edit. H. Hatanaka), Nishimura, Niigata, Japan (1986) 298-300.
4. Kobayashi T. and K. Kanda, Nucl. Instr. Meth. 204 (1983) 525-531.
5. Kobayashi T., K. Kanda, Y. Ujeno and M.R. Ishida, Neutron Beam Design, Development and Performance for Neutron Capture Therapy, (Edit. O.K. Harling), Plenum, NY (1990) 321-339.
6. Kobayashi T., K. Kanda and Y. Mishima, Strahlentherapie und Onkologie 165 (1989) 104-106.

TREATMENT PLANNING FOR NEUTRON CAPTURE THERAPY OF GLIO-BLASTOMA MULTIFORME USING AN EPITHERMAL NEUTRON BEAM FROM THE MITR-II RESEARCH REACTOR AND MONTE CARLO SIMULATION

R. Zamenhof[1], J. Brenner[1], J. Yanch, D. Wazer[1], H. Madoc-Jones[1], S. Saris[1], O. Harling[2]

[1]Tufts University School of Medicine and New England Medical Center Hospitals, Boston, MA 02111, USA
[2]Massachusetts Institute of Technology, Cambridge, MA 02139, USA

INTRODUCTION

This paper describes the practical implementation of treatment planning procedures we have developed for the proposed clinical trial of neutron capture therapy (NCT) at NEMC and MIT in the Fall of 1991. Proper treatment planning for any form of radiation therapy is beneficial not only for the safety and optimal management of the patient, but can provide a valuable tool for performing radiological/pathological correlation in those patients who ultimately fail NCT.

MATERIALS AND METHODS

A previous paper[1] has described in detail the techniques and supporting software that we utilize for NCT treatment planning. A schematic overview is shown in Fig. 1. For the examples to be shown, the patient's CT scans were obtained on a Siemens DR-3 CT scanner using 125 kVp, 480 mAs, 2 mm contiguous transverse scans parallel to the base of the skull, and a hardware zoom factor of 2X. The scans were performed with nonionic contrast. The patient had cytoreductive surgery for a grade III/IV astrocytoma in the occipital region, and at the time of the acquisition of the CT scans had been implanted with high-activity ^{125}I seeds.

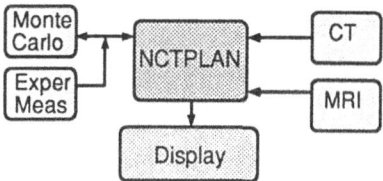

Fig. 1.   Schematic overview of the NCT treatment planning code NCTPLAN.

RESULTS

Based on preliminary results of a biodistribution and pharmacokinetic study of *p*-boronophenylalanine (BPA) in patients with glioblastoma multiforme currently in progress at NEMC, a ^{10}B concentration of 50 ppm (by weight) is assumed for tumor, and a conservative tumor-to-normal brain ^{10}B ratio of 3:1. Additionally, based on recommendations of experts in the field[2], the RBE factors applied to the various radiation components are: 2.3 for the ^{10}B dose, 1.6 for neutron dose, and 0.5 for gamma dose (the latter factor is our own choice, based upon the assumption that NCT treatments will be delivered in 5-6 daily fractions).

Fig. 2 shows isodose contours computed by MCNP and NCTPLAN for an anatomical plane corresponding to the widest level of the brain, which in this case does not contain tumor. The 18 cm diameter currently installed MITR-II epithermal neutron beam (M-055) is incident laterally on the patient's head. The thick elliptically shaped contour (labelled "AD") is the planar advantage depth contour. Definitions of NCT treatment planning parameters such as advantage depth, regional and global advantage ratio, and advantage depth dose rate have been published elsewhere[1]. If the maximum dose to normal structures is designated 100% (or the AD contour), then the contours inside the AD contour represent the corresponding doses to tumor (100%, 120%, 140%, 160%, and 180%), while the contours outside the AD contour represent the corresponding doses to normal structures (100%, 60%, 40%, and 20%) Tumor isodose contours outside the AD contour and normal structure isodose contours inside the AD contour have been omitted for clarity of presentation. It may be observed that a superficial tumor in the left hemisphere would receive a dose of at least 100%, whereas distant occult tumor cells in the right hemisphere would receive substantially lower dose. The total integral dose to tumor divided by the total integral dose to normal structures has been previously defined as the global advantage ratio (GAR)[1], and has a value of 1.75 under the present treatment configuration.

Fig. 3 shows a similar display to Fig. 2 except that a two-beam, equally weighted, parallel-opposed (POP) irradiation is assumed. Since the maximum normal structure dose is a global maximum, the % values assigned to the contours in this figure and subsequent figures are all internally consistent. With POP irradiation a much larger region of the brain is encompassed by the AD contour, showing that the M-055 epithermal neutron beam is suited to treating identifiable disease and occult tumor cells essentially anywhere within the brain in this anatomical plane.

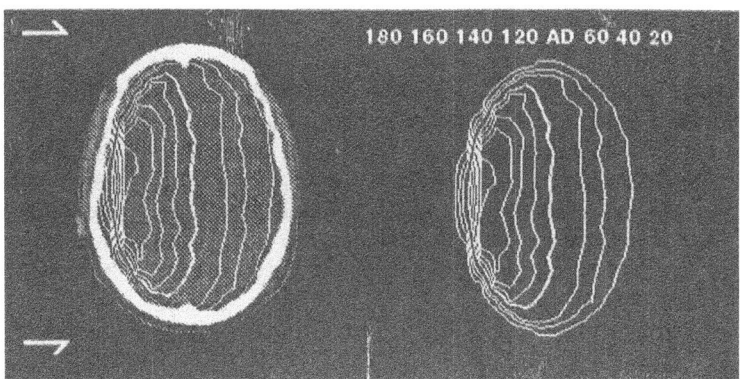

Fig. 2. Transverse CT scan through widest plane of the brain (no tumor visible). Epithermal neutron beam is incident from left. Isodoses inside thick AD contour are tumor isodoses (100, 120, 140, 160, and 180%), and those outside AD contour are normal structure isodoses (100, 60, 40, and 20%).

Figure 4 shows a transverse dose plane through the residual enhancing tumor mass and its associated edema. Once again a POP irradiation is assumed and the AD contour is seen as encompassing essentially the whole brain in this anatomical plane.

Figure 5 shows a sagittal anatomical plane passing through the pituitary and thebrainstem. Hatanaka has reported[3] that some of his patients treated for grade III/IV astrocytomas who received elevated radiation doses to the deeper intracranial structures developed transient diabetes insipidus, thus implicating some degree of transient radiation

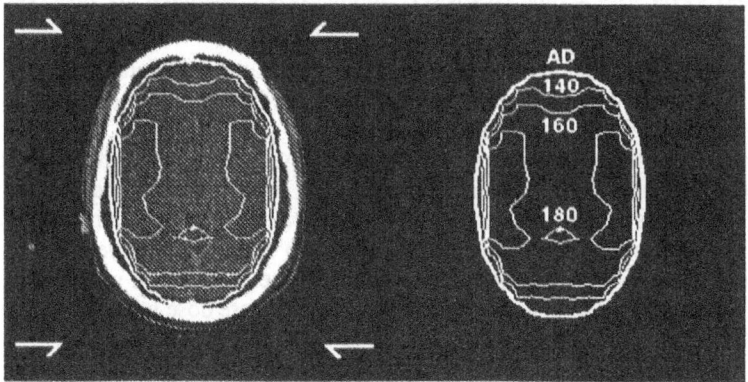

Fig. 3. Similar to Fig. 2, except that two POP beams are used. AD contour encompasses essentially the entire brain. No normal structure isodoses are shown.

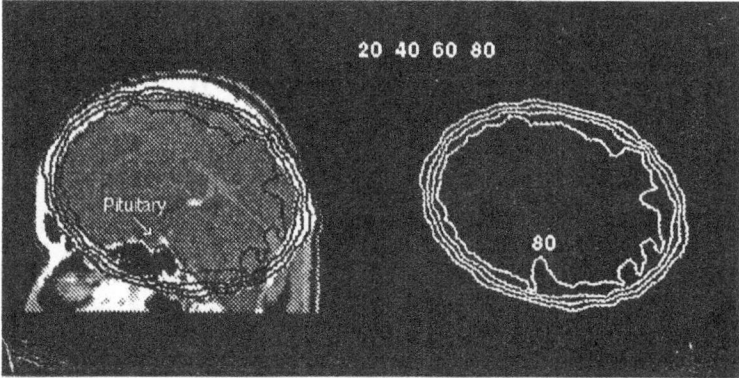

Fig. 4. Tumor isodoses for POP fields through plane which includes tumor. Residual tumor is essentially enclosed by AD contour (100% tumor isodose), while area of edema is essentially enclosed by 140% tumor isodose.

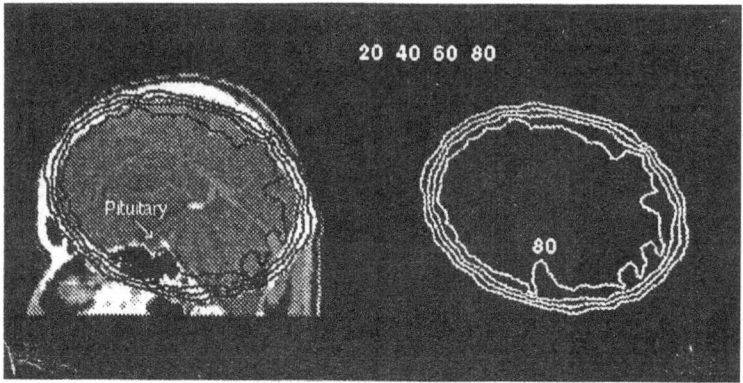

Fig. 5. Reformatted sagittal anatomical plane through brain midline showing pituitary and brainstem. Normal brain isodoses are for POP lateral fields.

injury to the pituitary. With the deeper penetration of an epithermal neutron beam, such sequelae may occur with greater frequency. In the present example, the dose received by the pituitary is 80%.

As is well recognized in conventional radiation therapy, the tolerance of brain tissue and its vasculature depends not only on absolute dose but also on the volume of tissue receiving that dose. Normal brain dose histograms are produced by NCTPLAN to aid in the assessment of this effect on brain tolerance . Figure 6 shows a planar differential normal brain dose histogram for this patient . It can be seen that the normal brain dose (using POP fields) is rather uniform, shown by the peak of the histogram "pointing" to a relatively narrow band of dose values. Normalized to equal cumulative areas under the histograms (i.e., equal integral doses) such an even dose distribution would result in the ability to deliver more dose to tumor than if there were severe dose inhomogeneities in the normal brain.

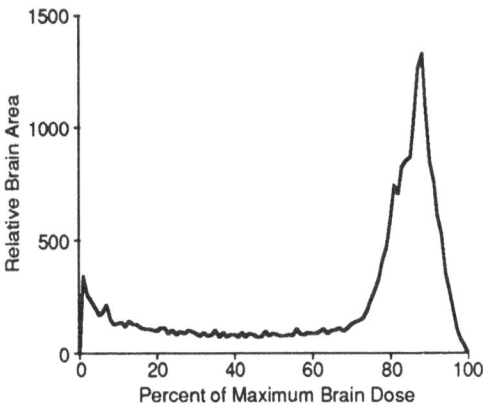

Fig. 6. Planar differential normal brain dose histogram for treatment configuration shown in Fig. 3. A majority of normal brain dose is seen to fall in the 75%-100% range.

SUMMARY

We have illustrated the NCT treatment planning capabilities that have been developed at NEMC in anticipation of NCT clinical trials for the treatment of grade III/IV astrocytomas in the Fall of 1991. We have shown the application of concepts such as advantage depth, advantage ratio, and normal brain differential dose histograms to NCT treatment planning, and have demonstrated the value of superimposing isodose contours on diagnostic CT scans of corresponding anatomical planes to permit both tumor and normal structure doses to be more accurately assessed.

Recent developments in NCTPLAN enable the Monte Carlo anatomical model to be automatically specified from the CT scan data, thereby customizing the treatment plan to each individual patient.

ACKNOWLEDGMENTS

This research has been partly supported by U.S. DOE Grant No. DE-FG02-87ER6060.

REFERENCES

1. R. G. Zamenhof, S. D. Clement, O. K. Harling, J. F. Brenner, D. E. Wazer, H. Madoc-Jones, and J. C. Yanch, "Monte Carlo Based Dosimetry and Treatment Planning for Neutron Capture Therapy of Brain Tumors," In: Neutron Beam Design, Development, and Performance for Neutron Capture Therapy, Plenum Press, NY (1990).

2. O. K. Harling, J. Bernard, R. G. Zamenhof, (Eds.) "Introduction," In: Neutron Beam Design, Development, and Performance for Neutron Capture Therapy, Plenum Press, New York (1990).

3. Dr. H. Hatanaka, personal communication.

ENHANCEMENT OF TUMOR DOSE BY THE GADOLINIUM NEUTRON CAPTURE REACTION IN Cf-252 BRACHYTHERAPY

J. Wierzbicki[1], Y. Maruyama[1], R. Martin[2]

[1]University of Kentucky Medical Center, Lexington, KY USA
[2]Peter MacCallum Cancer Institute, Melbourne, Victoria, Australia

Neutron capture therapy (NCT) applied by means of an external neutron beam has been extensively studied in the last 3 decades. Another option for the neutron capture (NC) reaction, the enhancement of tumor dose by interstitial Californium-252 implant, has been proposed recently[9]. Most sigmoid dose response curves for neutron irradiation are very steep and therefore even a small (few %) enhancement of tumor dose may dramatically change the clinical outcome. The potential of boron-10 as a capture agent is very well known but new methods of selective delivery of other isotopes into tumor cells may make them useful in NCT.

In this paper we address the potential of Gadolinium-157 to be used for neutron capture enhancement in Cf-252 implant. Neutron capture by Gd-157 has a large cross section (255,000 barns), produces gamma rays and is therefore considered to be of lesser importance for NCT. However, the majority of photons produced in this reaction are of low energy and are accompanied by emission of low energy conversion, Auger and Coster-Kronig electrons.

Radiative thermal neutron capture in Gd-157 nuclei has been studied in a number of laboratories[1]. Spectroscopy of gamma radiation and conversion electrons have been summarized in collaborative papers[2].

The decay of the compound nucleus Gd-158 of 7.937 MeV excitation energy may be divided into two groups; primary high energy transitions (7.857 MeV to 3.7 MeV) and secondary low energy transitions (79.5 keV to 2.2 MeV). Almost all de-exciting transitions go through the two lowest levels (79.5 keV and 261.44 keV) of Gd-158 and transition from the 261.44 keV level to ground level is forbidden by selection rules. Therefore, the intensity of 79.5 keV and 181.93 keV lines are the highest.

An alternative way of de-excitation is internal conversion. In this process the energy of the excited nucleus is transferred to the electron and the electron leaves the atom with the energy, $E_{exc} - E_B$, where E_B is binding energy of the electron in the atom. The relative probability of electron conversion is described by the internal conversion yields:

$$\alpha = \frac{\text{number of conversions in a given shell}}{\text{number of } \gamma \text{ transitions}}$$

*Supported in part by funds from the Physician Service Plan
Awarded by the College of Medicine
University of Kentucky

Conversion yield decreases with increasing transition energy and that means that internal conversion plays a significant role only for very low energies. For primary, high energy transitions (3.7 - 7.9 MeV) in Gd-158, emission of conversion electrons is negligibly small, $\alpha = 10^{-5}$, but for de-excitation of the two lowest states in the K and L shells, internal conversion plays an important role. For the first excited state 79.51 keV, the probability of electron emission is about 6 times higher than the probability of γ ray emission.

Approximately 0.76 conversion electrons[4] are emitted per neutron capture. More than 90% of them are K electrons de-exciting the first energy level of Gd-157. The binding energy of K and L electrons in Gd-158 is 50.1 keV and 8.3 keV respectively. Therefore, K and L conversion electrons will be emitted with energies of 30 keV and 71 keV respectively. As a result of conversions, we have an empty place in the atomic K or L shell. Further de-excitation of such atoms may proceed by emission of a cascade of Auger and Coster-Kronig electrons. Energies of these electrons are $E_{klm} = 40$ keV, $E_{lmn} = 7$ keV, $E_{mno} = 3$ keV and smaller.

Cf-252 As A Source Of Thermal Neutrons

Cf-252 brachytherapy is based on interactions of fast neutrons with tissue nuclei. Fast neutrons lose their energy by multiple scattering on tissue nuclei (mainly by hydrogen) and finally become thermalized. These thermal neutrons do not play any role in radiotherapy. They may interact with hydrogen or with nitrogen nuclei but the cell killing effect of these reactions is negligibly small compared to cell killing by recoiled protons or by primary photons. Our project is aimed at evaluating Gd-157 compounds to enhance Cf-252 implants by utilizing the thermalized neutrons, which otherwise make virtually no contribution to dose. To evaluate the neutron capture contribution to tumor dose, one has to know the thermal neutron flux in the vicinity of implanted Cf-252 sources. Flux measurements in the center of a volume implanted by four 21 μg Cf sources give values of about 2×10^6 n/cm^{2}s.

Gd-157 Dose Calculations

We assumed for our calculations that the tumor is a sphere with diameter of 6cm and that concentration of Gd-157 in tumor cells is 160μg/cm^3. The number of interactions of thermal neutrons with Gd-157 nuclei calculated for flux 2×10^6 n/cm^{2}s was 2.8×10^5cm^{-3}s^{-1}. In one

TABLE 1

THERMAL NEUTRON FLUX AND NEUTRON/
PHOTON DOSE RATES IN THE CENTRAL POINT
OF CIRCULATORY IMPLANTED (DIAMETER 6 cm)
Cf SOURCES 21 μg EACH

THERMAL FLUX	cm^{-2}s^{-1}	$2 \ 10^6$
FAST NEUTRON DOSE	cGy/hr	17
PHOTON DOSE	cGy/hr	9.76
Gd-NEUTRON CAPTURE DOSE (160 μg Gd/cm^3)	cGy/hr	9

reaction almost 8 MeV of gamma radiation is released. A significant part of this energy, about 0.5 MeV, is released in the tumor. That gives us a gamma dose rate from the gadolinium-neutron-capture equal to about 9 cGy/hr.

This dose rate doubles the gamma dose rate in a volume implant (see Table 1). It has been pointed out in numerous experimental and theoretical studies[7,8] that the biological effectiveness of gamma irradiation has a strong dose rate dependence. Therefore, doubling the gamma dose rate may mean increased biological dose, and for this radiation, the location of the Gd reaction in the cell is not important.

Conversion Electrons

The number of conversion electrons released per cm^3 of the implant volume will be about 7.7×10^8 cm^{-3} hr^{-1} and the average energy released in internal conversion followed by a cascade of Auger and Coster-Kronig electrons will be less than 80keV. Simple calculations gives us a dose rate produced by these electrons less than 0.9cGy/hr.

This dose rate is so small that if centers of reactions are distributed isotropically in the cell, then electron radiation may not play any role in cell killing.

This prediction is supported by the results of thermal neutron capture experiments which investigated the effects of including Gadolinium citrate during thermal neutron irradiation of V79 cells. Concentrations of more than 1mM Gd citrate, are required for significant enhancement of cell kill, as determined by clonogenic survival[6,10].

Auger and KK Electrons

However, the biological effectiveness of conversion, Auger and Coster-Kronig electrons from Gd-157 neutron capture will be much greater if the Gd-157 is DNA-bound. In particular, DNA double-strand breaks are observed[5], as would be expected from the well established vacancy cascade effects of the decay of DNA-bound I-125[6]. If the biological effectiveness of the DNA-associated events are similar for Gd-157 NC and I-125 decay, then a D_{37} for Gd-NC on DNA will be the order of 50 events per genome. A Gd-157 labelled-DNA ligand could be used to ensure the Gd-NC events were DNA associated. At a thermal neutron flux of 2×10^6 cm^{-2} s^{-1} a 10 hour exposure would yield 2×10^{-8} Gd NC reactions per Gd-157 atom. Thus, in order to achieve a D_{37} dose, about 2.5×10^8 Gd-157 atoms will be required per cell. This approaches saturation binding by a DNA ligand, given that the diploid human chromosome corresponds with 6.6×10^9 bp. This in turn implies a requirement for a Gd-157 labelled DNA ligand that is bio-chemically non-toxic at saturation levels of binding to nuclear DNA.

Conclusion

There is potential to exploit the high thermal neutron capture cross section of Gd-157 to enhance Cf-252 brachytherapy. The gamma component of Gd-157 NC would effectively double the gamma dose rate for a typical Cf-252 implant, if the concentration of the Gd enhancer in the tumor was 160μg/g. Exploitation of low energy electrons that are emitted as a consequence of internal conversion during the Gd NC event will require the development of suitable Gd-157-labelled DNA ligands. The extent of enhancement that might be obtained depends on the biological effectiveness of the DNA-associated Gd NC event, which is yet to be determined.

REFERENCES

1. Groshev, L.V., et al, 1968. Comparison Of Thermal-Neutron-Capture γ Ray Measurements, Part II: Z=47 to Z=67 (Ag to Ho). Nuclear Data Tables, A5, 1-242.

2. Greenwood, R.C., et al, 1978. Collective and Two-Quasiparticle States In ^{158}Gd Observed Through Radiation Neutron Capture in ^{157}Gd. Nuclear Physics. A304:327-428.

3. Wierzbicki, J., Alexander, C.W., Yaes, R.J., Maruyama. Y. Boron-Neutron-Capture Enhancement In Californium Brachytherapy. Radiology. 173:362, 1989.

4. Charlton, D.E. and Humm, J.L. A method of calculating initial DNA strand breakage following the decay of incorporated ^{125}I. Int. Radiat. Biol., Vol. 53, No. 3:353-365, 1988.

5. Martin, R.F., D'Cunha, G., Pardee, M., Allen, B.J. Induction of double-strand breaks following neutron capture by DNA-bound ^{157}Gd. Int. Radiat. Biol., Vol. 54, No. 2:205-208, 1988.

6. Martin, R.F., D'Cunha, G., Pardee, M., Whittaker, A., Kelly, D.P., Allen, B.J. These Proceedings.

7. Orton, C.G., Brit. J. Radiol. 47:603, 1974.

8. Dutreix, J. Expression of the Dose Rate Effect in Clinical Curietherapy. Radiotherapy and Oncol. 15:25-37, 1989.

9. Wierzbicki, J.G., Yaes, R.J., Maruyama, Y. Role of Thermal Neutrons in Californium-252 Brachytherapy. International Neutron Therapy Workshop, Lexington, Kentucky, Nucl. Sci. Appl. (in press), 1991.

10. Akine, Y., Tokita, N., Matsumoto, T., Oyama, H., Egawa, S., Aizawa, O. Cell Survival Studies on Gadolinium Neutron Capture Reactions. International Neutron Therapy Workshop, Lexington, Kentucky, Nucl. Sci. Appl. (in press), (1991).

GADOLINIUM AS A NEUTRON CAPTURE THERAPY AGENT

J.A. Shih and R.M. Brugger

Nuclear Engineering Program and Research Reactor, University of
Missouri-Columbia, Columbia, MO 65211, USA

The isotope ^{157}Gd has been evaluated at the University of Missouri-
Columbia (MU) as an alternative neutron capture therapy (NCT) agent to ^{10}B.
The studies were directed to the following three major portions: the
evaluation of Gd Neutron Capture Therapy (GdNCT), the combination of NCT
and brachytherapy and the development of neutron autoradiography for Gd.

GADOLINIUM NEUTRON CAPTURE THERAPY. Chemicals that are used to
enhance MRI may be effective for GdNCT. It is estimated that a tumor
concentration of up to 300 μg ^{157}Gd/g tumor can be achieved with the
injection of 0.5 mmole/kg body weight of Gd-DTPA or Gd-DOTA.[1] Monte
Carlo calculations with MCNP show that GdNCT can deliver at least 2,000 cGy
of Gd prompt gamma dose to a tumor of 2 cm diameter or larger with 250 μg
^{157}Gd/g of tumor. To verify the calculations, gamma dose in plastic
phantoms was measured with Kodak Industrex M2 films. The code MCNP
calculates Kerma while the measurements assessed absorbed dose. These
results are both presented as doses.

The measurements were done with a thermal neutron beam at the
Missouri University Research Reactor (MURR) and with an epithermal neutron
beam at the Brookhaven Medical Research Reactor (BMRR). Two sets of the
film measurements were made. One set was made with ready-packed films
which were covered by a light-tight paper cover. The other set was made
with bare films and the entire phantom was enclosed in a light-tight paper
box. The first set of measurements provided the information of Gd prompt
gamma exposure only and the second set revealed the combined effect of
prompt gammas and the Auger electrons.[2,3]

The optical density (OD) on the films were converted to dose by using
a characteristic curve of Gd prompt gammas. This curve was obtained by
extrapolating the characteristic curves of ^{60}Co and ^{125}I by their mass
absorption coefficients of AgBr. The measurements agree with the
calculations. The results of the phantom containing the 3.5 cm diameter
tumor phantom and the MURR beam are compared in Figure 1.a. The higher
curve in the figure shows that the Auger electrons deposit energy to the
tumor phantom. The Auger effect should enhance the therapeutic effect of
GdNCT. The difference between the two curves is an Auger electron effect.
The "Auger Dose" was translated directly from the OD's with the gamma dose
calibration curve.

Calculations were done with MCNP to compare the dose distributions of GdNCT and BNCT. The model used was a tissue equivalent phantom of 20 x 20 x 20 cm^3 with a 4 cm long cylindrical tumor of 4 cm diameter buried 3 cm behind the incident surface of the neutrons. The axis of the cylinder is on the axis of the neutron beam which has a cross section of 20 x 20 cm^2 and most of the neutrons are epithermal. No NCT agents were distributed in the phantom other than the tumor. The result is shown in Figure 1.b. The dose of BNCT drops rapidly at the edges of the tumor but the dose of GdNCT also decreases rapidly due to the inverse square factor. Some effect of neutron flux suppression is observed on the back side of the tumor which also contributes to the dose drop-off of GdNCT. Gadolinium NCT shows comparable dose distribution to BNCT.

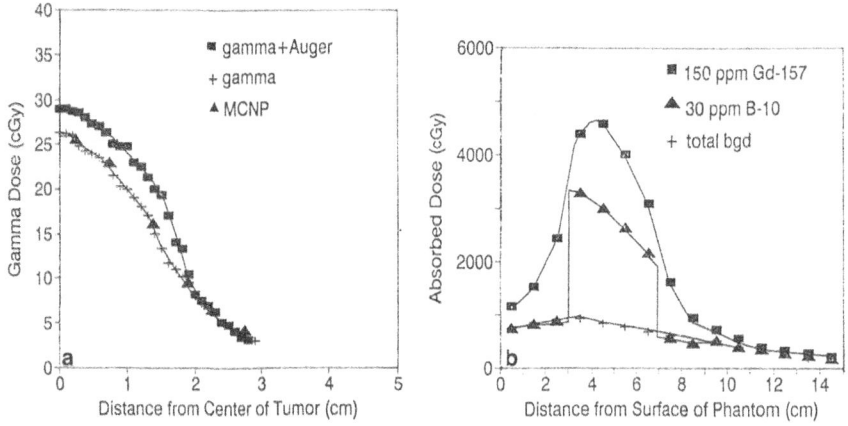

Figure 1 a) Calculated and measured results of a 3.5 cm diameter tumor containing 162.5 ppm ^{157}Gd irradiated with the MURR beam 5.2 x 10^{10} n/cm^2; b) dose distributions of BNCT and GdNCT with T/N=∞, 5 x 10^{12} source neutrons/cm^2

NEUTRON INDUCED BRACHYTHERAPY (NIB). Gadolinium NCT with solid Gd sources bears interesting properties. It reduces the personnel dose, its dose rate is controllable and fractionation can be easily applied. Monte Carlo based treatment planning indicates that at least 5,000 cGy of Gd prompt gamma dose can be delivered to a treatment volume of 40 cm^3 with a 3-plane implant of a total of nine 5 cm long Gd needles. The dose drop-off is similar to that of ^{60}Co implants. Figure 2.a shows the isodose curves of this case. Dose measurements similar to those described above were performed to verify these calculations. The results match well with the calculations (Figure 2.b). Gadolinium NIB can be used to treat most solid tumors that are suitable for brachytherapy. Larger treatment volumes can be treated with longer needles. Calculations show that longer Gd needles not only cover a bigger volume but deliver higher dose to the volume. This method alleviates the difficulty of delivering the NCT agent into the tumor. Neutron induced brachytherapy appears to be a promising therapeutic technique.

NEUTRON AUTORADIOGRAPHY. An imaging technique that displays and quantifies the distribution of ^{157}Gd is important for studying GdNCT. Neutron autoradiography has been developed to meet this criterium. Neutron autoradiographs of sliced samples containing stable Gd were obtained by placing the samples in a cassette next to Kodak Industrex SR film and irradiated with neutrons. The Auger electrons emitted in the Gd neutron capture reactions exposed the film. The OD's can be converted to concentrations of ^{157}Gd by comparing with a calibration curve obtained with

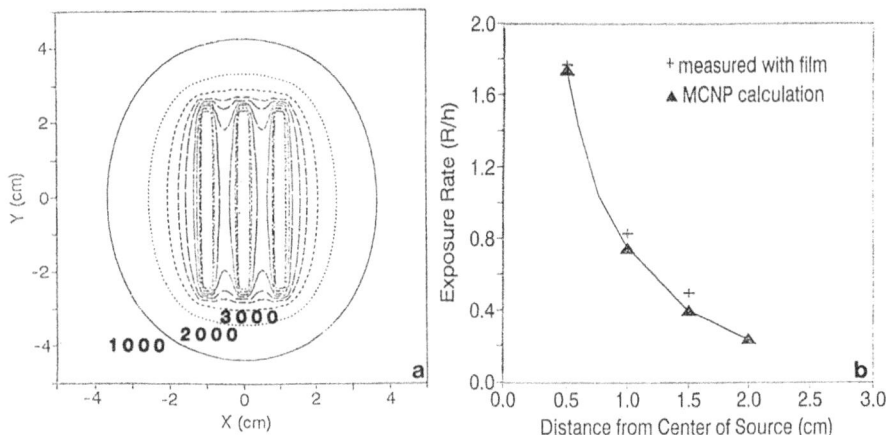

Figure 2 a) The isodose curves of a 3-plane implant of a total of 9 Gd needles (5 cm long and 0.1 cm diameter) with 5×10^{12} n/cm^2 source neutrons; b) calculated and measured results of a 2.5 cm long needle with 0.1 cm x 0.06 cm cross section irradiated with the MURR beam, 5×10^6 n/cm^2 sec.

Figure 3 - A neutron autoradiography of a rat bone sample containing Gd taken with the MURR beam.

standard samples. A neutron autoradiograph of a rat femur sample containing Gd is show in Figure 3. The intrinsic spatial resolution of this system used at MU is 70 μm. The technique is able to determine ^{157}Gd concentration ranges from 20 to 500 ppm. A neutron beam which has a neutron to gamma ratio of 10^8 n·hr/cm^2·sec·R is required to obtain high quality images.

Monte Carlo calculations show that GdNCT and NIB provide high tumor dose and good healthy tissue sparing. Measurements in phantoms verified the calculations. Gadolinium appears to be a promising alternate of B as a NCT agent.

ACKNOWLEDGEMENTS

The authors thank the MURR and the BNL for support during this research.

REFERENCES

[1] J.A. Shih, "Gadolinium as a Neutron Capture Therapy Agent", PhD dissertation, University of Missouri-Columbia, May 1991

[2] R.M. Brugger and J.A. Shih, "Evaluation of ^{157}Gd as a Neutron Capture Therapy Agent", Strahlentherapie und Onkologie, Proceedings of the 3rd International Symposium on Neutron Capture Therapy, Bremen, FRG, 1988, Urban and Vogel, FRG, 1989

[3] R.F. Martin, G. d'Cunha, M. Pardee, and B.J. Allen, "Induction of Double-Strand Breaks Following Neutron Capture by DNA-Bound Gd-157", Int. J. Rad. Biol. Phys. Chem. Med., accepted 1987

BORON NEUTRON CAPTURE ENHANCEMENT IN CF-252 BRACHYTHERAPY

J. Wierzbicki[1], Y. Maruyama[1], C. Alexander[2]

[1]University of Kentucky Medical Center, Lexington, KY USA
[2]Oak Ridge National Laboratory, Oak Ridge, TN USA

Supported in part by funds from the Physician Service Plan Awarded
by the College of Medicine, University of Kentucky

In this paper we address the potential of Cf-252 for neutron capture
therapy in brachytherapy where capture agents are used to enhance
treatment efficacy.

Total dose in Cf-252 (Cf) therapy is the sum of neutron and photon
dose, and may be calculated using along and away tables[1,2,3]. Biological
dose requires adjustments for biological effects of neutrons and is
prescribed in dose-equivalents i.e., Gy-eq. It follows the formula:

$$D_{Gy-eq} = RBE\ D_n + D_\gamma$$

where RBE is the relative biological effectiveness (RBE) of the Cf
neutrons. RBE depends on dose rate and type of cells or biological
system under study. To obtain reliable values for clinical use, one
ultimately has to evaluate clinical data about tumor control and normal
tissue complications. At the University of Kentucky, the RBE values for
Cf neutrons used in the carcinoma of the cervix trials[4] were 6 and were
based on estimates of normal tissue tolerance to the fast neutron
components of the radiation. The contribution of photons to the total
biological dose is small for two reasons; 1) low dose rate that causes
repairable biological effects, and 2) the very high RBE of neutrons.
Therefore, almost all (90%) of the biologically effective dose in Cf
implants is a result of the neutron component of the radiation.

The dominant mechanism of interaction of Cf neutrons with tissue is
elastic scattering of nuclei, mainly hydrogen. The scattered neutron
loses part of its energy and this energy is released as kinetic energy of
the recoiled nucleus. The recoil nuclei have high LET and have a very
short range in tissue (i.e., a few microns). This means that all energy
lost by neutrons may be dissipated in the cell where the reaction was
induced. This energy which is a few tens of keV or higher can lead to
reproductive death if released in the cell.

By multiple scattering, neutrons lose their energy and eventually
become thermalized and in energetic equilibrium with tissue atoms with an
average energy of 0.025 eV. They do not play any role in radiotherapy.

These thermal neutrons may interact with hydrogen or nitrogen nuclei, but the cell killing effects by these reaction products are negligible compared to the elastic scattering by fast neutrons emitted by Californium. Nonetheless, these thermal neutrons are still potentially usable for boron neutron capture (BNC) therapy and may enhance Cf brachytherapy effects. To evaluate potential enhancement, one must know the thermal neutron flux in the vicinity of Cf sources implanted in the brain. We have studied this problem in head phantoms. Pilot studies have been conducted at the University of Kentucky in collaboration with the Chemical Technology Division at Oak Ridge National Laboratory. The thermal neutron flux was measured by means of the gold foil method with the gold foils positioned in the head phantom around Cf sources. We irradiated thin gold foils (60 mg/cm^2) twice, with and without 0.5mm thick cadmium envelopes. (Self-shielding corrections were negligible).

TABLE 1. Thermal neutron flux, fast neutron, photon and BNC dose rates measured in geometry from Figure 1 in three planes. Accuracy of these values is about 10%.

Plane	Point #	1	2	3	4	5
Central Plane	Thermal Neutron Flux 10^6 s^{-1} cm^{-2}	1.82	1.74	1.67	1.45	1.14
	Neutron Dose	17.69	19.50	21.9	18.28	10.35
	Photon Dose cGy/hr	9.76	10.83	11.37	9.16	6.24
	BNC Dose cGy/hr	2.8	2.6	2.5	2.2	1.7
Plane Crossing Ends of Tubes	Thermal Neutron Flux 10^6 s^{-1} cm^{-2}	1.81	1.82	1.66	1.46	1.10
	Neutron Dose	14.53	16.16	17.37	14.78	8.94
	Photon Dose cGy/hr	8.94	9.55	9.56	8.33	5.85
	BNC Dose cGy/hr	2.8	2.6	2.5	2.2	1.7
Plane 1 cm Below Tubes	Thermal Neutron Flux 10^6 s^{-1} cm^{-2}	1.49	1.57	1.54	1.39	1.09
	Neutron Dose	10.79	11.27	11.55	10.0	6.69
	Photon Dose cGy/hr	6.99	7.16	6.93	6.01	4.75
	BNC Dose cGy/hr	2.3	2.4	2.3	2.1	1.6

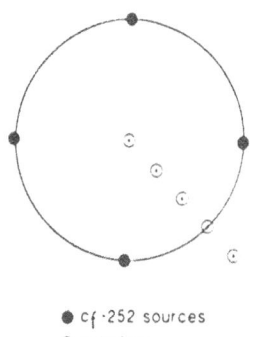

● Cf-252 sources
Ⓒ gold foils

FIGURE 1 Top view of Cf-252 sources and gold foils experimental arrangement.

We have used four 19 μg Cf tubes (2.3 cm long, 0.28 cm diameter), arranged in a circle of diameter 6 cm in a water phantom. We used cylinders which were 20 cm in height and 15 cm in diameter in the preliminary studies. A top view of our experimental arrangement is shown in Figure 1. One to five gold foils were placed in a plane crossing the centers of the Cf tubes. Thermal neutron flux values in three planes i.e., crossing centers of Cf-252 tubes, crossing ends of tubes, and 1 cm below ends of tubes are shown in Table I. The doses for boron neutron capture (BNC) have been calculated using the experimental values of the thermal neutron flux and assuming a concentration of 50 μg of B-10 in a cm^3 tissue. In Table I BNC doses, as well as fast neutron doses and photon doses, are presented.

The data in Table I indicates that BNC may be very useful in brain implants for the following:

- BNC appears to give a 10 to 20% enhancement of total local dose at a B-10 concentration of 50μg/cc.

- There appears to be higher enhancement of dose on the periphery of the implant volume.

- BNC radiation is high LET and thus can be effective against radioresistant tumor cells.

- BNC added to Cf therapy may offer a therapeutic gain in Cf brachytherapy by enhancing high LET tumor dose.

A large more homogeneous therapeutic dose distribution may improve outcome of therapy. Likewise, the enhancement of dose at the periphery of the target volume represents a region where it is desirable that dose be enhanced since this is the region at high risk of microscopic tumor spread. The above conclusions encourage us to continue these studies. We plan to measure thermal neutron flux at many points around different Cf tube arrangements and activities to determine along-away tables that can be used for treatment planning for BNC-enhanced Californium implant therapy.

REFERENCES

1. Colvett, R.E., Rossi, H.J., Krishnaswamy, V: Dose distributions around a Californium-252 needle. Physics. Med. Biology, 17:356, (1972).
2. Anderson, L.L.: Cf-252 physics and dosimetry. Nuclear Science Applications, 2:273, (1986).
3. Wierzbicki, J., Beach, L.J., Maruyama, Y.: Dose distribution in stereotactic brain implant with cf-252 sources. Medical Physics, 17:3, (1990).
4. Maruyama, Y., Feola, J., Wierzbicki, J., van Nagell, J.R., Powsell, D., Yoneda, J.: Clinical study of relative biological effectiveness for cervical carcinoma tested by Cf-252 neutrons and assessed by histological tumor erradication. Brit. J. Radiol., 63:270-277, (1990).

COMPARISON OF DOSE DISTRIBUTIONS WITH [10]BORON AUGMENTED SOURCES OF [252]CF OBTAINED BY MONTE CARLO SIMULATION AND BY EXPERIMENTAL MEASUREMENT

J.C. Yanch[1], R.G. Zamenhof[2], J. Wierzbicki[3] and Y. Maruyama[3]

[1]Department of Nuclear Engineering and Whitaker College of Health Sciences and Technology, Massachusetts Institute of Technology, Cambridge, MA, USA

[2]Tufts-New England Medical Center, Boston, MA 02111, USA

[3]University of Kentucky Medical Center, Lexington, KY, 40536, USA

INTRODUCTION

Intracavity and interstitial ^{252}Cf implants have been used to treat a number of tumor types including gynecological tumors and glioblastoma[1,2,3], the former with encouraging results. As a neutron source, ^{252}Cf offers certain theoretical advantages over photon therapy (i.e., in treating tumors with significant hypoxic or necrotic components). With the recent availability of ^{10}B-labelled tumor seeking compounds, the usefulness of ^{252}Cf may be further improved by augmenting the ^{252}Cf dose to tumor with an additional dose due to the fission (following thermal neutron capture) of ^{10}B located in the tumor itself. While the high mean neutron energy permits ^{252}Cf to deliver a high LET, low OER dose to tumor on a macroscopic scale, thermalization of neutrons followed by ^{10}B capture may augment this dose at the cellular level if adequate loading of tumor cells with ^{10}B is possible. This paper presents results of a Monte Carlo simulation study which investigates the dosimetric characteristics of linear ^{252}Cf sources and the quantitative increase in tumor dose possible with the addition of ^{10}B. Comparison of the presented Monte Carlo results with experimental and analytic dosimetry data presented in the literature will also be made.

Since 1973, the entire supply of ^{252}Cf in the western world has been produced at the High Flux Isotope Reactor at Oak Ridge National Laboratory in the United States. Although production and purification is a lengthy process it is anticipated that approximately 1.5 g/yr could become available if the demand exists[4]. Properties of ^{252}Cf decay and neutron emissions are given in Table 1. A schematic drawing of a medical ^{252}Cf source, as considered for the present calculations, is shown in Figure 1. Such sources have been used for fast neutron brachytherapy at the University of Kentucky Medical Center for many years, and it has recently been proposed that the addition of ^{10}B in the tumor could provide further clinical advantage.

Table 1. Emission and decay properties of ^{252}Californium[4].

Half-life	2.645 years
Specific Activity	536.3 Ci/g
Branching Fraction	α: 96.908 % S.F.: 3.092 %
Neutron Emission	2.31 x 10^{12} n/s/g
Mean Fission Neutron Energy	2.14 MeV
Average Prompt Gamma Energy	0.8 MeV

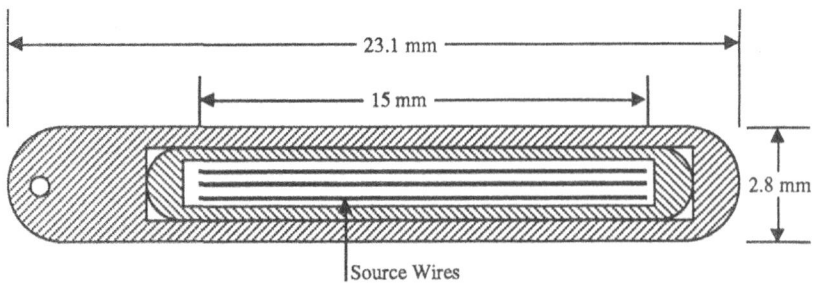

Figure 1. Medical ^{252}Cf linear source consisting of wires of californium oxide in a palladium matrix, doubly encased in a platinum (10% iridium) assembly.

MATERIAL AND METHODS

The Monte Carlo simulation code employed for this work was MCNP, a coupled neutron photon code developed at Los Alamos Scientific Laboratory[5]. For the current study, MCNP version 3b was run on SUN workstations at the Whitaker College Biomedical Imaging and Computation Laboratory at MIT.

The active portion of the ^{252}Cf implant was modelled as a single 0.8 mm diameter wire with a length of 15 mm. Because of limited cross-sections available with MCNP version 3b, the regions of the source constructed of platinum and iridium were represented by bismuth having the appropriately weighted densities of these elements. This material substitution was believed to be acceptable considering the low attenuation of gammas and neutrons that would occur in the walls of the actual source.

A single ^{252}Cf capsule was modelled as centrally positioned within a cylinder (60 cm diameter x 60 cm length) of water. Photons and neutrons were emitted isotropically from the source; energy spectra were obtained from Mannhart[6]. Particle flux measurements of all components including fast neutron, thermal neutron, induced gamma and source gammas were obtained in concentric cylinders of 2 mm separation near the source with the sampling grid separation becoming progressively more coarse with increasing distance from the source. Neutron and photon dose rates were calculated using flux-to-KERMA conversion factors for water calculated from Caswell et. al.[7] and Hubbel et. al.[8]. The increased dose to a tumor located at different distances from the ^{252}Cf source, for various concentrations of ^{10}B, was calculated using ^{10}B flux-to-KERMA conversion factors from Zamenhof et. al.[9]

RESULTS

The individual dose components and total tumor dose for a 50 ppm tumor concentration of ^{10}B is shown in Figure 2. The distance axis is perpendicular to, and at the centre of, the active region of the source. The increase in tumor dose with the addition of ^{10}B is shown in Table 2.

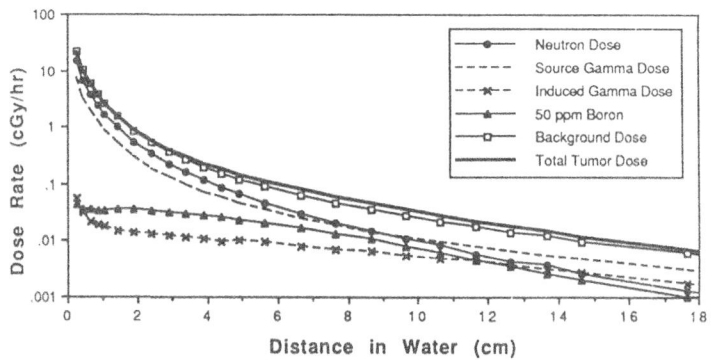

Figure 2. Dose (cGy/hr) vs. depth for all dose components (50 ppm ^{10}B in tumor is assumed) for a 1 μg source of ^{252}Cf.

Table 2. Percent increase in tumor dose due to presence of ^{10}B.

Distance from Source (cm)	ppm ^{10}B				
	1	5	10	50	100
1.0	0.0	0.1	0.3	1.3	2.6
5.0	0.4	1.8	3.6	15.8	27.3
10.0	0.5	2.2	4.3	18.3	31.0
15.0	0.4	1.9	3.7	16.2	27.9
25.0	0.2	0.8	1.6	8.2	16.4

DISCUSSION

It has been shown that the addition of ^{10}B can result in clinically significant augmentation of dose to tumor. The level of dose increase depends on the concentration of ^{10}B and on the distance away from the source. Maximum increase appears to occur at a distance of roughly 10 cm, since closer to the source any additional dose from ^{10}B is minor in comparison with the neutron and source gamma doses. At distances greater than 10 cm, the additional ^{10}B dose again becomes small relative to the total dose. With a boron concentration of 50 ppm, a 18 % increase in tumor dose is achieved at a distance of roughly 10 cm from the source. Using TCD (Tumour Control Dose) curves for mouse mammary tumors[10], and assuming a tumor to normal tissue ^{10}B ratio of 4:1, an approximately 40 % increase in tumor control might be achieved with no increase in complications.

Table 3 compares results of this study with results of experimental and analytical dosimetry (at 3.0 cm from the ^{252}Cf source) reported in the literature[11-15]. Comparison indicates that the Monte Carlo is in good agreement with all dose components, including the ^{10}B dose.

The results of this study indicate that ^{10}B can provide clinically useful increases in tumor dose at distances of 5 - 15 cm away from a ^{252}Cf source. Results also predict that the simulation data presented here will be suitable for use in treatment planning calculations with or without ^{10}B augmentation.

Table 3. Comparison of Monte Carlo results with experimental and analytical results reported in the literature. Doses (cGy/hr) are obtained in water at a distance of 3.0 cm from a 1 µg source of ^{252}Cf.

	Neutron Dose	Total Gamma	Source Gamma	Induced Gamma	Total Background	^{10}B (50 ppm) Dose
Current Study	2.17	1.36	1.24	0.12	3.50	0.31
Wierzbicki	—	—	—	—	—	0.37
Colvett, et. al.[11]	2.33	1.29	—	—	3.62	—
Krishnaswamy[12]	2.07	1.22	—	—	3.29	—
Fairchild[13]	2.00	1.30	—	—	3.30	—
Oliver[14]	1.39	1.30	—	—	2.70	—
Keller[15]	—	—	—	—	—	0.45

REFERENCES

1. Maruyama, Y., Californium-252: new radioisotope for human cancer therapy, *Endocurtherapy/Hyperthermia Oncology*, **2**:171-187 (1986).
2. Patchell, R.A., Y. Maruyama, P.A. Tibbs, J.L. Beach, R.J. Kryscio and A.B. Young, Neutron interstitial brachytherapy for malignant gliomas: a pilot study, *J. Neurol.*, **68**:67-72 (1988).
3. Chin, H.W., Y. Maruyama, A.B. Young, J.L. Beach, P. Tibbs and W. Markesbery, [252]Cf Brain implantation for malignant glioma, *Nucl. Sci. Appl.*, **2**:585-598 (1986).
4. Knauer, J.B., C.W. Alexander and J.E. Bigelow, [252]Cf: Properties, production, source fabrication and procurement, *Proceedings of the Workshop on [252]Cf Neutron Therapy*, Lexington, KY, May 1990.
5. Briesmeister, J.F., MCNP - A general Monte Carlo code for neutron and photon transport, *Los Alamos National Laboratory, LA7396-M Rev. 2* (1986).
6. Mannhart, IAEA - TEDOC - 410 (1987).
7. Caswell, R.S., J.J. Coyne and M.L. Randolph, Kerma factors of elements and compounds for neutron energies below 30 MeV, *Int. J. Appl. Radiat. Isot.*, 33: 1227-1262 (1982).
8. Hubbel, J.H., Photon mass attenuation and energy-absorption coefficients from 1 keV to 20 MeV, *Int. J. Appl. Rad. Isot.*, 33: 1269, 1982.
9. Zamenhof, R.G., B.W. Murray, G.L. Brownell, G.R. Wellum and E.I. Tolpin, Boron neutron capture therapy for the treatment of cerebral gliomas. 1: Theoretical evaluation of the efficacy of various neutron beams, *Med. Phys.*, **2**: 47-60, 1975.
10. Hall, E.J., *Radiobiology for the Radiologist*, J.B. Lippincott Co., Philadelphia, (1988).
11. Colvett, R.D., H.H. Rossi and V. Krishnaswamy, Dose distribution around a [252]Cf needle, *Phys. Med. Biol.*, **17**: 356-364 (1972).
12. Krishnaswamy, V., Calculation of the dose distribution about [252]Cf needles in tissue, *Radiol.*, **98**: 155-160 (1971).
13. Fairchild, R.G., N.B.S. U.S. Document (1969)
14. Oliver, G.D. and C.N. Wright, Dosimetry of an implantable [252]Cf source, *Radiol.*, **92**: 143-147 (1969)
15. Keller, U.S. AEC CONF - 6711 (1968).

[Research supported in part by U.S. Department of Energy, Grant No. DE-FG02-87ER6060]

BORON NEUTRON CAPTURE ENHANCEMENT OF THE TUMOR DOSE IN FAST NEUTRON THERAPY BEAMS

P. Wootton, R. Risler, J. Livesey, S. Brossard,
G. Laramore, T. Griffin

University of Washington Medical Center
Seattle, Washington 98195

The moderation of fast neutron beams by patients' tissue, combined with developments in tumor affinic boron carriers,[1] may allow supplementation of fast neutron beam therapy by boron neutron capture (BNC) reactions. This has the potential to enlarge the "radiation therapeutic window" in some types of tumors, e.g. prostate, and/or permit the development of such a window in the radiation response of others, e.g. brain. The work reported here extends from the studies made by others in fast neutron beams with average energies less than 10 MeV[2,3] to beams with average energies up to 24 MeV such as are generated by the p(50.5 MeV) + Be(26MeV) reaction.

The University of Washington Clinical Fast Neutron Therapy System (CNTS) has been described previously.[4,5] Its design permits the study of the influence of particle type and energy, target thickness

Table 1

"filter" conditions and collimator construction philosophy on the expected BNC enhancement of the tumor dose in fast neutron beams, all in one treatment head configuration.

Particle	Particle Energy (MeV)	Energy Loss in Target (MeV)	Filter	$\frac{1}{2}D_{N+\gamma}$ max Depth (cm)	① $D_B$max Depth (cm)	① D_B max (x10⁵) (cGy/μC)	② $\dfrac{D_B}{D_{N+\gamma}}$ max Depth (cm)	② $\dfrac{D_B}{D_{N+\gamma}}$ max (x10³)
d	16	16	none	9.2	6.25	.38	11	1.1
d	20.5	20.5	none	9.75	6.25	.61	11	0.75
p	50.5	50.5	#2 iron	12.8	4.5	1.5	6	0.97
p	50.5	26	none	14.5	5.0	1.26	7	0.66
p	50.5	26	5 cm Perspex	16.0	4.0	0.59	5.5	0.46
p	50.5	26	#2 Iron③	14.8	4.5	1.07	6.0	0.77
p	50.5	26	#2 Iron④	14.8	4.5	0.85	6.0	0.66

Table Notes
① D_B expressed as cGy per μg ^{10}B per gm tissue normalized to target charge (μC).
② D_B expressed as cGy per μg ^{10}B per gm tissue normalized to FNB dose (cGy).
③ 95% by weight iron powder + plastic binder collimator converges upstream target face.
④ Multivane iron collimator with plastic inclusions converges downstream target face.

Progress in Neutron Capture Therapy for Cancer
Edited by B.J. Allen *et al.*, Plenum Press, New York, 1992

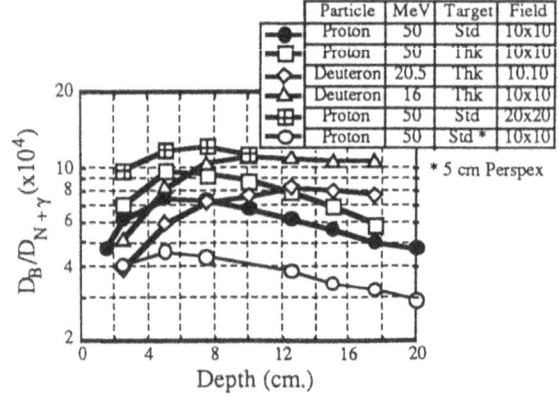

Particle	MeV	Target	Field
Proton	50	Std	10x10
Proton	50	Thk	10x10
Deuteron	20.5	Thk	10.10
Deuteron	16	Thk	10x10
Proton	50	Std	20x20
Proton	50	Std *	10x10

* 5 cm Perspex

Figure 1

Fast neutron beam total dose, $D_{n+\gamma}$, was measured in a water phantom according to the European/U.S. protocol[6] for beams generated under a range of conditions summarized in Table 1. Following the formalism of Waterman et al[2], activation of sodium in jig supported 1 cc aliquots of an $NaNO_3$ solution (350 gm/liter) along and orthogonal to the fast neutron beam axis in phantom was combined with a knowledge of the relevant cross-sections to estimate the neutron capture events that would have occurred in ^{10}B similarly exposed. The dose from BNC, D_B, expressed as cGy per microgram of ^{10}B per gram of tissue was calculated from the energetics of that capture process.

Table 2

Side of Field (cm)	$\dfrac{D_B(S)}{D_{N+\gamma}}$ / $\dfrac{D_B(10)}{D_{N+\gamma}}$	
	Filter #2	Filter #1
5.0	0.45	
7.5	0.73	
10.0	1.00	1.00
16.5	1.72	1.50
20.5	2.03	1.74
30.0		1.91

The observed dependence of D_B on depth along the fast neutron beam axis normalized to (1) the generating charge on target, (2) the fast neutron dose $D_{n+\gamma}$ at the same location is summarized in Table 1 for seven beam conditions. Normalizations to $D_{n+\gamma}$ are the more relevant when considering dose enhancement, and are graphed in Fig. 1. The observed values of D_B were not influenced by insertion of a 0.5 mm cadmium sheet centered on the beam. The ratio of the maximum value of $D_B/D_{n+\gamma}$ for a square field of side S to that for a 10x10 cm field in our standard p(50.5 MeV) + Be(26 MeV) beam is shown in Table 2 for the two filter shapes. In fields less than 12.5x12.5 cm, the orthogonal profile of D_B falls rapidly from a maximum on axis to 65% of that maximum at the fast neutron beam edge. In large fields, eg. 30x30 cm, D_B was constant over the central 18 cm falling to 70% of that value at the beam edge (Fig. 2). These data were used to

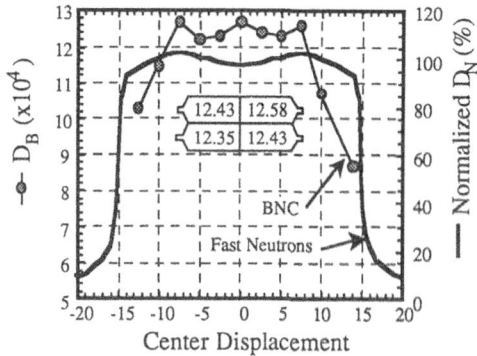

Figure 2

design an irradiation condition, p(50.5) + Be(26) #1 shape, 23 mm iron filter[4], 30x30 cm field at 5.6 cm depth in a 40x40x30 cm phantom, where D_B and $D_{n+\gamma}$ were constant to within 3% over the area of four culture flasks (Fig. 2).

The biological effect of this enhanced dose was estimated by determining the survival decrement of cells irradiated in the moderated beam. V-79 cells were grown in tissue culture plastic flasks in Eagles basal medium supplemented with 10% fetal bovine serum. Cells were treated while attached to their growth surface with either (a) cesium mercapto-undecahydro-closo-dodecaborate (99% ^{10}B, 0.8 mM, 42 hours) or (b) boric acid (99+% ^{10}B 14 or 28 mM, 1 hour). These treatments if assumed to provide uniform distribution of ^{10}B throughout the cells achieved a concentration of 100, 250, 500 µg ^{10}B per gram of cell material. Irradiation in the presence of boronated compounds at a depth of 5.6 cm in the previously specified field and subsequent plating of the cells for colony forming efficiency allowed construction of the survival curves shown in Fig 3. The dose modifying factors for these treatments are 1.88 and 1.19 for 500 and 100 µg ^{10}B/g tissue, respectively. Model calculations based on the approach of Gabel et al[7] predict the main features of these measurements.

From these data, it appears that boron neutron capture can be an effective boost to the tumoricidal effects of fast neutron beams.

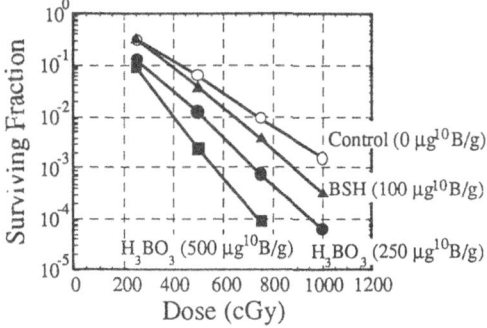

Figure 3

REFERENCES

1. R. F. Barth, A. H. Soloway and R. G. Fairchild, Boron neutron capture therapy of cancer. Cancer Res. 50:1061 (1990).

2. F. M. Waterman, F. T. Kuchnir, L. S. Skaggs, D. K. Bewley, B. C. Page and F. H. Attix, The use of 10-B to enhance the tumor dose in fast neutron therapy. Phys. Med. and Biol. 23:592 (1978).

3. W. Sauerwein, W. Ziegler, K. Olthoff, C. Streffer, J. Rassow and H. Sack, Neutron capture therapy using a fast neutron beam: clinical considerations and physical aspects, Strahlenther. Onkol. 165:208 (1989).

4. A. Brahme, J. Eenmaa, S. Lindback, A. Montelius and P. Wootton, Neutron beam characteristics from 50 MeV protons on beryllium using a continuously variable multi-leaf collimator, Radiother. and Oncol. 1:65 (1983).

5. R. Risler, J. Eenmaa, J. Jacky, I. Kalet, P. Wootton and S. Lindback, Installation of the cyclotron based clinical neutron therapy system in Seattle, in: 10th Int. Conf. on Cyclotrons and Their Applications, Michigan State University, East Lansing, Michigan, F. Marti, ed., IEEE Cat. #84CH1996-3 (1984).

6. B. J. Mihnheer, P. Wootton, J. R. Williams, J. Eenmaa and D. J. Parnell, Uniformity in dosimetry protocols for the therapeutic applications of fast neutron beams, Med. Phys. 14:1020 (1987).

7. D. Gabel, S. Foster and R. G. Fairchild, The Monte Carlo simulation of the biological effect of the $^{10}B(n,a)^7Li$ reaction in cells and tissue and its implication for boron neutron capture therapy, Radiat. Res. 111:14 (1987).

NEUTRON CAPTURE REACTIONS IN A d(14)+Be FAST NEUTRON BEAM

W. Sauerwein, I. Heselmann, F.Pöller, J. Rassow, H. Szypniewski,
C. Streffer, H. Sack

Radiologisches Zentrum, Universitätsklinikum Essen, Germany

INTRODUCTION

Since 1978 at the Essen University Hospital a compact cyclotron has been used for fast neutron therapy with neutrons produced by 14 MeV deuterons incident on a beryllium target. The poor depth dose distribution of this beam (median energy 5.7 MeV) limits the treatment of deep seated tumors (Fig 1). During fast neutron therapy, low energy neutrons are present in tissue. An enhancement of the dose at depth could be obtained by neutron capture reactions if there is a sufficient flux of thermalized neutrons derived from fast neutrons after slowing down in tissue (1).

PHYSICAL ASPECTS

The slowing down of the fast neutrons by a target, resulting in a thermal flux peaking at 6 cm depth for a tissue equivalent phantom, has been computed in a Monte Carlo model. This model, which includes a deep seated tumor, was experimentally verified for different phantom materials by 1) neutron flux measurements from gold foil activation and 2) γ-dose measurements by TLD's. The differential γ-dose in a phantom with and without boronated tumor model gives the total dose from the $^{10}B(n,\alpha)^{7}Li(\gamma)$ reaction and therefore demonstrates the effect of neutron capture as a booster for fast neutron therapy.

When non-boronated polystyrene and water phantoms were irradiated to a total dose of 1 Gy for a detector point at 6 cm depth, the thermal neutron fluences at this detector point were found to be 1.43×10^{10} cm^{-2} and 2.0×10^{10} cm^{-2}, respectively. Adding boron to the water phantom yielded an enhancement of the total absorbed dose at the same dose point of approx. 17 % per 100 ppm ^{10}B. The field size was 10 cm x 10 cm.

The depth distribution in the irradiated volume of thermalized neutrons from a fast neutron beam is different from the depth distribution using a thermal beam (Fig 2). Fast neutrons slow down to thermal energies at each point in the irradiated volume. Hence in a large tumor with a high ^{10}B concentration, the depression of the thermal fluence rate due to neutron capture is not significant (Fig 2). Beside the normal Neutron Capture Therapy effect which needs ^{10}B concentrated in the tumor, the described technique has an additional advantage. The relative contribution of the NCT reactions to the total dose is higher at depth than at the surface even for a homogenous ^{10}B distribution. Hence the total absorbed dose at depth can be boosted even without a tumor specific boron compound.

Progress in Neutron Capture Therapy for Cancer
Edited by B.J. Allen *et al.*, Plenum Press, New York, 1992

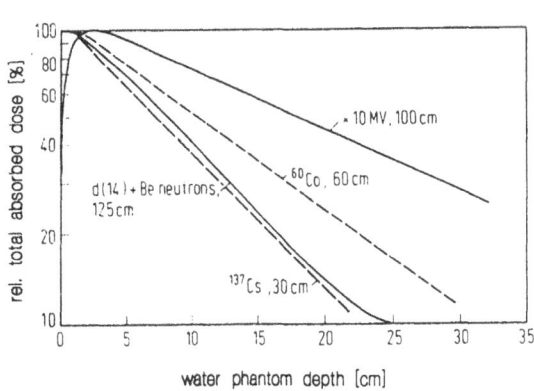

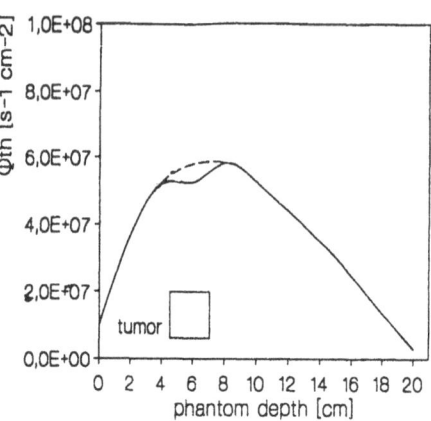

Fig 1. Depth dose curves for d(14)+Be neutrons, ^{137}Cs, ^{60}Co and 10 MV-photons, radiation source to skin distances are indicated (field size 10 x 10 cm)

Fig 2. Monte Carlo simulation of the thermal neutron fluence rate (Φth) in a water phantom in presence or absence of 100 μg/g ^{10}B in a deep seated tumor (2 cm x 2 cm x 2 cm)

EFFECTS IN BIOLOGICAL SYSTEMS

Exponentially growing human tumor cells were irradiated as monolayers in a tissue equivalent phantom at a depth of 5 cm in the presence or absence of ^{10}B (2). The 2 melanoma cell lines MeWo and Be 11 and a head and neck squamous cell carcinoma PECA 4451 were used. The cells were plated after irradiation for colony formation. Borate alone was not cytotoxic up to 16 hours in a concentration of 4 mg/ml. The presence of 4 mg/ml (10)borate greatly enhances cell kill compared to neutron irradiation alone. The effect of 0.8 mg/ml (10)borate was equal to the effect of 4 mg/ml naturally occuring borate containing 20% ^{10}B (Fig 3). This proves that the enhanced cell kill results solely from ^{10}B(n,α)^{7}Li reaction and is not due to an increase in radiosensitivity by some chemical or pharmacological mechanism. Cell survival depends on the ^{10}B concentration and Φth at the depth in the phantom where the monolayers were irradiated (Fig 4). The enhancement of cell kill by neutron capture reactions was also seen in cells irradiated under hypoxic conditions (2). Similar results were obtained using ^{6}Li (LiCl, Fig 5). No effect was observed in the presence of ^{157}Gd (Magnevist®). Harding Passey melanoma bearing BALB/c mice were locally irradiated after intraperitoneal injection of L-BPA or intratumoral injection of boric acid (H$_3$BO$_3$). In both experiments a significantly better cure rate was obtained by neutron capture reactions (Table 1).

Table 1. Harding Passey Melanoma bearing BALB/c mice experiment

	neutrons(8.4 Gy) + (H$_3$^{10}BO$_3$ vs H$_3$^{11}BO$_3$) (intratumoral injection)		neutrons(7.5 Gy) + L-BPA (30 mg i.p.) vs (control, L-BPA, n(7.5 Gy))			
	^{10}B	^{11}B	control	L-BPA	n(7.5 Gy)	n(7.5 Gy) + L-BPA
No. of animals	55	56	31	28	35	35
no tumor after 4 months 6 months	- 39	- 20	2 -	1 -	10 -	21 -

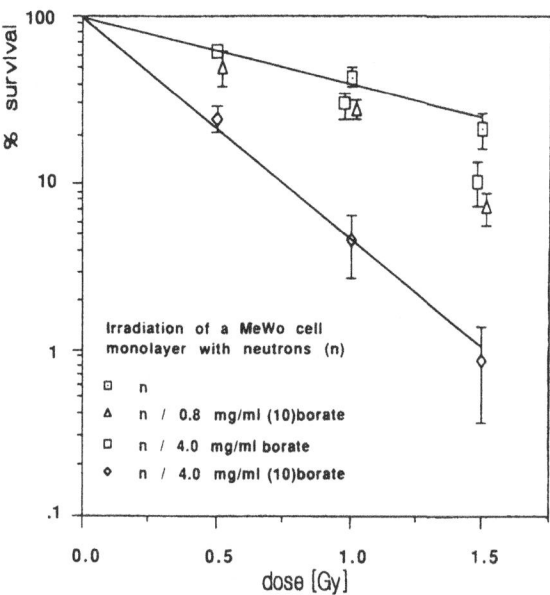

Fig 3. Irradiation of MeWo cell monolayers in
the presence or absence of borate.

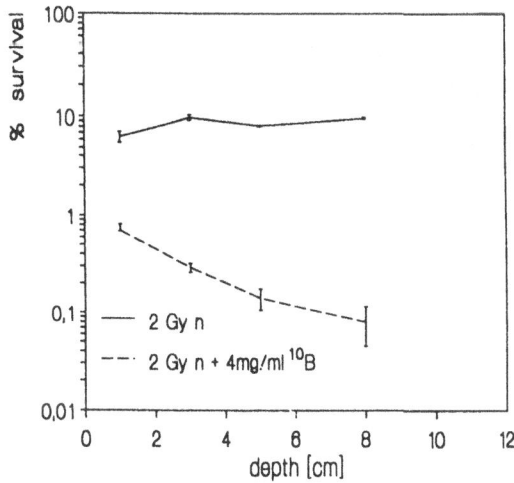

Fig 4. Irradiation of McWo cells in a phantom
at different depths.

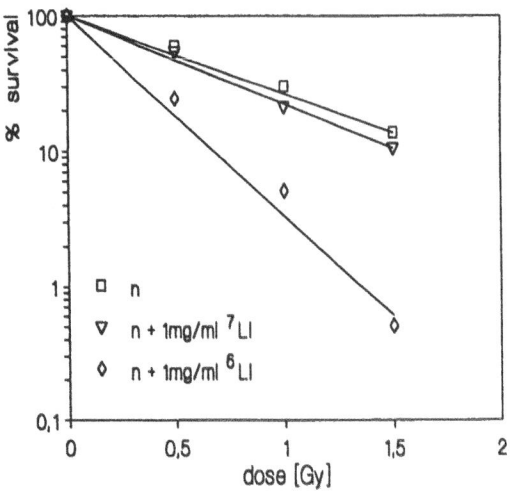

Fig 5. Effect of neutron (n) irradiation on McWo
cells in presence of ^{6}Li.

CONCLUSION

These results suggest a therapeutic gain by enhancing tumor dose using neutron capture in fast neutron therapy. Clinical studies of neutron capture assisted fast neutron therapy can be undertaken if a suitable ^{10}B containing drug is available for humans.

ACKNOWLEDGEMENT: This work has been supported in part by the DFG (Deutsche Forschungsgemcinschaft)

REFERENCES

1. Sauerwein W., W.Ziegler, K.Olthoff-Münter, C.Streffer, J.Rassow, H.Sack: Neutron capture therapy using a fast neutron beam: Clinical considerations and physical aspects. Strahlenther.Onkol.165 (1989),208-210.
2. Sauerwein W., W. Ziegler, H. Szypniewski, C. Streffer: Boron neutron capture therapy (BNCT) using fast neutrons: Effects in two human tumor cell lines. Strahlenther.Onkol.166 (1990), 26-29.
3. Pöller F., W. Sauerwein, D.Rau, F.M.Wagner, K. Olthoff, J. Rassow, H. Sack: Neutronenfluenzmessungen im d(14)+Be-Neutronenstrahlungsfeld des Zyklotrons in Essen. Strahlenther. Onkol. 166 (1990), 426-429.

THE POTENTIAL OF INTERNAL NEUTRON SOURCES IN CAPTURE THERAPY

J. F. Crawford

Paul Scherrer Institute, CH-5232 Villigen, Switzerland

The use of high intensity accelerators as neutron sources for neutron capture therapy (NCT) is discussed elsewhere in this Symposium[1]. It is the purpose of the present paper to draw attention to another possible use of accelerators, of much lower power, in this field.

In stereotactic neuro-surgery, it is standard practice to insert, directly into the brain, tubes of diameter perhaps 5 mm. Now it is also perfectly practicable to focus a beam of charged particles down such a tube, to hit a suitable neutron production target at the end. We can therefore contemplate making an intense, controllable source of neutrons inside a tumour, in the brain or elsewhere. Ways of generating suitable proton beams will be discussed later.

Using the well-known code MCNP[2], a set of calculations has been done on what dose rates and distributions might be expected. These calculations were made for a neutron source at the centre of a spherical phantom, under the following assumptions:

- The neutron source was taken to be monoenergetic and isotropic. The neutron energy, different in each calculation, was chosen to cover the lower part of a spallation or fission spectrum, from a few keV to 1 MeV; these energies are readily accessible with a low energy proton beam and a ^7Li target, or with a spallation target.

- The phantom was 20 cm in diameter, containing 10.6% H, 14% C, 1.84% N and 72.6% O; differences between brain, muscle tissue, etc. were neglected for the purposes of this preliminary study.

- No attempt was made to estimate biological effects; quoted results are physical doses only.

- The phantom contained 30 ppm of ^{10}B uniformly distributed.

Some results are shown in Figure 1, both for ^{10}B-loaded and normal tissue. It can be seen that doses of the order of Gy result from the emission of 10^{13} neutrons from the source, which corresponds to a 10 μgram Californium source implanted for about four days. As the initial neutron energy is reduced, there is a considerable improvement in the dose advantage conferred by the ^{10}B, and a reduction in the very high dose near the target. There is therefore a clear advantage in going to as low neutron energies as possible. All this reflects the fact that fast neutrons, which do not distinguish between boronated and normal tissue, will deliver dose to both while they are slowing down; they are therefore less useful than slower neutrons.

If the intense dose near the source is intolerable, some kind of inert moderator could be inserted with the source. This is clearly practicable in such locations as the uterus or rectum; the experience that the Kentucky and Thai groups will develop in the course of their work with Californium may well be very relevant[3,4,5,6,7]. In brain tumours, of more immediate interest here, this is much harder. However, it may be possible to develop some kind of

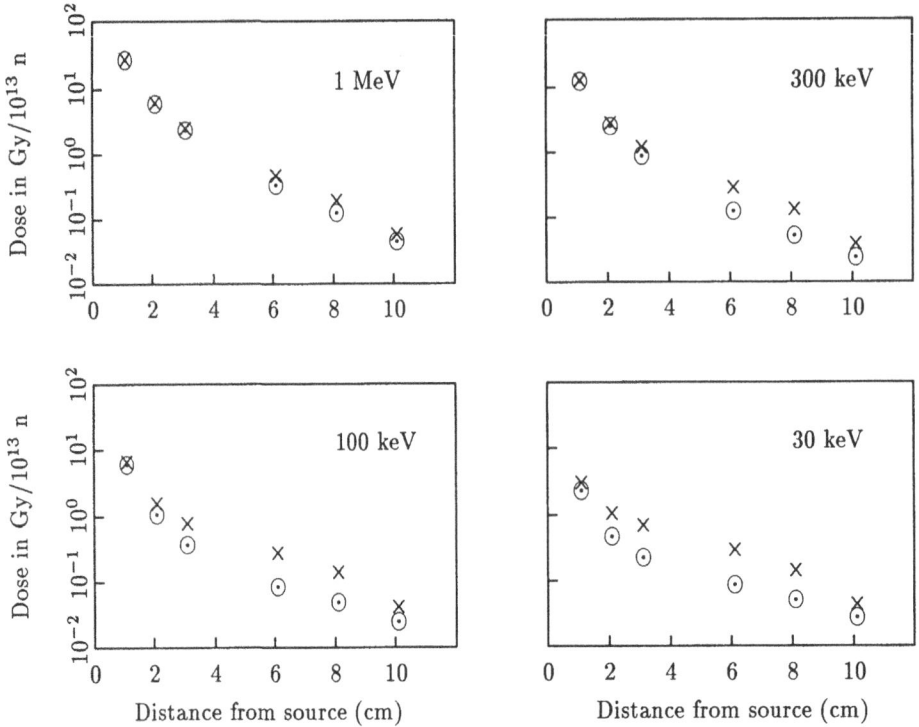

Figure 1. Dose in ^{10}B-loaded and normal tissue, for various initial neutron energies, shown on each plot. The horizontal scale shows the distance from the phantom centre in cm. The vertical (logarithmic) scale shows the dose in Gy for 10^{13} neutrons emitted.

⊙: sum of dose from neutrons and γs; ×: same plus ^{10}B dose.

Statistical errors from MCNP are a few percent.

balloon which could be inserted with the tube, and later inflated with moderator to expand into the cavity which is formed by surgical debulking, and which is frequently of centimetre size. Devices similar to this are in routine use in vascular surgery[8].

There seem to be two ways of generating suitable proton beams:

- With a 72 MeV beam, such as is routinely available at the Paul Scherrer Institute (PSI), about five protons are required to liberate each neutron by spallation from a heavy target such as tungsten[1]. Then for a total neutron emission of 10^{13} neutrons, some 5×10^{13} protons, or about 8 μC, would be needed. This corresponds to the deposition in the target of 72 MeV $\times$ 8 μC, or 600 J, of heat. This seems tolerable even without a special cooling system, given that the brain's glucose consumption[9] implies that the brain dissipates about 20 W of heat, and assuming that the irradiation would last for (say) 15 minutes.

- A better alternative might be to use a much lower energy proton beam, derived perhaps from the kind of small accelerators described at this and previous meetings[10,11,12,13,14], operating at 2-3 MeV; a ^{7}Li target would be required. The advantage here would be that the neutrons are released by an exchange process at a lower energy: from zero to a maximum of a few hundred keV, depending on the proton energy[15]. This compares favourably with an average energy of an MeV or more from a spallation or fission reaction. The disadvantage is that the neutron yield per proton is some hundreds of times less, and more beam current is needed. Specifically, an energy of 2.5 MeV requires about 7800 protons per neutron[12]. While this presents no difficulty from the point of view of accelerator technology, the production target now has to bear a significant heat load, which becomes 35 watt if 10^{13} neutrons are emitted in 15 minutes. Some kind of cooling circuit, capable of supplying a few grams of cooling water per second, would have to be built into the beam tube.

Some additional points are perhaps worth stressing:

- The neutron source is very effectively located: spallation sources deliver typically 1-2 neutrons to a treatment position for every 10^5 neutrons liberated from the target[1]; the corresponding figure for reactors is even lower. But in the present concept, essentially all neutrons are potentially usable, and a correspondingly less intense source is needed.

- Since neutrons are well shielded from neighbouring healthy tissue, ^{10}B load there is less important. This may allow higher ^{10}B loads, itself a considerable advantage.

- Neutrons from a ^7Li target are not isotropic; this may be useful in sparing healthy tissues near a tumour.

- By modern standards, accelerators for both scenarios are low current devices, and can be expected to be both budget- and user-friendly. With reference to the second scenario, for example, the SRL/MIT group[13,14] intends to build a 2×1.25 MeV tandem linac based on solid-state high voltage generating techniques, which would be capable of two orders of magnitude more current than required here, and which is projected to cost US$500,000[16].

- The concept could also be useful for superficial tumours.

It is a pleasure to acknowledge useful discussions with K. Elmgren, who carried out the computations, and with H. Fankhauser, B. Larsson and L. Salford.

REFERENCES

[1] J. F. Crawford, H. Condé, K. Elmgren, E. Grusell, B. Larsson, B. Nilsson, O. Pettersson, H. Reist, T. Rönnqvist, G. Russell and P. Strömberg, these proceedings.

[2] J. F. Briesmeister (Ed), 'MCNP - A General Monte Carlo Code for Neutron and Photon Transport, Version 3A' Los Alamos National Laboratory, LA-7396-M, Rev. 2 (1986).

[3] Y. Maruyama and J. G. Wierzbicki, these proceedings.

[4] J. G. Wierzbicki, Y. Maruyama and R. Martin, these proceedings.

[5] J. G. Wierzbicki, C. W. Alexander and Y. Maruyama, these proceedings.

[6] J. C. Yanch, R. G. Zamenhof, J. G. Wierzbicki and Y. Maruyama, these proceedings.

[7] Ch. Wongwiechintana, S. Choonchartpreset, S. Tampitak and S. Prachayasittigul, Strahlentherapie und Onkologie 165, 125-126 (1989).

[8] Dr. H. Fankhauser, CHUV, CH-1011 Lausanne, Switzerland; private communication.

[9] The Cecil Textbook of Medicine, edited by P. B. Beeson, W. McDermott and J. B. Wyngaarden, p646; W. B. Saunders Co., Philadelphia, 1979.

[10] R. E. Shefer, R. E. Klinkowstein, J. C. Yanch and G. L. Brownell, in 'Neutron Beam Design, Development and Performance for Neutron Capture Therapy', Eds O. K. Harling, J. A. Bernard and R. G. Zamenhof, Plenum Press, New York (1990).

[11] C. K. Wang, T. E. Blue and J. W. Blue, in 'Neutron Beam Design, Development and Performance for Neutron Capture Therapy', Eds O. K. Harling, J. A. Bernard and R. G. Zamenhof, Plenum Press, New York (1990).

[12] Ch. K. Wang, Th. E. Blue and R. A. Gahbauer, Strahlentherapie und Onkologie 165, 75-78 (1989).

[13] R. E. Shefer, R. E. Klinkowstein, J. C. Yanch and G. L. Brownell, these proceedings.

[14] J. C. Yanch, X.-L. Zhou, R. E. Shefer, R. E. Klinkowstein, and G. L. Brownell, these proceedings.

[15] J. B. Marion & J. L. Fowler (Eds.), Fast Neutron Physics, Interscience Publishers, New York, 1960, p133-176.

[16] J. C. Yanch, private communication.

CARBORANYL PRECURSORS OF NUCLEIC ACIDS--

POTENTIAL DNA PROBES FOR BNCT

A.H. Soloway, A.K.M. Anisuzzaman, L. Liu, R.F. Barth, F.
Alam and W. Tjarks

The Ohio State University
500 W. 12th Avenue
Columbus, Ohio 43210

Introduction

It has been determined that the biological effectiveness of BNCT
will be maximized if the capture reaction were to occur in the cell
nucleus in comparison with the cytoplasm, on cell membrane or in
extracellular spaces.[1-2] This has been the basis for the ongoing
synthesis of boron compounds which are chemically similar to the building
blocks of the nucleic acids. Initially, the approach concentrated on the
preparation of purine and pyrimidine bases which contain boron.[3-7] The
rationale was that such structures might emulate the naturally-occurring
purine and pyrimidine bases and become more selectively incorporated into
tumor cell nuclei in comparison to normal cells due to the higher
proliferative rates of the former. Of the different boron compounds
which were initially synthesized, many were unstable, toxic or failed to
become incorporated into nucleic acids. One structure which resembled
more closely its natural counterpart was 5-dihydroxyboryluracil.[8] Its
synthesis encouraged Schinazi and Prusoff to prepare the first boron-
containing pyrimidine nucleoside.[9]

Conversion to the corresponding nucleotide by cellular kinases could
result in the compound's entrapment and thereby retention in rapidly
proliferating malignant cells. Additional selectivity could be attained
if such boron-containing nucleotides were ultimately incorporated into
the tumor cell's nucleic acids by action of appropriate kinases and
polynucleotide ligases/polymerases. Interest in borononucleosides led to
the synthesis of cyanoborane adducts of 2'-deoxynucleosides[10] and to the
development of a method for synthesizing such compounds from halogenated
nucleoside derivatives.[11] These structures possess a single boron atom.
The insertion of a carboranyl group having 10 boron atoms into a
nucleoside could offer clear advantages for BNCT since such compounds
would possess a tenfold increase in the number of boron atoms per
nucleoside. We have succeeded in synthesizing the first carboranyl
nucleoside with the boron cluster on the 2' position of the carbohydrate
portion of the compound, 2'-O-(o-carboran-1-ylmethyl)uridine.[12] Placement
of the carborane moiety on the carbohydrate portion of the nucleoside was
done so as to minimize any conformational and electronic changes in the
base portion of the nucleoside. Insertion of pendant groups attached to
the 2' position of nucleosides which were subsequently incorporated into

sequence-specific oligonucleotides did not compromise the latter's ability to hybridize strongly with its complementary RNA and DNA sequences.[13]

<u>Cellular</u> <u>Uptake</u> <u>and</u> <u>Persistence</u>

Cellular uptake and persistence studies were performed with F98 rat glioma cells. Comparisons have been made between this carboranyluridine and boric acid and $Na_2B_{12}H_{11}SH$ (Figure 1). Tumor cells were cultured in the presence of the various boron compounds for 16 hrs. After incubation, some experiments were terminated and their cells, after washing, were analyzed for boron content by means of direct current plasma atomic emission spectroscopy. Compounds, with demonstrated cellular boron concentrations, were evaluated for persistence. Cultures of these cells were incubated in boron-free media for an additional 12, 24 or 48 hours and their cells analyzed for boron content. The results of these <u>in</u> <u>vitro</u> studies are shown in Table 1 and Figure 2. Additionally, fractionation studies were carried out to determine where in the cell the boron compounds are localized. From preliminary studies, approximately 30% is associated with the nucleus.[14]

Table 1

Uptake and Persistence Studies with F98 Glioma Cells

	Conc. in Incubating Media	Conc. in F98 Glioma Cells 16 hrs incubation	Persistence Studies		
			12 hrs	24 hrs	48 hrs
$Na_2B_{12}H_{11}SH$	14.6	4.3	3.1†	.4†	*
$Na_2B_{12}H_{11}SH$	58.0	7.2	2.8†	.8†	*
$Na_2B_{12}H_{11}SH$	116.0	26.7	3.4†	1.8†	*
Carboranyl Uridine	13.5	88.9	23.9	19.3	10.5
Carboranyl Uridine	40.5	98.2	24.1	22.0	12.7

#All values are in μg boron/g or ml.

*Not measured.

†These approximate the blank value for cells, the average DCP reading being 1.3 (range .4 - 3.0).

While there is no data as yet regarding the conversion of the carboranyluridine to its nucleotide, these preliminary studies demonstrate significant glioma uptake of this compound and long persistence times. These results raise the important question as to the nature of the boron compound trapped within the cell if moving the carboranylmethoxy group to the 3' and 5' position affects cellular retention and is the pyrimidine part of the molecule required? An important goal of this research is to begin to correlate chemical structure with tumor cell penetration and persistence. This is the basis for the synthesis of the <u>nido</u> analogue of 2'-O-(o-carboran-1-ylmethyl)uridine, the corresponding <u>closo</u> nucleotide and the carboranylglucose. The objective is twofold, namely: to develop boron compounds which serve as the vehicle for achieving selectivity between tumor and normal cells; and (2) to determine the physicochemical parameters required to maximize tumor cell incorporation on the one hand and yet retain solubility in aqueous systems. In essence, a suitable amphipathic balance must be attained. In Figure 3 are presented the various structures which have now been synthesized and are in the process of being evaluated.

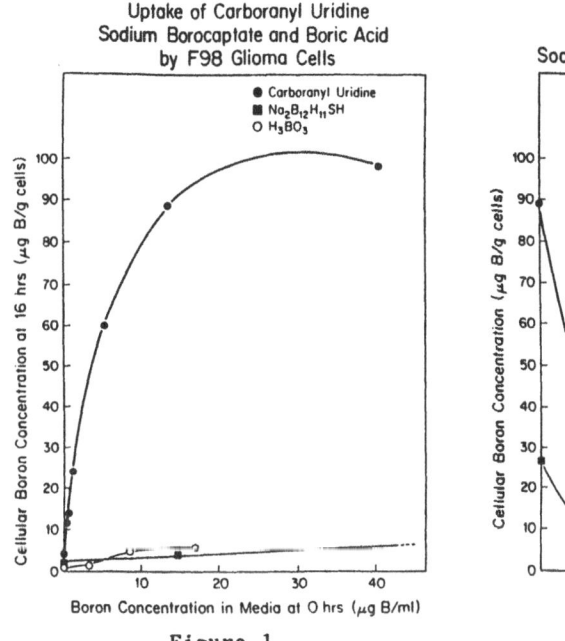

Figure 1

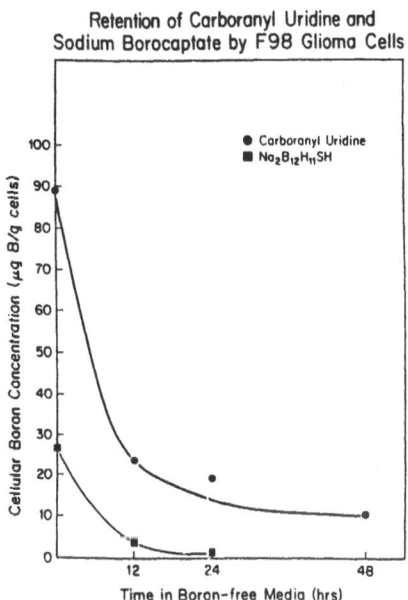

Figure 2

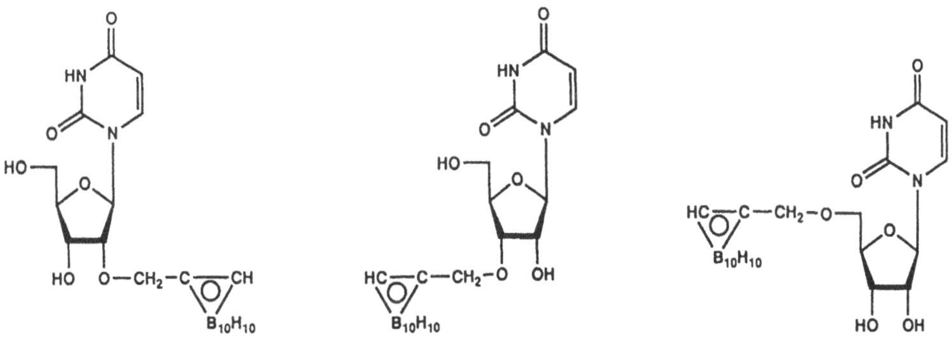

Figure 3. Carboranyl Derivatives

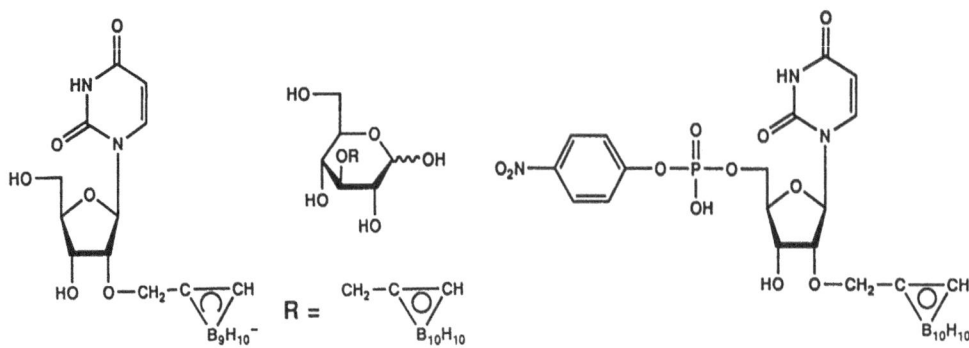

Figure 3. Carboranyl Derivatives (cont.)

Acknowledgements

The authors wish to acknowledge support for their research by the United States Department of Energy and the National Cancer Institute.

References

1. T. Kobayashi and K. Kanda, Analytical calculation of boron-10 dosage in cell nucleus for neutron capture therapy, Radiat. Res. 91:77 (1982).
2. D. Gabel, B. Larsson, and W.R. Rowe, The biological effect of the $^{10}B(n,\alpha)^{7}Li$ reaction and its simulation by Monte Carlo calculations, Proc. 1st Intl. Symp. on Neutron Capture Therapy, October 12-13 (1983).
3. S.S. Chissick, M.J.S. Dewar, and P.M. Maitlis, A boron-containing purine analog, J. Am. Chem. Soc. 81:6329 (1959).
4. H. Zimmer, A.D. Sill, and E.R. Andrews, Functional organoboron compounds, Naturwissenschaften 47:378 (1960).
5. S.S. Chissick, M.J.S. Dewar, and P.M. Maitlis, New heteroaromatic compounds. XIV. Boron-containing analogs of purine, quinazoline and pyrimidine, J. Am. Chem. Soc. 83:2708 (1961).
6. D.S. Matteson, A.H. Soloway, D.W. Tomlinson, J.D. Campbell, and G.A. Nixon, Synthesis and biological evaluation of water-soluble 2-boronoethylthio compounds, J. Med. Chem. 7:640 (1964).
7. A. Maitra, Boron analog of uracil, Indian J. Chem. 16B:85 (1978).
8. T.K. Liao, E.G. Pondrebarac, and C.C. Cheng, Boron substituted pyrimidines, J. Am. Chem. Soc. 86:1869 (1964).
9. R.F. Schinazi and W.H. Prusoff, Synthesis of 5-(dihydroxylboryl)-2'deoxyuridine and related boron-containing pyrimidines, J. Org. Chem. 50:841 (1985).
10. A. Sood, B.F. Spielvogel, and B.R. Shaw, Boron-containing nucleic acids: Synthesis of cyanoborane adducts of 2'-deoxynucleosides, J. Am. Chem. Soc. 111:9234 (1989).
11. Y. Yamamoto, T. Seko, and H. Nemoto, New method for the synthesis of boron-10 containing nucleoside derivatives for neutron-capture therapy via palladium-catalyzed reaction, J. Org. Chem. 54:4734 (1989).
12. A.K.M. Anisuzzaman, F. Alam, and A.H. Soloway, Synthesis of a carboranyl nucleoside for potential use in neutron capture therapy of cancer, Polyhedron 9:891 (1990).
13. P.D. Cook, personal communication.
14. G.H. Morrison, personal communication.

BORON CONTAINING NUCLEIC ACIDS

B.F. Spielvogel[1,2], A. Sood[1,2], B.R. Shaw[2], I.H. Hall[3],
R.G. Fairchild[4], B.H. Laster[4], C. Gordon[4]

[1]Boron Biologicals, Inc., 2811 O'Berry St., Raleigh, NC, USA
27607 [2]Gross Chemical Laboratory, Duke University, Durham,
NC, USA 27706 [3]Division of Medicinal Chemistry and Natural
Products, School of Pharmacy, University of North Carolina,
Chapel Hill, NC, USA 27599 [4]Brookhaven National Laboratory,
Upton, NY, USA 11973

INTRODUCTION

The radiobiological effectiveness of the neutron capture reaction is
thought to be twice as great if it occurs in the cell nucleus rather than in
the cytoplasm.[1,2] To enhance the probability of localization in the cell
nucleus, we have been carrying out the synthesis of a variety of boronated
nucleic acids.

Boronated nucleic acids may also be useful in slowing tumor growth by
interference with metabolic processes of tumor cells. Ultimately, boronated
oligonucleotides may be designed to specifically inhibit (tumor, viral,
etc.) gene expression by an "antisense" mechanism.[3,4]

Along these lines, we have prepared boronated nucleosides with
boronation on the purine or pyrimidine base[5] and boronated nucleotides in
which a borane group (BH_3) is attached to the phosphorus backbone.[6]

SYNTHESIS - BORONATED NUCLEOSIDES

The boronated (BH_2CN) nucleosides were prepared by an exchange
reaction of silylated nucleosides with triphenylphosphine-cyanoborane
followed by deprotection of the silylated products.[5] The compounds prepared
and characterized are shown in Figure 1.

SYNTHESIS - BORONATED OLIGONUCLEOTIDES

The "boranophosphate" oligonucleotides are prepared by formation of an
intermediate phosphite which is then converted into the boranophosphate by
reaction with Me_2SBH_3.

The hydrolytic and nuclease stability is of considerable importance
for use of these species in antisense therapy and for BNCT. We have found
that the internucleotide boranophosphate group is remarkably stable to basic
and acidic hydrolysis and is also quite stable to nucleases.[6]

TABLE 1.   CYTOTOXICITY OF BORONATED NUCLEOSIDES AND NUCLEOTIDES
μg/mL ED_{50} Values

| Cpd* # | Murine | | Human | | | | | |
	L1210	P388	Tmolt$_3$	Colorectal Adeno Car- cinoma SW480	KB	Lung Bronchogenic	Hela-S$_3$	Glioma
Ino*	4.00	7.21	1.73	3.86	3.45	4.93	2.41	8.49
Ade*	3.68	5.96	1.36	2.82	3.12	5.26	2.35	6.88
Cyt*	2.61	3.17	1.13	2.96	5.46	3.73	3.37	4.39
1	3.21	--	2.04	3.53	3.51	4.60	3.10	4.72
2		--	3.16	0.875			1.88	1.77
3	3.45	--	3.89	1.48	0.61	6.53	1.92	
Standards								
5FU	1.41	3.72	2.14	3.09	1.25	5.64	2.47	
ara-C	2.76	4.06	2.67	3.42	2.54	4.60	2.13	

-- not tested
*Structures are given in Fig. 1.

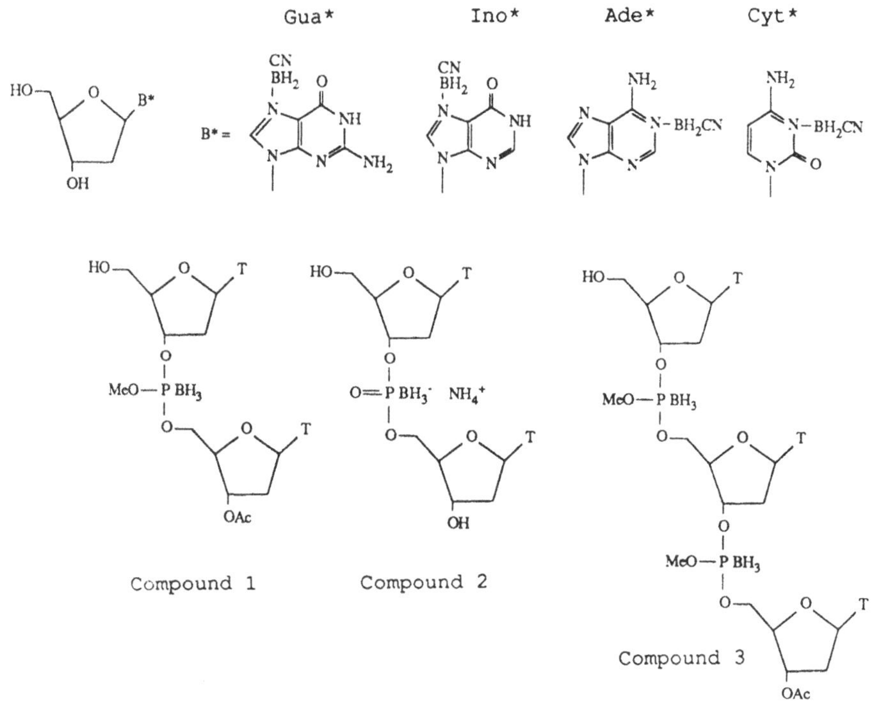

Figure 1

CYTOTOXICITY

Investigation of the inherent antitumor activity has demonstrated significant cytotoxicity in murine and human tumor screens. However, for the five boronated nucleosides tested so far, both silylated and deprotected, <u>overall</u> toxicity was not observed, with LD_{50} values in mice all over 1000 mg/kg.

BIOLOGICAL EFFICACY FOR BNCT

Preliminary biological efficacy has been evaluated by *in vitro* comparative survival assays of V-79 Chinese hamster cells, which have been exposed to a boronated compound compared with unboronated control cells irradiated at the thermal neutron beam at the Brookhaven Medical Research Reactor (BMRR).[7] Cell viability after irradiation was measured by a survival curve. Cells were exposed to 6 and 100 μm solutions of Cyt* (Figure 1) and 200 μM of Gua* (Figure 1) and washed three times before irradiation. The survival assay of these two compounds gave no indication of incorporation into the cells. When a similar experiment was conducted with 50 μM of compound 1 (and washed three times), a dose enhancement of about 1.1 was obtained in spite of a concentration of $1.8 \times 10^{-10}g$ ^{10}B/ml in the growth medium. Although an effect was observed, the significance must be established and experiments with B-10 enriched samples at higher concentrations are planned.

In a preliminary *in vivo* experiment (mouse, Ehrlich Ascites Carcinoma) with radiolabeled $[^{14}C]2'$-deoxycytidine-^{3}N-cyanoborane, a tumor/blood ratio of 4.2 after 2 hrs and 8.5 after 4 hrs was observed. Further testing of these species both *in vitro* and *in vivo* are underway.

REFERENCES

1. T. Kobayashi and K. Kanda, Analytical calculation of boron-10 dosage in cell nucleus for neutron capture therapy, <u>Radiat. Res.</u> 91:71 (1982).

2. D. Gabel, S. Foster, and R. G. Fairchild, The Monte-Carlo simulation of the biological effect of the $^{10}B(Nn\alpha)^7Li$ reaction in cells and tissue and its implication for boron neutron capture therapy, <u>Radiat. Res.</u> 111:14 (1987).

3. C.L. Brakel, ed., "Discoveries in Antisense Nucleic Acids," Gulf Publishing Co., Houston (1990).

4. J.S. Cohen, ed., "Oligodeoxynucleotides: Antisense Inhibitors of Gene Expression," CRC Press, Inc., Florida (1989).

5. A. Sood, B.R. Shaw, and B.F. Spielvogel, Boron containing nucleic acids: Synthesis of cyanoborane adducts of 2'-deoxynucleosides <u>J. Amer. Chem. Soc.</u> 111:9234 (1989).

6. A. Sood, B.R. Shaw, and B.F. Spielvogel, Boron containing nucleic acids 2: Synthesis of oligodeoxynucleoside boranophosphates, <u>J. Am. Chem. Soc.</u> 112:9000 (1990).

7. R.G. Fairchild, S.B. Kahl, B.H. Laster, J. Kalef-ezra, and E. Popenoe, <u>Cancer Research</u> 50:4860 (1990).

PREPARATION OF NEW BORON COMPOUNDS WITH POTENTIAL FOR APPLICATION IN ^{10}B NCT : DERIVATIVES OF MONOCARBON CARBORANES

John H Morris, Shah-Alam Khan, Francis Mair, and
Gavin Peters
Department of Pure and Applied Chemistry
University of Strathclyde
Glasgow, G1 1XL, U.K.

INTRODUCTION

Cluster compounds for application in ^{10}B NCT require a large number of boron atoms, should be kinetically stable to hydrolysis at biological pH, and should be water-soluble. Those that have been studied most have been derivatives of the anion $[B_{12}H_{12}]^{2-}$ and the neutral molecule $C_2B_{10}H_{12}$. In order to extend the range and versatility of boron clusters appropriate to NCT we have studied routes to derivatives of the anions 1-carba-*closo*-dodecahydrododecaborate-1, $[CB_{11}H_{12}]^-$, (I), and its synthetic precursor, 7-carba-*nido*-tridecahydroundecaborate-1, $[CB_{10}H_{13}]^-$, (II).

Substitution chemistry of *closo*-$[CB_{11}H_{12}]^-$ and its derivatives been examined previously primarily with respect to substituents at the C-atom.[1] The different isomeric sites of boron substitution, which have been much less studied, offer potential scope for subtle modification of properties of the substituted species. We have sought to prepare thiol substituted derivatives analogous to the widely studied species $[B_{12}H_{11}SH]^{2-}$. Our preliminary experiments to introduce the thiol substituent by routes analogous to those for the preparation of $[B_{12}H_{11}SH]^{2-}$ or 1- and 2-$[B_{10}H_9SH]^{2-}$ were unsuccessful. Therefore we considered routes involving prior substitution of either the precursor *nido*-$[CB_{10}H_{13}]^-$ and its derivatives, or the monoboron species used for boron insertion.

The neutral compound, *nido*-7-Me$_3$N-7-CB$_{10}$H$_{12}$, (III) has been substituted at positions B-4, B-8, or B-9 by a variety of groups.[2] Electrochemical chlorination resulted in 4-Cl-7-Me$_3$N-7-CB$_{10}$H$_{11}$, whereas treatment with HCl in the presence of AlCl$_3$ resulted in 9-Cl-7-Me$_3$N-7-CB$_{10}$H$_{11}$. (III), deprotonated with NaH in THF, yielded [8-HO-7-Me$_3$N-7-CB$_{10}$H$_{11}$]$^-$ on aqueous work-up, and treatment of the deprotonated intermediate with oxalyl chloride gave 9-OC-7-Me$_3$N-7-CB$_{10}$H$_{10}$. Oxidation of (III) with Tl^{3+} in the presence of Et$_3$N yielded 8-Et$_3$N-7-Me$_3$N-7-CB$_{10}$H$_{10}$.

RESULTS AND DISCUSSIONS

Nido-Carboranes

When (III) was treated with S$_2$Cl$_2$ in the presence of AlCl$_3$, it produced {4(6)-S-Me$_3$N-7-CB$_{10}$H$_{11}$}$_2$, (IV). (IV) was reduced by NaBH$_4$ to the thiol, 4(6)-HS-7-Me$_3$N-7-CB$_{10}$H$_{11}$, (V). Sulphur substitution at B-4(6) was also achieved with 2,4-(NO$_2$)$_2$C$_6$H$_3$SCl under Friedel-Crafts conditions (AlCl$_3$) to give 4(6)-{(NO$_2$)$_2$C$_6$H$_3$S}-7-Me$_3$N-7-CB$_{10}$H$_{11}$, (VI). Similar reactions with CH$_3$OSCl and CH$_3$SCl are also under investigation. These compounds have potential application in ^{10}BNCT.

Closo-Carboranes

Previously, (II) and (III) reacted with Et_3NBH_3 at high temperature to give the *closo*-derivatives (I) and $1\text{-}Me_3N\text{-}1\text{-}CB_{11}H_{11}$, (VII), although the latter compound is obtained via demethylated intermediates.[3] We observed that $4\text{-}Cl\text{-}7\text{-}Me_3N\text{-}7\text{-}CB_{10}H_{11}$ also gave (VII) via demethylated species, and the Cl-substituent was eliminated.[2]

When (IV) was heated with Et_3NBH_3 at 200°, the product was $[2\text{-}HS\text{-}1\text{-}Me_2N\text{-}1\text{-}CB_{11}H_{10}]^-$, (VIII), which on methylation with Me_2SO_4 gave $2\text{-}Me_2S\text{-}1\text{-}Me_2N\text{-}1\text{-}CB_{11}H_{10}$, (IX). Isomerism occurred during the course of the high-temperature reaction to give sulphur substitution at position B-7. These compounds also have potential application to $^{10}BNCT$.

The unsubstituted *nido*-cluster, (II), obtained from (III) through reaction with Na/NH_3, was further deprotonated with ^nBuLi to give the anion $[CB_{10}H_{10}]^{3-}$, (X), which underwent low temperature boron insertion reactions with $PhBCl_2$, $^tBuSBCl_2$, and $Et_2O.BF_3$ to yield $[2\text{-}Ph\text{-}1\text{-}CB_{11}H_{11}]^-$, (XI), $[2\text{-}^tBuS\text{-}1\text{-}CB_{11}H_{11}]^-$, (XII), and $[2\text{-}F\text{-}1\text{-}CB_{11}H_{11}]^-$, (XIII). This route therefore offers scope for the introduction of boron with a variety of functional groups suitable for neutron capture therapy into the kinetically stable icosahedral $\{CB_{11}\}$ cluster.

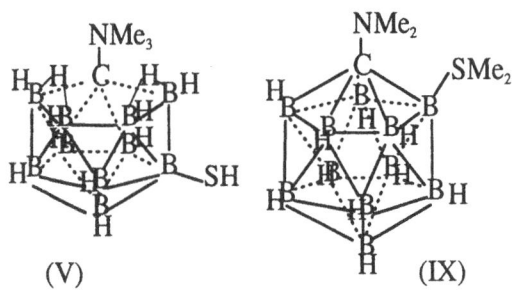

(V)   (IX)

EXPERIMENTAL

$\{4(6)\text{-}S\text{-}7\text{-}Me_3N\text{-}7\text{-}CB_{10}H_{11}\}_2$, (IV) and $4(6)\text{-}HS\text{-}7\text{-}Me_3N\text{-}7\text{-}CB_{10}H_{11}$, (V).- To a suspension of (III) (0.5g, 2.6mmol) and $AlCl_3$ (0.347g, 2.6mmol) under N_2 in CH_2Cl_2 ($40cm^3$) was added a solution of S_2Cl_2 (0.176g, 1.3mmol) in CH_2Cl_2 ($5cm^3$). After refluxing for 5hr, the mixture was treated with water ($100cm^3$) and the resulting solid (IV) separated by chromatography on SiO_2. (Found: C,22.1; H,8.9; N,6.5; S,14.1%. $C_8H_{40}B_{20}N_2S_2$ requires C,21.6; H,9.1; N,6.3; S,14.4%).
To a suspension of the isomer mixture (IV) (1.0g) in 2% NaOH in EtOH ($20cm^3$) was added $NaBH_4$ (0.68g) and the mixture stirred for 5hr. The solution was poured into water, saturated with CO_2, extracted with Et_2O, and the product (v) chromatographed on SiO_2. (Found: C,21.6; H,9,4; N,6.2; S,14.4%. $C_4H_{21}B_{10}NS$ requires C,21.5; H,9.5; N,6.3; S,14.4) Mass spectral cutoff at m/e 225 corresponding to $[^{11}B_{10}{}^{12}C_4{}^1H_{21}{}^{14}N^{32}S]^+$. ^{11}B nmr chemical shifts (ppm ref. Et_2OBF_3) (assignments) were: 4.9(5), -7.1(3), -8.4(2), -10.8(8), -14.6(11), -18.6(9), -20.4(10), -22.5(4,1), -30.8(6). Assignments were based on COSY correlations.

$4(6)\text{-}\{(NO_2)_2C_6H_3S\}\text{-}7\text{-}Me_3N\text{-}7\text{-}CB_{10}H_{11}$, (VI).- In a similar method, (III) (0.66g, 3.4mmol), $AlCl_3$ (0.53g, 4.0mmol) and $2,4\text{-}(NO_2)_2C_6H_3SCl$ (0.88g, 3.6mmol) were refluxed to give (VI) which was purified by chromatography on SiO_2. (Found: C,31.0; H,5.2; N,8.9% $C_{10}H_{23}B_{10}N_3O_4S$ requires C,30.8; H,5.9,; N,10.8%). ^{11}B nmr chemical shifts (ppm ref. Et_2OBF_3) (assignments) were: 2.5(5), -9.4(2,3), -12.9(8), -14.3(11), -21.6(4,9,10), -32.4(6).

$2\text{-}Me_2S\text{-}1\text{-}Me_2N\text{-}1\text{-}CB_{11}H_{10}$, (IX).- A mixture of (IV) (2.0g, 4.5mmol) and Et_3NBH_3 ($3.5cm^3$, 28mmol) was heated at 200° for 4.5hr. On cooling, the mixture was diluted with Et_2O, and the oily layer purified by chromatography on SiO_2 to give

[Et$_3$NMe][1-Me$_2$N-2-HS-1-CB$_{11}$H$_{10}$] (R$_f$ 0.3; 10%MeCN-90%CH$_2$Cl$_2$). (Found: C,35.6; H,10.6; N,8.5; S,9.4%. C$_{10}$H$_{35}$B$_{11}$N$_2$S requires: C,35.9; H,10.6; N,8.4; S,9.6%). This intermediate (0.5g, 1.5mmol) was treated with Et$_2$O (5cm^3) and dil. HCl (10cm^3). The ether layer was evaporated, the solid dissolved in 5% KOH (15cm^3)and treated with Me$_2$SO$_4$ (0.35cm^3, 3.7mmol). The filtered product (IX) was chromatographically purified. (Found: C,24.4, H,13.0; N,5.8; S,9.1% C$_5$H$_{22}$B$_{11}$NS requires: C,24.3; H,13.0; N,5.7; S,9.0%) The mass spectrum cutoff m/e 249 corresponding to [^{11}B$_{11}$^{12}C$_5$^{1}H$_{22}$^{14}N^{32}S]$^+$. ^{11}B nmr chemical shifts (ppm ref. Et$_2$OBF$_3$) (assignments) were: -5.7(2), -7.3(12), -10.7(7,11), -12.2(3,6), -13.7(4,5,8,10), -14.7(9). (Assignments were obtained from COSY correlations). The structure was confirmed from single crystal x-ray diffraction data.

[N^{n}Bu$_4$][2-Ph-1-CB$_{11}$H$_{11}$], (XI).- A solution of [Me$_3$NH]{CB$_{10}$H$_{13}$] (0.189g) in dry THF (6cm^3)was treated under Schlenk conditions with 1.6M ^{n}BuLi in hexane (2cm^3), and PhBCl$_2$ (1cm^3) was added. After removal of volatiles, the residue was digested with dil. NaOH; the crude product was precipitated on addition of [N^{n}Bu$_4$]Br (0.329g) . After chromatographic purification, (R$_f$ 0.8; 10%MeCN in CH$_2$Cl$_2$) the crystals of (XI) melted at 108-110°. (Found: C,59.8; H,11.8; N,3.1% C$_{23}$H$_{51}$B$_{11}$N requires: C,59.9; H,11.4; N,3.0%). ^{11}B nmr chemical shifts (ppm ref Et$_2$OBF$_3$) (multiplicity; rel. intensity) were: -5.2(d;1), -5.2(s;1), -10.7(d;2), -11.5(d;2), -12.9(d;2), -14.1(d;3).

[N(PPh$_3$)$_3$][2-^{t}BuS-1-CB$_{11}$H$_{11}$], (XII).- The procedure was similar to (XI) but used ^{t}BuSBCl$_2$ and [N(PPh$_3$)$_2$]Cl. (XII) showed ^{11}B nmr chemical shifts(ppm) of -3.5(d;1), -8.5(s;1), -9.6(d;3), -11.0(d;2), -13.2(d;2), -14.3(d;2).

[PhCH$_2$NMe$_3$][2-F-1-CB$_{11}$H$_{11}$] , (XIII).-The procedure was similar to (XI) but used Et$_2$OBF$_3$ and [PhCH$_2$NMe$_3$]OH. The product (XIII) melted at 226-227°. (Found: C,42.3; H,9.0; N,4.5% C$_{11}$H$_{27}$B$_{11}$NF requires: C,42.5; H,8.7; N,4.5%). ^{11}B nmr (ppm): 8.6(s;1), -3.7(d;1) -10.0(d;2), -10.85(d;4), -12.9(d;2), -17.2(d;1).

REFERENCES

1. T. Jelinek, J. Plesek, S. Hermanek, and B. Stibr, Collect. Czech. Chem. Commun. 51:819 (1986).
2. S.-A. Khan, J.H. Morris, and S. Siddiqui, J.Chem.Soc. Dalton Trans. 2053 (1990).
3. J. Plesek, T. Jelinek, E. Drdakova, S. Hermanek and B. Stibr, Collect. Czech. Chem. Commun. 49:1559 (1984).

MOLECULAR DESIGN AND SYNTHESIS OF B-10 CARRIERS FOR

NEUTRON CAPTURE THERAPY

Yoshinori Yamamoto, Hisao Nemoto, Toshiya Seko,
Satoshi Takamatsu, Feng Guang Rong

Department of Chemistry, Faculty of Science, Tohoku
University, Sendai 980, Japan

PREPARATION OF MONO-BORON CONTAINING CARRIERS

We have developed several new synthetic methods for B-10 containing bio-related molecules. (1) The palladium-catalyzed coupling reaction of halogenated nucleoside derivatives with the aryltin compound having a boronic moiety proceeded chemoselectively at the C-Sn bond rather than the C-B bond to give boron containing nucleoside derivatives in good yields (eq. 1)(ref. 1). The use of $Pd(PPh_3)_4$ as a catalyst, and the use of a less polar solvent such as toluene and a higher reaction temperature were essential to achieve the coupling. The use of acetonide and methoxymethyl as the sugar

$$R-X + Bu_3Sn-Ar-B(OR^1)_2 \xrightarrow{\text{Pd cat.}} R-Ar-B(OR^1)_2 \qquad \text{(eq 1)}$$

protecting groups, or conducting the reaction without protection gave poor results. The sterically bulky t-butyldimethylsilyl group afforded the coupling products in much higher yields.

One of the most often used procedures for preparation of ^{10}B carriers is the direct reaction of the carbanions YLi with trialkyl borates (substitution reaction)(ref. 2). However, the desired coupling does not take place in certain cases. (2) We anticipated that the 1,2-addition of YLi to the aldehyde group would proceed more readily and rapidly than the substitution reaction; YH=nucleoside derivatives. Actually, YLi reacted selectively with the aldehyde group in the presence of boronic groups, giving the boron containing biologically active compounds (eq. 2)(ref. 3). Here also, proper choice of the protecting group of the boronic acid was

(eq 2)

important for obtaining the coupling product in high yield.   Use of N-methyldiethanolamine gave the best result.

PREPARATION OF POLY-BORON CONTAINING CARRIERS

We next examined the preparation of decaborane containing uridine and guanosine derivatives (ref. 4). It is known that the reaction of acety-lenic derivatives with decaborane produces 1,2-dicarba-closo-dodecaborane (12)(ref. 5). Our strategy is shown in eq 3. The acetylene derivatives of nucleosides, derived from the palladium catalyzed coupling between acetylene and RX(R: nucleoside), were treated with $B_{10}H_{14}$ in the presence of CH_3CN, giving the desired products in good yields. The compounds prepared by this method are shown in Scheme 1. An application of the carbanion condensation method mentioned in eq 2 to the aldehyde having an ortho-carborane moiety was also examined (ref. 6). The reaction of YLi with the R-substituted aldehyde proceeded smoothly, giving the desired product (eq 4). If R was hydrogen, that is, if the un-substituted aldehyde was used, the condensation did not take place. Presumably, the hydrogen abstraction by YLi took place, giving polymerized materials. The compounds prepared by this procedure are also shown in Scheme 1.

The palladium catalyzed reaction of 1,2-dicarbora-closo-docecaboranes (o-carboranes) with allyl ethyl carbonate gave 2-allylated o-carboranes in good to excellent yields (ref. 7). The allylated carboranes could be converted to the corresponding diols upon treatment with OsO_4, which were soluble in water and thus could be utilized as carriers for ^{10}BNCT (Scheme 2).

HYDROPHILICITY AND LIPOPHILICITY INVESTIGATION OF CARRIERS

Hydrophilic character is required for B-10 carriers in order to be delivered to cancer cells. On the other hand, lipophilic character is needed to penetrate cell membrane. Accordingly, an amphiphilic character-istic is essential for an ideal carrier. We intended to prepare such compounds, and a typical example is shown in Scheme 3 (ref.8). The reaction of methyl p-bromobenzoate with ethynyltrimethylsilane in the presence of catalytic amounts of $Pd(OAc)_2$ and Ph_3P in THF gave methyl p-trimethylsilylethynylbenzoate in 93% yield. Subsequent treatment with tetrabutylammonium fluoride produced methyl p-ethynylbenzoate in 55% yield. The reaction of acetylenic compound with decaborane gave the corresponding carborane in 69% yield. Hydrolysis with NaOH afforded p-carboxyphenyl-o-carborane. The condensation of the carborane with t-butoxycarbonyl-N-butyl(N-(2S, 3S)-2,3,4-tris(benzyloxy)butyl-L-asparaginamide) was carried out as described in Scheme 3: HOBt=1-hydroxybenzotriazole, EDC·HCl=1-ethyl-3-[3-(dimethylamino)propylcarbodiimide]·hydrochloride. The chain length of hydrocarbon part, and a liphophilic part, can be changed at will. The length of the alcohol (after debenzylation) chain (a hydrophilic part) also can be changed. The two chains were combined via the amide bonds. The carrier is connected to the carborane moiety again via the amide bond.

The partition coefficient of the carriers (m=1 and n=4, or m=1 and n=8) was investigated. The result is shown in Scheme 4. When the length of lipophilic part increased, needless to say, the solubility to the organic solvents increased. The compound with m=1 and n=8 was soluble both in water and in organic solvents. So, we are now in a position to have an amphiphilic carrier.

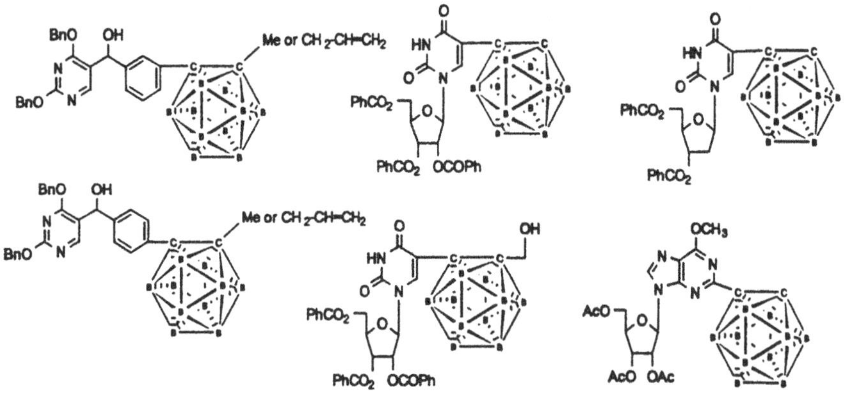

Scheme 1

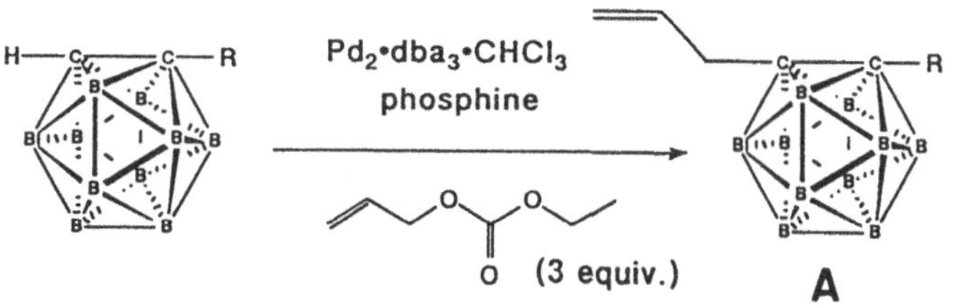

a: R = -C$_6$H$_4$-m-CHO   b: R = -C$_6$H$_4$-m-CO$_2$Me,   c: R = -C$_6$H$_4$-p-CO$_2$Me
d: R = -CO$_2$Me,   e: R = -CH$_2$OCOCH$_3$ f: R = -CH$_2$OH

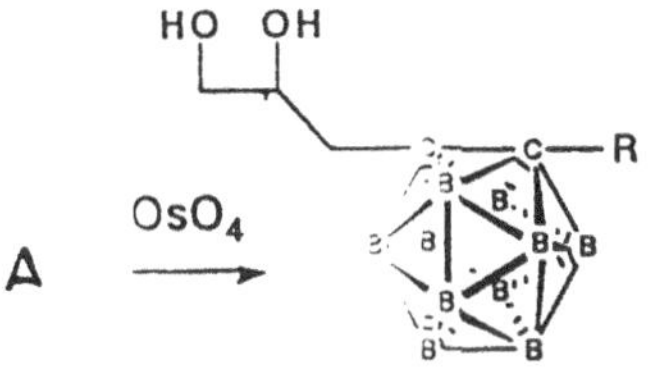

Scheme 2

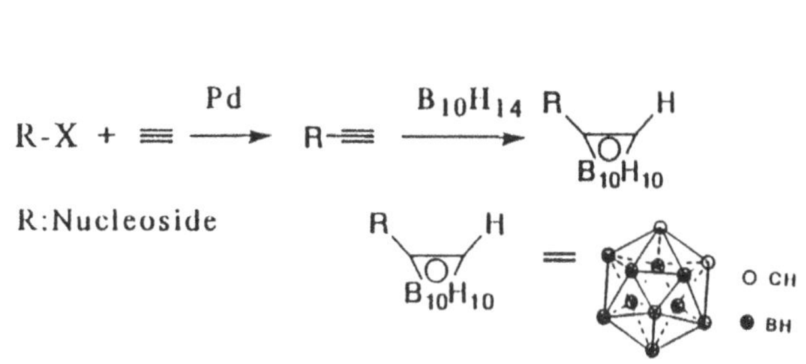

eq 3

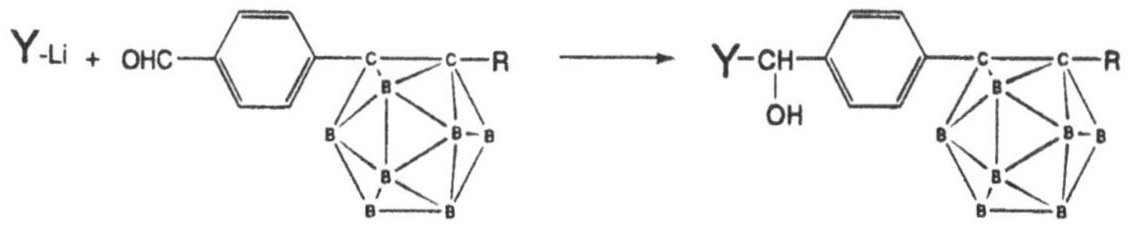

eq 4

An Amphiphilic Carrier

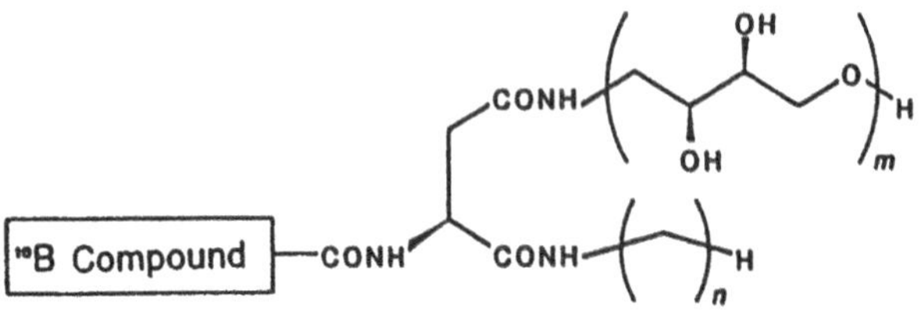

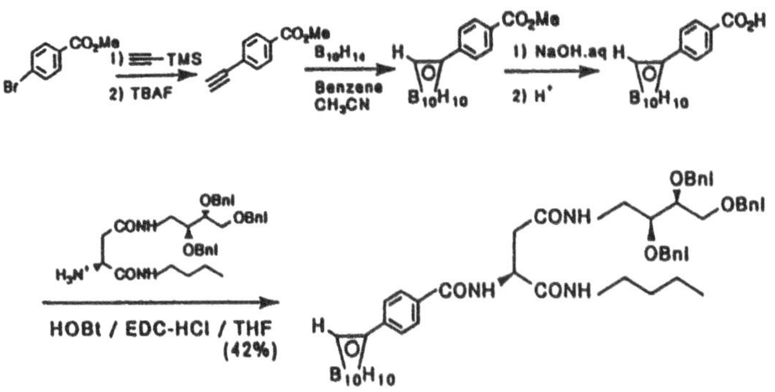

Scheme 3

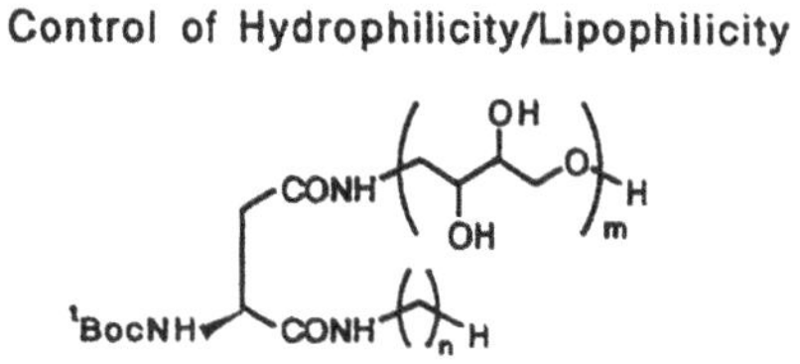

Control of Hydrophilicity/Lipophilicity

Partition Coefficient: Pow=Corg / Cwater

m	n	$CHCl_3$	C_6H_6	$C_8H_{17}OH$
1	4	0.061	0.022	1.5
1	8	0.44	0.29	

Scheme 4

REFERENCES

1. Y. Yamamoto, T. Seko, H. Nemoto, J. Org. Chem., 54, 4734 (1989).
2. R. F. Schinazi, W. H. Prusoff, J. Org. Chem., 50, 841 (1985).
3. Y. Yamamoto, T. Seko, F. G. Rong, H. Nemoto, Tetrahedron Lett., 30, 7191 (1989).
4. Y. Yamamoto, H. Nemoto, T. Seko, unpublished results, from the master thesis of Seko (1989).
5. (a) T. L. Heying, J. W. Ager, Jr, S. L. Clark, D. J. Mangold, H. L. Goldstein M. Hillman, R. J. Polak, J. W. Szymanski, Inorg. Chem., 2, 1089 (1963). (b) M. M. Fein, J. Bobinski, N. Maves, N. Schwartz, M. Cohen, Inorg. Chem., 2, 1111 (1963).
6. Y. Yamamoto, H. Nemoto, F. G. Rong, unpublished results, form the doctor thesis of Rong (1989).
7. H. Nemoto, F. G. Rong, Y. Yamamoto, J. Org. Chem., 55, 6065 (1990).
8. Y. Yamamoto, H. Nemoto, S. Takamatsu, unpublished results, from the master thesis of Takamatsu (1989).

SYNTHESIS AND PROPERTIES OF TETRAKIS-CARBORANE-CARBOXYLATE

ESTERS OF 2,4-BIS-(α,β-DIHYDROXYETHYL) DEUTEROPORPHYRIN IX

Stephen B. Kahl and Myoung-Seo Koo

Department of Pharmaceutical Chemistry
University of California
San Francisco, CA 94143

INTRODUCTION

Porphyrins and other macrocyclic nitrogen heterocycles have long been known to accumulate in a wide variety of solid tumors, although the precise biochemical mechanism for the phenomenon remains unclear.[1] In this paper we report the synthesis of a new type of water-soluble boronated porphyrin (which we call BOPP) in which four closo-carborane cages are appended to the porphyrin macrocycle by acid-resistant ester linkages. Water solubility is achieved by selective deprotection of the dipropionic acid methyl esters followed by ion exchange to the dipotassium salt. The overall yield of BOPP starting from readily available protoporphyrin dimethyl ester is usually 90% or better. Spectroscopic evidence supporting a most novel structure for BOPP is presented. Octanol/water partition coefficients determined for BOPP over a range of near-physiologic pH's suggest that the closo-carborane cages confer nearly ideal hydrophobicity to BOPP while the two propionic acid side groups maintain exceptional aqueous solubility. Its ideal combination of high boron content, ease and yield of synthesis, and excellent physicochemical properties, together with its exceptional tumor localizing ability as discussed by others at this Symposium, make BOPP a strong candidate for human NCT localization studies.

MATERIALS AND METHODS

The carborane ester (1) was prepared in 85-90% yield by room temperature reaction of 4.5 equiv. of the carborane carboxylic acid chloride with 2,4-di(α,β-dihydroxyethyl) deuteroporphyrin IX dimethyl ester in dry CH_2Cl_2 in the presence of p-dimethylamino-pyridine. Traces of a bis-carboranyl ester are also formed, suggesting that the reaction proceeds *via* initial acylation of the b-primary alcohols. Initial acylation of the 1° (β) alcohols with the sterically demanding carborane group may result in a side chain conformation which exposes the 2° (α) hydroxyls to acylation. Support for this type of mechanistic activation comes from our observation that the 2° hydroxyl groups of hematoporphyrin resist acylation under these conditions. Isolation of (1) is easily accomplished by washing the dichloromethane solution with 0.5 M HCl and 0.1M $NaHCO_3$ followed by filtration through a silica gel pad and removal of the solvent *in vacuo*. Further purification may be accomplished by recrystallization from hexane-CH_2Cl_2. Incubation of an ether solution (1) with an equal amount 25% aq. HCl overnight results in cleavage of the dimethyl esters to give the tetracarboranyl porphyrin diacid (2) in quantitative yield with no evidence of carboranyl ester cleavage. Esters of carborane carboxylic acid are known to be extremely resistant to acid-catalyzed cleavage despite the strongly electropositive nature of the carborane cage.[2] Passage of a THF-H$_2$O solution (4:3) of the porphyrin diacid through a Dowex 50x2-400 ion exchange resin in the K$^+$ form produces the highly water-soluble dipotassium salt (3) after lyophilization of the eluate.

RESULTS AND DISCUSSION

Evidence in support of structures (1-3) comes from mass spectrometric and spectroscopic sources. The liquid selected ion (LSI) mass spectrum of (1) in a tetraethylene glycol matrix shows a molecular ion cluster (MH$^+$) at nominal mass 1341 corresponding to the formula C$_{48}$H$_{83}$B$_{40}$N$_4$O$_{12}$. The shape of the theoretical molecular ion cluster of this formula is nearly identical to the 15-peak ion cluster observed at 1341. Similarly, LSIMS of the free acid (2) produces a molecular ion cluster at nominal mass 1321 corresponding to the formula C$_{46}$H$_{79}$B$_{40}$N$_4$O$_{12}$ and whose shape is almost identical to the theoretical molecular ion cluster. In both mass spectra, four successive losses of B$_{10}$H$_{11}$C$_3$O$_2$ fragments are observed corresponding to loss of the carborane carboxylate. The visible spectrum of (1) in CH$_2$Cl$_2$ (10 µM) consists of peaks at 404 (Soret), 502, 536, 572 and 624 nm.

A summary of the 300 MHz proton n.m.r. data for (1) is presented in Table 1. The lack of a molecular C$_2$ axis is clearly demonstrated by the presence of four, distinct resonances for the meso-H and β-CH$_3$ groups. This makes difficult a detailed analysis of the spectrum, especially the conformation of the carboranyl ester-bearing side chains. Nevertheless, several features are apparent. At least two distinct and equivalent carborane CH environments are present, perhaps a reflection of the primary and secondary alcohol ester functions. Three resonances are assigned to the two-carbon side chain protons, a chiral methine (H$_\alpha$) and pro-chiral methylene (H$_\beta$). The H$_\alpha$ assigned to 7.68 ppm is strongly deshielded by virtue of its being bound to a carbon bearing two strongly deshielding groups: the porphyrin (ring current) and carboranyl acyl (σ effects). The two H$_\beta$ resonance have significant (0.7 ppm) chemical shift difference which might arise if the most stable configuration forces one of the H$_\beta$ protons into a position over the porphyrin ring where it is subject to ring current deshielding relative to the other.

As reported elsewhere in this Proceedings, the dipotassium salt BOPP is an excellent and selective tumor localizer and is strongly retained in one or more cytoplasmic organelle fractions for very prolonged periods. It has also been found to have an *in vitro* uptake and

Table 1. Proton chemical shift data for (1)[a]

δ	multiplicity	assignment
10.27, 10.23, 10.16, 10.14	s, 4H	meso H
7.68	m, 2H	α CH
5.68; 4.99	m, 4H	β CH$_2$
4.41	m, 4H	Por-CH$_2$
4.17; 4.10	s, 4H	carborane CH
3.81; 3.80	s, 6H	CO$_2$CH$_3$
3.68; 3.64	s, 12H	β-CH$_3$
3.63; 3.61		
3.30	m, 4H	-CH$_2$CO$_2$R
-3.65	s, 2H	NH

[a]   N.M.R. spectrum was recorded in CDCl$_3$ (ca. 5x10^{-3}M) at 300 MHz at ambient temperature with TMS internal reference.

retention ~20 times that of BSH and ~4 times that of BSSB.[3] The compound has low systemic toxicity, in contrast to the nido (open cage) porphyrin known as BTPP which has previously been reported by us.[4] The difference in toxicity may be related to the differing nature of the carborane cages in the two compounds. In BOPP all four cages are of the closo variety which are known to have very low toxicities whereas the four nido carborane cages of the BTPP species provide a reactive site for metabolic enzymes. Alternatively, the BTPP compound is a tetraphenyl porphyrin derivative while BOPP is a hematoporphyrin-like compound. Determination of the precise features leading to lowered toxicity in BOPP requires careful toxicological studies which are currently underway.

In an attempt to gain insight into the molecular architectural features of BOPP and other tumor-localizing porphyrins which lead to tumor uptake and retention, we determined the octanol/buffer partition coefficients of twenty-five porphyrins at four near-physiologic pH's. Table 2 tabulates our results with nine of the most interesting porphyrins, including BOPP. Interestingly, compounds 1-3 and 5-8 are all potent tumor localizers and each appears to localize intracellularly. Thus we suggest that porphyrins having octanol/water partition coefficients at physiologic pH (7.4) in the range from ~0.5 to ~10 may be desirable design targets for new photodynamic and neutron capture therapy agents. We predict on this basis that compound 4 will be an excellent tumor localizing agent. The relationship between hydrophobicity and tumor uptake has been noted previously. Moan *et al.* and Kessel have recently demonstrated that the more hydrophobic fractions of the photosensitizer hematoporphyrin derivative (HPD) are bound more strongly to low density lipoproteins (LDL) and are better tumor localizers.[5,6] Gabel *et al.* have found a strong correlation between cell uptake and partition coefficient *in vitro* at pH 7.5.[7]

The pH dependence of partition coefficients is noteworthy and potentially significant. Both BOPP and TPP (p-COOH)$_4$ undergo at least an order of magnitude increase in hydrophobicity over the pH range studied, while the other tumor-localizing porphyrins show much smaller increases as the pH drops. It has been observed that the interstitial pH in the immediate vicinity of tumor cells is significantly lowered, in some cases to as low as 6.5, and that pretreatment of animals with glucose significantly enhances tumor porphyrin

Table 2

	Compound	pH 7.4	7.2	7.0	6.8
1.	TPPS$_2$ (trans)	8.69	10.01	10.07	9.94
2.	BOPP	6.22	14.08	21.98	69.00
3.	hematoporphyrin	2.15	3.60	6.40	9.74
4.	TPP (p-COOH)$_4$	1.88	7.43	15.29	50.78
5.	chlorine$_6$	0.72	1.30	1.86	4.04
6.	photofrin (II)	0.48	0.65	1.97	2.54
7.	2,4-(2-hydroxyethyl)DP IX	0.43	0.56	0.99	2.20
8.	TPPS$_3$	0.34	0.33	0.28	0.26
9.	2,4-(1,2-dihydroxyethyl)DP IX	0.01	0.16	0.21	0.39

uptake.[8,9] Such a local decrease may result in protonation of the carboxylate residues of sensitive porphyrins to produce a higher fraction of neutral species which may then either diffuse across tumor cell membranes or into plasma lipoproteins which are subsequently taken up by receptor-mediated endocytosis.

ACKNOWLEDGMENTS

This work was supported by the National Institutes of Health, National Cancer Institute under grant CA 37961. We also wish to acknowledge the Mass Spectrometry Facility, University of California, San Francisco, for performing the mass spectral analyses. The Mass Spectrometry Facility is supported by the NIH Division of Research Resources Grant RR01614.

REFERENCES

1. T.F. Delaney and E. Glatstein, *Comp. Therapy* **14**:43 (1989).
2. D. Grafstein, J. Bobinski, J. Dvorak, H. Smith, N. Schwartz, M.S. Cohen and M.M. Fein, *Inorg. Chem.* **2**:1120 (1963).
3. R.G. Fairchild, S.B. Kahl, B.H.Laster, J. Kalef-Ezra, and E.A. Popenoe, *Cancer Res.* **50**:4860 (1990).
4. S.B. Kahl, D.D. Joel, M.M.Nawrocky, P.L. Micca, K.P. Tran, G.C. Finkel and D.N. Slatkin, *Proc. Natl. Acad. Sci. USA* **87**:7265 (1990).
5. M. Kongshang, J. Moan and S.B. Brown, *Br. J. Cancer* **59**:184 (1989).
6. D. Kessel, *Cancer Res.* **41**:1318 (1981).
7. G. Oenbrink, P. Jurgenlimke and D. Gabel, *Photochem. Photobiol.* **48**:451 (1988).
8. R.M. Bohmer and G. Morstyn, *Cancer Res.* **45**:5328 (1985).
9. J.P. Thomas and A.W. Girotti, *Photochem. Photobiol.* **49**:241 (1989).

CARBORANE COMPOUNDS FOR NEUTRON CAPTURE THERAPY OF MALIGNANT MELANOMA

J Gerald Wilson[1]

[1]Biomedicine and Health Program, Australian Nuclear Science and
Technology Organisation PMB 1 Menai NSW 2234 Australia

THIOURACIL-CARBORANES

The possibility of using thiouracil as a vehicle for stable nuclei such
as ^{10}B for neutron capture therapy (NCT) of melanoma was first discussed by
Fairchild and co-workers[1] in 1982. Since then a number of boron-containing
thiouracils have been synthesized and investigated.[2,3] Our research has been
directed towards the design and synthesis of a number of
o-carboranyl-thiouracils, the ten boron atoms of the carborane cage having a
clear advantage for NCT. Our first step was the preparation, previously
reported, of thiouracils bearing an alkyl group containing a triple bond for
later elaboration to a carborane.[4] The present paper describes the
continuation of this work with the preparation of the carboranes of this
series and its extension to the synthesis of a thiouracil in which a
carboranylalkyl group is attached to the nitrogen in the 3-position.

The carboranes, **DBTU-1 (1)**, **DBTU2 (2)** and **DBTU-3 (3)** (Scheme 1) were
prepared from the corresponding acetylenic alkyl thiouracils by reaction with
the decaborane-acetonitrile adduct *via* their *bis*-trimethylsilyl derivatives.[4]
The three carboranes are high melting crystalline solids and their spectra
are in complete agreement with the proposed structures.

To prepare a thiouracil bearing an alkyl group on one of the nitrogens
requires prior protection of the sulphur by a group capable of later removal
and alkylation under mild conditions. When alkylation was carried out by
stirring S-benzylthiouracil (4) and propargyl bromide in DMSO at ambient
temperature in the presence of potassium carbonate, two products were formed.
These were separated by flash chromatography and have been assigned the
structures (5) and (6) (Scheme 1) on the basis of spectral evidence.
N-3-propargyl-S-benzylthiouracil (6) was converted to the carborane (7) by
reaction with the decaborane-acetonitrile adduct in toluene or benzene in
reasonable yield (30%). The benzyl group was smoothly removed with anhydrous
aluminium bromide in toluene to give **DBTU-4 (8)** in 60% yield. The structures
of these four thiouracil carboranes were fully supported by spectral data
(IR, ^{1}H-NMR, FAB-MS) and elemental analysis (C, H & N). (Scheme 1).

DBTU-1 was found to accumulate in certain melanoma lines to give a boron
concentration 11 times that of the monoborono-thiouracil, BTU-1.[5] It also
showed good selectivity in kinetic studies with murine and human melanoma
xenografts in nude mice.[6] Poor solubility was overcome by formulation with
phospholipids, a process known as liposome entrapment, which in the case of
DBTU-1 and **DBTU-2** resulted in increased concentrations of these compounds in
several melanoma lines.[7] When tested in nude mice bearing the Harding-Passey

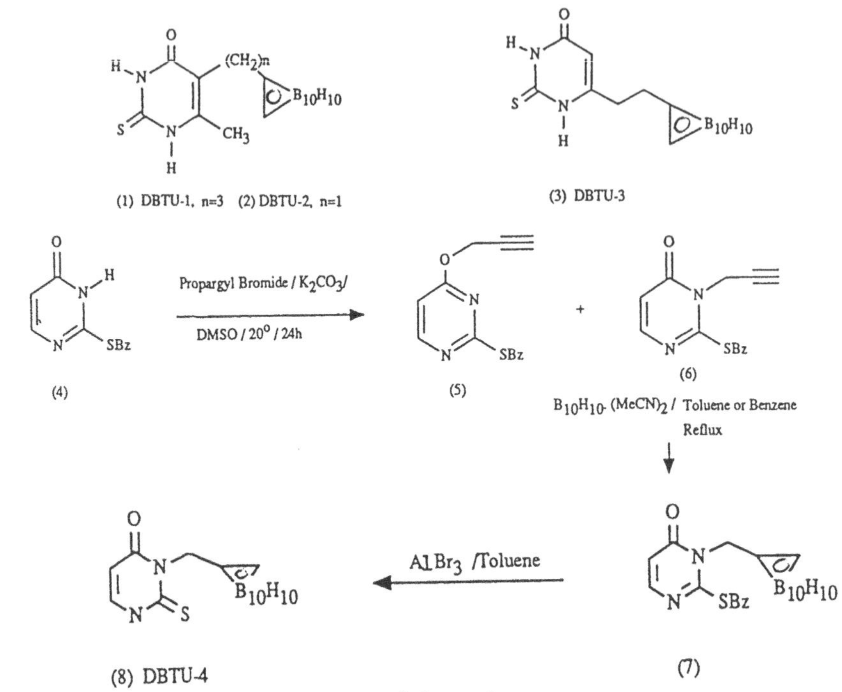

(1) DBTU-1, n=3   (2) DBTU-2, n=1

(3) DBTU-3

Propargyl Bromide / K$_2$CO$_3$/

DMSO / 20^0 / 24h

(4)

(5)

+

(6)

B$_{10}$H$_{10}$· (MeCN)$_2$ / Toluene or Benzene
Reflux

Al Br$_3$ /Toluene

(8) DBTU-4

(7)

Scheme 1

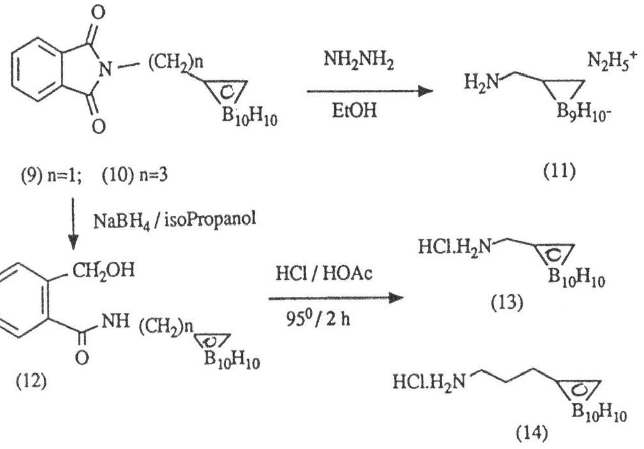

NH$_2$NH$_2$

EtOH

(9) n=1;   (10) n=3

(11)

NaBH$_4$ / isoPropanol

HCl / HOAc

95^0/ 2 h

(13)

(12)

(14)

Scheme 2

(15)

(16)

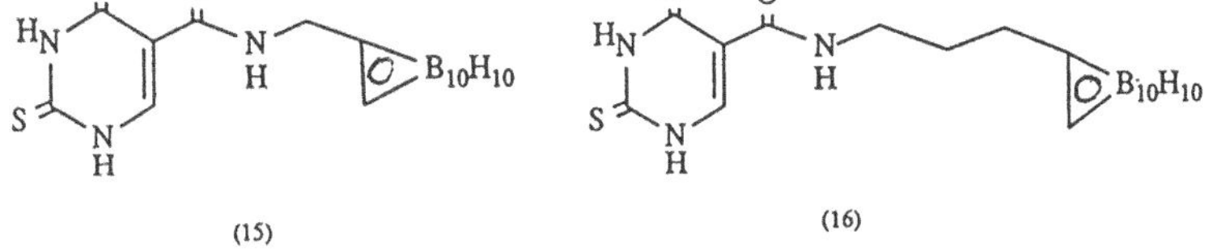

Scheme 3

228

melanoma, **DBTU-4** proved to be rather toxic. At a dose at which the animals survived, biodistribution studies indicated a level of 12 µg/g of tumour, about half the concentration required for effective BNCT.

AMINOALKYLCARBORANES

A carborane synthon consisting of a carborane cage bearing a reactive functional group capable of covalent attachment to a variety of other moieties, particularly those of interest to BNCT, has been an attractive synthetic goal for some time.

In our synthesis of a reagent of this type we chose the amino functionality as the reactive group for attachment to other structures. Our first objective, was the parent aminomethylcarborane **(13)**, aminoalkylcarborane. The preparation of this compound from phthalimidomethylcarborane **(9)** by the action of hydrazine in the usual way was reported in 1970[8], but on reinvestigation the product of this reaction was found to be not **(13)** but the hydrazinium salt of the **nido** structure **(11)** (scheme 2). This resulted from abstraction of a boron atom from the carborane cage by the action of hydrazine. Strong bases are known to degrade the carborane cage to the corresponding **nido** dicarbaundecarborate.[9] The compound was characterised as its tetramethylammonium salt.

A recent method[10] for removing the phthaloyl group from amino acid derivatives was then investigated. This method employs sodium borohydride in isopropanol to open the phthaloyl ring to give an o-hydroxymethylbenzoyl derivative **(12)** which is then converted by acid to phthalide and the amine hydrochloride. In this way phthalimidomethylcarborane **(9)** was converted *via* **(12)** to **aminomethylcarborane hydrochloride (13)** in good yield. In the same way **aminopropylcarborane hydrochloride (14)** was prepared from phthalimido-propylcarborane **(10)**. The structures of these two compounds are supported by spectral evidence (Scheme 2).

To provide derivatives of potential utility for BNCT, these two compounds were converted into the **amides of thiouracil-5-carboxylic acid, (15) and (16)**, in excellent yield by the mixed anhydride method. Physical data are in agreement with the proposed structures (Scheme 3). These amides are novel compounds and illustrate another way of linking a carborane moiety to thiouracil to produce boron derivatives that show potential for selectively concentrating in melanoma cells. They are awaiting biological evaluation.

Work directed towards the attachment of **(13)** and **(14)** to phenylalanine by joining the amino acid moiety to the carborane by means of a thiourea bridge is in progress. The presence of the amino acid in the product is expected to assist in overcoming solubility problems.

REFERENCES

1.   R.G. Fairchild, S. Packer, D. Greenberg, P. Som, A.B. Brill, I. Fand and W.P. McNally. Cancer Res., 1982, *42*, 5126.

2.   A. Roberto and B.S. Larsson. Strahlenther. Onkol., 1989, 165-167.

3.   W. Tjarks. Dissertation, University of Bremen, 1989.

4.   J.G. Wilson. Pigment Cell Res., 1989, 2, 297.

5.   S. Corderoy-Buck, B.J. Allen, J.G. Wilson, J.K. Brown, M.H. Mountford, W. Tjarks, D. Gabel, D. Barkla, A. Patwardhan, A.K. Chandler and D.E. Moore. Proc 6th Internat. Symp. Radiopharmacology, Sydney, Aug. 24-26th, 1989, p.14.

6. S. Corderoy-Buck, J.G. Wilson, D. Gabel, W. Tjarks, D.E. Moore and A.K. Chandler. Proc 4th Aust-Japan Workshop for Malignant Melanoma, Kobe, Japan, Feb. 13-16, 1990, p. 51.

7. S. Corderoy-Buck, J.G. Wilson, D.E. Moore, A.K. Chandler and B.J. Allen. Proc. 4th Internat. Symp. NCT.

8. T. Nakagawa, H. Watanabe and T. Yoshizaki. Japan Patent, 7, 031, 940; Chem. Abstr., 1970, $\underline{74}$, 100213[t].

9. M.F. Hawthorne, D.C. Young, P.M. Garrett, D.A. Owen, S.G. Schwerin, F.N. Tebbe, and P.A. Wegner. J. Amer. Chem. Soc., 1968, $\underline{90}$, 862.

10. J.O. Osby, M.G. Martin and B. Ganem. Tet. Letts., 1984, $\underline{25}$, 2093.

SYNTHESIS OF ^{10}B- AND ^{157}Gd-LABELLED DNA LIGANDS FOR NEUTRON

CAPTURE THERAPY

A.D. Whittaker, D.P. Kelly
Department of Chemistry, University of Melbourne

M. Pardee and R.F. Martin
Peter MacCallum Cancer Institute, Melbourne Australia

Introduction

Experiments with plasmid DNA have demonstrated that neutron capture by DNA-associated ^{157}Gd induces DNA double-strand breaks, presumably mediated by the Auger electron emission accompanying internal conversion, which in turn is associated with the n, gamma reaction[1]. Those experiments involved use of $GdCl_3$ in a low ionic strength buffer, which allowed ionic association of the Gd^{3+} with phosphate groups on the DNA. Dissociation of the Gd^{3+}/DNA complex by inclusion of EDTA markedly decreased the DNA damage induced by thermal neutron irradiation, reflecting the limited range of Auger electrons. Given the established[2] radiobiological toxicity of DNA-associated decay of Auger-emitting isotopes such as ^{125}I, and the high thermal neutron capture cross-section of ^{157}Gd, there is obvious potential to exploit ^{157}GdNC for NCT. However, a stable Gd-DNA association is a clear pre-requisite, and we have therefore undertaken the synthesis of Gd-labelled DNA ligands.

Desirable characteristics of a Gd-labelled DNA ligand designed to evaluate potential application to NCT include:-

(i)   a stable association of the ligand with DNA,

(ii) a Gd-chelate that is stable under physiological
       conditions,

(iii) appropriate solubility and lipophilicity
       characteristics, enabling uptake of the ligand
       by cells in culture, and

(iv) low cytotoxicity at concentrations at which
       appreciable ligand binding to nuclear DNA
       is achieved

After the failure of cell culture experiments with some DNA ligands with innate metal-chelating ability - these failed criteria (ii) - we embarked on the approach of conjugating a

Progress in Neutron Capture Therapy for Cancer
Edited by B.J. Allen *et al.*, Plenum Press, New York, 1992

known Gd-chelating moiety with a known DNA ligand. We chose bibenzimidazoles as the DNA ligand part because of their favourable uptake/toxicity properties established with the application of Hoechst 33342 to cytofluorograph studies, and because of our experience with ligands of this sort[3-4]. Diethylene triaminepentaacetic acid (DTPA) was chosen for the Gd-chelating moiety largely for convenience, the anhydride is available and provides a facile route to amide conjugates. It was recognised that with only one of the acetic acid groups involved in such an amide, the Gd^{III}-chelate moiety would have a residual negative charge, and hence compromise requirement (iii), but we proceeded because such a ligand would nevertheless provide the opportunity for NC experiments with purified DNA.

We have also synthesised a bibenzimidazole phenylboronic acid, to provide a "control" for the Gd-labelled ligands, so that the radiobiological efficacy of the ^{10}B-NC and ^{157}Gd-NC events in DNA could be compared directly. ^{10}B-labelled DNA ligands also have interesting potential for BNCT[5].

Experimental and Results

The bibenzimidazoles were synthesised essentially as originally described by Loewe and Urbaniet[6]; details will be reported elsewhere. Each benzimidazole ring system is formed by reacting a phenyl iminoether (derived from the corresponding benzonitrile) with an aryl o-diamine.

I

II

The required intermediate for boroHoechst(**I**), 4-cyanophenylboronic, was prepared from the bromobenzonitrile by reaction with n-butyllithium[7] and then tributoxyborane[8]. The aminoethylbibenzimidazole used for conjugation with DTPA anhydride to yield **II**, was prepared from the nitroethyl analogue. The corresponding benzonitrile was obtained by NaBH$_4$ reduction of 3-(2-nitroethenyl)benzonitrile, which in turn was prepared from 3-cyanobenzaldehyde and nitromethane.

Both compounds were purified by HPLC on a reverse phase C-18 column. In general, methanol/water mixtures containing 0.1% TFA was used as the mobile phase. However, the aminoethylHoechst/DTPA anhydride reaction mixture was metallated with $GdCl_3$ prior to HPLC. It was found that the chelate was unstable in TFA, so it was purified using methanol/water mixtures with 0.1% acetic acid and 0.1% sodium hexane sulphonate. In the initial experiments, HPLC was monitored using samples that were trace-labelled with [153]Gd. The major product Gd-DTPA monoHoechst was characterised as **II**; a later eluting Gd-chelate was the bisamide - a conjugate between two aminoethyl bisbenzimidazoles and Gd-DTPA referred to as Gd-DTPA, bisHoechst.

Discussion

In the evaluation of the three compounds described[5], the boroHoechst is particularly interesting, and we will be proceeding directly to cell culture experiments. The uptake of both Gd-ligands is suboptimal, although the dimer is better. Both compound will be useful for NC experiments with purified DNA. We are now exploring further approaches to synthesise a Gd-labelled DNA ligands with improved uptake characteristics.

Acknowledgements   Tony Whittaker is supported by a Postgraduate Award from the Anti-Cancer Council of Victoria.

References

1. Martin, R.F., D'Cunha, G., Pardee, M., and Allen, B.J., Induction of double-strand breaks following neutron capture by DNA-bound [157]Gd. Int. J. Radiat. Biol. 54: 205 (1988).
2. Baverstock, K.F., and Charlton, D.E., DNA Damage by Auger Emitters. Taylor and Francis (1988).
3. Martin, R.F., Pardee, M., Mack, P., and Kelly, D.P., Synthesis and characterization of 2-iodo-4-[5"-(4"'-methylpiperazin-1"'-yl)-2",5'bi-1H-benzimidazol-2'-yl]phenol (iodoHoechst 33258) and 2,5-disubstituted benzimidazole model compounds. Aust. Jour. of Chem. 39: 373 (1985).
4. Martin,, R.F. Murray, V., D'Cunha, G., Pardee, M., Kampouris, E., Haigh, A., Kelly, D.P., and Hodgson, G.S., Radiation sensitisation by an iodine-labelled DNA ligand. Int. J. Radiat. Biol. 57: 939 (1990).
5. Martin, R.F., Haigh, A., Monger, C., Pardee, M., Whittaker, A., Kelly, D.P., and Allen, B.J. [157]Gd-Neutron Capture. Potential of [157]Gd-labelled DNA ligands for neutron capture therapy. These proceedings
6. Loewe, von H,. and Urbanietz, J., Basisch substituierte 2,6-Bis-benzimidazolderivate, eine neue chemotherapeutisch aktive Korperklasse. Arzneim. Forch. 24: 1927 (1974).
7. Parham, W.E., and Jones, L.D., Elaboration of bromoarylnitriles. J. Org. Chem. 41: 1187 (1976).
8. Thompson, W.J., and Gaudino, J., A general synthesis of 5-aryl nicotinates. J. Org. Chem. 49: 5237 (1984).

BEHAVIOUR OF THE BIOLOGICALLY ACTIVE SULFHYDRYL GROUP OF

MERCAPTOUNDECAHYDRO-*closo*-DODECABORATE(2-)(Mercaptoborate)

STUDIED BY ESR AND POLAROGRAPHY

O. Štrouf[1], P. Stopka[1], J. Velická[1], S. Bednářová[1]
J. Krupička[2], F. Jelen[3], E. Paleček[3] and L. Šerák[4]

Czechoslovak Academy of Sciences, Czechoslovakia
[1]Institute of Inorganic Chemistry, Prague
[2]Institute of Organic Chemistry and Biochemistry, Prague
[3]Institute of Biophysics, Brno
[4]J. Heyrovský Institute of Physical Chemistry and
Electrochemistry, Prague

Introduction

Mercaptoundecahydro-*closo*-dodecaborate(2-) (mercaptoborate) (**I**)
[B(12)H(11)SH](2-) is preferentially accumulated in cancerous
tissues in contrast to the surrounding ones; the mechanism of
this prolonged accumulation is not clear as yet. A possible
role of the sulfhydryl group present in this dianion was
postulated [1]. On the other hand, the presence of the
sulfhydryl group leads to the easy autoxidation of
mercaptoborate and thus to a significant instability of the
drug containing this dianion. In connection with this problem,
we have examined the ESR spectrum of mercaptoborate and its
polarographic behaviour.

Method

a) ESR spectra of mercaptoborate [2]

The superoxide anion-radicals (g = 2.0339 and g = 2.0039) are
generated by the ultraviolet irradiation (high-pressure
discharge mercury lamp HBO-200) of air- or oxygen-saturated
aqueous solutions of tetramethylammonium mercaptoundecahydro
-*closo*-dodecaborate(2-) at 77K. The superoxide anion-radicals
are probably formed from the activated oxygen molecule
coordinated on the mercaptoundecahydro-*closo*-dodecaborate
dianion in the complex **II** (see the Scheme), because in the
absence of this dianion no superoxide anion-radicals are
generated. By the irradiation in the presence of hydrogen
peroxide the formation of these anion-radicals is more
effective than in the presence of oxygen only. Simultaneously
the corresponding thiol radical **III** are formed from
mercaptoborate. These radicals give μ-disulfido-bis(undeca-

Progress in Neutron Capture Therapy for Cancer
Edited by B.J. Allen *et al.*, Plenum Press, New York, 1992

hydro-*closo*-dodecaborate)(4-)(IV). Under UV irradiation, this disulfide compound can give the anionic radical V [3]. In aqueous solutions this unstable radical is in equilibrium with a proposed double disulfide derivative VI [4,5]. Alternatively, the disulfide radical V gives with superoxide anion-radical the corresponding disulfoxide VII as a final product of autoxidation. The formation of sulfur-centered radicals from mercaptoborate is a principal key to a solution of autoxidation mechanism which can proceed according to the following scheme:

$$2 \ [B_{12}H_{11}SH]^{2-} \xrightarrow{\quad O_2 \quad} 2 \ \{[B_{12}H_{11}SH]^{2-} \cdot O_2\}$$
$$\underset{I}{} \qquad\qquad\qquad\qquad \underset{II}{}$$
$$\downarrow h\nu$$

$$[B_{12}H_{11}S\text{-}S_{12}H_{11}]^{4-} + 4 \ H^+ \longleftarrow 2 \ [B_{12}H_{11}\overset{\cdot}{S}H]^{2-} + 2 \ \overset{\cdot}{O_2^-}$$
$$\underset{IV}{} \qquad\qquad\qquad\qquad \underset{III}{}$$
$$\downarrow h\nu$$

$$[B_{12}H_{11}\overset{\cdot+}{S}\text{-}SB_{12}H_{11}]^{3-} \xrightarrow{\quad \overset{\cdot}{O_2^-} \quad} [B_{12}H_{11}S(O)\text{-}SB_{12}H_{11}]^{4-}$$
$$\underset{V}{} \qquad\qquad\qquad\qquad \underset{VII}{}$$
$$\updownarrow$$
$$[B_{12}H_{11}\overset{+}{S}\text{-}SB_{12}H_{11}]_2^{6-}$$
$$\underset{VI}{}$$

b) Differential pulse polarography [6]

Sodium and tetramethylammonium salts of I produce sparingly soluble compounds with mercury and can be determined using differential pulse polarography (DPP) at a dropping mercury electrode in the concentration range 0.5-15 μM (Ep = -0.62 V, in 0.05 M aqueous borax solution). Detection limits below 0.005 μM i.e. 0.6 ng B per mL can be attained with stripping voltammetry (Ep =-0.55 V) using relatively short deposition times (120 sec.). The latter electrochemical analysis has comparable sensitivity with the very sophisticated track etch/TLC method [7]. Moreover, it is selective for the sulfhydryl group present in the mercaptoborate and can be used irrespective of its isotopic composition.

c) TAST polarography [8]

TAST polarography can be used for the simultaneous determination of mercaptoborate and its oxidation product IV. In 0.1 N sulfuric acid this method yields the anodic wave of I (Fig.1) as well as the cathodic wave of the oxidation product IV (Fig.2). The most positive wave [E(1/2) ~ + 0.12 V] probably is due to the reduction of the adduct II. Its position is shifted below the current zero line due to the anodic current of the mercury salt of the mercaptoborate formed at the surface of the dropping mercury electrode [E(1/2) ~ -0.27 V]. The height of this anodic wave is linearly proportional to the mercaptoborate in the concentration range 1 to 500 μM. The cathodic branch of the wave corresponds to the disulfide product IV. In the strongly oxidized solutions of mercaptoborate which contain the products of oxidation VI and VII according to TLC analysis [5], the more negative polarographic waves can be formed [8].

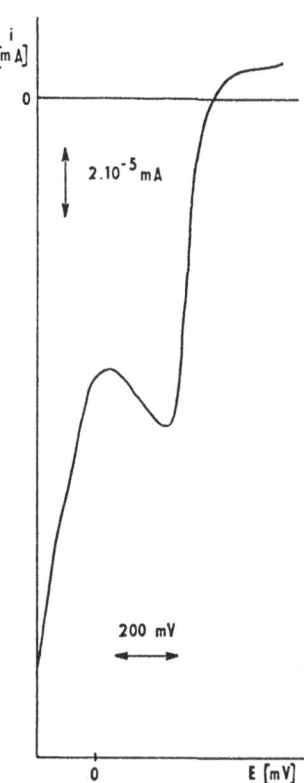

Fig.1 TAST POLAROGRAMS OF 20 μM SOLUTION OF MERCAPTOBORATE

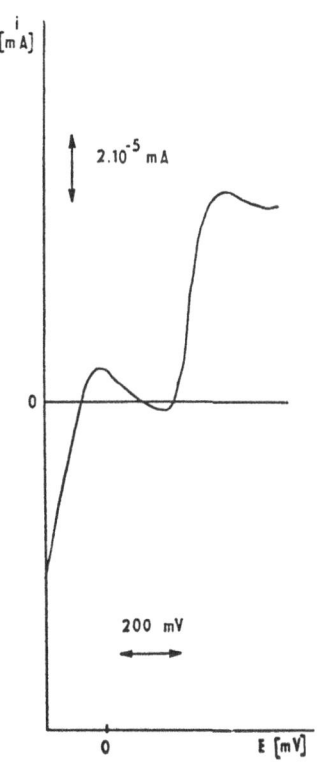

Fig.2 μ-DISULFIDO-BIS(UNDECAHYDRO-*closo*-DODECABORATE)(4-)
    ($E_{initial}$= +200 mV, supporting electrolyte 0.1 N H_2SO_4)

Conclusions

TAST polarography is suitable for the rapid analysis of the pharmaceutical preparations of the mercaptoborate and the DPP method is convenient for the assessment of trace amounts of this compound in a biological material such as urine [9]. The electrochemical methods represent highly versatile tools for the checking of autoxidation transformations of $\underline{I}$ which proceed probably by the above proposed mechanism.

REFERENCES

1. Soloway, A.H., Hatanaka, H., Davis, M.A. 1967, Penetration of brain tumor. VII. Tumor-binding sulfhydryl boron compounds, J. Med. Chem. 10:714-717.
2. Stopka, P., Štrouf, O. 1991, An ESR study of UV-irradiated solutions of tetramethylammonium mercaptoundecahydro-*closo*-dodecaborate(2-) at 77K, Coll. Czech. Chem. Commun., 56:657-662 and references therein.
3. Wellum, G.R., Tolpin, E.I., Soloway, A.H., Kaczmarczyk, A. 1977, Synthesis of μ-disulfido-bis(undecahydro-*closo*-dodecaborate)(4-) and of a derived free radical, Inorg. Chem., 16:2120-2122.
4. Ikeuchi, I., Amano, T. 1987, Quantitation of sodium mercaptoundecahydrododecaborate capillary isotachophoresis, J. Chromatogr. 396:273-279.
5. Štrouf, O., Bednářová, S., unpublished results.
6. Jelen, F., Štrouf, O., Paleček, E. 1991, Polarography and voltammetry of mercaptoundecahydro-*closo*-dodecaborate(2-), Electroanalysis 3:97:102 and references therein.
7. Schremmer, J.M., Noonan, D.J. 1987, Advances in analytical techniques for neutron capture therapy: thin layer chromatography matrix and track etch thin layer chromatography methods for boron-10 analysis, Med. Phys. 14:818-824
8. Velická,J., Krupička, J., Šerák, L., Štrouf, O.,unpublished results.
9. Štrouf, O.,unpublished results.

SYNTHESIS AND BIOLOGICAL PROPERTIES OF BORONATED THIOUREAS AS

HIGHLY SELECTIVE TUMOR SEEKERS FOR MELANOMA

Werner Tjarks, Hartmut Ketz, and Detlef Gabel

Dept. of Chemistry, University of Bremen, Bremen, FR Germany

INTRODUCTION

The success of boron neutron capture therapy (BNCT) depends to a very large extent upon the availability of boronated molecules with sufficient tumor selectivity and sufficient tumor uptake.

In targeting compounds to a tumor, several different mechanisms might be useful. They can be classified as relying on structural or on functional differences, and for each of these, qualitative or quantitative differences between the tumor and its environment could be utilized.

As an example of a qualitative structural difference, the use of tumor-specific surface antigens for binding specific antibodies might be quoted. An example of a quantitative structural difference would be the melanin contents in the case of melanoma, which might be utilized for accumulating melanin-binding substances. For the same tumor, the functional difference from its environment, namely the formation of melanin, might be used by offering false precursors of melanin.

Boron compounds might be tumor-seeking or tumor-retained as such. An example is $Na_2B_{12}H_{11}SH$ (BSH). For this compound, the targeting principle has not yet been identified. More frequent, however, are compounds which possess a tumor specificity on their own, and to which boron is attached chemically. In this paper, thioureas are described. Boronated thioureas, especially boronated thiouracils, have been proposed as melanoma seekers for BNCT [1]. The chemical preparation of the compounds, their stability, and their biological properties are described.

DEMANDS ON TUMOR SELECTIVITY

In the development of boronated tumor seekers, it is in principle possible to obtain compounds high tumor specificity (with uptake ratios of over 10 between healthy and tumor tissue), but with a low absolute concentration in the tumor. Other compounds are only moderately tumor specific (with uptake ratios of below 10 between healthy and tumor tissue), but with high absolute concentration in the tumor.

In previous discussions of tumor uptake of boron compounds (see, e.g., [2]) the absolute uptake of boron in the tumor necessary for successful therapy has been estimated to be around 30 $\mu g/g$ (30 ppm), with a tumor-to-blood ratio of 10 (i.e. a blood concentration of 3 ppm). Many calculations for epithermal neutron beams in BNCT have been based on these numbers (see, e.g., [3]).

The usefulness of each compound will be determined by its tumor specificity in combination with its uptake. Because BNCT is a bimodal therapy, the usefulness of a compound will be determined mostly by its uptake in the healthy tissue immediately surrounding the tumor, but not by its uptake in non-exposed parts of the body.

Whereas it might be tempting to assume that high specificity of tumor uptake might be of greater value than the absolute concentration that can be obtained, this is not so. In BNCT, and especially in BNCT of deeper-seated tumors, the healthy tissue (as well as the tumor tissue) will receive radiation dose contributions not only from the $^{10}B(n,\alpha)^7Li$ reaction, but also from other unavoidable sources. Therefore, less optimal tumor selectivity can be more than compensated for by high absolute uptake.

As an example, assume that in the absence of boron, a relative dose rate of 1 is found, but if the boron increases to 5 ppm, then a relative dose rate of 2 is observed. Then, for the tumor, a dose differential of 2 (i.e. a 100 % increase in dose) is found when 5 ppm are present in the tumor, and no boron in the healthy tissue (concentration ratio tumor/healthy tissue >> 10). If the same compound is present in the tumor in a concentration of 25 ppm, a dose differential of 2 would be obtained with 10 ppm boron in the healthy tissue (ratio = 2.5). For 50 ppm boron in the tumor, the same dose differential would be obtained with as much as 22.5 ppm boron in the healthy tissue (ratio = 2.22).

It is on this basis that less selective tumor seekers, but which show a robust uptake in the tumor, might be attractive. Such compounds include porphyrins, amino acids, and antibodies against receptors commonly found in excess on rapidly proliferating cells.

SYNTHESIS AND STABILITY OF BORONATED THIOUREAS

A number of boronated thiourea derivatives have been described recently [4, 5]. They contain either the dihydroxyboryl group (DHB) or the nido-1,2-dicarbaundecaborate (nido-carborate) cage.

Synthesis of DHB-containing compounds could be carried out from corresponding bromo compounds with butyl lithium and subsequently tributylborate. It was important to control the temperature during this reaction. Only between -100 and -85 °C could satisfactory yields be obtained. In this manner, the thiouracil compounds 1 to 4 of Fig. 1 could be obtained.

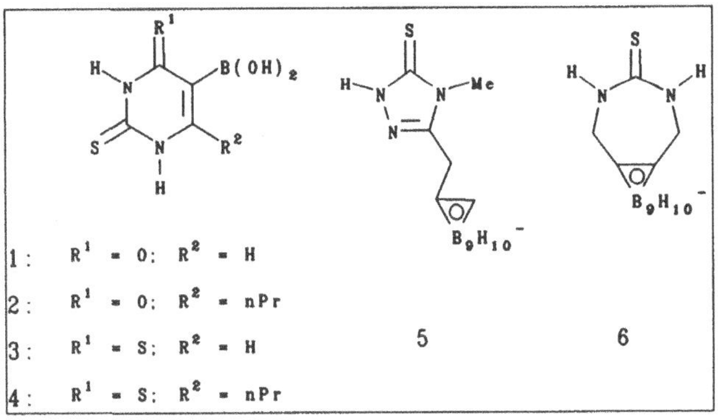

Fig. 1. Boron-containing thiourea derivatives prepared. Compounds 1 through 4 are described by Tjarks [5], compounds 5 and 6 by Ketz [4].

Whereas the synthesis of 2-thiouracil derivatives with a dihydroxyboryl group in 5-position led to stable products, it was found that other DHB derivatives were not stable to physiological conditions. This was especially true for the DHB derivative of methimazol, a melanoma seeker superior to 2-thiouracil [6]. Instability of the DHB group has been observed by others as well [7, 8]. The 5-DHB compounds prepared by us were reasonably stable in water, but could be hydrolyzed rapidly by base and by acid [5]. During the synthesis of 4-DHB methimazole, we could isolate the S-benzyl derivative and prove its identity with mass spectrometry. In the freezer, the compound could be kept for some days. However, at room temperature, it decomposed rapidly to S-benzyl methimazole and (presumably) boric acid.

We therefore speculated that the instability was caused by the attack of water (hydroxyl ions) on the sp^2 hybridized boron of the DHB group. This attack would yield an sp^3 hybridized boron atom, which allows the DHB group to leave as boric acid or borate. The remaining carbon would then be present initially as a carbanion. The probability of hydrolysis could therefore be influenced by the electron density and conjugation of the DHB group with its neighboring carbon atom, by the electron distribution in the tetrahedral transition compound, or in the stability of the carbanion formed.

Initial MNDO calculations were performed on the DHB compounds shown in Fig. 2. The results indicate that the electron density of the carbon atom linked to the boron is of crucial importance for the stability of the resulting bond. The electron density of the boron atom does not appear to greatly influence the stability of the compound.

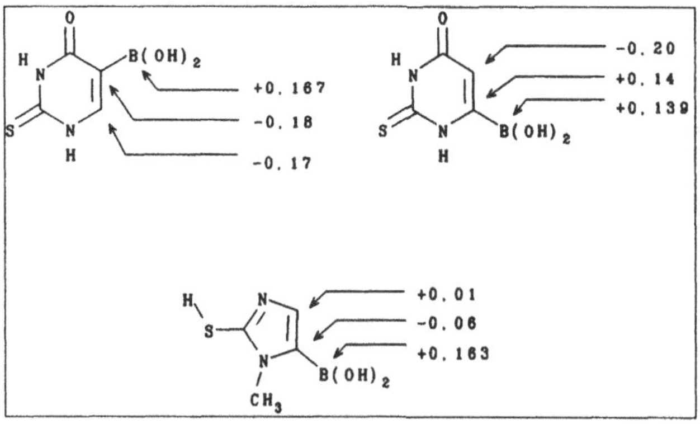

Fig. 2. Partial charges for the boron and carbon atoms of stable (5-dihydroxyboryl-2-thiouracil) and instable dihydroxyboryl compounds. Charges were calculated with the MOPAC program.

The synthesis of nido-carborate compounds could be achieved more easily. The known instability of the closo-cage to base was found not to be so great that no synthetic procedures in the presence of base could be performed without opening it. Instead, by careful control of the degree of alkalinity, closo compounds could be obtained [4].

BIODISTRIBUTION OF BORONATED THIOUREAS

Biodistribution was carried out in C57 black mice carrying the B16 pigmented melanoma. Compounds were given intraperitoneally. Boron was determined by quantitative neutron capture radiography [9]. The results are summarized in Table 1.

All 5-DHB substituted thiouracils showed good tumor selectivity. Compounds 1 and 2, with oxygen in the 4-position showed also good absolute tumor uptake in melanoma, whereas compound 3 with sulfur in this position did so to a much lesser degree, although it showed the greatest selectivity of tumor over blood of these compounds.

Compounds 1 through 3 showed moderate to low toxicity even after chronic administration, whereas compound 4 was toxic even at lower doses.

Compounds 5 and 6 with the nido-carborate cage showed only greatly reduced selectivity of tumor over blood, and instead accumulated in the liver and other organs. The concentrations in the liver exceeded those in the tumor, and also other organs showed higher uptake than the tumor. Unspecific binding of nido-carborate compounds to biological material has been found before [10].

Table 1

Distribution of boron-containing thioureas in C57 mice with B16 tumors

Compound	Amount (μg B/gbw)	Time (h)	Tumor (ppm ^{10}B)	Tumor/ Blood
1	15.6	4	32	4
		13	15	31
2	9.5	4	29	7
3	14.0	3.5	1.7	>15
5	4.0	5	13	1.4
6	4.2	5	7	1.8

CONCLUSIONS

The synthesis of highly specific compounds for melanoma is possible. It could be demonstrated that all of these compounds would accumulate in tumors over blood. However, the degree of selectivity of the uptake in tumor over other organs was greatly influenced by different chemical structures. The highest tumor selectivity of >15 could be obtained with compound 3, 5-dihydroxyboryl-2,4-dithiouracil. The absolute uptake per mole administered was, however, much larger for less selective compounds such as 5-dihydroxyboryl-2-thiouracil (compound 1) and its 6-propyl analogue 2. For the choice of a tumor-seeking compound for BNCT, these compounds demonstrate the need to consider not only selectivity ratios, but also the equally important level of uptake.

ACKNOWLEDGMENTS

This work was supported by the Deutsche Forschungsgemeinschaft, the Deutsche Krebshilfe Mildred Scheel Stiftung, the Fonds der Chemischen Industrie, and the North Atlantic Treaty Organization. The work of the European Collaboration on Boron Neutron Capture Therapy is supported by the Commission of the European Communities.

REFERENCES

[1] Fairchild, R.G., Packer, S., Greenberg, D., Som, P., Brill, A.B. Cancer Res. 42, 5126 (1982).
[2] Fairchild, R.G., Bond, V.P. Int. J. Radiat. Oncol. Biol. Phys. 11, 831 (1985).
[3] Clement, S.D., Choi, J.R., Zamenhof, R.G., Yanch, J.C., Harling, O.K. Neutron Beam Design, Development, and Performance for Neutron Capture Therapy, Plenum Press, NY, 51 (1990).
[4] Ketz, H., Tjarks, W., Gabel, D. Tetrahedron Lett. 31, 4003 (1990).
[5] Tjarks, W., Gabel, D. J. Med. Chem. 34, 315 (1990).
[6] Dencker, L., Larsson, B., Olander, K., Ullberg, S., Yokota, M. Br. J. Cancer 39, 449 (1979).
[7] Yamamoto, Y., Seko, T., Nemoto, H. J. Org. Chem. 54, 4734 (1989a).
[8] Yamamoto, Y., Seko, T., FengGoang, R., Nemoto, H. Tetrahedron Lett 30, 7191 (1989b).
[9] Gabel, D., Holstein, H., Larsson, B., Gille, L., Ericson, G., Som, P., Fairchild, R.G. Cancer Res. 47, 5451 (1987).
[10] Pettersson, M.L., Courel, M.-N., Girard, N., Abraham, R., Gabel, D., Thellier, M., Delpech, B., J. Immunol. Meth. 126, 95 (1990).

COMPLEX FORMATION OF PHENYLBORONIC ACID DERIVATIVES WITH ALDOPENTOSES AND OLIGOSACCHARIDES

Y. Kinoshita[1], K. Yoshino[1], Y. Mori[1], H. Kakihana[2], and Y. Mishima[3]

[1] Department of Chemistry, Faculty of Science, Shinshu University
Asahi, Matsumoto 390, Japan

[2] Department of Chemistry, Faculty of Science and Engineering
Sophia University, Kioi-cho, Chiyoda-ku Tokyo 102, Japan

[3] Department of Dermatology, Kobe University School of Medicine
Kusunoki-cho, Chuo-ku, Kobe 650, Japan

INTRODUCTION

p-Boronophenylalanine (p-bpa) has been studied for use in neutron capture therapy for melanoma [1,2,3,4]. The solubility of p-bpa is only 1.6 g/L in water, which is too small for medical uses. It is desirable and necessary to find a method to increase the solubility of p-bpa at the pH value of blood (pH 7.4).

It is well known that boric acid reacts with some sugars to form an anionic complex. Therefore, it was expected that the boronic acid group of p-bpa would react with sugars to form a soluble complex, as indicated in eq. (1).

$$p\text{-BPA} + \text{SUGAR} = \text{COMPLEX} \qquad (1)$$

Therefore we have studied this process and found that the solubility of p-bpa is increased by complex formation with aldohexoses [5]. Since D-fructose has the largest complex formation constant, the p-bpa/D-fructose complex was chosen for neutron capture therapy of malignant melanoma [6]. We have now investigated the complex formation of phenylboronic acid derivatives with monosaccharides (other than aldohexoses) and with oligosaccharides, and to estimate the stability constants of those complexes.

EXPERIMENTAL

To confirm complex formation and to estimate stability constants, the ^{11}B-NMR method [5] was used as described previously. D-ribose, D- and L-arabinose, D-xylose and D-lyxose were used as examples of aldopentoses, and maltose, lactose and sucrose were used as representative oligosaccharides.

11B-NMR Method. Solutions were prepared (i) containing 0.04 M of p-bpa with the same concentration of each sugar and (ii) containing 0.05 M of phenylboronic acid with 0.1 M of each sugar were prepared. The pH value of each solution was kept at 7.4. ^{11}B-NMR spectra were obtained by JEOL FX-90Q with resonance frequency at 27.8 MHz. During the measurements, the temperature of the solution was kept at 29°C.

RESULTS AND DISCUSSION

The complexation of aldopentoses with p-bpa or with phenylboronic acid was confirmed from ^{11}B-NMR spectra. In the cases of solutions containing phenylboronic acid derivatives with aldopentoses, there were two signals (8 ppm and 28 ppm, BF_3OEt_2). The difference between the chemical shifts is due to the electronic environment around the boron atom, for example, whether it is uncomplexed or complexed. Since the value of the chemical shift of an uncomplexed boron atom in a solution of pH 7.4 was about 28 ppm, the signal at 8 ppm was deduced to correspond to the complexed boronic acid group.

The complex formation constants were calculated from the area ratio of the two signals by using a computer simulation method [7] (see table 1). For both p-bpa and phenylboronic acid, the rank order of the complex formation constants of the aldopentoses was D-ribose > D-arabinose = L-arabinose = D-lyxose > D-xylose. Most of the values of log K for p-bpa were smaller (by 0.2 - 0.4) compared to those for phenylboronic acid.

In the cases of lactose and maltose, complexation was also confirmed by existence of two signals in the experimental conditions of high mole ratio (5:1 or 10:1) of sugars against phenylboronic derivatives. The complex formation constants were estimated by the same method as used for the aldopentoses. The complex formation constants with both sugars with p-bpa or phenylboronic acid were nearly equal (Table 1). In the case of sucrose, the signal of the complex could not be observed at up to 10:1 sugar-boron mole ratio solutions.

Table 2 shows the amounts of each sugar required to prepare 100 mL solutions containing 1 to 10 gram of p-bpa at pH 7.4. The sugar amount was obtained using the equilibrium constant in equation 1 (see Appendix).

It is important in respect to solutions to be used for injection into humans that the amount of sugar used to complex with p-bpa is small. From this point of view, it seemed that D-fructose, D-mannitol and D-sorbitol are suitable for complexation with p-bpa.

Appendix

The equilibrium constant of equation 1 is

$$K = [X] / \{([B_0] - [X]([S_0] - [X])\} \tag{2}$$

where [X] is the concentration of p-bpa-sugar complex, [B] and $[S_0]$ are the initial concentrations of p-bpa and sugar respectively. Since the solubility of p-bpa is $7.68*10^{-3}$ M in neutral pH, the concentration of uncomplexed p-bpa, $[B_0]-[X]$, is replaced by $7.68*10^{-3}$.

Thus equation 2 is rewritten as

$$[S_0] = \{ [B_0] - 7.68*10^{-3}\} / \{1 + 7.68*10^3 . K^{-1}\} \tag{3}$$

244

Table 1. Complex formation constants of various sugars
          with phenylboronic acid (ϕ-B) and p-bpa at pH 7.5

log K	ribose	arabinose	glucose	mannose	galactose	maltose
ϕ-B p-bpa	2.1 1.8	1.9 1.6	1.8 1.0	1.5 1.1	1.8 1.4	0.68 0.44

log K	xylose	lyxose	fructose	mannitol	sorbitol	lactose
ϕ-B p-pba	1.6 1.4	1.9 1.5	2.7 2.4	2.9 2.5	3.2 3.4	0.67 0.44

Table 2. Amounts (grams) of sugar required to prepare 100 mL solutions
          containing 1 to 10 grams of p-bpa at pH 7.4

p-bpa g	ribose g	arabinose g	glucose g	mannose g	galactose g	maltose g
1	1.9	2.6	10	8.3	4.5	70
2	4.1	5.7	22	18	9.9	150
3	6.3	8.8	35	28	15	240
4	8.5	12	47	38	21	320
5	11	15	59	48	27	400
10	22	31	120	97	53	824

p-bpa	xylose g	lyxose g	fructose g	mannitol g	sorbitol g	lactose g
1	3.8	3.1	1.1	1.0	0.77	70
2	8.2	6.8	2.1	2.3	1.7	150
3	13	11	3.7	3.5	2.6	240
4	17	14	5.0	4.7	3.5	320
5	22	18	6.4	5.9	4.4	400
10	44	36	13	12	9.0	824

References

1. J.A. Coderre, J.D. Glass, R.G. Fairchild, U. Roy, S. Cohen, I. Fand: Selective targeting of boronophenylalanine to melanoma in BALB/c mice for neutron capture therapy. *Cancer Res.* 47 (1987) 6377-6383.

2. M.Ichihashi, T. Nakanishi, Y. Mishima: Specific killing effect of [10]B-para-boronophenylanlanine in thermal neutron cappture therapy of malignant melanoma: In vitro radiobiological evauations. *J. Invest. Dermatol.* 78 (1982) 215-218.

3. Y. Mishima, M. Ichihashi, M. Ueda, S. Hatta, T. Nakagawa, C. Tanaka, K. Taniyama, T. Suzuki: Prerequisites of first clinical trial for melanoma selective thermal neutron capture therapy. *Proc. of the 2nd International Symposium on Boron Neutron Capture Therapy*, 1985, p 230-236.

4. K. Yoshino, M. Okamoto, H. Kakihana, Y. Mori, Y. Mishima, M. Ichihashi, M. Tsuji, T. Nakanishi: Chemical assay of boron and its distribution in melanoma-bearing subjects. *Proc. of the 2nd International Symposium on Neutron Capture Therapy*, 1985, p 291-302.

5. K. Yoshino, A. Suzuki, Y. Mori, H. Kakihana, C. Honda, Y. Mishima, T. Kobayashi, K. Kanda: Improvement of solubility of p-boronophenylalanine by complex formation with monosaccharides. *Strahlenther. Onkol.* 165 (1989) 127-129 (Nr. 2/3).

6. Y. Mishama, C. Honda, M. Ichihashi, H. Obara, J. Hiratsuka, H. Fukuda, H. Karashima, T. Kobayashi, K. Kanda, K. Yoshino: Treatment of malignant melanoma by single thermal neutron cpature therapy with melanoma-seeking [10]B-compound. *The Lancet*, Aug. 12 (1989) 388-389.

7. Y. Kato, K. Ando and A. Nishioka: Quantitative analysis of NMR spectra by computer simulation methods. *Kobunshi Ronbunshu*, 32 (1975) 200-206 (in Japanese).

OPTICAL PURITY DETERMINATION OF D,L-BORONOPHENYLALANINE BY

HIGH PERFORMANCE LIQUID CHROMATOGRAPHY WITH A CHIRAL MOBILE PHASE

Anita K. Gianotto and William F. Bauer

PBF/BNCT Research Programs, Idaho National Engineering
Laboratory, Idaho Falls, ID   83415-3519

INTRODUCTION

To effectively use p-boronophenylalanine (BPA) as a tumor-specific
agent for Boron Neutron Capture Therapy (BNCT) and to accurately interpret
the data from experiments utilizing BPA, the purity and enantiomeric
purity of the drug must be known.   The enantiomeric composition of the
drug must be known, since apparently only the L form of the drug is
biologically active[1].

A procedure utilizing reverse phase-high performance liquid
chromatography (RP-HPLC) with a chiral selective mobile phase has been
developed.   This type of ligand exchange chromatography has been known for
some time[2] and is based on the formation and subsequent separation of
diastereomeric, mixed-metal, chelate complexes.   These metal chelate
complexes are formed in the mobile phase and consist of a metal ion, a
chiral selector molecule, and the D or L form of the analyte.   In the
procedure used in this study, the metal ion is Cu(II) and the chiral
selector is L-proline.   There are many other chiral selectors, including
N-alkyl-L-Amino Acids,[3,4] that have been used to achieve similar separations of chiral molecules.   While this technique may not be suitable for
preparative scale separations because of the presence of the metal ions
and chiral selector molecules, it is a very nice technique for analytical
determinations of purity and optical purity.

Table I   Chromatographic Parameters Used for Separation
of BPA Enantiomers.

Column:	ET 300/8/4 Nucleosil® 10 C_{18} - Machery-Nagel
Eluent:	0.8 mM $Cu(CH_3COO)_2$, 3.0 mM L-Proline, pH 3.8
Flowrate:	1.0 mL/min - Rainin Rabbit HPLC Pump
Injection:	20 µL with a Rheodyne 8082 Injection Valve
Temperature:	Ambient to 60 °C
Detection:	Waters 991 Photodiode Array, UV-Vis, 200-300 nm, 2 nm resolution, quantitation at 215 nm

The chromatographic conditions outlined in Table I provide a more than adequate separation of the D and L isomers of BPA, tyrosine (Tyr), and phenylalanine (Phe). The elution order (Figures 1-3) under these conditions is D-Tyr, L-Tyr, D-BPA, L-BPA, D-Phe, and L-Phe. Several parameters were found to have an effect on the chromatographic resolution of the enantiomeric pairs and the amino acids themselves, including mobile phase pH, column temperature, and organic modifiers.

The effects of eluent pH can be quite dramatic. As is demonstrated by the k' values plotted in Figure 1, at pH values greater than 4, the retention times become excessively long and the separation between L-Tyr

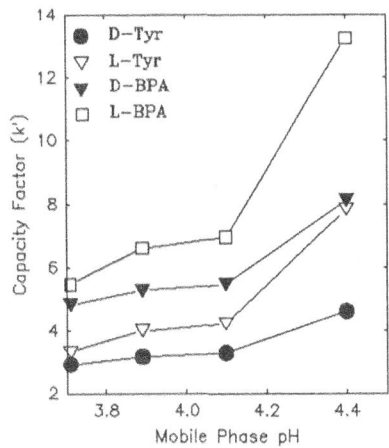
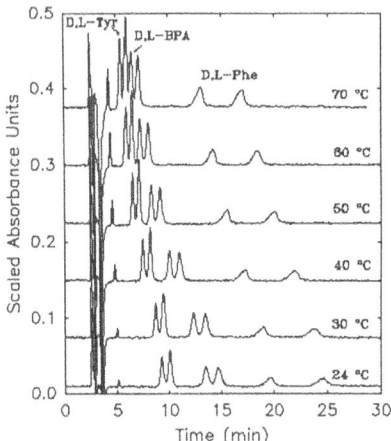

Figure 1. Effects of mobile phase pH on retention (k') of D,L isomers of BPA and related amino acids.

Figure 2. Effects of temperature on separation of D,L-BPA and related amino acids.

and D-BPA is completely lost by pH 4.4 (α = 1.04). At high pH values, phenylalanine fails to elute within 40 minutes. Similar results are obtained if N,N-di-n-propyl-L-alanine is used as the chiral selector.

The effects of temperature on the separation of the enantiomeric amino acid pairs are shown in Figure 2. Retention times are significantly shortened and peak shapes are somewhat improved at higher temperatures. The improvement in peak shape is particularly apparent for Phe and is because of an improvement in the kinetics of complex formation at higher temperatures. Resolution of all components can be maintained from ambient temperature to 60°C at a mobile phase pH of 3.8.

Similar effects on retention can be obtained with the addition of an organic modifier such as methanol or acetonitrile (Figures 3a and 3b) to the mobile phase. Resolution of D,L-Tyr and D,L-BPA is almost completely lost with only a 5% addition of an organic modifier to the mobile phase.

Because of the dramatic effects of an organic mobile phase modifier on the chromatography, temperature is considered a much more effective and useful parameter for controlling retention times while maintaining adequate resolution.

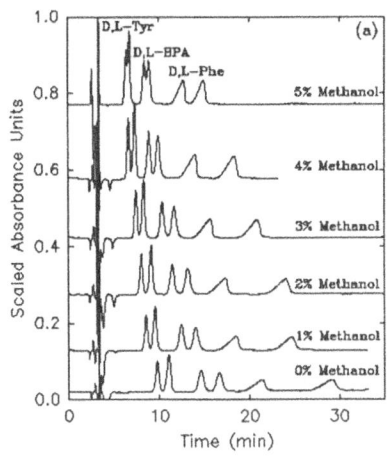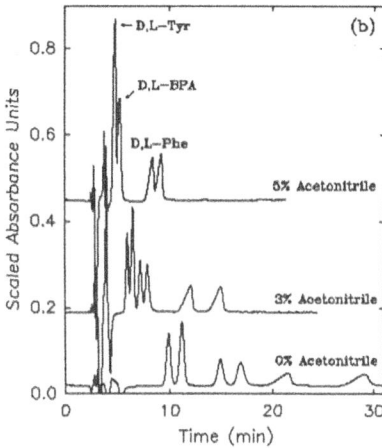

Figure 3. Effects on separation of D,L-BPA and related analogs caused by addition of methanol (a) and acetonitrile (b) to a pH 3.8 mobile phase.

The ligand exchange chromatographic method described here is quite linear, as demonstrated by the data in Table II. Detection limits were determined as three times the standard deviation of the Y-intercept from the calibration curve. Typical detection limits for each of the isomers of Tyr, BPA, and Phe are less than 0.1 mM and the response appears to be linear to well beyond 10 mM.

Table II. Typical Calibration Data for Quantitative Determinations of D,L-BPA, D,L-Tyr, and D,L-Phe.

Sample	Slope (AU/mM)	Y-Intercept (AU)	R^2	Detection Limit (mM)
D-Tyr	0.142 ± 0.004	−0.003 ± 0.002	0.996	0.05
L-Tyr	0.146 ± 0.008	−0.002 ± 0.006	0.988	0.1
D-BPA	0.15 ± 0.03	−0.001 ± 0.002	0.997	0.04
L-BPA	0.155 ± 0.004	0.001 ± 0.002	0.997	0.05
D-Phe	0.102 ± 0.004	0.000 ± 0.002	0.995	0.04
L-Phe	0.111 + 0.001	−0.0012 + 0.0009	0.999	0.02

CONCLUSIONS

A simple and reliable chromatographic method has been developed to separate BPA from other related amino acids and simultaneously separate the D and L forms of each of the amino acids. Separation can be easily controlled by adjustments to the mobile phase pH, column temperature, and addition of an organic modifier to the mobile phase. Other chiral selectors such a N,N-di-n-propyl-L-alanine can also be used in the mobile phase to achieve similar separations. The chromatographic technique described above demonstrates a linear response curve and can be used to determine drug purity as well as physiologic BPA levels. For the latter purpose, a method for extracting and concentrating BPA from biological samples using a solid phase extraction technique is being developed in conjunction with Dr. Eric Jarvi at Idaho State University.

REFERENCES

1. Coderre, J. A., J. D. Glass, R. G. Fairchild, P. Micca, and J. Kalef-Ezra, "Boronophenylalanine for Neutron Capture Therapy of Melanoma," in: Proceedings of the Workshop on Boron Compounds Suitable for Neutron Capture Therapy for the Treatment of Cancer, NCI, Bethesda, MD (1988).

2. Wainer, I. W., "Comparison of LC Approaches to Resolution of Enantiomeric Compounds, "Chromatography Forum 1: (4) 55 (1986).

3. Davankov, V. A., A. S. Bochkov, A. A. Kurganov, P. Roumeliotis, and K. K. Unger, "Separation of Unmodified α-Amino Acid Eenantiomers by Reverse Phase HPLC," Chromatographia 13: 677 (1980).

4. Duchateau, A., M. Crombach, M. Aussems and J. Bongers, "Determination of the Enantiomers of α-Amino Acids and α-Amino Acid Amides by High Performance Liquid Chromatography with a Chiral Mobile Phase," J. Chromatogr. 461: 419 (1989).

ENANTIOSELECTIVE SYNTHESIS OF L-(-)-4-BORONOPHENYLALANINE
(L-BPA) BY ASYMMETRIC CATALYTIC HYDROGENATION

Edward G. Samsel[1] and Brenda M. Simpson[2]

[1]Present Address: Ethyl Technical Center, Baton, Rouge, LA
[2]PBF/BNCT Research Programs, EG&G Idaho, Inc.
Idaho National Engineering Laboratory
Idaho Falls, ID 83415-3519

INTRODUCTION

Boronophenylalanine (BPA) currently has United States (U.S.) Food and Drug Administration (FDA) Investigational New Drug (IND) status in the U.S. and is being extensively investigated in the U.S. and abroad for the Boron Neutron Capture Therapy (BNCT) treatment of metastatic melanomas and other tumors. It has been used to cure melanomas in Japan.[1] The rationale for its use is that BPA can be a mock biosynthetic precursor for melanin, which is normally made by the enzyme tyrosinase from dopa and tyrosine. It is widely believed that the pure enantiomer, L-BPA, possessing S configuration, is more biologically active than is the D,L racemate.

The traditional synthetic route to D,L-BPA was developed by Snyder, et.al.[2] in 1958. Pure L-BPA has been prepared by Kemp, et.al.[3] by resolving the racemic product of Snyder's synthesis. Thus, D,L-BPA was esterified and enantioselectively hydrolysed using the enzyme α chymotrypsin. More recently, Glass, et.al.[4] have reported the selective hydrolysis of the N-acetamide derivative. All methods of resolution suffer from the inherent disadvantage that, at most, only 50% of the racemic material can be recovered as a pure enantiomer. At least 50% of the ^{10}B isotope is discarded during resolution.

METHODS

We have developed a direct enantioselective synthesis of L-BPA utilizing the asymmetric hydrogenation of a prochiral olefin using a chiral 1,2-diphosphine complex of rhodium.[5] This technique was originally developed at Monsanto Corporation by Knowles, et.al.[6] and was used for the manufacture of L-DOPA. The optimal diphosphine (called DIPAMP) is not commercially available, so in our research we screened those diphophines that are available for their ability to induce chirality in the reduciton of our substrate. The ligand called R-Prophos, originally developed by Bosnich,[7,13] was found to be adequate for the large-scale preparation of L-BPA, described below.

The use of cationic rhodium diphosphine complex in catalytic hydrogenations is well established.[8] To our knowledge, however, this is the first example in which a boronic acid group has been present on the olefin, and it is well tolerated by the catalyst. The methodology described here should be adaptable to the synthesis of other α-amino acids containing this functionality. Moreover, the tolerance for this group suggests that other boron-containing moieties, such as carboranes or closoborane dianions, could also be tolerated.

The route developed is outlined in the scheme. All compounds were characterized by high-field nuclear magnetic resonance (NMR) (^{1}H, ^{13}C, ^{11}B) and by infrared spectroscopy. New compounds were also characterized by combustion analysis (C, H, N). In the first step, 4-boronobenzaldehyde 2 was prepared in 93% yield from the ethylene glycol acetal of 4-bromobenzaldehyde 1 by a Grignard reaction with tributyl borate (^{10}B-enriched material may be used). The hydrolysis must be performed at low temperature to produce 2 in high efficiency. Direct reaction of aldehyde 2 with uric or hippuric acid by the conventional procedure[9] is not possible, as all attempts resulted in B-C cleavage. Therefore, the boronic acid group was protected[10] by esterification with diethanolamine, giving compound 3. Since the B-C cleavage described above probably resulted from reaction of the aryl boronic acid and ester with acetic anhydride, we prepared 2-phenyl-2-oxaxolin-5-one[11] and achieved the preparation of azlactone 4 in 62% yield by refluxing in dioxane. Boiling yellow 4 in 1% KOH-H$_2$O for 15 minutes produces a colorless solution which, upon acidification, precipitates white N-benzoylamido-4-boronocinnamic acid 5 in 87% yield. The product is the desired Z isomer, as evidenced by its vinyl resonance at δ 7.44; the undesirable E isomer should resonate at δ 8.66, by analogy with its unboronated analogue,[12] but no E isomer was observed.

The ability of the various chiral diphosphines to induce asymmetry in the hydrogenation of 5 was not previously known; nor was the stability of the catalyst to the boronic acid group known. An in-situ screening method was devised to evaluate the effectiveness of the phosphines and the configuration of their products. The optical rotations were measured and are shown in Table I. The specific rotation of optically pure 6 is not known, but the measured values are indicative of relative effectiveness. Subsequent hydrolysis of the product 6 formed with R-Prophos was shown to be L-BPA by comparison with authentic material, so the sign of rotation of 6 bearing the S configuration is (+). Of the phosphines tested, only R-Prophos gives (+) and this ligand also produced the highest optical yield of either configuration. The most significant aspect of this screening is that the results in Table I closely parallel the literature results[14] for hydrogenation of N-benzoylamidocinnamic acid without a boronic acid substituent. The catalyst is insensitive to the presence of this group in the para position. Therefore, those phosphines that are known to be superior to R-Prophos (i.e., DIPAMP, Norphos) could be used to good effect in this reaction, should they become available.

TABLE I.   Results of Chiral Diphosphine Screening

Diphosphine	Optical Rotation $[\alpha]^D_{23}$
(S,S)-Chiraphos	O (N,R)*
(R)-Prophos	+ 50 °
(S,S)-BDPP	− 40 °
(S,S)-DIOP	− 23 °

* No reaction, unreacted 5 recovered

Preparative hydrogenations were conducted with the preformed (1,5-COD)(Prophos)Rh(I) cationic complex shown in Figure 1. This type of catalyst was developed by Schrock and Osborn[8] and is readily prepared from [(1,5-COD)RhCl]$_2$ or its norbornadiene analogue.[15] The hydrogenations proceed at 45 psi and 50 °C in excellent chemical yield.

The optical yield of the hydrogenation reactions depend on the ratio of catalyst to substrate. For example, the use of 1/500 equivalents produce L-(+)-6 with 88% enantiomeric excess (ee), while the use of 1/1000 equivalents of catalyst gave product with only 76% ee. These values of ee were determined for L-BPA, obtained by hydrolysis of the hydrogenation products 6 and before crystallization of the L-BPA. The method used was developed at the Idaho National Engineering Laboratory (Bauer and Gianotto, this symposium) and involves chiral high-performance liquid chromatography (HPLC) analysis. Measurement of ee values by polarimetry is precluded by the unknown specific rotation of optically pure 6 and by the low specific rotation of L-BPA.

Although optical yields are less than 90%, enantiomerically pure L-BPA is readily isolated by crystallizing the product of the hydrolysis of 6. During crystallization, the crude L-BPA resolves itself to give product with greater than 96% ee and enantiomerically impure mother liquor. Such self resolution is a very common phenomenon during crystallization of materials that are highly enriched in one enantiomer. The isolated yield (67%) of pure L-BPA suffers, however, and would be greater if higher optical yields were obtained in the hydrogenation step.

CONCLUSIONS

The procedures described here constitute the first practical route for the bulk preparation of pure L-BPA. The product is prepared in 23% overall yield from 4-bromobenzaldehyde as opposed to less than 5% overall yield from 4-bromotoluene by the conventional method of enzymatic hydrolysis of BPA-ethyl ester. The high cost of rhodium is offset by its high catalytic efficiency and the rhodium can be recovered and recycled by conventional methods.

Synthetic Scheme

REFERENCES

1. Mishima, Y., et.al., "First Human Clinical Trial of Melanoma Neutron Capture: Diagnosis and Therapy," Strahlentherapie und Onkologie 165: (2/3) 251-254 (February/March 1989).

2. Snyder, et.al., "Synthesis of Aromatic Boronic Acids/Aldehydo Boronic Acids and a Boronic Acid Analog of Tyrosine," J. Am. Chem. Soc. 80: 835 (1958).

3. Roberts, B. C., et.al., "Pluripotential Amino Acids I. (L)-p-Dihydroxyborylphenylalanine (L-BPH) as a Precursor of L-Phe and L-Tyr Containing Peptides; Specific Tritiation of L-Phe Containing Peptides at a Final Step in Synthesis," Tett. Lett., 21: 3534 (1980).

4. Glass, J. A., "p-Borono-L-phenylalanine," Proc. First Intl. Symposium on Neutron Capture Therapy, Cambridge, MA (1983).

5. "Asymmetric Synthesis," Volume 5, L. D. Morrison (ed), Academic Press, NY (1985).

6. Knowles, W. S., et.al., "Asymmetric Hydrogenation with a Complex of Rhodium and a Chiral Bisphosphine," J. Am. Chem. Soc. 97: 2567 (1975); B. D. Vineyard, et.al., "α-Amino Acids by Catalytic Asymetric Hydrogenation," J. Molec. Catal. 19: 159 (1983).

7. Fryzuk, M. D., et.al., "Asymmetric Synthesis. Preparation of Chiral Methyl Chiral Lactic Acid by Catalytic Hydrogenation," J. Am. Chem. Soc. 101: 3043 (1979).

8. Schrock, R. R., et.al., "Catalytic Hydrogenation Using Cationic Rhodium Complexes I. Evolution of the Catalytic System and the Hydrogenation of Olefins," J. Am. Chem. Soc. 98: 2134 (1978); R. R. Schrock, et.al., "Preparation and Properties of Some Cationic Complexes of Rhodium (I) and Rhodium (II)," J. Am. Chem. Soc. 93: 2397 (1971).

9. Harbst, R. M., et.al., "α-Acetaminocinnamic Acid, in: Organic Synthesis, Col. Vol. II, p. 1, A. Gillman and A. H. Blatt (eds), John Wiley and Sons, NY (1943)

10. Yamamoto, Y., et.al., "New Method for the Synthesis of Boron-10 Containing Nucleoside Derivatives for Neutron-Capture Therapy via Palladium Catalyzed Reactions," J. Org. Chem. 54: 4734 (1989).

11. Crawford, M., et.al., "The Erlenmeyer Reaction with Aliphatic Aldehydes, 2-Phenyloxazol-5-one Being Used Instead of Hippuric Acid," J. Chem. Soc. 729 (1959).

12. Vineyard, B. D., et.al., "Asymmetric Hydrogenation. A Rhodium Chiral Bisphosphine Catalyst," J. Am. Chem. Soc. 99: 5946 (1977).

13. Fryzik, M. D., et.al., "Asymmetric Synthesis. Production to Optically Active Amino Acids by Catalytic Hydrogenation," J. Am. Chem. Soc. 99: 6262 (1977).

14. Koenig, K. E., Chapter 3, "The Applicability of Asymmetric Homogeneous Catalytic Hydrogenation," in: Asymmetric Synthesis, L. D. Morrison (ed), Volume 5, pp 71-103, Academic Press, NY (1985).

15. Abel, E. W., et.al., "Norbornadiene - Metal Complexes and Some Related Compounds," J. Chem. Soc. 3178 (1959).

COPYRIGHT

COMPLETE SEPARATION OF RACEMIC p-BORONOPHENYLALANINE BY HIGH PERFORMANCE LIQUID CHROMATOGRAPHY WITH CROWN ETHER-COATED REVERSED-PHASE PACKINGS

K.Yoshino[1], S. Mieda[1], T. Maruyama[1], Y. Mori[1], Y. Mishima[2], M. Ichihashi[2],

[1]Department of Chemistry, Faculty of Science, Shinshu University, Asahi, Matsumoto, 390, Japan

[2]Department of Dermatology, Kobe University School of Medicine, Kusunoki-cyo, Chuo-ku, Kobe 650, Japan

INTRODUCTION

Since the L-form of p-boronophenylalanine (p-bpa) has been shown to be more efficiently incorporated into melanoma cells than racemic p-bpa[1,2] separation of racemic p-bpa into its stereoisomers is an important subject.

One of the preparative methods used to resolve racemic p-bpa involves the use of α-chymotrypsin[3]. However, there has been a problem in that optical purity of resolved L- or D-p-bpa products was not easily determined.

In this paper, we describe a method which can be used to confirm the optical purity of p-bpa using high performance liquid chromatography (HPLC) with crown ether coated reversed-phase packings.

EXPERIMENTAL

The column with crown ether-coated reversed-phase packings (0.46 x 15 cm) was used. A liquid chromatograph pump (LC9A; Shimadzu, Kyoto) was equipped with an injector, an UV spectrometer (SPD6A; Shimadzu, Kyoto), and an integrator (CR6A; Shimadzu, Kyoto). The volume of the sample loop was 20 μl. The eluents were aqueous pH 1.5 $HClO_4$ solution. The flow-rate was 1 mL/min. The resolved enantiomers were detected using UV absorption at 270 nm.

RESULTS AND DISCUSSION

Figure 1 shows typical chromatograms obtained for p-bpa. The column parameters are given in Table 1. The capacity factors k_D and k_L for the D- and L-p-bpa respectively were calculated in the usual manner. The separation coefficient, α, and the resolution factor, R_S, were defined as

$$\alpha = k_L / k_D$$

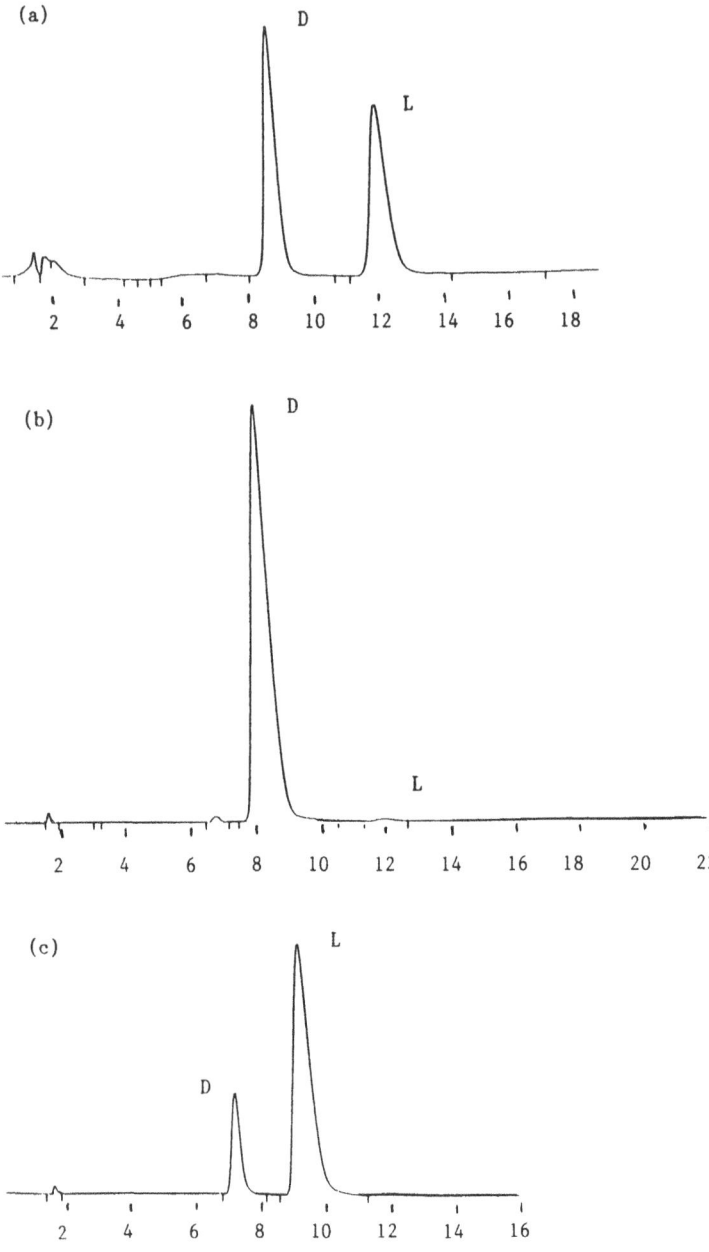

Figure 1. Separation of p-bpa on a reversed-phase packing coated with
crown-ether: (a)racemic p-bpa, 0.54mg/ml, at 20℃ ; (b)D-p-bpa, 1.1mg/ml,
at 19℃ ; (c)L-riched p-bpa ,1.0mg/ml, at 25℃ . Elution sequence: D = D-
p-bpa; L = L-p-bpa.

Table 1   Capacity Factors and Enantioselectivity for p-bpa on Crown Ether-coated Reversed-phase Packing

Run	p-pba	Temp.°C	k_D	k_L	α	R_S
(a)	racemic	20	4.1	6.1	1.5	4.5
(b)	D-enriched	19	3.9	6.2	1.6	-
(c)	L-enriched	25	3.4	4.5	1.3	2.9

Column: 150 x 4 mm; Eluent : pH 1.5 perchloric acid;
Flow-rate: 1mL/min. Detection: 260 or 270nm.
The run numbers (a) (b) and (c) correspond to those in Figure 1.

$$R_S = 2(V_L - V_D)/(W_L + W_D)$$

$$= 1.18(V_L - V_D)/(W_{hL} + W_{hD})$$

where V, W and W_h are the retention volume, the base peakwidth, and the width at half-height respectively, and the subscripts D and L refer to the D- and L-enantiomers. Since the obtained R_S value was more than 2.9, it could be concluded that racemic p-bpa is completely resolved into its enantiomers.

This method has the advantage that the procedure is simple, with complete resolution obtained at room temperature within 15 minutes. Therefore, this method is suitable for routine work to confirm the optical purity of resolved D- or L-p-bpa.

The column with crown ether reversed-phase packings also shows the ability to completely resolve racemic phenylalanine and tyrosine.[4] It will therefore be used to investigate the stability of L-, D- or racemic p-bpa.

References

1. J.A. Coderre, J.D. Glass, R.G. Fairchild, U. Roy, S. Cohen, I. Fand: Selective targeting of boronophenylalanine to melanoma in BALB/c mice for neutron capture therapy. *Cancer Res.* 47, 6377-6383 (1987).

2. M.Ichihashi, M. Shiono, K. Yamamura, A. Komura, Y. Mishima, K. Yoshino, T. Kobayashi, K. Kanda, and H. Fukuda: Further *in vitro* radiobiological analysis on [10]B-BPA BNCT of malignant melanoma: correlation of determined [10]B-content and cell killing effect. This symposium proceedings.

3. D.C. Roberts, K. Suda, J. Samanen, and D.S. Kemp: Pluripotential amino acids I. (L)-p-Dihydroxyborylphenylalanine(L-Bpa) as a precursor of L-Phe and L-Tyr containing peptides; specific tritiation of L-Phe containing peptides at a final step in synthesis. *Tetrahedron Lett.* 21, 3435-3438 (1980).

4. T. Shinbo, T. Yamaguchi, K. Nishimura, and M. Sugiura: Chromatographic separation of racemic amino acids by use of chiral crown ether-coated reversed-phase packing. *J. Chromatogr.* 405, 145-153 (1987).

LIPOSOMAL DELIVERY OF BORON FOR BNCT

Kenneth Shelly,* M. Frederick Hawthorne,* and Paul G. Schmidt[†]

*Department of Chemistry and Biochemistry   [†]Vestar, Inc.
University of California at Los Angeles   650 Cliffside Drive
Los Angeles, CA 90024 U.S.A.   San Dimas, CA 91773 U.S.A.

INTRODUCTION

The development of effective targeting strategies for the selective transport of boron to cancer cells has been the single most urgent problem in the area of BNCT. Successful therapy requires the site-specific delivery of relatively large amounts of boron to tumors. Strategies employed have included the use of boron compounds with some natural affinity for tumors such as 4-(dihydroxyboryl)phenylalanine (BPA)[1] or $B_{12}H_{11}SH^{2-}$,[2] the attachment of boron species to other molecules such as porphyrins,[3] and the conjugation of boron compounds with tumor-specific monoclonal antibodies.[4] In any targeting strategy, the primary difficulties are delivering therapeutic quantities of boron, lack of specificity, and loss of specificity after incorporating useful amounts of boron in the targeting agent.

Liposomes represent a new approach to these problems. While liposomes, in general, do not concentrate specifically in tumors, Vestar, Inc. has shown that certain liposomes can be made to accumulate in tumors in high concentration relative to normal tissue, including blood. Further, liposomes can encapsulate a wide variety of water soluble species in significant amounts. We have been investigating these liposomes as specific carriers of boron compounds to cancerous cells.

LIPOSOMES

Lipid vesicles (liposomes) are spheroidal bilayers, enclosing an aqueous core, which are composed of phospholipids (fatty acid esters of phosphatidic acid). They may be comprised of one bilayer or several bilayers (unilamellar or multilamellar), and their size can range from twenty to several hundreds of nanometers. The utility of liposomes as drug carriers arises from their ability to encapsulate water-soluble species in the aqueous core, or to dissolve hydrophobic compounds within the lipid membrane.

There have been numerous attempts, generally unsuccessful, to target lipid vesicles to tumors in vivo.[5] Many previous studies have been hindered by the use of lipids of varying chemical composition or inappropriate size. Inhomogeneity of phospholipid components can adversely affect the stability of the liposome in serum,[6] and the surface presented by the lipid is related to its interaction with cells and serum components and therefore its specificity. The size of the vesicle is related to its clearance from the bloodstream by the reticuloendothelial system as well as its ability to diffuse into tissues.[7]

Research at Vestar, Inc., utilizing pure synthetic phospholipids, has produced useful vesicles of relatively small size, 50 - 100 nm. These liposomes have been shown to preferentially deliver their contents to tumor cells in animals[8] and humans[9] such that the tumor levels of effector molecules are five to ten times that of normal tissue, including blood.

One such useful liposome system is diagrammed in Figure 1. The phospholipid bilayer has been prepared with added cholesterol to increase the stability of the membrane, and nitrilotriacetic acid (NTA) has been encapsulated. Embedded in the bilayer is a small amount of the ionophore A23187 to facilitate the passage of ions through the membrane.[10] Upon treatment with a solution of radioactive $^{111}In^{3+}$, the metal cation is transported via the ionophore to the vesicle interior where it is complexed by the NTA. After i.v. injection the indium may be followed by gamma camera scanning. About 25 - 30% of the dose is taken up in the liver within 2 h in humans. However, because of the enhanced stability of this membrane[11] the remaining dose continues to circulate with a half-life of 4 - 10 h during which time tumors internalize the liposomes. As the vesicles are endocytosed, the $^{111}In^{3+}$ is released and binds to intracellular proteins such as transferrin. In Vestar, Inc.'s clinical trials[9,12] of the liposomal tumor imaging agent described above (trade name VesCan), over 230 patients have been imaged and a wide variety of cancers were detected in diverse sites such as soft tissue, lung, lymph node, bone, and liver.

Because they are made from natural body constituents, these liposomes are safe — no adverse reactions have been seen in the clinical trials and no toxicity was detected in the pre-clinical animal toxicity tests of VesCan. Since the targeting characteristics of the liposomes are essentially independent of their contents, we have examined the amount of boron that could be delivered to tumors using a similar liposomal preparation.

PROCEDURES

The boron hydrides employed were made by published methods.[13-15] Borocaptate sodium was a gift from the Callery Chemical Company. All murine biodistribution studies employed female Balb/c mice (approximately fifty days old, 16 - 20 g), with EMT6 tumors implanted in the flank 7 -10 days prior to the experiment. Tumor mass at time of sacrifice was 125 - 350 mg. Injections of liposomal solutions (200 μL) were made in the tail vein. Each data point represents the average of five mice. For clarity, error bars are not shown in the graphical data; standard deviations were typically 5 - 15% of the average values. Boron analyses were performed by ICP-AES[16] except for the liposomal $Na_2B_{10}H_{10}$ which was determined colorimetrically in vitro and by scintillation counting of animal tissue (*vide infra*).

Liposomes were prepared by probe sonication of the phospholipid, cholesterol, and the hydrating solution (typically 5 mL, 250 - 300 mM in the borane salt) at 65° C for 15 - 30 min. After cooling, the vesicles were separated from the remaining free borane salt by passage through a column of Sephadex G25-M which had been equilibrated with either phosphate- buffered saline (PBS, 5 mM sodium phosphate in 0.9% NaCl, pH 7.4) or phosphate-buffered lactose (PBL, 5 mM sodium phosphate in 9% lactose, pH 7.4). The vesicles eluted in the void volume of the column and were diluted with the appropriate buffer to a lipid concentration of 23 - 24 mg/mL. Liposomal preparations were sterilized by successive filtrations through Millipore membranes (first 0.45 μm and then 0.22 μm pore size).

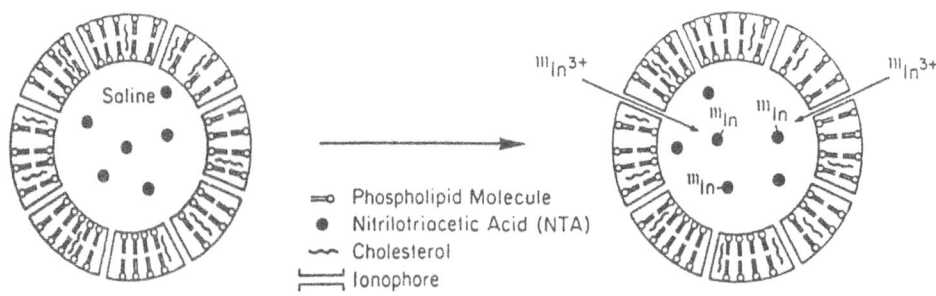

Figure 1. Schematic diagram of a precursor liposome and loading of In-111 for tumor imaging.

The decahydrodecaborate ion was selected for the initial investigation for several reasons. The triethyammonium salt is conveniently prepared in high yield in one step from decaborane (Eq. 1),[17] which, in turn, can be converted to the sodium salt by treatment with two equivalents of NaOH followed by extraction of the liberated triethylamine with hexane. This sodium salt is relatively inert and known to be non-toxic.[18] The $B_{10}H_{10}^{2-}$ ion also reacts quantitatively with phenyldiazonium cation[19] to produce an intensely colored red azo dye (Eq. 2). This reaction was used to determine decahydrodecaborate concentrations in vitro. For in vivo analysis the anion was tritiated by an acid-catalyzed hydrogen exchange process[20] which is rapid at pH < 1 (Eq. 3).

$$B_{10}H_{14} + 2\,Et_3N \rightarrow [Et_3NH]_2B_{10}H_{10} + H_2 \qquad \text{(Eq. 1)}$$

$$B_{10}H_{10}^{2-} + C_6H_5N_2^+ \rightarrow 1\text{-}B_{10}H_9NH{=}NC_6H_5^- \qquad \text{(Eq. 2)}$$

$$B_{10}H_{10}^{2-} + T_2O \rightarrow B_{10}H_9T^{2-} + HTO \qquad \text{(Eq. 3)}$$

The mean vesicle diameter of the liposomes containing $Na_2B_{10}H_{10}$ was determined by dynamic light scattering and found to be 70 nm. The concentration of the borane salt in the liposomal solution, as determined by the colorimetric method, was 4.8 mM (95% of which is encapsulated). This represents an encapsulation efficiency (before dilution) of <4%, which is typical for liposomes made in this manner. It should be noted that the remainder of the borane salt is recoverable. After 3.5 months storage at room temperature, only about 6% of the original contents had escaped from the liposomes. This is a clear indication of the stability of the bilayer, since the entrapped solution has an osmolarity 2.5 times that of the external buffer.

The biodistribution of vesicles loaded with tritiated $B_{10}H_{10}^{2-}$ is presented in Fig. 2A. As expected, the liver and spleen rapidly take up some of the injected dose, and the blood clears at a reasonable rate. Although good tumor uptake usually depends upon a long circulation period and liposomes with longer lifetimes could be produced, experience at Vestar indicates that optimal tumor to blood ratios usually appear between thirty and forty-eight hours post-injection. The tumor initially accumulates boron, but the dose that is delivered quickly washes out of the tumor (46% loss between 6 and 24 h) and the ultimate concentration of boron remains below the therapeutic level. The blood boron concentration does not drop below that of the tumor until late in the 48-hr experiment when the tumor boron concentration is too low to be useful. In fact, all tissues rapidly lose their delivered dose as time progresses. We interpreted this early experiment as indicating that the liposomes could be used to deliver a non-specific species to tumors, but what was required was a different boron compound that would have a propensity to remain within the tumor cells once it was delivered.

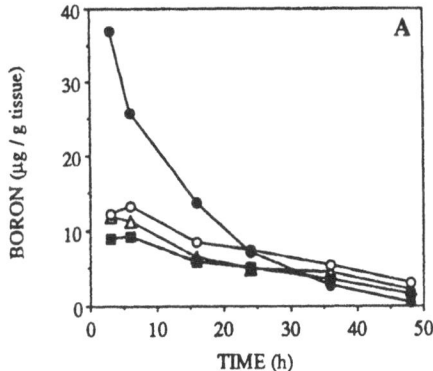 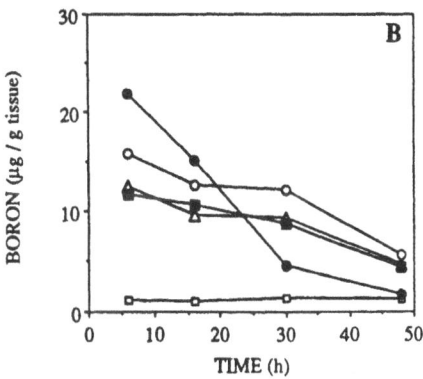

Figure 2. Biodistribution of liposomal boron in mice. A) $Na_2B_{10}H_{10}$, inj. dose 110 µg boron (~6 mg/kg); B) $Na_2B_{12}H_{11}SH$, inj. dose 126 µg boron (~7 mg/kg). Legend: ● = Blood; ■ = Tumor; ○ = Liver; △ = Spleen; □ = Muscle.

For this purpose we next examined borocaptate sodium, $Na_2B_{12}H_{11}SH$, a compound known to have some affinity for tumors. Liposomes loaded with this species exhibited the biodistribution displayed in Figure 2B. Here the blood is cleared at the same rate as in the case of $B_{10}H_{10}^{2-}$, but because the boron species escapes from the tumor cells at a lower rate (25% loss between 6 and 30 h) the results are more favorable. Blood boron concentrations have dropped below those of tumor 24 h post-injection and at 30 h the tumor/blood ratio is nearly 2 with a tumor boron concentration of 8.8 μg/g. As tissue levels continue to fall, the tumor/blood ratio reaches 2.6 at 48 h. While these results do not represent therapeutically useful values, the injected doses we have used for the screening of compounds in liposomes are quite low, in this case 7 mg/kg body weight. Further studies will be performed using higher liposomal concentrations, larger dose volumes, and an investigation of the dimer of borocaptate, $B_{12}H_{11}SSB_{12}H_{11}^{2-}$.

In search of a species that would persist in the tumor cells for an even longer period, we turned our attention to $B_{20}H_{18}^{2-}$, the oxidatively coupled dimer of decahydrodecaborate. This species is conveniently prepared[21] from $B_{10}H_{10}^{2-}$ by the ferric ion oxidation shown in Eq. 4. This anion offers two advantages. First, it doubles the number of boron atoms per particle, allowing an increase in the boron concentration without increasing the demand on the liposome bilayer to contain a hyperosmotic solution. The second advantage is the reactivity of this anion.

$$2 \, B_{10}H_{10}^{2-} + 4 \, Fe^{3+} \quad \rightarrow \quad B_{20}H_{18}^{2-} + 4 \, Fe^{2+} + 2 \, H^+ \tag{Eq. 4}$$

The two B_{10} cages in $B_{20}H_{18}^{2-}$ are linked by a pair of 3-center 2-electron bonds between boron atoms.[22] This portion of the anion is electron deficient and reacts readily with nucleophiles[23] as illustrated in Figure 3A for hydroxide ion. The initial product of this reaction, $B_{20}H_{18}OH^{3-}$, is reversibly deprotonated ($pK_a = 6.8$) to form $B_{20}H_{17}OH^{4-}$. The ^{11}B nmr of this product is presented in Figure 3B. In the low field region, where resonances for apical boron atom resonances occur, there are three doublets arising from the three unsubstituted apical boron atoms. The apical boron bonded to the other cage gives rise to a singlet, and the remaining low-field peak is due to the hydroxy-substituted equatorial boron. It was expected that a similar reaction by $B_{20}H_{18}^{2-}$ could occur with a protein residue (such as an amino group) once the anion had been deposited within a cell. This reaction would covalently bond the borane species within the cell and prevent its rapid loss from the tumor.

Another facet of $B_{20}H_{18}^{2-}$ chemistry is its photochemical reactivity. The product from Eq. 4 (hereinafter referred to as n-$B_{20}H_{18}^{2-}$) rearranges upon exposure to ultraviolet light to produce a photoisomer[15] (referred to as i-$B_{20}H_{18}^{2-}$) as shown in Figure 4. This isomerization can be reversed by prolonged thermal soaking. In the photoisomer, the two B_{10} cages are linked by a pair of B-H-B bridges.[24] This bonding arrangement is also reactive toward nucleophiles, and produces other isomers of $B_{20}H_{17}OH^{4-}$ in its reaction with hydroxide ion.

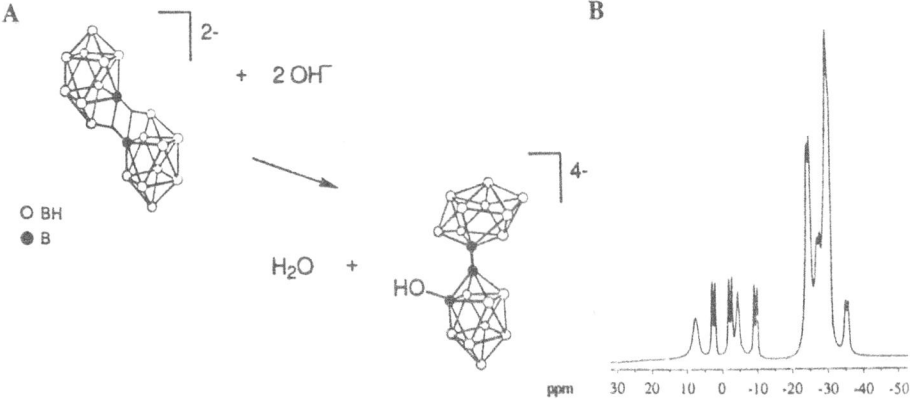

Figure 3. A) Nucleophilic reaction of n-$B_{20}H_{18}^{2-}$ with a hydroxide ion. B) 160 MHz ^{11}B nmr of the product of this reaction, $K_4B_{20}H_{17}OH$, in H_2O.

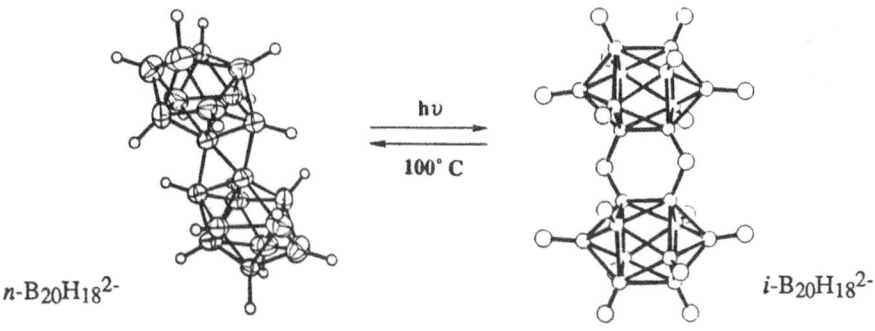

Figure 4. Photochemical and thermal isomerization of the structural isomers of $B_{20}H_{18}^{2-}$.

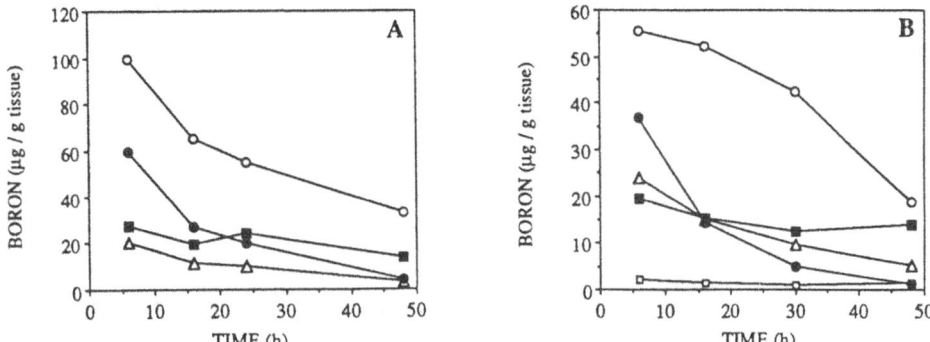

Figure 5. Biodistribution of liposomal boron in mice. A) $Na_2(n-B_{20}H_{18})$, inj. dose 273 µg boron (~15 mg/kg); B) $Na_2(i-B_{20}H_{18})$, inj. dose 206 µg boron(~11 mg/kg). Legend:● = Blood; ■ = Tumor; ○ = Liver; △ = Spleen; □ = Muscle.

The biodistribution of the liposomes containing $Na_2(n-B_{20}H_{18})$ is displayed in Figure 5A. As expected, using a twenty-boron atom species has significantly raised the boron dose delivered to tissue. This is most noticeable in the liver values, which at 6 h represent about 35% inj. dose/g. However, while the blood and liver clear rapidly, the tumor level remains fairly constant, decreasing only 11% between 6 and 24 h. At this point the tumor/blood ratio is 1.2 with 24.1 µg B/g in tumor. The ratio increases to 3.3 at 48 h while the tumor level has dropped to 13.6 µg/g.

Even more promising results were obtained with the photoisomer entrapped in liposomes. Using this species the tumor boron concentration persists quite well; the tumor boron concentration at 48 h (13.9 µg/g) is still 71% of the value at 6 h. This long retention allows time for the blood boron concentration to fall to very low levels resulting in a tumor/blood ratio of 11.7. This repesents a potentially therapeutically useful accumulation of boron in the tumor with an extremely low blood boron concentration (1.2 ppm).

The results obtained to this point suggest that small unilamellar liposomes of appropriate size and composition are a viable modality for the delivery of therapeutic concentrations of boron in tumors, in the presence of low normal tissue boron concentrations, for BNCT. Further studies are directed towards the discovery of other boron species with the ability to persist in tumor cells, determination of the biodistribution of larger or more concentrated dosages, investigation of the effect of various injection modes (e.g., multiple injection or route of administration), and the extension of these methods to other tumor models.

REFERENCES

1. Y. Mishima, C. Honda, M. Ichihashi, H. Obara, J. Hiratsuka, H. Fukuda, H. Karashima, T. Koboyashi, K. Kanda, and K. Yoshino, Treatment of malignant melanoma by single thermal neutron capture therapy with melanoma-seeking ^{10}B-compound, Lancet 2:388 (1989).

2. H. Hatanaka, Introduction, in: "Boron Neutron Capture Therapy for Tumors," H. Hatanaka, ed., Nishimura Co., Ltd., Niigata, Japan (1986).

3. S.B. Kahl, Boronated porphyrins for NCT, in: "Abstracts of Papers: Fourth International Symposium on Neutron Capture Therapy for Cancer," Sydney, Australia, 3-7 Dec, 1990, Abstr. 16.2.

4. E.A. Mizusawa, M.R. Thompson, and M.F. Hawthorne, Synthesis and anti-body labeling studies with the p-isothiocyanatobenzene derivatives of 1,2-dicarba-closo-dodecaborane(12) and the dodecahydro-7,8-dicarba-nido-undecaborate(1-) ion for neutron capture therapy of human cancer, Inorg. Chem. 24:1911 (1985).

5. E. Mayhew and D. Papahadjopoulos, Therapeutic applications of liposomes, in: "Liposomes," M.J. Ostro, ed., Marcel Dekker, Inc., New York (1983).

6. R.H. Wallingford and L.E. Williams, Is stability a key parameter in the accumulation of phospholipid vesicles in tumors? J. Nucl. Med. 26:1180 (1985).

7. K.J. Hwang, Liposome pharmacokinetics, in: "Liposomes: from biophysics to therapeutics," M.J. Ostro, ed., Marcel Dekker, Inc., New York (1987).

8. R.T. Proffitt, L.E. Williams, C.A. Presant, G.W. Tin, J.A. Uliana, R.C. Gamble, and J.D. Baldeschwieler, Tumor imaging potential of liposomes loaded with In-111-NTA: Biodistribution in Mice, J. Nucl. Med. 24:45 (1983); R.T. Proffit, L.E. Williams, C.A. Presant, G.W. Tin, J.A. Uliana, R.C. Gamble, and J.D. Baldeschwieler, Liposomal blockade of the reticuloendothelial system: Improved tumor imaging with small unilamellar vesicles, Science 220:502 (1983).

9. C.A. Presant, R.T. Proffitt, A.F. Turner, L.E. Williams, D. Winsor, J.L. Werner, P. Kennedy, C. Wiseman, K. Gala, R.J. McKenna, J.D. Smith, S.A. Bouzaglou, R.A. Callahan, J.D. Baldeschwieler, and R.J. Crossley, Successful imaging of human cancer with In-111-labeled phospholipid vesicles, Cancer 62:905 (1988).

10. M.R. Mauk and R.C. Gamble, Preparation of lipid vesicles containing high levels of entrapped radioactive cations, Anal. Biochem. 94:302 (1979).

11. M.R. Mauk and R.C. Gamble, Stability of lipid vesicles in tissues of the mouse: A γ-ray perturbed angular correlation study, Proc. Natl. Acad. Sci. USA 76:765 (1979).

12. C.A. Presant, D. Blayney, R.T. Proffitt, A.F. Turner, L.E. Williams, H.I. Nadel, P. Kennedy, C. Wiseman, K. Gala, R.J. Crossley, S.J. Preiss, G.E. Ksionski, and S.L. Presant, Preliminary report: imaging of Kaposi sarcoma and lymphoma in AIDS with indium-111-labeled liposomes, Lancet 335:1307 (1990).

13. M.F. Hawthorne and R.L. Pilling, Bis(triethylammonium) decahydrodecaborate(2-), Inorg. Synth. 9:16 (1967).

14. M.F. Hawthorne, R.L. Pilling, and P.F. Stokely, The preparation and rearrangement of the three isomeric $B_{20}H_{18}^{4-}$ ions, J. Am. Chem. Soc. 87:1893 (1965).

15. M.F. Hawthorne and R.L. Pilling, Photoisomerization of the $B_{20}H_{18}^{2-}$ ion, J. Am. Chem. Soc. 88:3873 (1966).

16. S.R. Tamat, D.E. Moore, and B.J. Allen, Determination of boron in biological tissues by inductively coupled plasma atomic emission spectroscopy, Anal. Chem. 59:2161 (1987).

17. M.F. Hawthorne and A.R. Pitochelli, The reactions of bis(acetonitrile) decaborane with amines, J. Am. Chem. Soc. 81:5519 (1959).

18. W.H. Sweet, A.H. Soloway, and R.L. Wright, Evaluation of boron compounds for use in neutron capture therapy of brain tumors. II. Studies in man, J. Pharm. Exp. Therapy 137:263 (1962).

19. M.F. Hawthorne and F.P. Olsen, Reaction of $B_{10}H_{10}^{2-}$ with aryldiazonium salts, J. Am. Chem. Soc. 87:2366 (1965).

20. E.L. Muetterties, J.H. Balthis, Y.T. Chia, W.H. Knoth, and H.C. Miller, Chemistry of boranes. VIII. Salts and acids of $B_{10}H_{10}^{2-}$ and $B_{12}H_{12}^{2-}$, Inorg. Chem. 3:444 (1964).

21. B.L. Chamberland and E.L. Muetterties, Chemistry of boranes. XVIII. Oxidation of $B_{10}H_{10}^{2-}$ and its derivatives, Inorg. Chem. 3:1450 (1964).

22. R.L. Pilling, M.F. Hawthorne, and E.A. Pier, The boron-11 nuclear magnetic resonance spectrum of $B_{20}H_{18}^{2-}$ at 60 Mc./sec, J. Am. Chem. Soc. 86:3568 (1964).

23. M.F. Hawthorne, R.L. Pilling, and P.M. Garrett, A study of the reaction of hydroxide ion with $B_{20}H_{18}^{2-}$, J. Am. Chem. Soc. 87:4740 (1965).

24. B.G. DeBoer, A. Zalkin, and D.H. Templeton, The crystal structure of the rubidium salt of an octadeca-hydroeicosoborate(2-) photoisomer, Inorg. Chem. 7:1085 (1968); S.E. Johnson, K. Shelly, and M.F. Hawthorne, unpublished results.

DELIVERY OF BORON-10 FOR NEUTRON CAPTURE THERAPY BY MEANS OF

MONOCLONAL ANTIBODY - STARBURST DENDRIMER IMMUNOCONJUGATES

Rolf F. Barth[1], Albert H. Soloway[2], Dianne M. Adams[1], and Fazlul Alam[3]

[1]Department of Pathology and [2]College of Pharmacy, The Ohio State University, Columbus, Ohio 43210, U.S.A. and [3]U.S. Borax, Anaheim, California 92801, U.S.A.

Introduction

The use of monoclonal antibodies (MoAbs) for the delivery of radionuclides, drugs and toxins for therapeutic purposes has been the subject of intensive investigation over the past decade. A few investigators, including ourselves, have focused on the possible use of MoAbs directed against tumor associated antigens (TAA) for targeting boron-10 to tumors[1,2]. Using a high molecular weight macromolecule, poly-DL-lysine and a methyl isocyanato-polyhedral borane, $Na(CH_3)_3 NB_{10}H_8NCO$, we have prepared a boronated polylysine (BPL) containing 23% boron by weight and having >1700 boron atoms per polymeric unit[3]. This boronated macromolecule was then attached to MoAbs utilizing two heterobifunctional reagents N-succinimidyl 3-(2 pyridyldithio) propionate (SPDP), which was used to introduce potential sulfhydryl groups into proteins, and sulfo m-maleimidobenzoyl-N-hydroxysuccinimide ester (sMBS), which was used to introduce maleimido groups on MoAbs[4]. The resulting immunoconjugates retained a high degree of in vitro immunoreactivity but had lost their in vivo tumor localizing properties[5]. It became apparent that an alternative approach was required to produce boron containing immunoconjugates that would retain both their immunoreactivity and in vivo tumor localizing properties[6]. The purpose of the present report is to describe our most recent efforts to prepare boron containing immunoconjugates using a neutrally charged precision macromolecule consisting of repetitive polyamido amino groups(PAMAM) arranged in a starburst pattern ("starburst" dendrimers)[7].

Materials and Methods

Boronation of starburst dendrimer

Starburst dendrimers are composed of repetitive PAMAMs consisting of an inner core, interior layers of repetitive monomeric units and an outer functional group surface (Fig. 1). We have used a "fifth generation" dendrimer (Polysciences, Inc., Warrington, PA) having a molecular weight of 10,633 with 48 reactive amino end groups. $Na(CH_3)_3 NB_{10}H_8NCO$, synthesized in our laboratory[3], was used as the boronating species. All reactions were carried out at ambient temperature unless indicated otherwise. Fifteen mg of this and 100 μL of acetone were added to 1 mL of the dendrimer suspension, and pH was adjusted to 9 by the addition of Na_2CO_3. The mixture was stirred continuously for 7-10 days following which 1 mg of sulfo-MBS (Sigma Chemicals, St. Louis, MO) was added. After 30 minutes the mixture was passed through a Sephadex G-25 column (0.8 x 40 cm) and eluted with 0.1M TRIS buffer, pH 8.5, in 0.2 M NaCl. Fractions were collected, protein concentrations were determined by measuring absorbance at 280 nm, and boron values were determined by direct current plasma-atomic emission spectroscopy (DCP-AES), as described elsewhere[8]. From these data the boronated dendrimer fractions were located and pooled (Fig. 2).

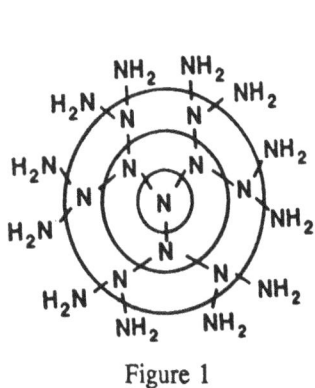

Figure 1

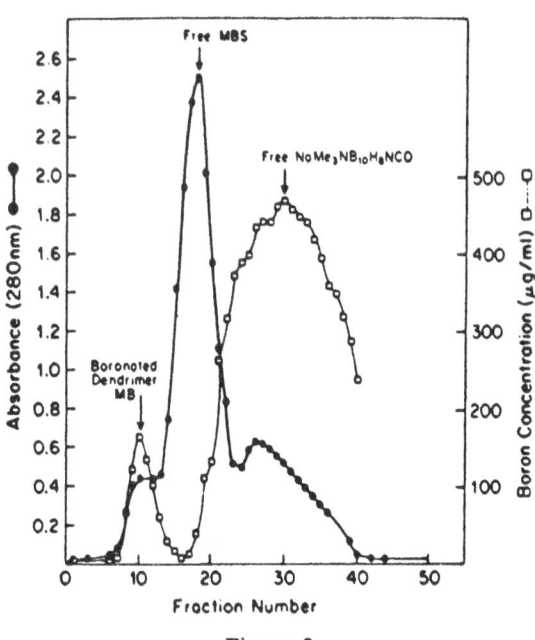

Figure 2

Conjugation of antibody

The MoAb IB16-6 is directed against a surface membrane antigen expressed on the murine B16 melanoma[9]. To a stirred solution containing 5mg of IB16-6 in phosphate buffered saline (PBS), pH 7.2, were added 2.5 mg of SPDP over a 2 hour period. Following this, it was dialyzed against PBS, treated with 3 mg of dithiothreitol (DTT) for 90 minutes at 37°C in order to cleave the disulfide bond, and dialyzed first against PBS and then 0.1 TRIS buffer, pH 8.5 in 0.2M NaCl.

The boronated starburst dendrimer (BSD) was combined with the derivatized MoAb, allowed to stand for 24 hours, and then loaded on to a Sephacryl S-300 column (1.2 x 19cm) and eluted with 0.1M TRIS buffer in 0.2 M NaCl. The synthetic scheme is summarized in Fig. 3. Protein concentrations were determined by the Lowry[10] method and by radial immunodiffusion, and boron concentrations were determined by DCP-AES. Immunoreactivity of the boronated IB16-6 was determined by means of ELISA, as previously described[3].

Results and Discussion

Two immunoconjugates were produced and these were shown to contain 1840 and 2200 atoms of boron per molecule of antibody. As determined by ELISA, the immunoreactivity of the boronated IB16-6 ranged from 77% to 82% of that of the native antibody. These results indicate that boron containing immunoconjugates containing the large numbers of boron atoms required for sustaining a lethal n, α reaction at the cellular level, and at the same time retaining their in vitro immunoreactivity, can be produced by using starburst dendrimers as the spacer molecule. Studies currently in progress should determine whether or not these immunoconjugates retain their in vivo tumor localizing properties.

A number of problems relating to the potential use of antibodies for targeting tumoricidal agents have been identified. It is beyond the scope of this article to discuss

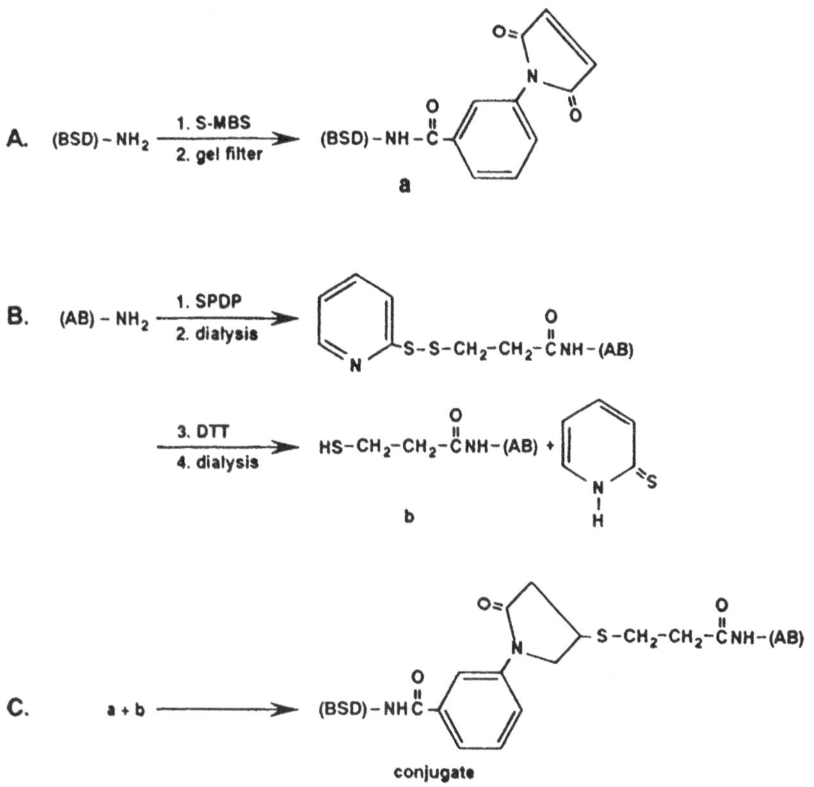

Figure 3

these, but it should be clear that the use of MoAbs for targeting ^{10}B to tumors represents a significant challenge. New developments in hybridoma technology may help to solve some of these problems. The production of recombinant antibody molecules that have two combining sites, one specific for a tumor associate antigen and the other for a boron containing macromolecule might have applicability to BNCT. Further advances in immunoconjugate chemistry, especially the ability to increase the distance between the combining site for the tumor associated antigens (TAA) and the boronated macromolecule, and the development of more stable chemical linkers would alleviate many of the problems associated with antibodies and immunoconjugates. The production of antibodies recognizing more universally expressed TAA might solve a number of the problems relating to the antigens. Problems intrinsic to the tumor itself might be reduced by using capillary disruptive agents together with low molecular weight, tumor-localizing, boron containing compounds. In summary, antibodies should be viewed as one among a number of different delivery systems that would be used in combination with one another. Using them exclusively to deliver ^{10}B to tumors is not only unreasonable, but also unworkable.

Acknowledgements

This work was supported by grant 5R01CA41288 from the National Cancer Institute, contract DE-ACC02-76CH000616 and grant DE-FG02-90ER60972 from the Department of Energy.

References

1. R.F. Barth, C.W. Johnson, W-Z Wei, W.E. Carey, A.H. Soloway and J. McGuire: Neutron capture using boronated monoclonal antibody directed against tumor-associated antigens. Cancer Detect and Prevent, 5:315-323, (1982).

2. E. Mizusawa, H.L. Dahlman, S.J. Bennett, D.M. Goldenberg and M.F. Hawthorne: Neutron capture therapy of human cancer: In vivo results on the preparation of boron-labeled antibodies to carcinoembryonic antigen. Proc Natl Acad Sci, 79:3011-3014, (1982).

3. A. Alam, A.H. Soloway, R.F. Barth, N. Mafune, D.M. Adams and W.H. Knoth, Boron neutron capture therapy: linkage of a boronated macromolecule to monoclonal antibodies directed against tumor associated antigens. J of Med Chem 32:2326-2330, (1989).

4. R.F. Barth, F. Alam, A.H. Soloway, D. Adams and Z. Steplewski, Boronated monoclonal antibody 17-1A for potential neutron capture therapy of colorectal cancer. Hybridoma 5:Suppl 1:S43-S50, (1986).

5. R.F. Barth, N. Mafune, F. Alam, D.M. Adams, A.H. Soloway, T.E. Blue and Z. Steplewski, Conjugation, purification and characterization of boronated monoclonal antibodies for use in neutron capture therapy. Strahlenther und Onkologie, 165:142-145, (1989).

6. F. Alam, R.F. Barth and A.H. Soloway, Boron containing immunoconjugates for neutron capture therapy of cancer for immunocytochemistry. Antibody Immunoconj and Radiopharm, 2:145-163, (1989).

7. J.C. Roberts, Y.E. Adams, D.E. Tomalia, J.A. Mercer-Smith and D.K. Lavallee, Using starburst dendrimers as linker molecules to radiolabel antibodies. Bioconjugate Chem 1, 305-308 (1990).

8. R.F. Barth, D.M. Adams, A.H. Soloway, E.B. Mechetner, F. Alam, and A.K.M. Anisuzzaman, Determination of boron in tissues and cells using direct-current plasma atomic emission spectroscopy. Anal Chem 63,4, 890-893, (1991).

9. C.W. Johnson, R.F. Barth, D. Adams, B. Holman, J.E. Price and I. Sautins, Phenotypic diversity of murine B16 melanoma detected by anti B-16 monoclonal antibodies. Cancer Res, 47:1111-1117, (1987).

10. O.H. Lowry, N.J. Rosebrough, A.L. Farr and R.J. Randall, Protein measurement with the Folin phenol reagent. J. Biol. Chem., 193:265-275, (1951).

ANTIBODY TARGETING OF BORON COMPOUNDS

V. A. Ferro, J. H. Morris and W. H. Stimson

Departments of Immunology and Pure and Applied
Chemistry
University of Strathclyde
Glasgow, Scotland, U. K.

INTRODUCTION

Success of ^{10}BNCT depends on localising sufficient ^{10}B (around 20µg/g of tumour) at the site of the tumour. One approach is to direct boronated monoclonal antibodies to specific tumour antigens. The method is dependent on the requirements that (i) each antibody carries 1000-2000 ^{10}B atoms, (ii) the specific immunoreactivity of the antibody is retained, (iii) the boronated antibody is water-soluble and stable under physiological conditions.

Previously, problems were encountered with the retention of activity of heavily boronated antibodies due to structural modifications around the binding sites. Recently, boronation of antibodies has been achieved using boron-carrying macromolecules including homoaminoacids.[1] We have chosen to boronate a heteroaminoacid, the random copolymer of D-glutamic acid, L-lysine (poly-GL), since the lysine groups provide a suitable functional group for boronation with $[B_{12}H_{11}SH]^{2-}$ and the glutamate groups allow for increased solubility. However, direct conjugation of this polymer onto antibody still results in a high degree of loss of immunoreactivity. Therefore we have tried to overcome this by indirectly linking the polymer to the antibody via a carrier molecule.

The biotin-streptavidin system is particularly useful since the interaction between these molecules is the strongest, non-covalent biological recognition known between protein and ligand ($K_a = 10^{15}$ M^{-1}).[2] The bond formation is very rapid and is unaffected by extremes of pH, organic solvents and other denaturing reagents. The biotin molecule which is extremely small (<500 daltons) can be coupled to antibodies or antigens with little structural alteration to the proteins and so their binding activity is retained. On the other hand, streptavidin is a tetramer of 60,000 daltons, which can also be easily conjugated with large molecules. In addition, each subunit of the tetramer can bind one molecule of biotin which is particularly useful for bridging associations.

METHODS

Firstly, we boronated poly-GL (average molecular weight 50,000 daltons; glutamate:lysine ratio 6:4) with $[B_{12}H_{11}SH]^{2-}$, using m-maleimidobenzoyl-N-hydroxysulphosuccinimide ester (S-MBS) as a linker agent.[3] Boronated polymer was then coupled to streptavidin using a N-hydroxysulphosuccinimide ester (S-NHS) enhanced carbodiimide reaction.[4] The boron-loaded streptavidin was then used in association with a biotinylated monoclonal antibody, specific to the N417 lung cancer cell line, in cell kill experimentation.

In a further experiment, in addition to biotinylating the antibody we also biotinylated poly-GL prior to boronation. In this way, using a free streptavidin molecule as an

Progress in Neutron Capture Therapy for Cancer
Edited by B.J. Allen *et al.*, Plenum Press, New York, 1992

intermediate (in a bridging association), three boronated polymers were able to bind indirectly to the monoclonal antibody.

These two interactions were tested for their ability to cause cell damage following thermal neutron activation. The cells, were irradiated at the Reactor Centre, East Kilbride, Scotland and fluxes determined using gold foils.

1) Boronation of poly-GL

Poly-GL was dissolved in a small volume of 0.1M NaHCO$_3$ buffer, pH7.5. S-MBS in 10x molar ratio was incubated with the polymer at room temperature for 45min. $[B_{12}H_{11}SH]^{2-}$ in 30x molar ratio to the polymer was added and incubated for 2hr at 37^{0}C. In order to remove excess reagent and $[B_{12}H_{11}SH]^{2-}$, the mixture was dialysed overnight against phosphate-buffered saline, pH7.5. The extent of boronation was assessed by ICP mass spectrometry.

2) Conjugation of boronated poly-GL to streptavidin

The boronated polymer was incubated with S-NHS and 1-ethyl-3(3-dimethylaminopropyl)carbodiimide (EDC) in 10x molar ratios for 45min at room temperature. Streptavidin in 0.5x molar ratio to the polymer was added and left overnight at room temperature. Separation of the boronated streptavidin from the rest of the components was achieved using gel filtration with G-75 Sephadex.

3) Biotinylation of antibody and poly-GL

Biotinylation was carried out using a kit from Amersham International, U.K. Following biotinylation of the poly-GL, boronation was carried as described above.

4) Cell kill experimentation

In order to work out suitable irradiation conditions, N417 cells, supplied by D. Carney (Department of Medical Oncology, Glasgow), were grown in complete RPMI 1640 medium containing 50μg/ml $[B_{12}H_{11}SH]^{2-}$ for 24hr. The cells were washed with medium only, resuspended to 1×10^6 cells/ml and 1ml was placed into a small plastic bijoux. Six bijoux could be placed into a graphite block for irradiating purposes. Irradiation for 30min at 52.6kW and at a flux of 5×10^{12}ncm^{-2} was found to be the least damaging to non-boron treated cells (3% cell kill) and so these conditions were chosen for subsequent experimentation.

Cells (1×10^6) were incubated with 100μg/ml biotinylated antibody for 2hr at 37^{0}C, washed with medium and then incubated with 1μg/ml boron-coupled streptavidin for 30min at 37^{0}C. The cells were washed prior to irradiation.

In the bridging experiments, the cells were incubated with biotinylated antibody, followed by free streptavidin (1μg/ml) for 30min at 37^{0}C and then with the biotinylated boronated poly-GL (1μg/ml) for 30min at 37^{0}C. The cells were washed at each stage and prior to irradiation. Cell counts were taken before and after irradiation and viability was determined using trypan blue dye exclusion. Controls were run concurrently of cells without antibody and cells without the boronated complexes.

RESULTS AND DISCUSSION

Boronation of poly-GL resulted in 360 ^{10}B atoms per polymer. When this was coupled indirectly to biotinylated antibody via boronated streptavidin and via a bridging association through streptavidin, 720 and 1090 ^{10}B atoms respectively were loaded onto each antibody molecule. In both systems of indirect boronation, the antibody activity as determined by ELISA, was retained. The cell system is viable to BSH in the absence of neutron irradiation.

Assessment of cell kill following neutron irradiation was carried out. In the case of cells exposed to $[B_{12}H_{11}SH]^{2-}$, 60% of the cells were killed, as opposed to 3% in the case of untreated cells. Although such a large proportion of cells were killed due to neutron irradiation after treatment with $[B_{12}H_{11}SH]^{2-}$, cell death was non-specific. Survival by 40% of the population may be due to the fact that as the cells grow in clusters, the $[B_{12}H_{11}SH]^{2-}$ is unable to penetrate through to the inner cells.

Similarly, cells treated only with biotinylated antibody or with the boronated

270

complexes in the absence of the antibody, showed 3% cell death. However, cells treated with biotinylated antibody and boronated streptavidin showed 25% cell death. Cells treated with biotinylated antibody, free streptavidin and biotinylated boronated polymer showed 40% cell death.

These results show that an increase in boron content results in an increase in cell death. The reasons for the low results may be due to the cluster formation of the cells. We were able to demonstrate this by staining the cells with 10D2 antibody, followed by an anti-mouse fluoroscein conjugated antibody. The outer cells in the clusters were heavily stained but the inner cells showed reduced fluoresence as the antibodies had been unable to penetrate the clusters. We are presently in the process of trying multiple treatments and irradiations to see if a greater cell kill can be achieved. Another way of increasing cell kill efficency may be to internalise the boronated complexes into the cells and we are currently considering a range of drugs which have this potential.

ACKNOWLEDGEMENTS

This study was supported by the Medical Research Council.

REFERENCES

1 H. Hatanaka (ed.), "Boron Neutron Capture Therapy for Tumours", Nishima, Tokyo (1986).
2 L. Chaiet and F. Wolf, Arch. Biochem. Biophys. **106**:1 (1964).
3 H. N. Aithal, J. Immunol. Meth. **112**:63 (1988).
4 J. V. Staros, R. W. Wright and D. M. Swingle, Anal. Biochem. **156**:220 (1986)

APPLICATION OF BORONATED ANTI-CEA IMMUNOLIPOSOME TO BORON NEUTRON

CAPTURE THERAPY

H. Yanagie,[1] Y. Fujii,[1] T. Tomita,[2] H. Nariuchi,[3]
M. Sekiguchi[1] and H. Kobayashi[4]

[1]Department of Clinical Oncology, [2]Laboratory of Biological
Product, [3]Department of Allergy, Institute of Medical
Science, University of Tokyo, Tokyo, and [4]Institute for
Atomic Energy, Rikkyo University, Yokosuka, Japan

INTRODUCTION

Boron neutron capture therapy (BNCT) is based on irradiation of a tumour
with thermal neutrons after accumulation of a large amount of boron-
10(^{10}B) atoms on the target tumour cells. ^{10}B captures neutrons and
produces α- and ^{7}Li particles through the reaction ^{10}B(n,α)^{7}Li. This
reaction is very efficient in cell killing.[1] BNCT has been applied to
the treatment of malignant brain tumours or melanoma by using ^{10}B-
compounds selectively taken up by tumour cells.[2]   Alam *et al* reported
that 1300 boron atoms had been conjugated to a molecule of monoclonal
antibody.[3] However, in these experiments, antibody was shown to lose
activity by the direct conjugation with ^{10}B-compound.

Recently, liposomes have attracted attention as drug delivery systems.[4]
It is possible to carry a large amount of ^{10}B-compound in a liposome and,
therefore, the liposome could deliver a large amount of the ^{10}B-compound
to a tumour cell, if it bears an antibody specifically raised against the
cell-surface associated antigens.

In the present experiments, we prepared liposomes containing a ^{10}B-
compound and to which were conjugated an anti-carcinoembryonic antigen
(CEA) monoclonal antibody. The immunoliposome was shown to deliver the
^{10}B-compound to the specific target tumour cells and to inhibit tumour
cell growth *in vitro* following thermal neutron irradiation.

MATERIALS AND METHODS

Target tumour cells: Human pancreatic carcinoma cell line AsPC-1
producing carcinoembryonic antigen (CEA) was maintained in RPMI 1640
medium supplemented with 10% foetal calf serum and 100 μg/mL kanamycin.

^{10}*B-compound*: The cesium salt of undecahydro-mercapto-*closo*-dodeca-
borate (Cs$_2$^{10}B$_{12}$H$_{11}$SH) was kindly supplied by Shionogi Research
Laboratories Co. Ltd. (Tokyo, Japan).

Preparation of immunolipsosomes containing ^{10}B-compound: Egg yolk
phosphatidylcholine (5 μmoles), cholesterol (5 μmoles) and 3-(2-pyridyl-
dithio)propionyl-dipalmitoyl-phosphatidylethanolamine (DTP-DPPE)
(0.25 μmoles) dissolved in chloroform-methanol (2:1) were mixed in a
conical flask. After evaporation, 25, 100, or 250 mM ^{10}B-compound
($Cs_2{}^{10}B_{12}H_{11}SH$) solution was added to the dried lipid film, and then
multilamellar vesicles were prepared by vortex dispersion (mean diameter:
4 to 6 μm, determined by the dynamic light scattering method). The
boronated liposomes were then conjugated with anti-CEA monoclonal
antibody (0, 0.5, 1.0, or 4.0 mg/mL) using N-hydroxy-succinimidyl
3-(2-pyridyldithio)-propionate (SPDP).

Determination of ^{10}B-compound concentration entrapped in liposomes: The
amount of ^{10}B-compound entrapped in liposomes was determined by a
colorimetric method in the presence of curcumine.[6]

Thermal neutron irradiation: AsPC-1 cells, 5 x 10^4 cells/culture, were
incubated in the presence of immunoliposomes. After washing, the cells
were irradiated with thermal neutrons at the TRIGA-II atomic reactor of
Rikkyo University (5 x 10^{11} - 5 x 10^{12} n/cm^2). After irradiation, uptake
of ^3H-thymidine by the cells was estimated as a measure of cell viability
using a liquid scintillation spectrometer.

RESULTS

Concentration of ^{10}B entrapped in liposomes: The amounts of ^{10}B in
immunoliposomes prepared with 100 mM and 250 mM ^{10}B compound were 178 ±
33 and 623 ± 80 μg/mL liposome, respectively. Anti-CEA conjugated with
liposome was estimated to be 734.0 ± 37 μg/mL liposome. Thus, the
liposomes prepared with 100 mM and 250 mM ^{10}B-compound were calculated to
contain 5.0 x 10^3 and 1.3 x 10^4 atoms of ^{10}B for each antibody,
respectively.

Growth inhibition of AsPC-1 cells treated with immunoliposomes: AsPC-1
cells were treated with liposomes prepared with 250 mM ^{10}B-compound and 4
mg/mL anti-CEA or anti-DNP. After washing to remove free liposomes, the
cells were irradiated with various fluxes of thermal neutrons and
cultured *in vitro*. The cells treated with the anti-CEA immunmoliposomes
showed a reduction in growth by 50% (expressed as % of control thymidine
uptake) at 1 x 10^{12} flux or more of thermal neutrons. When AsPC-1 cells
were treated with anti-DNP immunoliposomes, they grew as well as
untreated cells.

Effect of ^{10}B-compound concentration in immunoliposomes on cytotoxicity:
Liposomes were prepared by using 0, 25, 100, or 250 mM ^{10}B-compound, and
were conjugated with various concentrations of anti-CEA. AsPC-1 cells
showed reduced growth at 1 x 10^{12} n/cm^2 and more of thermal neutron
flux as the increment of the antibody concentration used for the
preparation of immunoliposomes (for anti-CEA at 1 mg/mL, 56% effective
growth, for 4mg/mL, 50%).

Effect of gamma-rays generated by thermal neutrons: AsPC-1 cells
irradiated with thermal neutrons were also irradiated with various doses
of gamma-rays, which did not exert any inhibitory effect on the cell
growth (93% of control).

DISCUSSION

Antibody reactive to tumour cells is one of the most useful vehicles for
ensuring selective accumulation of boron in tumours.

It was estimated that at least 10^9 ^{10}B atoms are required to destroy one tumour cell in BNCT. According to Alam et al., an antibody has to be conjugated with 10^3 ^{10}B atoms to destroy a tumour cell with 10^6 epitopes on its surface. 1300 boron atoms were reported to be conjugated to a molecule of monoclonal antibody by using the bifunctional reagent SPDP and a polylysine bridge.[3]

A monoclonal antibody against *alpha*-foetoprotein was found to exert some cytotoxic effect on AH-66 tumour cells in BNCT *in vitro*. However, a heavy boronation of antibody has been shown to markedly reduce the antibody reactivity and the numbers of epitope on the tumour cell surface have been estimated to be at most 10^6 per cell. These results indicate that monoclonal antibody directly conjugated with ^{10}B-compound has limited application in BNCT.

A liposome is a vehicle which can be used to entrap various materials. In this work, a method of conjugating protein molecules on the surface by SPDP was developed. By this means, it is possible for liposomes to carry a large amount of substance to the target cell surface, if the substance is entrapped in the liposome conjugated with a monoclonal antibody which is specifically active against the cells.[4]

In the experiments reported here, immunoliposomes suppressed tumour cell growth *in vitro* after thermal neutron irradiation. Suppression was dependent upon the concentration of entrapped ^{10}B-compound and also upon the density of anti-CEA conjugated with liposome. These results of *in vitro* experiments suggest that an immunoliposome containing ^{10}B-compound could be applied in BNCT as an effective carrier of a ^{10}B-compound to the target cells.

REFERENCES

1. Kruger, P.G. 1940, Some biological effects of nuclear disintegration products on neoplastic tissue. *Proc. Natl. Acad. Sci. USA*, 26: 181.

2. Hatanaka, H. 1986, "Boron-Neutron Capture Therapy for Tumors", Nishimura Co. Ltd., Niigata. 11.

3. Alam, F. 1984, Boronation of polyclonal and monoclonal antibodies for neutron capture, *Brookhaven Natl Lab Report*, 51730: 229.

4. Konno, H. 1987, Anti-tumor effect of adriamycin entrapped in liposomes conjugated with anti-human fetoprotein monoclonal anti-body, *Cancer Res.*, 47: 4471.

5. Leserman, L.D. 1981, Cell-specific drug transfer from liposomes bearing monoclonal antibodies. *Nature*, 293: 226.

6. Ikeuchi, I. 1978, A colorimetric determination of boron in biological materials. *Chem. Pharm. Bull.*, 26: 2619.

STUDIES RELATED TO ANTIBODY-MEDIATED BORON DELIVERY FOR BNCT

M. Frederick Hawthorne[*], Aravamuthan Varadarajan[*], Raymond J. Paxton[†],
Barbara G. Beatty[†] and Frederick L. Curtis[†]

[*]Department of Chemistry and Biochemistry
The University of California at Los Angeles
Los Angeles, California 90024 U.S.A.

[†]Beckman Research Institute of the City of Hope and
The City of Hope National Medical Center
Duarte, California 91010 U.S. A.

Of the many methods of selective boron delivery to tumor presently under consideration, the use of boron-labeled tumor-targeted monoclonal antibodies (Mabs) and their immunoreactive fragments appears to offer the most general, but complex, approach.[1-4] Assuming that tumor cells generally carry 10^6 characteristic antigenic sites of any one type and that there are approximately 10^9 cells per gram of tumor, one calculates that about 600 ^{10}B atoms must be attached to each individual Mab molecule (if all antigenic sites are complexed) for each 10 ppm of ^{10}B supplied to tumor. Rather than randomly attack IgG Mab molecules with a large number of relatively small boron-containing conjugation reagent molecules we have chosen to assemble a series of discrete, precisely synthesized oligomeric reagents ("trailers") each of which contains a fixed number of B-atoms up to approximately 200. These

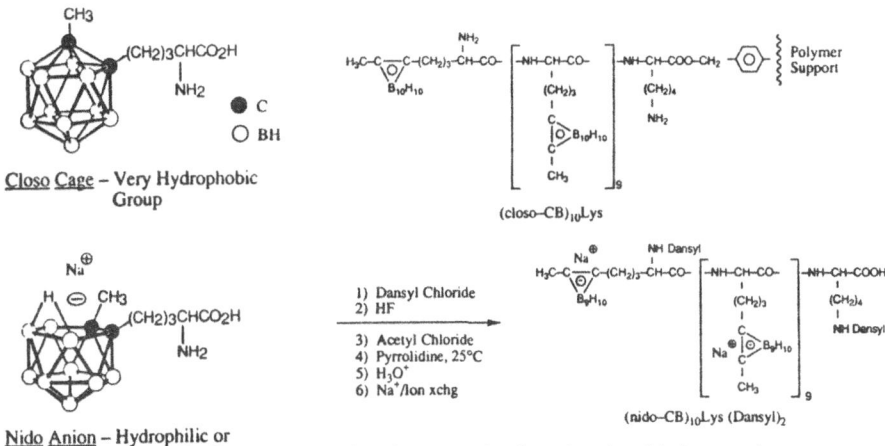

Fig. 1. Two boron-rich α-amino acids
employed in peptide synthesis
as their *t*-BOC derivatives.

Fig. 2. An undecapeptide trailer reagent synthesized
using the Merrifield method.

oligomeric reagents would carry a radioactive or fluorescent group for analytical purposes attached to a terminal-NH_2 group of their chain and the remaining -COOH terminus would be free for conjugation with the lysine ε-NH_2 groups of Mab protein. Two types of oligomeric trailer reagents are envisioned; hydrophilic peptides and polyamides. Both types of reagent are prepared using the solid-supported synthesis methods of Merrifield.[5] Figure 1 illustrates two typical α-amino acids which contain the hydrophobic closo-1,2-$C_2B_{10}H_{11}$-cage and the corresponding hydrophilic [nido-7,8-$C_2B_9H_{11}$-]-cage fragment. These amino acids are designated closo-CB and nido-CB, respectively, throughout this paper.

Having developed the synthesis of the essential α-amino acid, closo-CB, and its t-BOC derivative, the dansylated dipeptide (nido-CB)$_2$(dansyl) and the dansylated undecapeptide (nido-CB)$_{10}$ Lys(dansyl)$_2$ were constructed using standard Merrifield peptide synthesis conditions. The synthesis of the latter trailer is depicted in Figure 2. Both peptides were characterized by ^{11}B and ^{1}H FTNMR, mass spectra (as their closo derivatives prior to reaction with pyrrolidine), dansyl fluorescence intensities and HPLC chromatographic properties.

The IgG Mab selected for conjugation with the sodium salts of (nido-CB)$_2$(dansyl) and (nido-CB)$_{10}$Lys(dansyl)$_2$ was targeted for the carcinoembryonic antigen associated with LS174T human colon tumor xenografts employed in the biodistribution studies described below. For simplicity this Mab may hereafter be referred to by the abbreviated designation T84.

Conjugation of (nido-CB)$_2$(dansyl) to T84 Mab. A mixture of the dansylated anionic (nido-CB)$_2$ [hereafter (CB)$_2$] and N-hydroxysulfosuccinimide was treated with N,N-diisopropylcarbodiimide in dimethylformamide for one hour. The resulting active ester was incubated with T84 at pH 9.0 for 1h, with the molar ratio of (CB)$_2$ active ester to antibody being 10.5:1. A control reaction of T84 plus unactivated (CB)$_2$ was also prepared. Initial purifications were performed by Centricon-30 diafiltration. Final purifications of the T84-(CB)$_2$ conjugate and the control sample were by Superose 12 gel permeation chromatography.

The monomeric T84-(CB)$_2$ conjugate and the control sample were collected and used for fluorescence, electrophoretic, immunoreactivity, and tumor-targeting analyses. Based on the measured fluorescence intensity and protein concentration of the T84-(CB)$_2$ conjugate, an average of 3.5 (nido-CB)$_2$ peptides (63 B-atoms) were incorporated per antibody molecule. Enzyme immunoassay of the monomeric T84-(CB)$_2$ conjugate and an untreated sample of T84 Mab showed that they had identical immunoreactivities. For tumor-targeting analyses, aliquots of monomeric T84-(CB)$_2$ and untreated T84 were radioiodinated using Na^{125}I and chloramine-T.

Table 1 Biodistribution of ^{125}I-Labeled T84.66-CB2 in Nude Mice Bearing LS174T Xenografts [a]
% Injected Dose/Gram of Tissue [b]

Antibody	48h	72 h	120h	
Tissue:	T84.66-CB2	T84.66-CB2	T84.66-CB2	T84.66 (Control)
Blood (B)	7.35 ± 0.49	6.26 ± 0.75	0.43 ± 0.13	1.28 ± 0.38
Liver (L)	3.48 ± 0.15	2.99 ± 0.32	1.67 ± 0.17	0.87 ± 0.05
Spleen	1.77 ± 0.07	1.56 ± 0.16	0.69 ± 0.11	0.45 ± 0.02
Kidney	1.69 ± 0.05	1.58 ± 0.15	0.33 ± 0.07	0.41 ± 0.08
Lung	2.91 ± 0.22	2.40 ± 0.21	0.41 ± 0.11	0.64 ± 0.10
Tumor (T)	14.21 ± 0.81	14.50 ± 0.91	6.96 ± 0.57	9.87 ± 0.58
T/L	4.10 ± 0.30	4.93 ± 0.27	4.19 ± 0.07	11.57 ± 1.21
T/B	1.94 ± 0.08	2.40 ± 0.19	22.63 ± 5.47	9.26 ± 1.76
Tumor wt (g)	1.52 ± 0.06	1.74 ± 0.13	2.56 ± 0.20	2.15 ± 0.19

[a] 3 μCi (~0.4 μg) of ^{125}I-labeled T84.66-CB2 together with 92 μg unlabeled T84.66-CB2 was injected i.v. in nude mice bearing 14-day-old subcutaneous LS174T tumors. Equivalent amounts of ^{125}I-labeled and unlabeled T84.66 were used as a control. Groups of 4-5 mice were sacrificed at the indicated times after antibody injection, and the tumor and tissues were weighed and counted to determine the percent injected dose per gram tissue. [b] Values quoted are mean ± standard error.

Conjugation of (nido-CB)$_{10}$Lys(dansyl)$_2$ to T84 Mab. Preliminary studies with didansylated anionic (nido-CB)$_{10}$Lys [hereafter (CB)$_{10}$] suggested that the hydrophobic nature of the peptide led to its nonspecific binding to antibody, as well as incomplete recovery of the peptide and Mab-peptide conjugates during chromatographic procedures. Optimal results were obtained with Superose 12 in the presence of 0.05% Tween-20. The conjugation of (CB)$_{10}$ to T84 was carried out essentially as described above for (CB)$_2$, but at pH 8.5 with a molar ratio of peptide to antibody of 10:1. Control reactions of T84 alone and T84 plus unactivated (CB)$_{10}$ were also prepared. The conjugate and the two controls were brought to a final concentration of 0.05% Tween-20 and purified by Superose 12 chromatography. For the T84-(CB)$_{10}$ conjugate, a sharp, monomeric antibody peak was obtained with a sizeable peak due to a high molecular weight (HMW) species. A significant amount of fluorescence was associated with the T84-(CB)$_{10}$ conjugate relative to the unactivated (CB)$_{10}$ peptide control. The fluorescence was disproportionately associated with the HMW species. The HMW and monomeric antibody species were collected and analyzed separately. Quantitation of the nido-CB amino acid revealed that the HMW conjugate contained an average of 6.3 (CB)$_{10}$ peptides (570 boron atoms) per antibody. The monomeric conjugate averaged one peptide conjugation per antibody (90 boron atoms). Immunoreactivities for the HMW and monomeric conjugates were compared to untreated T84 Mab. The monomeric conjugate retained its native immunoreactivity while there was a slight decrease in the immunoreactivity of the HMW conjugate. For tumor-targeting analyses, aliquots of both the HMW and monomeric T84-(CB)$_{10}$ conjugates and untreated T84 Mab were radioiodinated as described above for the T84-(CB)$_2$ conjugate.

In progressing sequentially through the trailer reagent series (CB)$_2$ to (CB)$_{10}$, the number of boron atoms attached to T84 Mab increased from an average of about 60 to 600. Progression from (CB)$_2$ to (CB)$_{10}$ introduced the problem of nonspecific binding of Mab with peptide reagent, the formation of increased quantities of HMW species aided by a cascade conjugation reaction sequence and the enhancement of liver uptake of the conjugated Mabs relative to tumor. The nonspecific bonding of both activated and unactivated (CB)$_{10}$ with Mab T84 must arise from the interaction of hydrophobic regions of Mab with ambiphilic (CB)$_{10}$. Conjugation of (CB)$_2$ and (CB)$_{10}$ trailers with Mab led to a disproportionate amount of fluorescent label in the HMW species or aggregate accompanied by the formation of additional aggregate. Mechanistically, the initial lysine conjugation reaction appears to open the Mab structure exposing additional reactive sites which are attacked ever more rapidly as conjugation and the resulting structural perturbation proceeds. The result is a cascade reaction sequence. As the native Mab structure becomes more disarrayed by this process, the aggregate concentration will increase at the expense of monomeric Mab and its conjugates. Both the HMW and monomeric T84 Mab conjugates derived from (CB)$_{10}$ have good enzyme immunoassay responses and the reduction in tumor uptake is the apparent result of the very effective competitive loss of Mab and HMW conjugates to liver. Tumor/blood ratios were favorably high in all cases. These collected observations combined with the data of others[6-8]

Table 2 Biodistribution of ^{125}I-Labeled T84.66-CB10 in Nude Mice Bearing LS174T Xenografts [a]
% Injected Dose/Gram of Tissue [b]

Antibody	T84.66-CB10 (HMW)	T84.66-CB10 (Monomer)	T84.66 (Control)
Tissue:			
Blood (B)	1.20 ± 0.22	1.90 ± 0.12	7.93 ± 1.42
Liver (L)	43.84 ± 3.78	37.48 ± 1.73	2.89 ± 0.16
Spleen	13.98 ± 1.22	8.07 ± 0.65	1.65 ± 0.07
Kidney	2.30 ± 0.29	3.08 ± 0.18	1.86 ± 0.18
Lung	1.61 ± 0.15	2.36 ± 0.08	3.26 ± 0.26
Tumor (T)	4.35 ± 0.51	5.14 ± 0.33	23.19 ± 5.12
T/L	0.099 ± 0.008	0.139 ± 0.011	7.85 ± 1.23
T/B	3.79 ± 0.28	2.74 ± 0.19	2.91 ± 0.28
Tumor wt (g)	0.64 ± 0.18	0.57 ± 0.15	0.86 ± 0.21

[a] 7 µCi (~0.30 µg) of ^{125}I-labeled T84.66-CB10 samples together with 27 µg of the respective unlabeled T84.66-CB10 samples were injected i.v. in nude mice bearing 10-day-old subcutaneous LS174T tumors. Equivalent amounts of ^{125}I-labeled and unlabeled T84.66 was used as a control. Groups of 5-6 mice were sacrificed 2 days after antibody injection, and the tumor and tissues were weighed and counted to determine the percent injected dose per gram tissue. [b] Values quoted are mean ± standard error.

provide strong support to the conclusion that <u>random substitution</u> of full-sized Mab molecules with large, boron-rich conjugation reagents will become ever more complicated as the boron burden is increased. Therefore, if the splendid versatility of immunochemistry is to be applied to BNCT, radically different approaches will be required. Two such avenues of current research are briefly outlined below.

The results presented above suggest that the effective delivery of therapeutic quantities of ^{10}B to tumor might be achieved by (1) use of a greatly simplified chemically monofunctional FabSH antibody fragment related to T84.66 Mab and available by genetic engineering or (2) by synthesizing a bispecific (Fab'$_1$) (Fab'$_2$) antibody of the (Fab')$_2$ class which specifically binds tumor cell wall antigen (such as CEA) with one combining site, (Fab'$_1$), and with the other combining site, (Fab'$_2$), it binds a discrete, synthesized array of boron-rich oligomers based upon a 20-residue hydrophilic peptide or polyamide (20 mer species). In addition to these modifications of our attack upon the problem, the synthesis of very hydrophilic boron-rich α-amino acids equipped with polyhydroxy side chains is also underway.[9,10]

The ability of molecular engineering to provide monoclonal sources for species such as a simple antibody fragment, FabSH, suggests the adoption of strongly antigen-binding antibody fragments of this type which are monovalent with respect to cell wall antigen (CEA) complexation and monofunctional in the chemical sense (-SH group). Figure 3 illustrates how a simple FabSH species may be linked to a single large collection of boron-rich HOCO[Mer]$_{20}$NH(dansyl) peptide chains bonded, in turn, to a small manifold peptide, HOCOMF(NH$_2$)$_6$, rich in lysine residues. The numerals shown in this Figure depict the sequence of coupling reactions required to achieve the 1000 or so ^{10}B-atoms attached to the immunoreactive Fab. Advantages which accrue to this relatively simple BNCT reagent molecule are its low molecular weight giving enhanced mobility and clearance rates coupled with the complete control of the conjugation process since only one thiol function is available per Fab protein for reaction with the maleimide moiety linked to the boron-rich manifold conjugate. Complete structural control appears to be within our grasp. Research based upon this concept is in progress.

The concept of effector molecule delivery by use of a bispecific antibody, such as a (Fab'$_{CEA}$)(Fab'$_{Nido}$) species, which binds simultaneously to two different antigenic sites is relatively new[11,12] and has never been employed for the delivery of boron-containing arrays. One route to such systems, which is currently under investigation in our laboratory, may provide a method for binding cell wall antigens, such as CEA, to a large hapten [(nido-7,8-C$_2$B$_9$H$_{11}$-)$^-$]-bearing molecule such as the MF-[(Mer)$_{20}$]$_6$ illustrated in Figure 4. In practice the bispecific antibody would be injected, alone, into the tumor-bearing animal and then binds to tumor antigen with the Fab'$_{CEA}$ portion of its structure. After maximum tumor-loading has been achieved, the animal would then be innoculated with the hapten-bearing boron carrier having approximately 10^3 available ^{10}B-atoms. Binding of this large molecule to the free and uncomplexed (Fab'$_{Nido}$) arm of the already cell bound (Fab'$_{CEA}$)-(Fab'$_{Nido}$) should provide each involved cellular antigenic site with 10^3 ^{10}B-atoms without the use of conventional chemical bonds. Figure 4 displays the desired result viewed at a single cell

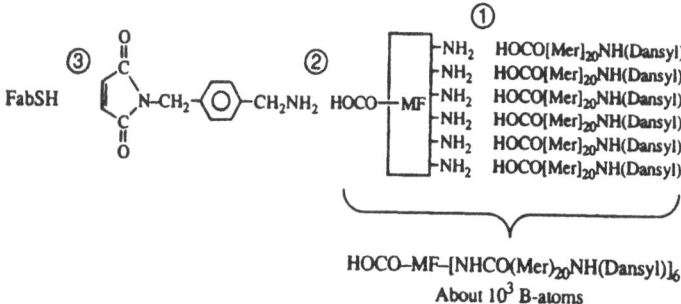

HOCO–MF–[NHCO(Mer)$_{20}$NH(Dansyl)]$_6$
About 10^3 B-atoms

Fig. 3. Sequence of reactions leading to immunodirected boron-rich oligomers. The HOCO(Mer)$_{20}$NH$_2$ precursor is a peptide or a polyamide with 20 boron-rich repeating units. The HOCO(MF)(NH$_2$)$_6$ species is a peptide manifold containing five lysine residues.

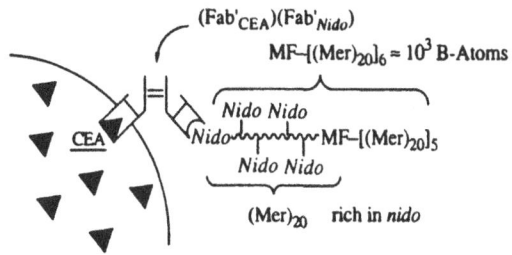

Fig. 4. The bispecific antibody binding hapten-containing boron-rich molecule to cell wall CEA.
The synthetic bispecific antibody is initially injected and binds to tumor cell wall CEA.
The manifold trailer MF-[(Mer)$_{20}$]$_6$ is injected later and the *Nido* hapten targets its specific antibody binding site now held to the cell wall by CEA antigen/antibody interaction.

antigen involved in dual host-guest bonding. The critical step in this sequence is the creation of a new hybridoma which produces the precursor IgG Nido-Mab which is targeted for the [*nido*-7,8-C$_2$B$_9$H$_{11}$-]$^-$ hapten. The isolation of such a hybridoma is in progress at the City of Hope National Medical Center, Duarte, California. With Nido-Mab in hand, enzymatic cleavage of this Mab and the chemical synthesis of (Fab'$_{CEA}$)(Fab'$_{Nido}$) using the similarly obtained Fab'$_{CEA}$ fragment should proceed without great difficulty. Use of bispecific antibody systems to carry boron to tumor will avoid the conjugation and product separation problems associated with conventional antibody delivery of effector species.

REFERENCES

1. Mizusawa, E. A.; Dahlman, H. L.; Bennett, S. J.; Hawthorne, M. F. *Proc. Natl. Acad. Sci. USA* **1982**, *79*, 3011.
2. Goldenberg, D. M.; Sharkey, R. M.; Primus, F. J.; Mizusawa, E. A.; Hawthorne, M. F. *Proc. Natl. Acad. Sci. USA* **1984**, *81*, 560.
3. Alam, F.; Soloway, A. H.; Barth, R. F.; Mafune, N.; Adams, D. M.; Knoth, W. H. *J. Med. Chem.* **1989**, *32*, 2326.
4. Wagener, C.; Yang, Y. H.; Crawford, F. G.; Shively, J. E. *J. Immunol.* **1983**, *130*, 2308.
5. Stewart, J. M.; Young, J. D. "Solid Phase Peptide Synthesis", 2nd Ed.; Pierce Chemical Co.: Rockford, Ill., 1984.
6. Alam, F.; Soloway, A. H.; Barth, R. F. *Appl. Radiat. Isol.* **1987**, *38*, 503.
7. Abraham, R.; Müller, R.; Gabel, D. *Strahlenther. Onkol.* **1989**, *165*, 148.
8. Tamat, S. R.; Patwardhan, A.; Moore, D. E.; Kabral, A.; Brodstock, K.; Hersey, P.; Allen, B. J. *Strahlenther. Onkol.* **1989**, *165*, 165.
9. Maurer, J. L.; Serino, A. J.; Hawthorne, M. F. *Organomet.* **1988**, *7*, 2519.
10. Maurer, J. L.; Berchier, F. B.; Serino, A. J.; Knobler, C. B.; Hawthorne, M. F. *J. Org. Chem.* **1990**, *55*, 838.
11. Chang, C. H.; Ahlem, C. N.; Wolfert, B.; Hochschwender, S. M.; Jue, R.; Frincke, J. M.; Carlo, D. J. *J. Nucl. Med.* **1986**, *27*, 1041.
12. Anderson, L. D.; Meyer, D. L.; Battersby, T. R.; Frincke, J. M.; Mackensen, D.; Lowe, S.; Connolly, P. *J. Nucl. Med.* **1988**, *29*, 835.

CONTINUOUS MEASUREMENT OF BORON-10 CONCENTRATION IN RABBIT BRAIN TISSUE AND

BLOOD USING PROMPT GAMMA-RAY SPECTROMETRY

Yoshinobu Nakagawa[1], Tooru Kobayashi[2], Youri Ueno[2], Hiroshi Hatanaka[3], Kanji Mukai[4], and Keizo Matsumoto[4]

1. Dept. of Neurosurgery, National Kagawa Children's Hospital, Kagawa 765
2. Research Reactor Institute, Kyoto University, Osaka 590-04
3. Dept. of Neurosurgery, Teikyo University, Tokyo 173
4. Dept. of Neurosurgery, Tokushima University, Tokushima 770

INTRODUCTION

One of the important factors which influences the efficacy of boron neutron capture therapy (BNCT) in patients with malignant brain tumour is the boron-10 concentrations in tumours. The boron-10 concentration in normal brain tissue and the tumour/blood concentration ratio are also valuable factors to decide the irradiation time and protect the normal tissue from radiation injury. Therefore, it is valuable to know the boron-10 concentration in the tumour, normal brain tissue and blood just before and during neutron irradiation. In this study we investigated continuously the boron-10 concentrations in the normal brain tissue of living rabbits and blood for 5 - 24 hours after injection of boron 10 compound using prompt gamma-ray spectrometry.

MATERIALS AND METHODS

New Zealand rabbits (n=6) weighing 3 - 3.5kg were used in this study. Under anaesthesia by intravenous injection of pentobarbital (30mg/kg iv), a small burr hole (ca. 7mm in diameter) was perforated in the right parietal region of the skull using a dental drill. The brain surface covered by duramatter was coagulated and the animals were fixed to the measuring system. This technique was developed by one of our authors and can measure boron-10 concentrations of ppm order. The detection limit of the system is 0.1 - 0.5ppm boron-10 concentration. The details of the prompt gamma-ray spectrometry were previously described (Kobayashi & Kannda 1981). The thermal neutron beam of 5mm in diameter from KUR E-3 neutron guide tube was delivered to the brain surface through the burr hole. Following intravenous injection of isotonic solution ($Na_2B_{12}H_{11}SH$ 50mg/kg) diluted in physiological saline, gamma emission from the target point on the surface of the brain was measured continuously. The measuring time was 600 seconds. Blood samples (1 ml) were intermittently drawn and was also studied. In 3 animals the atlanto-occipital membrane was exposed following the midline skin incision and cerebro-spinal fluid (CSF) was also obtained.

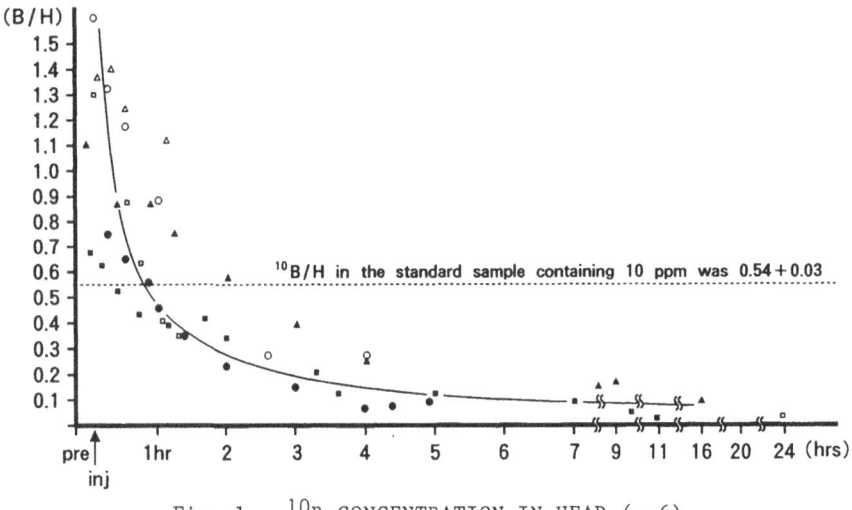

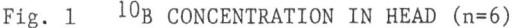

Fig. 1 ^{10}B CONCENTRATION IN HEAD (n=6)

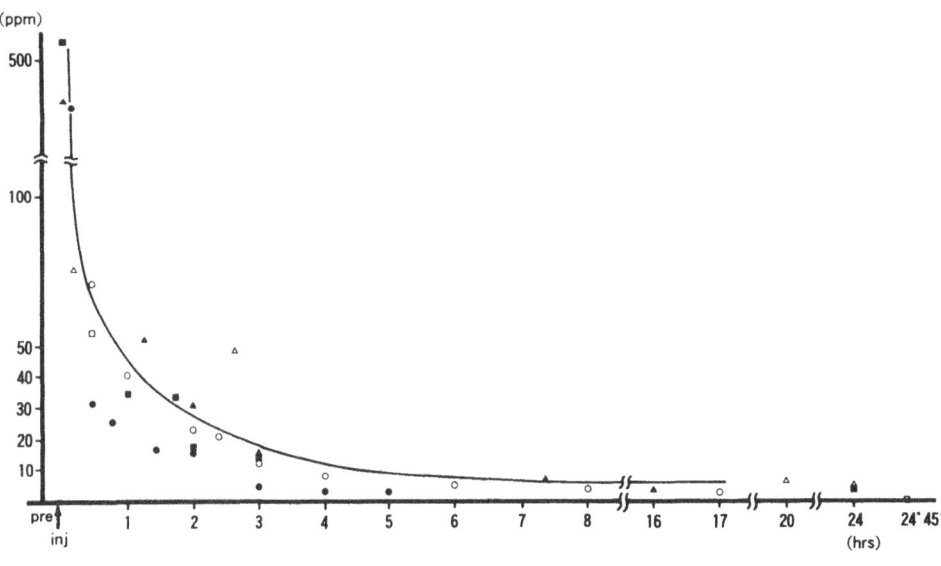

Fig. 2 ^{10}B CONCENTRATION IN BLOOD (n=6)

Table 1
^{10}B Concentration in the cerebro-spinal fluid (ppm)

Time (hours)	[B] ppm (n=3)
4	0.94
6	0.51
17	0
20	0.05
24	0.06
^{10}B compound was given by intravenous injection (50mg/kg) CSF was collected from cisterna magna	

Table 2
^{10}B Concentration in the brain (ppm) (n=6)

Post injection time (hours)	Cerebral cortex	Cerebellar cortex	Brain stem	Basal ganglia
5	0.88	1.14	2.96	0.98
8	0.43	0.36	0.72	0.22
9	0.95	0.16	0.27	0.08
23	0.04	0.26	0.51	0.06
^{10}B compound was given by intravenous injection (50mg/kg) The brain was removed immediately after venous injection of KCl (1Mole, 10ml) and the brain tissue sectioned.				

These materials were collected in a teflon tube for boron-10 analysis.
After all procedures, the animals were sacrificed at different time
intervals (5, 8, 9 and 23 hours after injection of the boron compound) by
venous injection of KCl (1 mole : 10 ml) and the brain was immediately
removed. The brain tissue was divided into four parts: cerebral cortex,
cerebellar cortex, brain stem and basal ganglia. These materials were
collected in pure teflon tubes and the boron-10 concentration of each area
was measured by the same method.

RESULTS

^{10}B/H (ratio of gamma radiation from boron-10 to gamma radiation from
hydrogen in tissue) in the standard sample containing 10 ppm was 0.5 ± 0.03
which was used to calculate the boron-10 concentration of all samples.
However, the boron-10 concentration of the brain tissue of living animals
was expressed in terms of ^{10}B/H (Fig.1). In 10 minutes after the injection
of the compound, the boron-10 concentration reached its peak. In 60
minutes the level of the boron-10 concentration rapidly decreased and then
a gradual decline was observed. At 3 hours, the value of ^{10}B/H was 0.2 -
0.4 and at 5 hours the ratio was 0.1 - 0.2. After 12 hours the mean ratio
of ^{10}B/H was below 0.1. Boron-10 concentration of blood showed similar
changes as in the brain tissue (Fig.2). In 10 minutes after the injection
of boron-10 compound, the level of boron-10 concentration reached the peak
of 400 - 500 ppm. In 60 minutes the level of boron-10 concentration in
blood rapidly decreased and afterwards a gradual decline was observed. The
value was 15 - 30 ppm at 3 hours after injection, 5 - 10 ppm at 6 hours and
2 - 5 ppm at 24 hours in the blood (Fig.1). On the other hand, boron-10
concentrations in the brain tissue of the sacrificed animals showed lower
levels than that of brain tissue studied in living animals (Table 1). The
value in the cerebral cortex was below 1 ppm 5 hours after injection of the
boron-10 compound. Boron-10 concentration in the cerebrospinal fluid was
also below 1 ppm in all samples (Table 2).

DISCUSSION

The in situ measurement of boron-10 concentration of brain tumour and
normal brain tissue around the tumour during the irradiation of patients
may be very interesting for BNCT. In this study we investigated the gamma
emission ratio ^{10}B/H of the brain tissue of living rabbits using prompt
gamma ray spectrometry and compared the value to that of blood. The time
course of the changes of boron-10 concentration was very similar for the
brain and blood. However, the concentration of the brain tissue was
demonstrated using ^{10}B/H and the absolute value was not obtained. In this
measuring system the boron-10 concentration was determined by comparison
with known sample data: ratio of ^{10}B to H. It is yet difficult to estimate
the accurate standard data for in vivo studies. When we compare the ratio
of ^{10}B/H in this study with that of the in vitro study, 10 ppm corresponded
to 0.54 ± 0.03 in ^{10}B/H. If so, the boron-10 concentration in the brain
tissue of a living animal was 3 - 5 ppm. However, the boron-10
concentration of the sacrificed brain tissue at the same interval was below
1 ppm. This discrepancy may be caused by the differences of blood volume
between the living brain and the sacrificed brain tissue. There are still
a few problems to make a control model. However, gamma-spectrometry is a
very useful method, not only for experimental use but also for clinical
trials.

ACKNOWLEDGEMENTS

This work has been carried out in part under the Visiting Researcher's Program of the Research Reactor Institute, Kyoto University.

REFERENCES

Kobayashi T. and Kanda K. 1983, Microanalysis system of ppm-order ^{10}B concentration in tissue for neutron capture therapy by prompt gamma-ray spectrometry, Nuclear Instruments and Methods 204:525-531.

BIOANALYTICAL INVESTIGATIONS ON EXPERIMENTAL BNCT WITH COLD NEUTRONS AT THE JÜLICH RESEARCH REACTOR FRJ-2, STATUS REPORT

M. Papaspyrou and L.E. Feinendegen

Institute of Medicine
Research Center Jülich
D-5170 Jülich, FRG

INTRODUCTION

Until recently "cold neutrons" with an average energy of 0.005 eV generated in Jülich were only used for [10]Boron micro-analysis of blood and tissue samples of tumor bearing mice using quantitative neutron capture radiography (QNCR). Because of the high quality of the pure cold neutron beam with respect to low core r-ray and fast neutron contamination, this neutron beam would constitute an exellent treatment modality for superficial tumors like malignant melanoma of the skin.

If one considers that living tissue contains 70 - 80 % water, the predominant interaction with neutrons is scattering by hydrogen atoms. The hydrogen scattering cross section for (0.005 eV) cold neutrons is 80 barn (1 barn = 10^{-24} cm^2) and the H-capture cross section is only 1 barn, so that the neutrons will be scattered many times before absorption. This leads to thermalization of the cold neutrons by collision with the room-temperature H atoms in the skin. The depth-dose distribution of a cold neutron beam in living tissue in regard to the half-value layer might be essentially the same as for a (0.025 eV) thermal neutron beam.

Thus, also, the number of [10]B (n,α) [7]Li reactions might be the same for cold as for thermal neutrons although the [10]B-neutron capture cross section for cold neutrons (8600 barn) is 2.24 times larger than for thermal neutrons (3840 barn).

COLD NEUTRONS IN JÜLICH

The FRJ-2 is a 23 MW, D_2O-cooled tank reactor. Neutrons from the core are moderated with liquid hydrogen in a cold source with a thermosyphon system which is located immediately after the reactor shielding. Then the neutrons are conducted by [58]Ni-coated guide tubes to an external neutron laboratory (ELLA, Fig. 1). A helium-cooled bismuth filter was installed between the cold source and the neutron guide system, in order to reduce the background of fast neutrons and γ-rays (1). The cold neutron flux (2.0 * 10^9 n/cm^2/s) was measured in the reactor hall past the bismuth filter close to the entrance of the guide system. Ten neutron instruments for various experiments are connected to the guide system, one experiment in the reactor hall and nine in the ELLA hall. The size of the neutron field at the end of the straight guide tube at the position EKN, as shown in Fig. 1, is 10 * 4.8 cm. The flux determined by gold foil activation is 1.1 * 10^8 n/cm^2/s. The γ-contamination contributed by the reactor core is in the range of 30 μSv/h and the background of fast neutrons is less than 10^3 n/cm^2/s.

EXPERIMENTAL SETUP FOR NEUTRON IRRADIATION OF CELL-CULTURES AND MELANOMA-BEARING MICE

To obtain a sufficiently high neutron flux for biomedical irradiation a focusing neutron guide segment (Fig. 2) was installed in the facility EKN between the end of the guide tube and the irradiation box. This neutron collimator is a

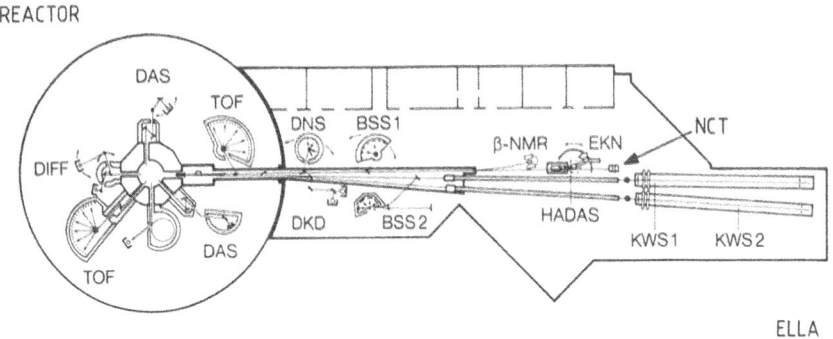

Fig. 1. Starting at the reactor core the neutrons are moderated and reach the entrance of the ELLA hall in separate guide tubes. At the end of the straight guide tube is a facility for cold neutron experiments (EKN) with a setup for experimental neutron capture therapy (NCT).

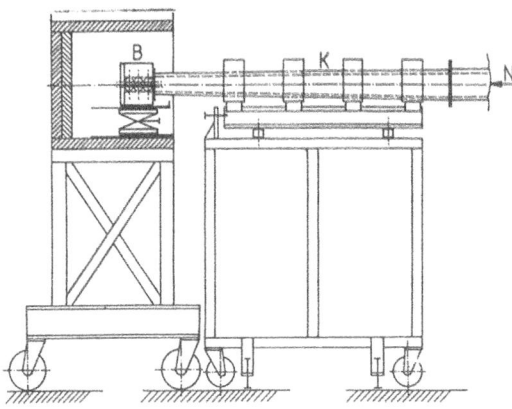

Fig. 2. Schematic view of the setup for experimental NCT. The neutron beam (N) is focused by the collimator (K) until it reaches the irradiation box (B), for exposure of either cultured tumor cells or tumor bearing mice.

tapering boron-silicate glass tube, 1.5 m in length, with an inner coating of alternating Ni and Ti layers. This coating has a higher critical angle of neutron reflection than the ^{58}Ni coating of the guide that precedes it. This leads to an enhancement of the neutron flux from $1.1 * 10^8$ to $2.8 * 10^8$ n/cm^2/s. The neutron field is reduced to 5.6 cm by 2.7 cm at the exit (1).

B16-mouse melanoma cells cultured in 96-well microplates can be irradiated with this horizontal beam because the surface tension of the cell culture medium permits tipping the microplate at an angle of 60° from the horizontal position without any leaking (2).

Six melanoma bearing mice can be positioned in a teflon box in front of the neutron collimator. The tumors had been transplanted subcutaneously into the hind legs of mice. Each mouse is placed in a single teflon tube which is inserted in a hole on one of the sides of the box. Three tubes can be accommodated on each side. Only the tumor bearing leg is situated in the beam. The tubes can be turned around so that no leg will be shielded by another (2).

The melanoma-seeking ^{10}B-compounds p-dihydroxyboryl-phenylalanine (^{10}BPA), 5-dihydroxyboryl-2-thiouracil (^{10}BPA) and 5-dihydroxyboryl-6-propyl-2-thiouracil (^{10}BPTU) are being used as capture agents in the cell cultures and in the animals (3,4). If these trials are successful, clinical trials for the treatment of primary human melanomas will be carried out in the near future.

CONCLUSION

The use of cold neutrons may represent a practical treatment modality in experimental NCT of cultured tumor cells or superficial tumors such as malignant melanomas. Because the beam is so clean, hardly any side effects resulting from core 𝛾-radiation or fast neutrons are expected.

REFERENCES

1. B. Alefeld, J. Duppich, O. Schärpf, A. Schirmer, T. Springer, and K. Werner, The new neutron guide laboratory at the FRJ-2 reactor in the KFA Jülich and its special beam forming devices, Thin-Film Neutron Optical Devices, 983:75 (1988).

2. M. Papaspyrou, and L. E. Feinendegen, Antrag auf Einbau- und Betriebsgenehmigung SV 5-EKN/ETT, RSA des Forschungszentrums Jülich, (1990).

3. Y. Mishima, C. Honda, M. Ishihashi, H. Obara, J. Hiratsuka, H. Fukuda, H. Karashima, T. Kobayashi, K. Kanda, and K. Yoshino, Treatment of malignant melanoma by single thermal neutron capture therapy with melanoma-seeking ^{10}B-compound, Lancet, 2:388 (1989).

4. W. Tjarks, and D. Gabel, Boron containing thiouracil derivatives for NCT of melanoma, J. Med. Chem., in press, (1990)

BORON CONCENTRATION MEASUREMENTS FOR THE PETTEN BNCT PROJECT

M. Konijnenberg[3], F. Stecher-Rasmussen[1], C.P.J. Raaymakers, R. Huiskamp[1],
R.L. Moss[2], A.C. Begg[3], L. Dewit[3], V.G.A. Gregoire[3] and B.J. Mijnheer[3]

[1]Netherlands Energy Research Foundation ECN,
        Petten, The Netherlands
[2]Commission of the European Communities, Joint Research Centre,
        Petten, The Netherlands
[3]Netherlands Cancer Institute, Amsterdam, The Netherlands

INTRODUCTION

In Petten two lines of BNCT research are conducted, one aiming at the development and
construction of a clinical facility at the High Flux Reactor (1-3), and the other one studying
the fundamental aspects of BNCT (3-5).   For both lines the measurement of boron
concentrations play a crucial role.   The precondition for the clinical application of BNCT,
high boron concentration in tumour cells and low concentration in normal tissue, requires
insight in the pharmacokinetics of the boron compound.   To understand the fundamental
mechanism of BNCT, knowledge about the macroscopic distribution of boron within a tumour
volume and the microscopic distribution at the cellular level are needed.

PROMPT-GAMMA RAY SPECTROSCOPY

Neutrons from a standard radial beamchannel (HB 7) of the HFR, located near the facility for
therapy, are filtered through a multireflecting focusing mirror system (6) before reaching the
target position (fig. 1).   Only thermal neutrons satisfy the condition for total reflection in the
neutron mirrors, the system being closed for direct transmission.   Epithermal neutrons and
gamma rays are attenuated by the bulk of the mirrors while the transmitted thermal neutrons
(mean energy 18 meV) are focused at the target.   This gives a flux density at the target
position of $\Phi_{th} = 2 \cdot 10^7$ cm$^{-2} \cdot$s^{-1} with a cadmium ratio of about 1000 and a gamma-ray
component in the beam of 1 cGy/h.   A collimator reduces the beam cross section over the
target to 2x2 cm^2.

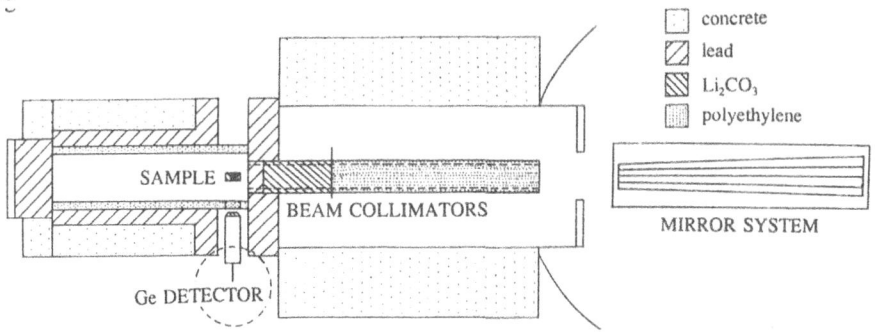

concrete
lead
Li$_2$CO$_3$
polyethylene

SAMPLE

BEAM COLLIMATORS

MIRROR SYSTEM

Ge DETECTOR

Fig. 1.   Geometry of prompt gamma setup at the HFR.   Source detector distance is 20 cm.

Progress in Neutron Capture Therapy for Cancer
Edited by B.J. Allen *et al.*, Plenum Press, New York, 1992

Samples are placed in 1 ml vials positioned in the focus plane of the beam. A Li_2CO_3 cylinder around the vial captures neutrons scattered from the target. One High Purity germanium spectrometer facing the target detects the photons released after the capture of neutrons. The recoiling ^7Li-particles from the $^{10}B(n,\alpha)^7Li$ reaction decay to the ground state emitting 478 keV photons. The photon intensity carries the information about the ^{10}B-concentration, as the surrounding shielding material has been stripped of any boron. Not only the boron but most of the other elements present in the sample emit photons after capture of neutrons. In this way the analysis of the γ-spectra give information about the composition of the sample, allowing the use of the γ-line from capture in hydrogen as internal calibration. For the registration of the spectra the signal from the Ge-spectrometer is processed by a ND851 ADC, transmitted to a ND66 MCA and stored on a VAX-750 computer for further analysis. In fig. 2 (upper curve) a part of a typical spectrum in the energy region around the boron line is shown. The content of the boron peak is here determined by fitting a proper function to the peak (lower part of fig. 2). However, the peak content can also be obtained from the measured boron spectrum by subtracting a background spectrum from a separate measurement with a non-boronated background sample. The two methods give identical results within the standard error.

Furthermore, by the Doppler-shift-attenuation the range of the Li-particles in the sample can be deduced from the analysis of the shape of the Doppler broadened peak.

INDUCTIVELY COUPLED PLASMA ATOMIC EMISSION SPECTROSCOPY

The ICP-AES equipment used in Petten, Jobin Yvon model JY 70 plus, located near the radiobiology unit, uses the 249.73 nm emission line and detects besides B, Fe and Ca. Zn is used as an internal standard.

The Inductively Coupled Plasma Atomic Emission Spectroscopy provides a lower detection limit than the prompt gamma technique, but the sample preparation is destructive and rather laborious. The destruction procedure involves digestion in a pressure controlled microwave system with an acid mixture consisting of nitric acid, perchloric acid and hydrofluoric acid (90:5:5 w/w). The detection limit (background) is 0.001-0.015 ppm B (mean +/- 3 st. dev.). For a 100 µl plasma sample this will result in a detection limit of 0.05-0.75 µg B and for a 300 mg tissue sample in a detection limit of 0.018-0.25 µg B.

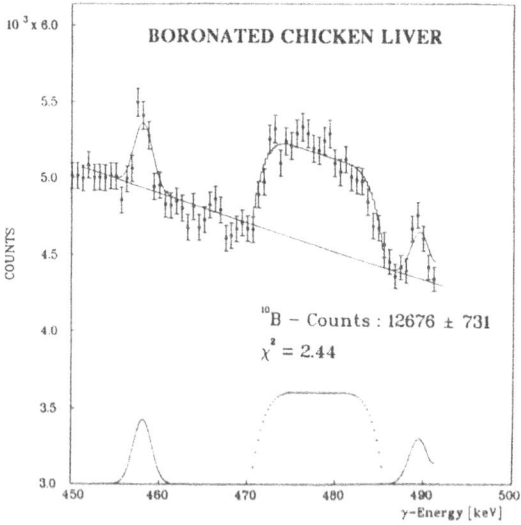

Fig. 2. Spectrum from 1 g chicken liver sample containing 20 ppm ^{10}B.
Measuring time: 15 min.

EXPERIMENTAL RESULTS

During the prompt gamma-ray analysis (PGRA) the content of the boron line (and the hydrogen line at 2223 kev) for an unknown sample is calibrated against standard samples with known boron (and hydrogen) concentration. A calibrated solution of 1000 µg/g natural B in demineralized water was diluted to obtain a set of standard samples with ^{10}B-concentrations in the range 1-200 µg/g. As inter-calibration between the prompt-gamma technique and ICP-AES is mandatory for the detection of eventual systematic errors, a series of samples has been measured by both methods. In fig. 3 the results from measurements of boronated chicken liver are presented. The dashed line indicates the expected 1:1 relation. At present a detection limit of ≤ 1 ppm ^{10}B in a 1 ml sample can be obtained with a measuring time of 20 min. The use of two Ge detectors instead of one will redcuce this time to 15 min.

The analysis of the Doppler-shift attenuation gives a range of 4.4 µm for Li-particles in chicken liver, which is equivalent to the range in water.

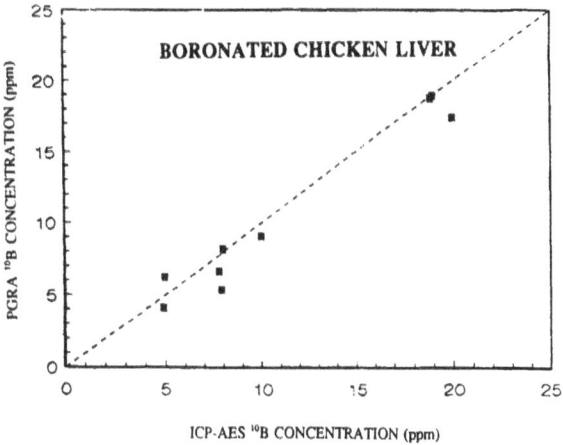

Fig. 3. Intercomparison of PGRA versus ICP-AES for chicken liver samples.

OTHER BORON DETECTION TECHNIQUES

With the Track Etch technique, neutron radiography based on tracking the alpha and lithium particles by a plastic sheet in contact with a thin slice of the sample, the boron distribution across the biological material (e.g. tumour) can be depicted. Basically this technique is of qualitative nature. However, by imbedding calibration samples adjacent to or in the tumour before slicing, quantitative information can be extracted with an image analysis system (Leitz texture analysis system). Sofar irradiation takes place in Studsvik, Sweden. The possibility for using the neutron facilities in Petten is under investigation.

On a cellular scale Electron Spectroscopic Imaging (ESI) is a promising approach for simultaneous imaging and concentration measurement of boron across one cell. A feasibility study is under preparation.

CONCLUSION

A method giving fast and accurate measurement of ^{10}B-concentration down to 1 ppm in a large number of samples (about 1 ml) of blood, urine and tissue is required for the clinical programme. For this purpose prompt-gamma is suited. The present setup, however, should be regarded as experimental and needs further improvement of shielding and geometry to reduce background.

For small samples and lower concentrations ICP is superior to prompt-gamma. Both methods will be used complementary in the Petten programme.

ACKNOWLEDGEMENT

This work was partly financially supported by the Netherlands Cancer Foundation under the project NKB grant NKI 90-03.

REFERENCES

1. R.L. Moss et al., Proceedings of the Fourth International Symposium on Neutron Capture Therapy for Cancer, Sydney December 1990, contribution 2.3, to be published
2. L. Dewit et al., ibid, contribution 18.1
3. D. Gabel, ibid, contribution 11.2
4. R. Huiskamp et al., ibid, contribution 12A1
5. V.G.A. Gregoire et al., ibid, contribution 14A3
6. F. Stecher-Rasmussen et al., Nucl. Phys. A181 (1972) 225

FLOW INJECTION FOR SAMPLE INTRODUCTION INTO INDUCTIVELY COUPLED PLASMA FOR THE DETERMINATION OF BORON IN BIOLOGICAL SAMPLES

W. F. Bauer, J. A. Wishard, C. Rae, and N. Lassahn

INEL BNCT Research Programs, Idaho National Engineering Laboratory, P.O. Box 1625, Idaho Falls, ID 83415-3519

INTRODUCTION

An important aspect of any BNCT program is the ability to rapidly and quantitatively determine boron in a variety of biological sample types. Inductively coupled plasma-atomic emission spectroscopy (ICP-AES) has proven to be well-suited for boron analysis in biological samples[1,2]. Detection limits for boron by ICP-AES are typically less than 0.010 μg boron/mL in the analytical solution (biological samples at 1 μg boron/g can be quantitated with dilution factors as large as 100) and the linear dynamic range is in the range of five to six orders of magnitude. The major limitation of boron determinations by ICP-AES is attributed to problems with carryover[3]. At the INEL BNCT laboratory, we have found that a rinse cycle utilizing both basic and acidic conditions helps to limit this problem. Unfortunately, the rinse procedure is time consuming and drives the total analysis time to 5-7 minutes per sample, depending upon the boron concentration of the previous sample. To limit the required rinse time, samples that are expected to have very high boron concentrations are diluted so the resulting analytical solution concentrations are less than 5 μg boron/mL.

To combat the carryover problems mentioned above and to simultaneously allow a much greater instrumental sample throughput, flow injection analysis (FIA) with ICP-AES detection (FIA ICP-AES) was investigated. Flow injection analysis[4] is a continuous flow analysis method in which a small volume of sample is reproducibly injected into a continuously flowing, nonsegmented stream. In the simplest case, the primary function of the stream is to carry a minimal amount of sample to a detector. In more elaborate systems, the sample can be diluted or modified online by the addition of reagents required for analysis. The only major disadvantage to FIA is that, in some cases, where extensive sample preparation is carried out online, detection limits can be adversely affected. A list of advantages of FIA would include very high reproducibility and accuracy, speed of analysis, the need for only small sample volumes, very short residence times (thus limiting carryover), and the potential for performing some sample preparation procedures online.

EXPERIMENTAL

All experiments and analyses were performed on an ARL Model 3520 ICP-AES instrument. Liquid argon provided the plasma torch gas supply under standard operating conditions. The instrument was operated for both conventional, continuous aspiration ICP-AES boron analysis and for FIA ICP-AES. In conventional ICP-AES, sample uptake was maintained at 2.6 mL/minute with a peristaltic pump. Quantitation was the result of three five-second integrations at both the 208.959 and 249.678 nm boron lines. In the FIA ICP-AES analysis mode, no modifications of the ICP sample introduction system were made other than to place a Rheodyne Model 5020 injection valve with a 200-μL sample loop into the carrier stream between the peristaltic pump and the nebulizer. The carrier stream consisted only of deionized water flowing at 3 mL/minute. Only 30 cm of 0.5 mm id Teflon™ tubing were used between the injection valve and the nebulizer; thus the sample plug reached the ICP almost immediately after injection. Quantitation for an FIA ICP-AES analysis was the result of a single 40-second integration which began immediately after injection. Emission intensity values were manual input to the calibration routines so replicate information was included in the calibration curve. Transient signals were recorded with a Perkin-Elmer LCI-100 recording integrator connected to the PMT output in the ICP-AES electronics with the instrument software operating in the "test" mode.

Blood serum and urine samples were prepared by dilution of 20-200 μL of sample to 10 mL with deionized water. Calibration standards were prepared from a commercial 1000 μg boron/mL solution (Fisher). Calibrations were checked with either a 0.5 or 2.5 μg boron/mL solution prepared from a 5 mg boron/mL NIST standard (SRM 3107).

DISCUSSION

The utility of FIA ICP-AES in boron analysis is demonstrated by the traces shown in Figure 1. The upper trace is representative of the time required for conventional, continuous aspiration ICP-AES analysis where two boron channels are monitored. This trace includes the aspiration time required to reach a steady state signal, to measure the two channels in triplicate, and to clear all of the connecting tubing of sample once the measurements have been made. The lower trace is of four 200-μL injections of the same 1 μg boron/mL solution made within the same timeframe as the upper trace. Reproducibility of these four injections is quite good (RSD = 2.3%) and the signal returns to the baseline much more quickly than for the continuous aspiration technique. Carryover problems with the continuous aspiration technique are enhanced at higher concentrations and when long (5 sec) integration times are used to average the noise observed in Figure 1. Generally, no carryover is noted at sampling frequencies up

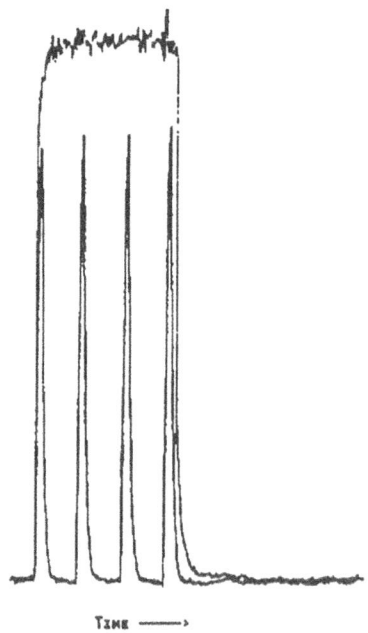

TIME ────>

Figure 1. Comparison of conventional, continuous aspiration ICP-AES and FIA ICP-AES for 1-μg boron/mL solution.

to and greater than one sample/minute with the FIA method. The calibration data ($r^2 = 0.998$) shown in Figure 2 and the subsequent sample analyses were aquired at an overall sampling rate of 1.17 samples/minute (51 manual injections in 43.5 minutes).

While the recording integrator is a very useful tool and can be used to determine the heights and areas of the FIA peaks, it is subject to integration errors caused by the periodic sampling of the natural flicker in the torch. Additionally, the integrator is unable to provide convenient feedback of concentration information to the analyst. A much betterz method of integration is performed by the ICP-AES instrument electronics when the entire signal is, in effect, collected and "integrated" for a period of 40 seconds. This latter method of sampling the torch output is more effective at averaging noise and provides more stable and precise instrumental output for quantitation.

Using the 40-second integration method, the instrument was calibrated and used to quantitate several prepared serum and urine samples by FIA-ICP-AES. Over a period of 3.6 hours, 120 manual injections were made, including triplicate injections of calibration and calibration check standards and 15 samples. An NIST boron standard, used as a calibration check, had a mean percent error of $0 \pm 2\%$ (n = 21). A blind standard and a matrix spike had recoveries of 101% and 95%, respectively. The mean relative standard deviation (percent RSD) for all injections made in triplicate was $1 \pm 1\%$ and the diluted sample concentrations ranged from 0.08-5.0 μg boron/mL. The detection limit, determined as three times the standard deviation, of the blank analyses was 0.012 μg boron/mL. In a separate experiment, a set of samples were run with both conventional ICP-AES and by FIA-ICP-AES with good agreement. The linear regression of the two techniques plotted against each other resulted in a line with a slope of 1.00 ± 0.01 and a y-intercept of 0 ± 4 and r^2 of 0.994.

The data presented above indicate that FIA, as a sample introduction method for ICP-AES analysis of boron, is accurate, very precise, and potentially very time efficient. The reproducibility is such that samples need not always be injected and run in triplicate and the throughput of samples can potentially be doubled or tripled over that of conventional ICP-AES.

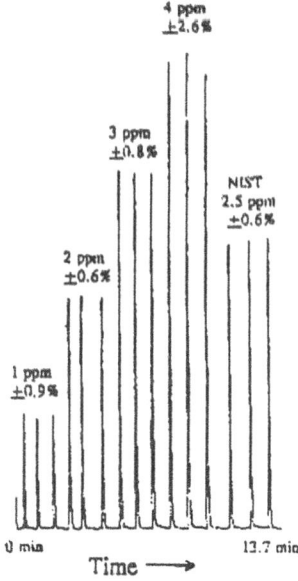

Figure 2. Typical calibration by FIA ICP-AES from 0-5 μg boron/mL (ppm) standards with NIST calibration check.

REFERENCES

1. Tamat, S. R., D. E. Moore, and B. J. Allen, "Determination of Boron in Biological Tissues by ICP-AES," Anal. Chem. 59: 2161 (1987).

2. Bauer, W. F., D. A. Johnson, S. M. Steele, K. Messick, D. L. Miller and W. A. Propp, "Gross Boron Determination in Biological Samples by ICP-AES," Strahlenther. Onkol. 165: (2/3) 176 (1989).

3. Mills, J. C., "An Acid Dissolution Procedure for the Determination of Boron in Coal Ash and Silicates by ICP-AES with Conventional Glass Nebulizers," Anal. Chim. Acta 183: 231 (1986).

4. Ruzicka, J. and E. H. Hansen, "Flow Injection Analysis: Principles, Applications and Trends " Anal. Chim. Acta 114: 19 (1980).

COPYRIGHT

BORON-10 PROMPT GAMMA ANALYSIS USING A DIFFRACTED NEUTRON BEAM

R. Rogus, O. K. Harling, I. Olmez and S. Wirdzek

Nuclear Reactor Laboratory, Massachusetts Institute of Technology

138 Albany Street, Cambridge, MA 02139, USA

INTRODUCTION

A prompt gamma neutron activation analysis (PGNAA) facility has been built at the 5 MW MITR-II Research Reactor to support our ongoing boron neutron capture therapy (NCT) program. This facility is used to determine the concentration of B-10 in NCT relevant samples such as blood and urine. The B-10 concentration is needed to determine the radiation doses that tumor and healthy brain receive during neutron irradiation of a patient (1). Assaying for B-10 by PGNAA has several advantages over conventional chemical methods. It is rapid, accurate, nondestructive (allowing for re-analysis), inexpensive, sensitive (ppm level), generally independent of the chemical or physical matrix of the B-10, and does not require chemical manipulations of the sample.

Our goal was to build an inexpensive facility with a suitably high thermal neutron flux for PGNAA and a low level of photon and fast neutron contamination. Our design is unique in that it uses a diffracted beam. Most prompt gamma facilities use direct beams; these beams have a high thermal flux ($> 10^7$ n/cm²-sec), but are heavily contaminated with photons and fast neutrons. Other prompt gamma facilities use totally reflecting guide tubes; these beams have little contamination, but are expensive. The high thermal flux of direct beam facilities might not be an advantage since the detector usually must be moved further away from the sample to avoid high dead times in the multichannel analyzer.

DESCRIPTION OF FACILITY

A schematic of the facility is shown in Figure 1. A tangential beam port from our reactor's D2O reflector tank was used. This port has a lower photon and fast neutron contamination than a radial port. The beam is filtered with a 15 cm long sapphire crystal; the crystal transmits 72% of the thermal neutrons, but scatters or absorbs roughly 95% of the epithermal neutrons, 75% of the fast neutrons (> 1 keV), and 70% of the photons. This filtered beam is then diffracted off the basal plane (002) of two slightly misaligned pyrolytic graphite crystals. The fraction of a degree misalignment permits more neutrons to satisfy the Bragg condition and be diffracted. Neutrons that satisfy the Bragg condition provide a relatively pure thermal ($E_n = 0.06 \pm 0.01$ eV) neutron beam. Soller slits were not used since our goal was to keep the thermal flux relatively high, not to limit the energy spread. The beam is collimated to a rectangular shape, 4.1 cm high x 1.5 cm wide, with blocks that contain $^6Li_2CO_3$ in epoxy. The detector is about 6.5 cm from the sample. The thermal flux averaged over the beam cross section at the sample is 3.5 x 10^6 n/cm²-sec. This intensity is about the maximum that can be used effectively for prompt gamma analysis of boron in aqueous samples of 3-5 ml volume and B-10 concentrations up to about 100 μg/g.

BORON-10 DETECTION SYSTEM

The nuclear reaction used to detect boron by PGNAA is B-10(n,α)Li-7. The recoiling Li-7, initially in an excited state, decays with 94% abundant Doppler broadened 478 keV prompt gammas (2). The peaks are Doppler broadened because the Li-7 nucleus is travelling at a high speed during emission of the gamma. These prompt gammas are detected with a lead and $^6Li_2CO_3$ shielded HPGE detector (Canberra Model GC 3020, 30.4% efficient relative to a 3" x 3" NaI

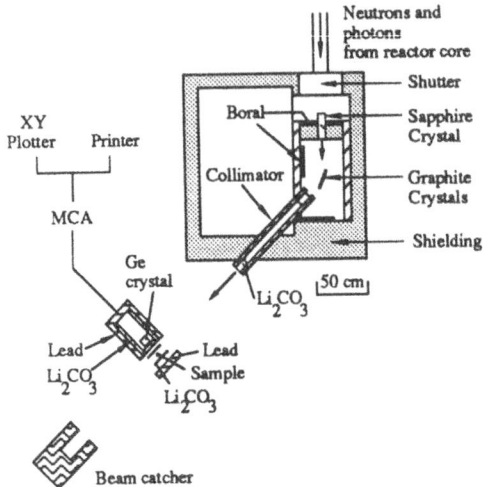

Figure 1. Schematic of the prompt gamma neutron activation analysis facility at the MITR-II.

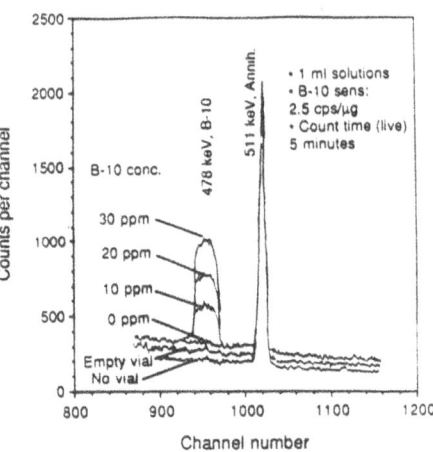

Figure 2. Pulse height spectra of several boric acid solutions. The solutions were in 1.5 ml polyethylene vials that were 6.5 cm from the detector. Reactor power was 4.5 MW.

crystal at 1332 keV), MCA (Canberra Series 85, Model 8505), and associated equipment (Canberra Model 3105 High Voltage Power Supply, Model 2022 Amplifier, and Model 8521 ADC/SCA). The gain is adjusted to obtain a spectrum over the 0 - 2300 keV range; this range includes the B-10 (478 keV) and H (2223. keV) prompt gammas. The total area of the B-10 peak is determined by summing the counts from 468 to 488 keV. The total area of the H peak is determined with the MCA's built-in peak search and gaussian peak fitting program. For both peaks, the net area is determined by subtracting the background using the straight line technique with 2 end point averaging.

METHOD

Samples such as blood, urine, or boric acid solutions are pipetted into polyethylene or Teflon vials and then positioned in the beam. The sample is surrounded by a 12 cm long four sided box with thin Teflon sheets to support a 0.5 cm thickness of $^6Li_2CO_3$ powder. Lithium-6 is a strong neutron absorber and has the interesting property of emitting a very low abundance of prompt gammas. These non-Doppler broadened 478 keV prompt gammas constitute a small correction that must be subtracted from the Doppler broadened B-10 peak. Using this neutron absorber around the sample reduces background in the pulse height spectrum that would be caused by prompt gammas resulting from neutrons scattered by the sample and absorbed in the surrounding materials. The B-10 sensitivity of aqueous solutions is 2-3 cps/μg, depending on the volume and geometry of the sample. For a relatively large 5 ml sample, the multichannel analyzer dead time is 15%; however, when the 0 - 450 keV part of the spectrum is discriminated against, dead time is reduced to 10%. Samples are counted long enough to obtain the desired statistical precision.

The B-10 sensitivity can be increased by moving the detector closer to the sample, but this would increase the dead time. Our ADC is a linear ramp converter (Wilkinson type, 100 MHz clock frequency) so the dead time remaining after the 0 - 450 keV discrimination is caused primarily by the relatively long conversion times of the higher channels. Dead times could be reduced by using a ramp converter with a faster clock (300 MHz) or by using the faster, successive approximation type of ADC. With a faster ADC, we could double the counting rate by moving the detector closer to the sample. This would cut the counting time in half. This might be useful in counting 3-5 ml samples of very low B-10 concentration (< 0.5 ppm). Typical NCT samples, however, have 1-50 ppm B-10 and can currently be counted in minutes to an hour. For small samples (< 1 ml), the current ADC would give reasonable dead times even with the detector moved closer to the sample.

The concentration of B-10 in the sample can be calculated by determining the B-10 reaction rate from the number of 478 keV gammas emitted. The B-10 concentration, however, is determined by using a calibration curve obtained with known concentrations of B-10. Standard solutions are prepared from boric acid crystals (Fisher Scientific Co., Certified A.C.S. Grade, Certified B-10 abundance). A calibration curve of B-10 count rate versus the known B-10 concentration could be made for a fixed reactor power. However, a slightly different approach is used that is more accurate since it accounts for the number of neutrons incident on the sample. The B-10 count rate is normalized to the H capture prompt gamma count rate. This eliminates any errors in the B-10 count rate that could result from changes in experimental conditions, such as fluctuations in reactor power, or more importantly, positioning of the sample in the beam or changes in the sample - detector distance.

RESULTS

Pulse height spectra for 5 minute counts of boric acid solutions are shown in Figure 2. Spectra are shown for 1 ml solutions with 0, 10, 20, and 30 ppm B-10. Spectra are also shown for just an empty vial and for nothing in the beam. Similar pulse height spectra for blood solutions are shown in Figure 3. These blood solutions had a lower B-10 concentration than the boric acid solutions and so were counted for a longer time. Pulse height spectra of blood solutions have a prompt gamma peak at 472 keV due to Na and a small non-Doppler broadened prompt gamma peak at 478 keV due to the ^{6}Li(n,γ) reaction, which increase the area under the Doppler broadened 478 keV peak of B-10. The area of these small peaks must be subtracted from the total area to determine the net B-10 count rate.

A B-10 calibration curve for boric acid solutions is shown in Figure 4. The ratio of B-10 to H prompt gamma counts (or ratio of count rates) is plotted against the known B-10 concentration. This curve has an excellent straight line association (correlation coefficient $r^2 \sim 1.0$, where a value of 1 indicates a perfect straight line relationship). A similar calibration curve for low levels of B-10 in blood is shown in Figure 5. Unknown solutions are run in a manner similar to the solutions used to prepare the calibration curves. The B-10 to H prompt gamma ratio is determined and the B-10 concentration is determined from the appropriate calibration curve. The unknown solutions and the standard solutions must have the same matrix (aqueous or blood, for example), be irradiated in the same type of sample vial, and have the same volume (for hydrogenous vials).

Solutions of increasingly lower concentrations of B-10 must be counted for longer times to obtain the same statistical precision (Figure 6). Recently, the B-10 sensitivity was increased by moving the detector closer to the sample. Background was reduced by adding lead shielding around the detector, adding the Li_2CO_3 shield, and using a lightweight Teflon sample vial. Also, a background level of B-10, caused primarily by boron in concrete adjacent to the detector, was eliminated by lead shielding. As a result, count times for NCT relevant samples (1-50 ppm B-10)

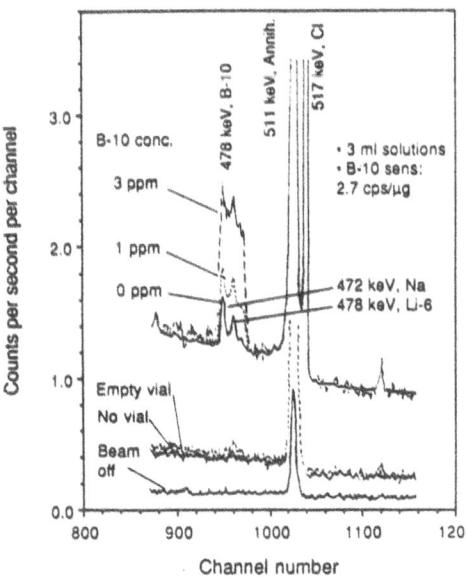

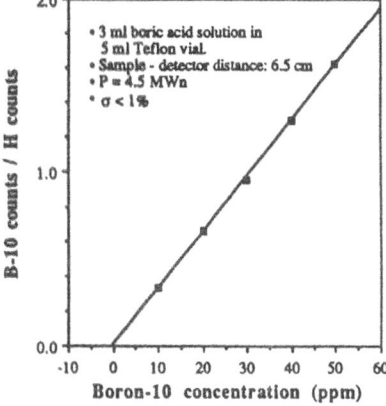

Figure 3. Pulse height spectra of several blood solutions. Count times were 2 hours for the 0 and 1 ppm samples, 15 minutes for the 3 ppm samples, and 8 minutes for the other samples.

Figure 4. Boron-10 calibration curve for boric acid solutions using the B-10/H ratio method. The curve is linear and shows very little background B-10 (intercept at 0.2 ppm).

have been significantly reduced. For a 1 ppm, 3 ml sample, a statistical precision of ±5% is obtained in 1 hour; a 10 ppm, 3 ml sample requires 1 minute for the same precision.

Our prompt gamma system has been intercalibrated with the prompt gamma system at BNL. The B-10 concentrations of several boric acid solutions were independently determined. Results agreed within the overall accuracy of the method.

DISCUSSION

For aqueous or tissue samples in the 1-3 ml volume range and B-10 concentrations $\geq$ 1 ppm, the current beam intensity is adequate and a significant increase would not be useful due to multichannel analyzer dead time. However, very small samples such as those obtained in needle biopsies would require higher intensities and smaller beam areas. Higher intensities with smaller beam areas can be achieved by using a focusing monochromator in place of the flat monochromator that we now use. An increase in intensity of one order of magnitude should be relatively easy to obtain, and one to two orders of magnitude increase may be feasible with a sophisticated monochromator and, of course, a proportionate decrease in beam area.

The performance of the MITR-II prompt gamma system is comparable to or better than other prompt gamma systems located on direct beams at reactors of comparable or higher power than that of the MITR-II. This system is being used extensively for blood, urine, and tissue analyses in support of the BNCT program at Tufts - New England Medical Center and MIT. The B-10 concentration of a patient's blood at the time of neutron irradiation will be essential for the safety of the patient when clinical trials are initiated. PGNAA will be used to provide this information. Similarly, the concentration of B-10 in blood, urine, and tumor of patients who are currently in a pharmacokinetic study of p-boronophenylalanine is being obtained with this facility.

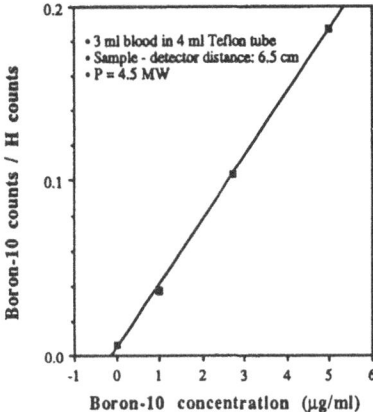
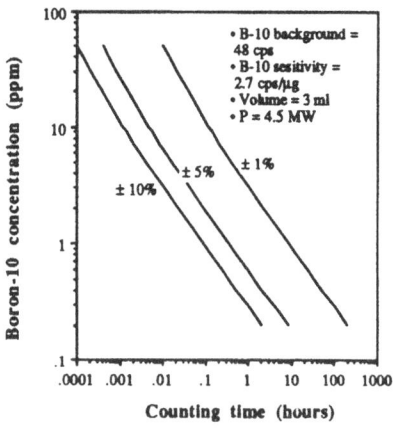

Figure 5. Boron-10 calibration curve for blood using the B-10/H ratio method.

Figure 6. The counting time necessary to achieve a desired statistical precision depends on the background level, B-10 sensitivity, volume of solution, and the B-10 concentration.

ACKNOWLEDGMENT

This research was funded by the U.S. Department of Energy, Office of Health and Human Assessments, under Grant No. DE-FG02-87ER-6060 and by a U.S. Department of Energy Reactor Sharing Grant awarded to the MIT Nuclear Reactor Laboratory.

REFERENCES

1. H. Madoc-Jones, D. E. Wazer, R.G. Zamenhof, O. K. Harling, J. A. Bernard, "Clinical Considerations for Neutron Capture Therapy of Brain Tumors," in Proceedings of an International Workshop on Neutron Beam Design, Development, and Performance for Neutron Capture Therapy, O. K. Harling, J. A. Bernard, R. G. Zamenhof, eds., Plenum Press, New York, (1990).

2. C. Lederer, J. Hollander, I. Perlman, Table of Isotopes, 6th ed, John Wiley & Sons, Inc., New York, (1967).

DETERMINATION OF BORON CONCENTRATION BY MEANS OF DIRECT CURRENT PLASMA - ATOMIC EMISSION SPECTROSCOPY

Rolf F. Barth[1], Albert H. Soloway[2], Dianne M. Adams[1], Fazlul Alam[2], and Abul K.M. Anisuzzaman[3]

[1]Department of Pathology, [2]College of Pharmacy, The Ohio State University, Columbus, Ohio 43210, U.S.A.

Introduction

The accurate measurement of total boron content in biological samples with a sensitivity in the ppm range is essential for evaluating the potential usefulness of various tumor localizing boron-containing compounds for Boron Neutron Capture Therapy (BNCT)[1]. Among the procedures that have been used are spectrophotometric analyses involving various complexing agents[2-4]. These methods are time consuming and require that the boron compounds can be oxidized to boric acid. Relatively low sensitivity and interference from various contaminants further limit their usefulness. Recently, inductively coupled plasma-atomic emission spectroscopy (ICP-AES) has been shown to be sensitive enough for the detection of microgram quantities of boron in biological samples[5,6], although the sensitivity is adversely affected by high concentrations of inorganic salts in the samples[7]. Since alkaline fusion is not suitable for use with ICP[8], samples were digested by exposure to either perchloric acid[5,6] or nitric acid[6]. There may be a danger of explosion with the former, and with the latter, it may be necessary to decompose the tissues in teflon-lined digestion bombs. Both procedures, therefore, have their limitations. The objectives of the present study were to determine whether DCP-AES could be used to quantify boron in a variety of chemical compounds including polyhedral boranes and carboranes, to improve the procedure for the digestion of tissue samples, to determine if this method could be used to quantify cellular uptake of boron, and finally to define the limits of boron detection in biologic samples by means of this method.

Materials and Methods

Direct Current Plasma Atomic Emission Spectroscopy

Instrumentation. A Spectraspan VB Direct Current Plasma-Atomic Emission Spectrometer, (Applied Research Laboratories, Brea, CA) was used for boron determinations. This instrument combines a high resolution spectrometer with a high resolution Echelle grating and prism.

Reagents and test compounds. All reagents were of analytical grade. Concentrated sulfuric acid and 70% hydrogen peroxide (E.I. Dupont de Nemours & Co., Wilmington, DE) were used for tissue digestion. A stock solution containing 1000 ppm of boron was prepared by dissolving weighed quantities of 95% enriched ^{10}B boric acid (Eagle Picher, Quapaw, OK) in a known volume of deionized, distilled water. The polyhedral boranes $Na_2B_{12}H_{11}SH$ and $Cs_2B_{12}H_{11}SH\cdot H_2O$ were generously provided by Callery Chemical Company, Callery, PA. The polyhedral borane $[(C_2H_5)_3NH]_3B_{12}H_{12}$ and the carborane $C_{15}H_{32}B_{10}O_6$ were synthesized in our laboratory.

Animal tumors. Male BALB/c mice, weighing ~20 gm, were purchased from Charles River Laboratories, Inc., (Wilmington, MA). Animals were injected intramuscularly into the flank with 1.5×10^6 Harding-Passey melanoma cells suspended in 0.2 mL of Hank's Balanced Salt Solution. Ten to 12 days later, when tumors had attained a size of ~1 cm^3, animals were bled via the retrorbital venous plexus and then killed. Tumor, liver, skin and muscle samples were removed and weighed. Known quantities of boric acid were added and the samples were processed for boron determination as described below.

Sample preparation for analysis. One to 2 mL of concentrated sulfuric acid, which was adequate for up to 1 g of tissue, were added to 150 x 16 mm Pyrex culture tubes, and these were placed in a mineral oil bath, heated to 100°C in an exhaust hood and stirred intermittently for one hour. Since no interference with the boron signal was found with the sulfuric acid-hydrogen peroxide cocktail, the amount of sulfuric acid used in digestions was determined by the ease of digestion for a particular sample, rather than by any specific ratio of sample weight to acid volume. Known quantities of H_3BO_3 were added to samples, either prior to or following tissue digestion in order to determine what effects, if any, the tissue matrix and digestion process had on boron detection. Samples were cooled to ambient temperature, and decolorized by adding carefully and slowly 1 mL of 70% H_2O_2 to avoid excess bubbling. The contents were quantitatively transferred to 15 mL graduated plastic tubes (Sarstedt, Newton, MA) and the volumes were then adjusted to 5 mL with distilled water. $C_{15}H_{32}B_{10}O_6$, which was insoluble in H_2SO_4, was dissolved in 2.5 mL of 90% methanol and an equal volume of 2N NaOH. Samples were heated in a mineral oil bath at 100°C for approximately one hour until the methanol was evaporated and then brought up to 5 mL with water to replace the methanol that had evaporated. $[C_2H_5)_3NH]_2 B_{12}H_{12}$ and $Cs_2B_{12}H_{11}SH\cdot H_2O$ were placed directly in 5 mL of 2N NaOH and heated at 100°C for one hour. Prior to DCP-AES analysis all samples that had been solubilized in NaOH were diluted at least tenfold with distilled water so that the final concentration of NaOH was no greater than 0.2N. Higher concentrations of NaOH produced high background readings. Samples were read against boric acid standards as well as the compound itself.

Results and Discussion

Direct Current Plasma Atomic Emission Spectroscopy

The level of agreement between the amount of boron added in the form of H_3BO_3 to varying amounts of liver and the amount of elemental boron detected by means of DCP-AES is summarized in Table I.

Microgram quantities of boron were measured with minimal interference at concentrations of up to 25 μg boron per ml (25 ppm) in tissue digests containing up to 500 mg of liver, and similar amounts of muscle, blood and tumor. In those tissues

Table I. Detection of Boron in the Form of Boric Acid in Liver.

boron (μg) added	Boron detected (μg) in varying amounts of liver*			
	50 mg	100 mg	200 mg	500 mg
0	0.05 ± 0.02	0.01 ± 0.02	0.06 ± 0.01	0.03 ± 0.01
1	1.03 ± 0.04	1.07 ± 0.19	0.89 ± 0.02	1.25 ± 0.07
5	4.73 ± 0.06	5.10 ± 0.17	5.00 ± 0.10	4.67 ± 0.06
10	10.16 ± 0.17	10.37 ± 0.80	9.93 ± 0.76	10.06 ± 0.23
15	15.53 ± 1.05	14.50 ± 0.96	14.87 ± 0.25	15.63 ± 0.38
25	26.20 ± 0.53	23.57 ± 0.90	25.23 ± 0.31	25.27 ± 0.57
50	51.67 ± 2.02	48.23 ± 1.60	46.63 ± 0.55	52.00 ± 2.04

*Values are reported as the mean of three replicate samples ± standard deviation.

samples weighing >1000 mg and containing >5.0 μg boron/mL there was a reduction in the amount of boron detected compared with the predicted value based on the amount of boron that was added. Since the majority of normal tissue samples to be analyzed would be expected to contain <50 μg boron/mL, a slight loss in sensitivity for those with >50 μg boron/mL would be of great significance. Furthermore, those samples containing >50 μg boron/mL can be diluted with water in order to obtain more accurate analytical results. Since many of the compounds that will be screened as potential agents for BNCT contain either polyhedral borane anions or carboranes, it was important to determine whether these boron clusters could be measured with similar sensitivity, precision and accuracy as boric acid standards. For this purpose, we have compared $[(C_2H_5)_3NH]_2 B_{12}H_{12}$, $Cs_2 B_{12}H_{11}SH \cdot H_2O$, $C_{15}H_{32}B_{10}O_6$ with H_3BO_3 standards. The results are tabulated in Table II and show that this analytical method is applicable to a variety of compounds with different chemical structures, including boron-containing clusters with a precision of < ± 5% deviation from the mean.

Table II. Detection of Different Boron Containing Compounds

boron added of μg compound	Boron detected (μg) with compound as standard*		
	$[(C_2H_5)_3NH]_2 B_{12}H_{12}$	$Cs_2B_{12}H_{11}SH \cdot H_2O$	$C_{15}H_{32}B_{10}O_6$
1.0	0.98 ± 0.04	0.98 ± 0.03	0.80 ± 0.02
2.0	2.04 ± 0.17	1.96 ± 0.13	1.90 ± 0.08
5.0	4.90 ± 0.19	4.86 ± 0.15	4.97 ± 0.20
10.0	9.88 ± 0.18	9.94 ± 0.15	10.00 ± 0.04

Some problems were noted with boron determinations of certain compounds, such as the ortho carborane $C_{15}H_{32}B_{10}O_6$, which was only soluble in methanol. These were obviated by dissolving the compound in methanol, adding 2 N NaOH, and then evaporating the methanol. Ease and safety of sample preparation is an important consideration for any analytical technique. The method that we have described utilizes a mixture of concentrated sulfuric acid and 70% H_2O_2 to solubilize tissues and cell samples without the need of high pressures and temperature. This method of solubilization avoids the explosive hazards of percholoric acid and the cumbersome use of nitric acid digestion with bombs. Furthermore, using our method, a large number of samples can be easily and safely processed in a short period of time. Previous reports have described the use of ICP-AES for boron determinations, and it has been suggested that this method is less subject to signal interference than DCP-AES[7]. Our experience, however, indicates that for biological samples, DCP-AES appears to be comparable to ICP-AES for the detection of boron, but that the ease of sample preparation may make DCP-AES the method of choice.

Acknowledgements

This work was supported by grant 5 RO1 CA 41288 and CA 53896 from the National Cancer Institute and grant DE-FG02-90ER60972 and contract DE-AC02-76CH00616 from the Department of Energy.

References

1. R.F. Barth, A.H. Soloway, R.G. Fairchild: Boron neutron capture therapy of cancer, Cancer Res 50, 1061-1070 (1990).

2. A.H. Soloway, J.R. Messer, Determination of Hydrolytically-stable boron hydrides in biological materials, Anal Chem 36, 433-434, (1964).

3. K. Yoshino, M. Okamoto, H. Kakihan, T. Nakanishi, M. Ichihashi, Y. Mishima: Spectrophotometric determination of trace boron in biological materials after alkali fusion decomposition. Anal Chem 56, 838-842, (1984).

4. J.W. Mair, H.G. Day: Curcumin method for spectrophotometric determination of boron extracted from radio frequency ashed animal tissues using 2-ethyl-1,3-hexanediol, Anal Chem, 44, 2015-2017, (1972).

5. S.R. Tamat, D.E. Moore, B. Allen: Determination of boron in biological tissues by inductively coupled plasma atomic emission spectrometry, Anal Chem 59, 2161-2164, (1987).

6. W.F. Bauer, D.A. Johnson, S.M. Steele, K. Messick, D.L. Miller, W.A. Propp: Gross boron determination in biological samples by inductively coupled plasma atomic emission spectroscopy, Stralenther Onkol 165, 176-179, (1989).

7. D.L. Mann, Analysis of boron in contaminated shrimp by inductively coupled plasma spectroscopy, Spectroscopy 3, 37-39, (1988).

8. M. Abe, K. Amano, K. Kitamura, J. Tateishi, H. Hatanaka: Boron distribution analysis by alpha-autoradiography, J Nucl Med 27, 677-684, (1986).

9. R.F. Barth, D.M. Adams, A.H. Soloway, E.B. Mechetner, F. Alam, and A.K.M. Anisuzzaman, Determination of boron in tissues and cells using direct-current plasma atomic emission spectroscopy. Anal Chem. 63, 4, 890-893, (1991).

RAPID SPECTROPHOTOMETRIC DETERMINATION OF BORON IN BIOLOGICAL TISSUE

WITH ALKALI FUSION DECOMPOSITION

K.Yoshino[1], C.Nishio[1], E.Ubukata[1], T.Maruyama[1], Y.Mori[1],
Y.Mishima[2], C.Honda[2], M.Shiono[2], N.Wadabayashi[2],
M.Ichihashi[2], T.Kobayashi[3], and K.Kanda[3]

[1]Department of Chemistry, Faculty of Science, Shinshu
University, Asahi, Matsumoto, 390, Japan
[2]Department of Dermatology, Kobe University School of
Medicine, Kusunoki-cyo, Cyuo-ku, Kobe 650, Japan
[3]Research Reactor Institute, Kyoto University, Kumatori-
cyo, Sennan-gun, Osaka, Japan

INTRODUCTION

During our clinical applications of neutron capture therapy (NCT),
after administration of ^{10}B-p-Boronophenylalanine (BPA), ^{10}B concentration in the melanoma and the skin near the melanoma are determined by the
prompt γ method. From the data obtained, it is possible to calculate
the boron concentration in melanoma during neutron irradiation, and irradiation time was determined. If the prompt γ method is not available,
it is difficult to estimate the concentration in melanoma at the time of
the irradiation.

However, if we could establish the time course of tumor/blood boron
concentration ratio after administration of BPA and if we knew the time
course of the boron concentration in blood before neutron irradiation at
a NCT treatment, we could estimate the boron concentration in tumor
during neutron irradiation. For success of this project, it is necessary
to be able to quickly determine the boron concentration in blood.

One of the fastest methods is acid decomposition with ICP-AES determination as developed by Tamat et al.[2]. In this method, samples are
decomposed with H_2O_2 and $HClO_4$ at 75°C for 1 hour. Kaczmarczyk et al.[3]
also used H_2O_2 for decomposition of tissue, and boron was determined by a
spectrophotometric method using dianthrimide dye. Alkali fusion is
another rapid decomposition procedure[4,5]. It takes about 10 minutes for
100mg sample. But, since alkali is used, the solution is not suitable
for ICP measurements. Therefore, we have used a spectrophotometric
method using methylene blue. This method does not require any special
equipment.

EXPERIMENTAL

Sample tissue, 0.1g, was placed in a platinum crucible, and 0.25mL
of 1.6N NaOH solution and 0.5mL of 53mg/5mL Na_2CO_3 solution were added.
The solution was evaporated to dryness on a hot plate with an infrared
lamp. After adding 0.4947g of Na_2CO_3 powder to the crucible, alkali fusion was carried out. After dissolving the alkali with 3.5mL of 4N sul-

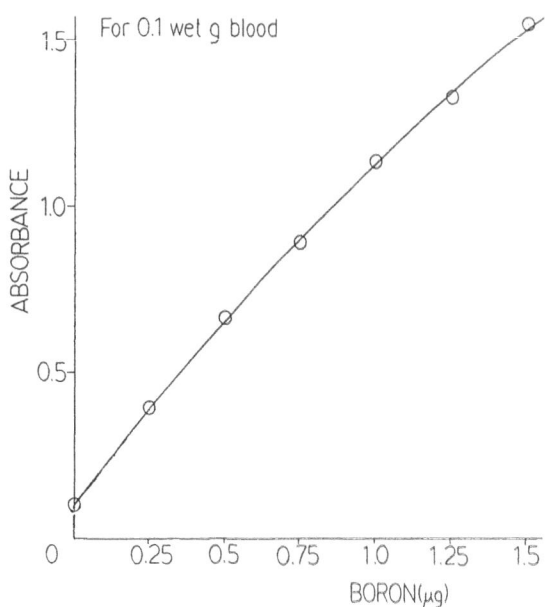

Figure 1 Calibration curve for assay of boron by methylene blue method. The curve was fitted to the equation, $ABS = an^2 + bn + c$, where ABS=absorbance, n=boron amount, a,b, and c are constants.

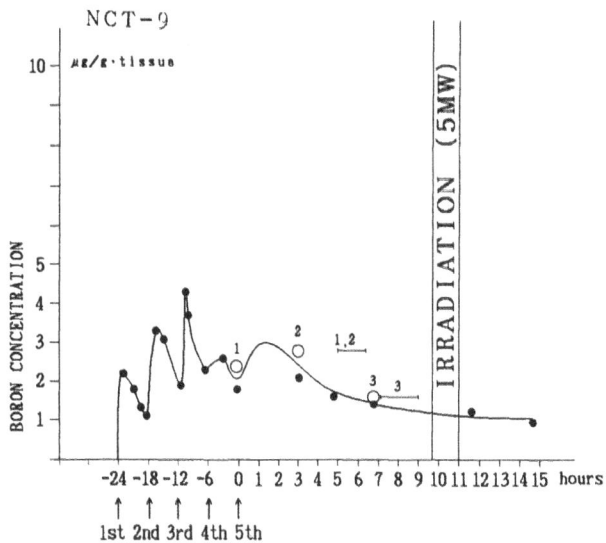

Injections of BPA-fuctose complex
(250mg BPA/Kg Body Weight)

Figure 2 A typical example of the rapid determination of boron in blood during the NCT performed on 19 November 1990 in Kyoto University Research Reactor. ○: results from this method, ●: results from the ICP-AES method which was carried out afterwards. Horizontal lines correspond to the time taken for completion of the method (the left edge is the beginning time and the right edge is the end time). The ^{10}B concentrations in the melanoma and the skin at 4 hours after the 5th injection were 9.8 and 7.5ppm respectively, and those at 6 hours after were 7.6 and 4.1ppm respectively. The results for the melanoma and the skin were obtained by the prompt γ method.

furic acid solution, the solution was transferred to a polypropyrene tube. Into the tube 1.5mL of 10% hydrofluoric acid (HF) solution was added, and H_2O was poured up to 10mL. After standing, 0.3mL of 0.01M methylene blue solution and 5mL of 1,2-dichloroethane were added. The tube was shaken by hand for one minute. To shorten the time for separation of water and organic phase, a centrifuge was used. The dichloroethane phase, which is below the water phase, was withdrawn by a syringe with a long needle, and transferred to another tube, which had 5mL of Ag_2SO_4 solution containig 1mg Ag^+. The mixed solution was shaken and separated with a centrifuge. The absorbance of the dichloroethane phase at 657nm was measured with a spectro-photometer.

RESULTS AND DISCUSSION

There are three points where the time can be reduced for more rapid determination of boron by the alkali fusion-methylene blue method. 1) Pre-treatment time for alkali fusion, 2) Time for conversion of boric acid to BF_4^-, 3) Waiting time to get two clear phases after extraction.

Pretreatment: Among the decomposition methods, alkali fusion seems to be the fastest method. Since alkali fusion is carried out at high temperature, there is some possibility for the boron to be lost by scattering. To solve the problem, we added alkaline solution and the solution was evaporated to dryness. To date the sample amount used was 1-2g, which took a relatively long time (overnight) for evaporation. To shorten time, the sample amount was reduced to 0.1g. Then, the evaporation time was reduced to 10 minutes. Alkali fusion time was also reduced to 10 minutes.

BF_4^- formation: In the methylene blue method, the BF_4^--methylene blue complex is extracted in the dichloroethane phase. After alkali fusion, the boron compound is converted to boric acid, and it must be then converted to BF_4^- by adding HF solution. It took a relatively long time for the conversion as reported by Isozaki et al.[6]. We have investigated the effect of the reaction temperature. Blood, 0.1g, was decomposed with and without 0.5 μg boron, and the methylene blue procedure was carried out. At 24°C, the absorbance for 0.5 μg become constant after 20 minutes standing, while at 35°C the absorbance become constant after 10 minutes standing, Thus, we could reduce the time for BF_4^- formation by warming the reaction solution.

Separation of the two phases; After extraction, the water and dichloroethane phases should be separated completely. However after shaking it took a considerable time to get clear phases. To solve the problem, we have used a centrifuge. One minute is enough for clear phases to be obtained.

The calibration curve was obtained by adding known amounts of boron as boric acid to 0.1g blood in the crucibles and carrying out the same procedure as that for the sample determination. A typical example is shown in Fig. 1.

The detection limit of this method for 0.1g blood was 0.15μg. The amount corresponds to $4\delta_{n-1}$, where δ_{n-1} is the standard deviation of the reagent blank, (n=5). The percent standard deviation for the four times measurements of the blood sample with 5ppm boron as boric acid was less than 2%.

By the modified procedure, we could achieve a measurement of the boron concentration in blood within 1-1.5hr. One of the examples of the application of the method to NCT is shown in Fig. 2.

REFERENCES

1. T.Kobayashi, K.Kanda, Y.Mishima: In situ measurement on ^{10}B

concentrations and absorbed dose estimations in human malignant melanoma treated by BNCT. Strahlenther. Onkol. 165 (1989), 104-106.

2. S.R.Tamat, D.E.Moore, B.J. Allen: Determination of boron in biological tissues by inductively coupled plasma atomic emission spectrometry. Anal. Chem. 59 (1987), 2161-2163.

3. A.Kaczmarczyk, J.R.Messer, C.E.Pierce: Rapid Method for Determination of Boron in Biological Materials. Anal. Chem. 43 (1971), 271-272.

4. K.Yoshino, M.Okamoto, H.Kakihana, T.Nakanishi, M.Ichihashi, Y.Mishima: Spectrophotometric determination of trace boron in biological materials after alkali fusion decomposition. Anal. Chem. 56 (1984), 839-842.

5. K.Yoshino, M.Okamoto, H.Kakihana, Y.Mori, Y.Mishima, M.Ichihashi, M.Tsuji, T.Nakanishi: Chemical assay of boron and its distribution in melanoma-bearing subjects. in: Neutron Capture Therapy, Proceedings of the second International Symposium on Neutron Capture Therapy. H. Hatanaka, ed. Nishimura Co., Ltd., Niigata, (1986), 291-302.

6. S.Utsumi, S.Ito, A.Isozaki: Extraction-spectrophotometric determination of trace boron (in Japanese). Nippon Kagaku Zasshi, 86 (1965), 921-925.

PHANTOM EXPERIMENT AND CALCULATION FOR IN VIVO ^{10}B ANALYSIS

BY PROMPT GAMMA-RAY SPECTROSCOPY AT THE MUSASHI REACTOR

Tetsuo Matsumoto and Otohiko Aizawa

Atomic Energy Research Laboratory, Musashi Institute of Technology
Ozenji 971, Asao-ku, Kawasaki-shi, 215 Japan

INTRODUCTION

In boron neutron capture therapy (BNCT), the tumor dose depends on ^{10}B concentration in tumor. Rapid assay of ^{10}B concentration in tissue is desirable so that dose to tumor and duration of irradiation time can be calculated before treatment. The most desirable method for practical application to patients is to determine ^{10}B concentrations in vivo. Prompt γ-ray facilities for in vitro ^{10}B analysis for BNCT have been developed by Kyoto University Reactor, Brookhaven National Laboratory and ourselves. The technique is based on detection of prompt γ-rays from the ^{10}B$(n,\alpha\gamma)^{7}$Li reaction. The 478 keV prompt γ-rays are emitted from the excited state of ^{7}Li in 93.5 % of the decays. This method is independent of the chemical form of boron and has the advantage of being nondestructive. This technique is employed for in vivo ^{10}B analysis as reported in this paper. We have examined the possibility of in vivo ^{10}B analysis using phantom experiments and calculations.

EXPERIMENTS

Figure 1 shows the positions of the phantom and detector. A relatively pure thermal neutron beam was extracted from the reactor core using a mono-crystal silicon filter. The phantom was made of polyethylene, 10 cm diameter x 10 cm long, with a simulated tumor located near the surface. ^{10}B concentrations in an actual tumor can be estimated from calibration curves generated by phantom experiments. Such calibration curves experimentally determined for simulated tumors with different volumes. Experiments to investigate ^{10}B distributions in a tumor and to distingush tumor with ^{10}B from normal tissue without ^{10}B were also carried out. The tumor region was divided into three concentric sections

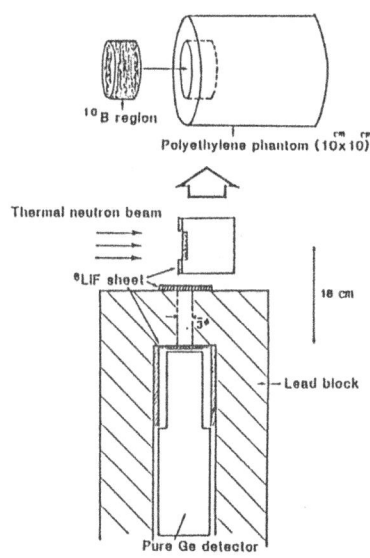

Fig.1 Experimental arrangement

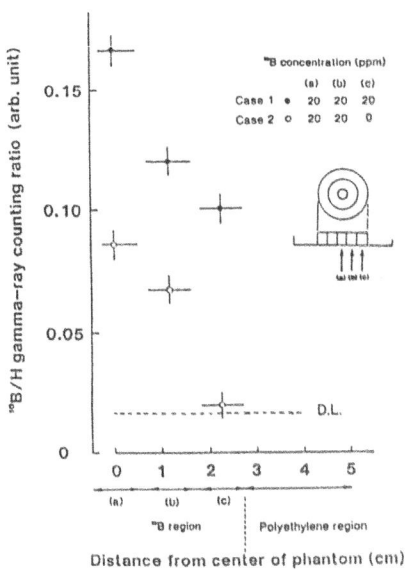

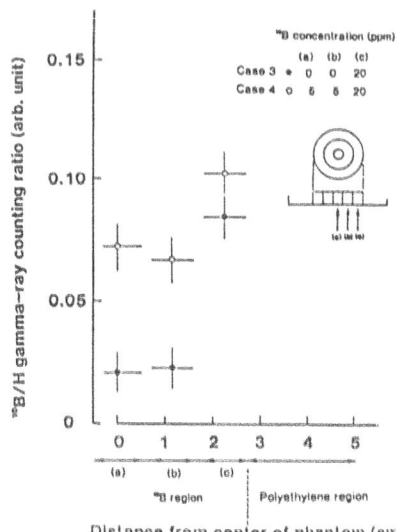

Fig. 2 Experimental conditions (cases 1,2,3 and 4) to distingush tumor with ^{10}B from normal tissue without and investigation results to distingush the ^{10}B distribution by ^{10}B/H γ-ray counting ratios.

and was irradiated by a thermal neutron beam collimated to 10 mm diameter (Fig. 2(a,b)). Four experimental conditions with various combination of the ^{10}B concentration were considered.

CALCULATIONS

A two-dimensional discrete ordinate transport code, DOT3.5, was employed for calculations of neutron flux distributions in a phantom. Figure 3 shows the analytical model to calculate the number of incidental γ-rays entering a detector. At first, we calculated the reaction rate in a small volume dV around a point X dependent on the local thermal neutron flux obtained by the DOT code. Then we estimated the number of γ-rays entering the detector by using below equation (1). The total γ-rays can be obtained by integrating over X.

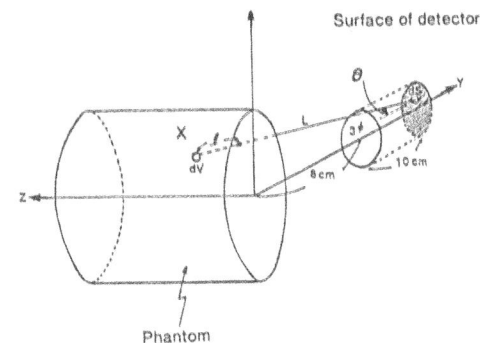

Fig. 2 Calculation model

$$N(X) = \Sigma a \quad \phi \ (X) \ e^{- K \ell} \ \frac{\cos \theta}{4 \pi L^2} \ dV \ dS \qquad (1)$$

Where, N(X) is the number of incidental γ-rays entering a detector, Σa are the macroscopic cross sections of ^{10}B(n,αγ)^{7}Li or ^{1}H(n,γ)^{2}H reactions (cm^{-1}), K is the attenuation coefficient of γ-rays in the phantom (cm^{-1}), ℓ is the γ-ray flight path in the phantom (cm), L is the distance between a small volume dV around a point X in the phantom and a small area dS on the surface of the detector (cm), θ is the angle between the Y axis and the γ-ray flight path (degrees).

RESULTS AND DISCUSSIONS

The calibration curves for various tumor sizes showed good linearity between the ^{10}B concentration and count rate normalized to the irradiated neutron fluence (^{10}B/H γ-ray counting ratio). We can estimate the ^{10}B concentration in the tumors by using these calibration curves depending on the tumor volume before actual treatment. A 10 ppm ^{10}B concentration of tumor size (30 mm diameter x 10 mm thick) can be determined to an accuracy of 8 % in counting time of 600 sec.

Figure 2a shows the results of the investigation to distingush the ^{10}B distributions for cases 1 and 2. The ^{10}B/H counting ratios showed different values although each sections contained same ^{10}B concentration of 20 ppm. This is because of interference between the divided sections. It was impossible to usefully estimate the ^{10}B distributions in a tumor. However, in the case of 2 (only c section without ^{10}B), the ^{10}B/H γ-ray counting ratio in c section showed a smaller value than those of sections a and b with ^{10}B. Figure 2b also shows the results for cases 3 and 4. In case 3, the ^{10}B/H γ-ray counting ratio in c section was clearly different from those of sections a and b, in contrast to the results of case 4 in which a small difference in the ^{10}B/H γ-ray counting ratios was observed. From these results, it appears that it is possible to distingush a tumor with ^{10}B from normal tissue without ^{10}B.

Thermal neutron flux distributions in the phantom with simulated tumor showed good agreement between experiment and calculation. Figure 4 shows the comparison of calculations with experimental results for ^{10}B/H γ-ray counting ratios. These were obtained at various diameters of simulated tumor containing 20 ppm of ^{10}B. The thickness of a tumor was chosen at 5 or 10 mm. The size of neutron beam was fixed at the same diameter as that of the tumor. The calculation results were in good agreement with the experiments. From these results, it seems that it is possible to estimate the ^{10}B concentration in a tumor by employing present methods. But the accuracy depends on the volume size, shape and position of tumor. The difference between the calculation and the experiment in the detector efficiency amounts to about 10 % within the tumor volume of 15

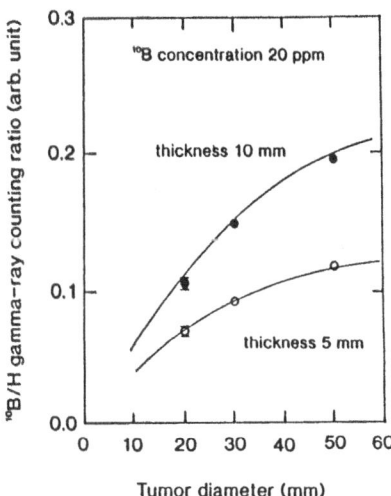

Fig. 4 ^{10}B/H γ-ray counting ratios

cm^3. Therefore, to obtain successful results, one has to obtain accuarte information about volume size, shape and position of a tumor and ^{10}B and hydrogen atoms in the tumor or normal tissue must be assumed to be uniformly distributed.

CONCLUSION

We conclude that it is possible to determine ^{10}B concentrations in vivo within acceptable accuracy (less 10 %) by a combination of phantom experiments and calculations.

DETERMINATION OF BORON CONCENTRATION IN TISSUES BY MEANS OF ALPHA AUTORADIOGRAPHY

Jeffrey E. Woollard[1], Yirun Jiang[1], James F. Curran[1], Thomas E. Blue[1], and Rolf F. Barth[2]

[1]Nuclear Engineering Program and [2]Department of Pathology, The Ohio State University, Columbus, Ohio 43210, U.S.A.

Introduction

The accurate measurement of total boron content in biological samples with a sensitivity in the ppm range is essential for evaluating the potential usefulness of various tumor localizing boron-containing compounds for Boron Neutron Capture Therapy (BNCT)[1]. A group of analytical procedures for boron quantitation are those involving nuclear methods. These include the detection of alpha particles resulting from the $^{10}B(n,\alpha,\gamma)^{7}Li$ reaction by means of alpha track autoradiography[2,3] and the measurement of gamma photons, by means of prompt gamma analysis[4]. The purpose of the present study was to develop alpha track autoradiography for microdistribution studies. It utilizes a solid state nuclear track detector (SSNTD), CR-39, which is composed of a polycarbonate resin, to record the charged products of the $^{10}B(n, \alpha)^{7}Li$ reaction.

Experimental Procedure

The first step in this technique was to construct an acrylic/tissue section/CR-39 sandwich. The tissue section which was analyzed was from a Fischer rat which was implanted intracerebrally with a D74 glioma[5]. The rat was killed 4 hours after the injection of 115 mg of boronophenylalanine (BPA).HCl in a solution which was made by diluting 115 mg of BPA.HCl in 3 mL of H_2O and adjusting the pH of the solution to 10. The brain was removed and frozen at $-80^{\circ}C$. The frozen brain was cut into 10 μm thick sections at 250 μm intervals. These sections were placed on 75 x 25 mm clear acrylic slides and air dried. Boron-coated tape pointers were then affixed to the slides with the ^{10}B side facing up. These pointers provided a means for aligning the tissue section images and the track density information. Next, 75 x 25 mm pieces of CR-39 were placed on top of the tissues and secured to the acrylic slides with slide tape. The acrylic/tissue section/CR-39 sandwiches were then irradiated in the thermal column of The Ohio State University Research Reactor (OSURR) to a fluence of 8×10^{11} neutrons/cm^2. A set of boron in Tissue Equivalent Liquid (TEL) standards were irradiated as liquids in wells in a paraffin gasket on a CR-39 slide along with the acrylic/tissue setion/CR-39 sandwiches. Details of our experimental procedure for analyzing liquid samples, such as the boron standards, are given in Ref. 6. Following irradiation, the acrylic and CR-39 slides which were taped together were separated and the boron tape alignment marks were covered with a thin layer of silicon sealant. This protected the pointers during the staining procedure. The tissue sections on the acrylic were then stained with hematoxylin and eosin (H&E) and coverslipped. Independently of this, the CR-39 slides, from both the boron standards and the tissues section, were etched in a 6.25 N NaOH solution at 70°C for 100 minutes using a high temperature etch bath.

Analysis

The tissue assay technique resulted in CR-39 slides containing spatial track density information and acrylic slides upon which tissue sections were mounted. The acrylic and CR-39 slides were analyzed separately. Chemical etching of the CR-39 revealed tracks that were visible with a light microscope. The track density (the number of tracks per field of view of the microscope) on the detector surface was related to the ^{10}B concentration of the sample that was on the detector. The SSNTD's were analyzed using our SARA (SSNTD Automatic Readout and Analysis) system for track counting. The SARA system included a contrast based automatic focusing system to maintain focus while counting large areas. A black and white video camera mounted on an American Optical Epistar industrial microscope provided the image signal for the SARA system. The tracks on the CR-39 detectors were counted in 80 x 80 μm fields along lines across the detectors, using the SARA system with a 100x microscope objective. The lines scanned on the CR-39 were chosen to correspond to lines across the tissue sections which pass through tumor and normal tissue. Tissue section imaging was carried out using a Macintosh Imaging System (MIS). This system consists of an Apple Macintosh II microcomputer with 8 megabytes of RAM, a Data Translation Quick Capture video frame grabber which resides inside the Macintosh II, a 140 megabyte hard disk for image storage, and a JVC TK-870U RGB color video camera. In order to image tissue sections, the black and white video camera, which provided input to the SARA system, was replaced with the RGB color video camera to provide separate red, green and blue video signals to the MIS system. The Macintosh controlled the stage as it stepped from frame to frame, and captured images until entire tissue sections were imaged. Alignment between the tissue images and the boron concentrations were established using the boron tape alignment marks. By placing the alignment marks on the image slides and on the corresponding CR-39 at identical coordinate locations of the stage controller when imaging and counting tracks, a common coordinate system was established. All counting and imaging were done in relation to the common coordinate system. Before the track density data was combined with its corresponding image, the track densities were converted to ^{10}B concentrations using the standard curve which is shown in Figure 1. This standard curve was obtained by analyzing the boron in TEL standards which were irradiated along with the tissue sections.

Results and Discussion

The tissue sections described above were analyzed as a realistic, preliminary test of our technique. The results from a representative section are shown in Figure 2. Four scan lines were analyzed across this tissue section. The straight horizontal lines indicate where the track density information was measured, and serve as the abscissas for the graphs of boron concentration. The ordinates of the graphs are the boron concentration. The dark region in the upper left corner of the section is the tumor. High track densities, and therefore high ^{10}B concentrations, were seen throughout the section. Possible explanations for the nearly uniform spatial ^{10}B concentrations across the section include non-selective delivery of the BPA to the tumor and/or high blood ^{10}B concentrations. Nevertheless, the technique showed good alignment and spatial resolution and that it potentially can be used to determine where boron containing compounds localize within a tumor. Space does not permit a discussion of spatial resolution in this paper. For a discussion of spatial resolution, especially its relationship with boron concentration, as well as discussions of threshold, sensitivity, and dynamic range the interested reader is referred to Ref 7.

The technique also can be used to determine ^{10}B concentrations in other types of tissues or across whole body cross sections in small rodents (i.e. mice or rats). Coupling this

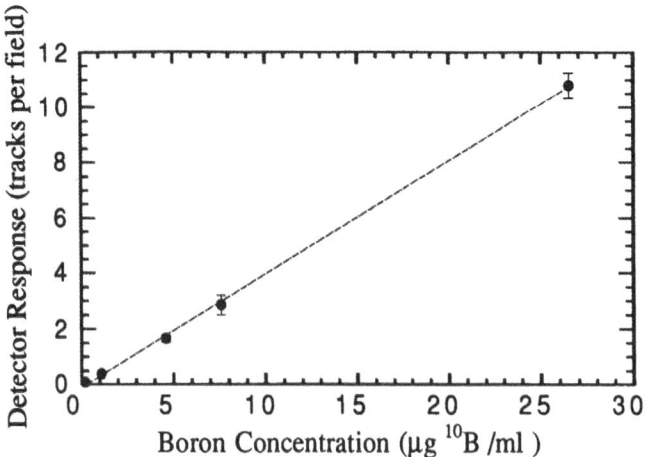

Figure 1.   Standards curve resulting from the analysis of the boron TEL standards.

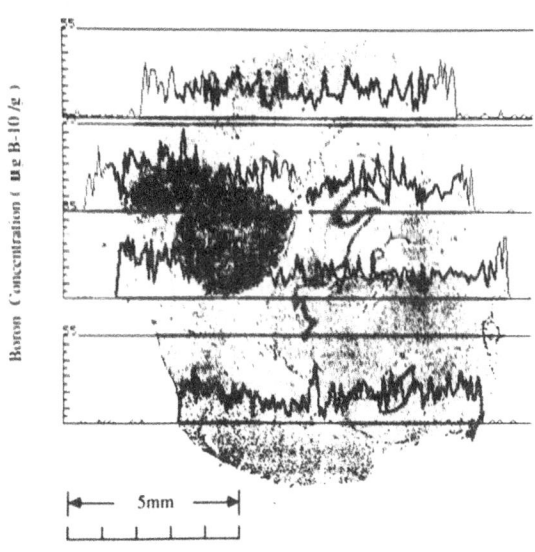

Figure 2.   A digital image of a tissue section with boron concentration distributions measured on four lines across the section.

technique with chemical analytical methods should permit the determination of ^{10}B concentrations in blood, tumor and normal tissues. Knowledge of their distributions is fundamental for the evaluation of ^{10}B delivery agents being developed for use in BNCT. Cellular uptake and localization on the other hand, which is very important in evaluating a boron compound's potential usefulness as a delivery system for BNCT, can best be detected by electron spectroscopic imaging and electron energy loss spectroscopy, as has been recently described by us[8], or by means of ion microscopy, as reported by Ausserer et al.[9]. It is now apparent that chemical analytical methods based on either inductively coupled plasma (ICP) or direct current plasma-atomic emission spectroscopy (DCP-AES)[10] will supplant nuclear techniques for routine determinations, if for no other reason than that the latter require either nuclear reactors of isotopic neutron sources, which are not readily available except at the most specialized centers. Nuclear techniques, on the other hand, should provide information as to the uptake in histologic sections, where spatial considerations are of paramount importance. Further refinements in alpha track autoradiography should permit a high degree of spatial resolution and thereby extend the usefulness of this technique.

Acknowledgements

This work was supported by the National Cancer Institute and grant DE-FG02-90ER60972 and contract DE-AC02-76CH00616 from the Department of Energy.

References

1. R.F. Barth, A.H. Soloway, R.G. Fairchild: Boron Neutron Capture Therapy of Cancer, Cancer Res. 50, 1061-1070 (1990).
2. M. Abe, K. Amano, K. Kitamura, J. Tateishi, H. Hatanaka: Boron Distribution Analysis by Alpha-Autoradiography, J. Nucl. Med. 27, 677-684 (1986).
3. D. Gabel, H. Holstein, B. Larsson, L. Gille, G. Erikson, D. Sacker, P. Som and R. G. Fairchild: Quantitative Neutron Capture Radiography for Studying the Biodistribution of Tumor-seeking Boron-containing Compounds, Cancer Res. 47, 5451-5456 (1987).
4. R.G. Fairchild, D. Gabel, B.H. Laster, D. Greenberg, W. Kiszenick, P.F. Micca: Microanalytical Techniques for Boron Analysis Using the ^{10}B(n, α)^{7}Li reaction, Med. Phys. 13, 50-56 (1986).
5. N.R. Clendenon, R.F. Barth, W.A. Gordon, J.H. Goodman, F. Alam, A.E. Staubus, C.P. Boesel, A.J. Yates, M.L. Moeschberger, R.G. Fairchild, J.A. Kalef-Ezra: Boron Neutron Capture Therapy of a Rat Glioma, Neurosurgery 26, 47-55 (1990).
6. J.E. Woollard, T.E. Blue, J.F. Curran, T.F. Mengers, R.F. Barth: An Alpha Autoradiographic Technique for Determination of ^{10}B Concentrations in Blood and Tissue. Nucl. Instr. and Meth. A 299, 600-605 (1990).
7. J.E. Woollard, T.E. Blue, J.F. Curran, M. C. Dobelbower, H. R. Busby: An Alpha Autoradiographic Technique for Spatial Quantification of Boron-10 Concentrations in Tissue, Nucl. Sci.and Eng.(in press).
8. M. Bendayan, R.F. Barth, D. Gingras, I. Londono, P.T. Robinson, F. Alam, D.M. Adams, L. Mattiazzi: Electron Spectroscopic Imaging for High Resolution Immunocytochemistry: Use of Boronated Protein A, J. Histochem Cytochem 37, 573-580 (1989).
9 . W.A. Ausserer, Y.C. Ling, S. Chandra, G.H. Morrison: Quantitative Imaging of Boron, Calcium, Magnesium, Potassium, and Sodium Distributions in Cultured Cells With Ion Microscopy, Anal. Chem. 61, 2690-2695 (1989).
10. R.F. Barth, D.M. Adams, A.H. Soloway, E.B. Mechetner, F. Alam and A.K.M. Anisuzzaman: Determination of Boron in Tissues and Cells Using Direct-Current Plasma Atomic Emission Spectroscopy, Anal. Chem. 63, 4 (1991).

A NEW BORON MRI METHOD FOR IMAGING BNCT AGENTS IN VIVO

G. W. Kabalka[*], Q. C. Cheng[*], P. Bendel[‡], D. N. Slatkin[∅], and P. L. Micca[∅]

[*]University of Tennessee Biomedical Imaging Center
Knoxville, TN 37996-1600, USA
[‡]Weizmann Institute of Science
Rehovot 76100, Israel
[∅]Brookhaven National Laboratory
Upton, New York 11973, USA

INTRODUCTION

In recent years, efforts have been made to develop boron-11 magnetic resonance imaging (MRI) and magnetic resonance spectroscopy (MRS) for use in boron neutron capture therapy (BNCT)[1-3] for noninvasive quantification and localization of BNCT agents such as the sodium salt of the closodecaboranyl mercaptide anion $B_{12}H_{11}SH^{-2}$ (BSH) and its dimer $B_{24}H_{22}S_2^{-4}$ (BSSB).[4] Generation of MR images for fast relaxing nuclei, such as boron-10 and boron-11, is often hampered by the fact that the transverse relaxation times (T_2) are considerably shorter than the available time-to-echo (TE). The minimal TE achievable in MR imaging is limited by the need to apply phase-encoding and dephasing/rephasing read-out gradients which have finite rise times imposed by the hardware limitations. Currently, echo times of 2.5 ms are attainable using conventional spin-warp imaging techniques and it may be possible to shorten TE to approximately 1 ms by reducing the resolution requirements. However, the transverse relaxation rate of the BNCT species is so short that even after 1 ms most of the signal has already decayed, resulting in an unacceptably low signal.

An alternate imaging method has been developed for boron nuclei and other elements with very short T_2 relaxation times.[1,5] The technique utilizes the FID, rather than the echo signal, but involves only phase-encoding of the signal without frequency encoding. The method was used to map the boron-11 distribution in an intact Fischer 344 rat infused with a therapeutic dose of a dimeric sulfhydryl dodecaborane agent which is currently used in boron-neutron-capture-therapy (BNCT)

EXPERIMENTAL

The MRI experiments were conducted using a Gyrex 2T, 90 cm bore, whole body MR unit (Elscint) operating at 26 MHz for

boron (81 MHz for hydrogen) and a home-built-six-turn
solenoidal radiofrequency coil of 10 cm diameter placed
horizontally along the y-axis, perpendicular to the long z-
axis of the magnet. Hydrogen survey images were obtained
using the standard body coil of the system.

The imaging protocol for the rat was described
previously[1]. For the image presented here, the phase encoding
period (between the end of the radiofrequency pulse and the
onset of data acquisition) was 180 μsec. 256 signal averages
were used at each of the 19 × 20 phase encoding steps, with a
repetition time of 36 msec, resulting in a total imaging time
of about 1 hour.

The animal used was a Fischer 344 male rat (Taconic
Farms, Germantown, New York). A 2 ml-capacity osmotic pump
was filled with a 48 mg/ml solution of $Na_4B_{24}H_{22}S_2$ (BSSB) with a
natural abundance (≈80 atom %) of [11]B. The pump was implanted
surgically[3,4] into the peritoneal cavity of a 260 g male
Fischer rat, which provided 224 μg B per gram body weight of
the rat. The rat was imaged about 25 hours after pump
removal. An image of the live rat was also taken three days
and one week post-infusion. All imaging experiments were
conducted at room temperature.

RESULTS

Figure 1 shows the hydrogen-1 survey image of the boron
infused rat (left) and the corresponding boron-11 image
(right). The superimposed rectangular region-of-interest
(ROI) corresponds to the same spatial extent (in the x-y
plane) in each image. The ROI are centered in the upper
abdominal region and roughly correspond to the liver which has
been shown to accumulate the BSSB agent.

The above results were obtained 25 hours after infusion
of the BNCT agent was complete. The orientation of the animal

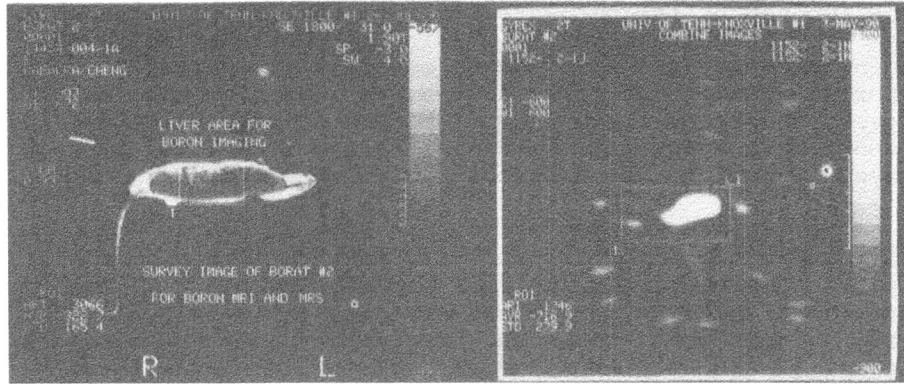

Fig. 1   Sagittal hydrogen-1 NMR survey image of the rat
          using a body coil with the boron-11 solenoid
          coil in place (left). [The region of interest
          (ROI) is marked.] Sagittal boron-11 NMR image
          of the rat 25 hours after infusion of the BNCT
          agent (right). [The same ROI is marked by the
          rectangle.]

is with the head-tail axis along the y-direction and the ventral-dorsal axis along the x-direction. The in-plane linear resolution on the boron image is about 1 cm. The boron-11 distribution is not resolved along the third dimension, so that the signal intensities represent integration along the z-axis, projected onto the x-y plane. The experiment was repeated three and six days later; no boron-11 image could be obtained in either instance.

DISCUSSION

The results demonstrate that the newly developed MRI technique[1,5] can be used to detect boron neutron capture agents _in vivo_. Since the technique can be used to monitor boron accumulation and clearance it could assist in establishing the optimum timing and duration of neutron irradiation following the infusion of a boron containing drug for BNCT.[6,7]

ACKNOWLEDGEMENTS

We thank the Department of Energy for support.

REFERENCES

1. P. Bendel, M. Davis, E. Berman, G. W. Kabalka, A method for imaging nuclei with short T_2 relaxation and its application to Boron-11 MR imaging of a BNCT agent in an intact rat. J. Magn. Res. 88:369-375 (1990).
2. T. L. Richards, K. M. Bradshaw, D. M. Freeman, C. H. Sotak, P. R. Gavin, Imaging with [11]B of intact tissues using magnetic resonance gradient echos. Strahlenther. Onkol. 165:179-183 (1989).
3. G. W. Kabalka, M. Davis, P. Bendel, Boron-11 MRI and MRS of intact animals infused with a boron neutron capture agent. Magn. Reson. Med. 8:231-237 (1988).
4. D. N. Slatkin, P. L. Micca, A. Forman, D. Gabel, L. Welopolski, R. Fairchild, Boron uptake in melanoma, cerebrum and blood from $Na_2B_{12}H_{11}SH$ and $Na_4B_{24}H_{22}S_2$ administered to mice. Biochem. Pharmacol. 35:1771-1776 (1986).
5. D. G. Cory, W. S. Veeman, Applications of line narrowing to 1-H NMR imaging of solids. J. Magn. Reson. 84:392-297 (1989).
6. G. W. Kabalka, P. Bendel, M. Davis, D. N. Slatkin, P. L. Micca, Boron-11 magnetic resonance and spectroscopy, tools for investigating pharmokinetics for boron neutron capture therapy, in "Clinical Aspects of Neutron Capture Therapy", R. G. Fairchild, V. P. Bond, and A. D. Woodhead, eds., Plenum Press, 243-249 (1989).
7. D. N. Slatkin, D. D. Joel, R. G. Fairchild, P. L. Micca, M. M. Nawrocky, B. H. Laster, J. A. Coderre, G. C. Finkel, C. E. Poletti, W. H. Sweet, Distributions of Sulfhydrylborane monomer and dimer in rodents and humans: boron neutron capture therapy of melanoma and glioma in boronated rodents, in "Clinical Aspects of Neutron Capture Therapy", R. G. Fairchild, V. P. Bond, and A. D. Woodhead, eds., Plenum Press, 179-191 (1989).

IN VIVO PHARMACOKINETIC EVALUATION OF BORON COMPOUNDS

USING MAGNETIC RESONANCE SPECTROSCOPY AND IMAGING

Kenneth M. Bradshaw,[1] Todd L. Richards,[2], and
Susan L. Kraft[3]

[1]Idaho National Engineering Laboratory, EG&G Idaho, Inc.,
Idaho Falls, ID 83415-3519
[2]Imaging Research Laboratory, University of Washington,
Seattle, WA 98195
[3]College of Veterinary Medicine, Washington State University,
Pullman, WA 99164-6610

INTRODUCTION

The success of Boron Neutron Capture Therapy (BNCT) will, in large
degree, depend upon knowing the kinetics of a boron compound and treating
when the optimum conditions have been reached. Before a potential boron
compound is administered to a human patient for treatment, the pharmacokinetics of the boron compound should be determined first with an animal
model and then with human studies. Until now, the accepted methods of
conducting pharmacokinetic studies have all been invasive. Magnetic
resonance (MR) spectroscopy and imaging is a new technology that has the
potential of measuring the concentration of selected nuclei in tissue
noninvasively. MR is presently being used to measure in-vivo concentration of chemical compounds containing ^{31}P, ^{19}F, and ^{23}Na.[1,2] The MR
techniques used to measure these compounds have been modified for boron,
but have not been used in conducting time studies.[3-5] The in-vivo MR
method proposed here provides a way to quantitate boron in tissue as a
function of time and location.

METHODS

All experiments were conducted on a GE Signa™, 1.5 Tesla, MR imaging
system that was modified to operate at the ^{11}B frequency of 20.5 Mhz.[6] For
the spectroscopy and chemical shift imaging (CSI) experiments described
herein, a 7-inch-diameter quadrature "birdcage" radiofrequency (RF) head
coil was developed.[7] The proton images for anatomical referencing were
taken with the resident clinical imaging head coil.

To observe the whole-head boron uptake and elimination, 1000 averages
of an ^{11}B free induction decay (FID) were obtained in two minutes. To
locate boron accumulation, CSI was performed with the following parameters: (1) spectral width of 10,000 Hz, (2) FID resolution of 256 points,
(3) in-plane resolution of 16x16 in eight slices, (4) repetition time of
80 msec, and (5) 10-20 averages per phase encode. A representation of the
pulse sequence using three-phase encoding gradients for the three-
dimensional CSI is shown in Figure 1. The resulting FID is sampled during
the A/D window. For a field of view of 24 cm, resolution of each voxel
(volume pixel) is 1.5x1.5x3.0 cm. The two-dimensional CSI uses only two
of the phase encoding gradients, resulting in an image with information in
only two dimensions over the entire volume. Scan time for the three-
dimensional CSI with 16 averages per phase encode was about 72 minutes.
The two-dimensional CSI is about eight times faster.

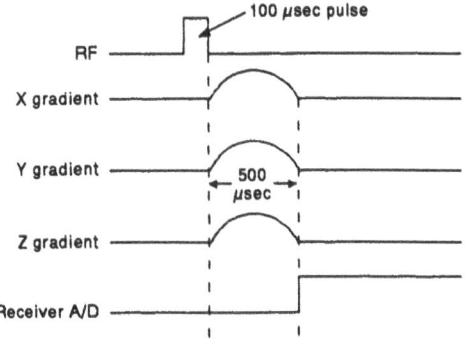

Figure 1

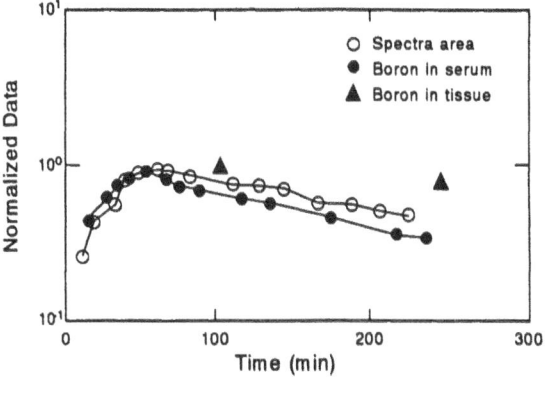

Figure 2

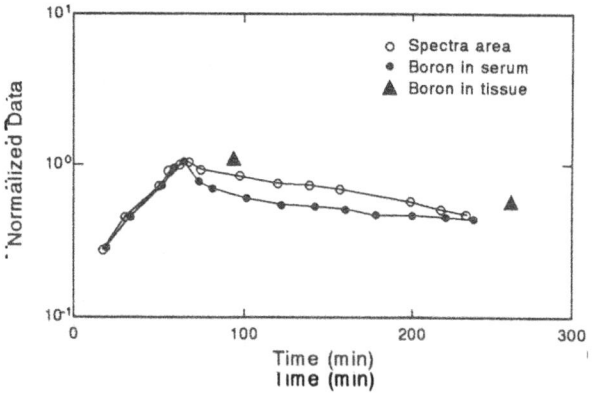

Figure 3   Boron spectroscopy for a 68-lb dog.

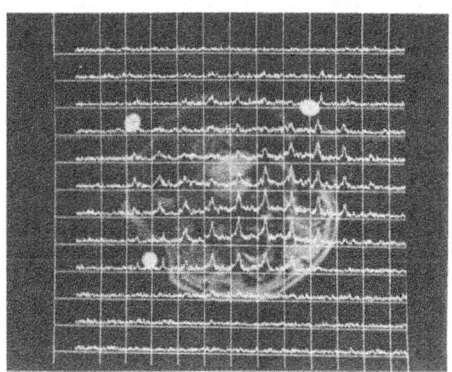

Figure 4   Three-dimensional, chemical-shift-imaging
data superimposed over proton image of
dog with coroid plexus papilloma.

Anesthesia is induced intravenously by an ultrashort-acting barbiturate and maintained by isoflurane (2%) gas anesthesia for the canine experiments. Borocaptate sodium ($Na_2B_{12}H_{11}SH$ or BSH) is administered intravenously over approximately 50 minutes into the saphenous or cephalic veins while the dog is positioned on the MR imaging patient table. The BSH compound is mixed by diluting 55 mg boron/kg into 11 ml/kg physiological saline solution. Whole-head spectroscopy acquisition was begun after ten minutes of BSH infusion. Spectra were acquired every ten minutes on uptake and every 20 minutes during elimination. CSI was obtained after a maximum in boron signal was observed. Blood and muscle biopsies (muscle from the thigh) were taken after each spectroscopy observation and were analyzed later by inductively coupled plasma-atomic emission spectroscopy (ICP-AES).

RESULTS

Figure 2 shows the pharmacokinetic data obtained from a 25-lb nontumor dog. The data for each parameter have been normalized to its maximum value. For reference, the maximum concentration for boron in serum was at 55 minutes (151.5 $\mu g/g$). The spectroscopy values are the results of an integration of each spectrum at that point in time. The maximum value for the boron spectra occurred at 61 minutes and are in arbitrary units. Tissue samples from the right rear thigh muscle were taken at 103 minutes (69.56 $\mu g/g$) and at 243 minutes (54.72 $\mu g/g$). The pharmacokinetic data obtained during the elimination phase from a 68-lb nontumor dog are displayed in Figure 3. The data are normalized to the maximum boron level in serum occurring at 63 minutes (245.9 $\mu g/g$) and the maximum boron signal occurring at 68 minutes. Tissue samples from the right rear thigh muscle were taken at 94 minutes (27.32 $\mu g/g$) and 260 minutes (15.4 $\mu g/g$).

Three-dimensional CSI scans were performed on three dogs with the results from a 53-lb dog with a coroid plexus papilloma shown in Figure 4. This three-dimensional CSI was begun about one hour after a 66-minute intravenous administration of BSH. The resulting data are superimposed over a proton image of the same 24-cm field of view. The three bright spots outside the dog's head are vials containing boric acid. These vials are used to align the CSI data to the proton image. Boric acid resonates 35 ppm downfield from BSH and is distinguishable in both the proton image and CSI data. Comparing the areas from the BSH spectra in Figure 4 reveals similar concentration between muscle and tumor, but a 10:1 tumor-to-brain boron-concentration ratio. With a known boric acid concentration, it should be possible to obtain absolute concentration of boron in tissue by comparing the boric acid spectra to the CSI spectra.[8]

DISCUSSION

The preliminary data shown in Figures 2 and 3 show a strong correlation during BSH uptake between the whole-head spectroscopy data and the serum analysis during uptake, but less correlation during the elimination phase, suggesting boron retention within the tissue. The whole-head spectroscopy signal contains contribution from both blood and tissue. No distinction can be made with boron MR between intracellular and extracellular boron in tissue at this time.

Even though the two-dimensional CSI scanning is much faster, the data in the three-dimensional CSI is more usable in obtaining pharmacokinetic information. The three-dimensional CSI of the 68-lb dog, even with the long time scan, showed a tumor-to-brain boron-concentration ratio for BSH comparable to the invasive studies that have an average ratio of 6:1. The scan time for the three-dimensional CSI has recently been reduced to 20 minutes, making it more useable to perform pharmacokinetic studies on the whole head.

In summary, we have shown that boron spectroscopy can yield reasonable pharmacokinetic information. Even with low spatial resolution, boron CSI can be used to image, *in-vivo*, the distribution of BSH in tissue. With a decrease in scan time, the three-dimensional CSI should be useful in observing the uptake of boron into different locations within the head.

REFERENCES

1. Tofts, P. S. and S. Wray, "A Critical Assessment of Methods of Measuring Metabolite Concentrations by NMR Spectroscopy," <u>NMR in Biomedicine 1:</u> 1 (1988).

2. Ra, J. B., et al., "An Algorithm for MR Imaging of the Short T2 Fraction of Sodium Using the FID Signal," <u>J. Comp. Asst. Tomo. 13:</u> 302-309 (March/April 1989).

3. Richards, T. L., et al., "Imaging With [11]B of Intact Tissues Using Magnetic Resonance Gradient Echoes," <u>Strahlentherapie Und Onkologie 165:</u> (2/3) 179-181 (February/March 1989).

4. Kabalka, G. W., et al., "^{11}B MRI and MRS of Intact Animals Infused with a Boron Neutron Capture Agent," <u>Mag. Reson. Med. 8:</u> 231-237 (1988).

5. Bendel, P., et al., "A Method for Imaging Nuclei with Short T2 Relaxation and Its Application to ^{11}B NMR Imging of a BNCT Agent in an Intact Rat," <u>J. Magn. Reson. 88:</u> 369-375 (1990).

6. Bradshaw, K. M., "Development of Magnetic Resonance Technology for Noninvasive Boron Quantification," U. S. Department of Energy formal report, EGG-2629 (1990).

7. Hayes, C. E., et al., "An Efficient, Highly Homogeneous Radiofrequency Coil for Whole-Body NMR Imaging at 1.5 T," <u>J. Magn. Reson. 63:</u> 622-628 (1985).

8. Richards, T. L., et al., "^{11}B NMR Spectroscopy of Excised Mouse Tissue After Infusion of Boron Compound Used in Neutron Capture Therapy," (abstract) <u>Radiology 165:</u> 346 (1987).

INTRACELLULAR BORON UPTAKE AND DISTRIBUTION OF BSH AND BPA

DETERMINED USING ION MICROSCOPY

Xiaohui Zha, Brian D. Bennett, Walter A. Ausserer[*], and George H. Morrison

Department of Chemistry
Cornell University, Ithaca, N.Y. 14853

[*]Cancer Biology SRI, 333
 Ravenwood Ave., Menlo Park, C.A. 94029

Introduction

An essential aspect of boron neutron capture therapy (BNCT) research is the synthesis of boronated compounds that demonstrate selective uptake into tumor cells. A corollary of this goal is the development of analytical methods for evaluating the uptake, localization, and retention of these compounds in biological test systems (cell culture and animal models). Quantification of boron at the level of individual cells allows direct comparison of drug uptake across various cell lines or tissue compartments. This ability would give direct evidence of selective drug uptake by targeted malignancies.

A new technique for single cell and subcellular elemental analysis, which shows considerable applicability to BNCT drugs is ion microscopy.[1-5] The technique is capable of quantitatively localizing any element or isotope with sensitivity in the low ppm range. Thus, it is applicable to isotopically labeled compounds such as boronated xenobiotics. Subcellular localization is possible since the lateral spatial resolution is on the order of 0.5 μm.

This paper describes some preliminary ion microscopic studies on the uptake of sodium borocaptate (BSH) and p-boronophenylalanine (BPA) in cell culture.

BSH Uptake

Four cell lines, U87 human glioblastoma, Hela human epitheloid carcinoma, 2408b mutant human skin fibroblast, and GM 3348 human skin fibroblast, have been used as models for in vitro boron uptake. Cells were incubated with BSH at four different concentrations for 6 hours (approximate drug half-life in animal studies[6]), then frozen, fractured, freeze-dried, and analyzed by ion microscopy. The intensity of the ion images is readily transformed into the corresponding elemental concentration using a charge coupled device (CCD) camera and the quantitation scheme developed previously in this lab.[7] The quantitative results for boron uptake are given in Table 1.

The results indicate that there is no obvious preferential uptake of BSH into tumor cells relative to the normal cells among the cell lines tested. The B (from BSH) was more concentrated in the cytoplasm than the nucleus. Also, the uptake in most cell lines shows a tendency to saturate, which suggests a carrier-mediated diffusion process.

Progress in Neutron Capture Therapy for Cancer
Edited by B.J. Allen *et al.*, Plenum Press, New York, 1992

Table 1. Comparison of BSH uptake; malignant vs. normal cell lines.

		U87	Hela	2408b	3348b
control	C	0	0	0	0
	N	0	0	0	0
100 µg/mL	C	136 (14)	240 (22)	146 (9)	186 (7)
	N	97 (12)	118 (9)	110 (13)	148 (5)
250 µg/mL	C	252 (20)	327 (18)	308 (13)	419 (20)
	N	167 (26)	274 (17)	231 (22)	366 (13)
500 µg/mL	C	691 (65)	486 (25)	422 (34)	644 (36)
	N	435 (57)	458 (40)	394 (37)	470 (32)

data are presented as µg B/g dry weight (S.E.M.)
C = cytoplasm; N = Nucleus

In order to examine the binding nature of BSH within the cell, a retention experiment has been performed on Hela cells. Cells were treated with 500 µg BSH/mL for 6 hours and then changed into fresh media. The elimination of B from loaded cells was monitored by ion microscopy The results are shown in Figure 1.

Figure 1 shows that the intracellular B (from BSH) is rapidly excluded from both nuclear and cytoplasmic regions once cells are moved into fresh media. The elimination data can be fit to the sum of two exponentials using nonlinear regression techniques. The results of this parameter estimation are:

$$Y = 365 * \exp(-1.6^*t) + 121 * \exp(-0.06^*t) : \quad \text{for the cytoplasm}$$

$$Y = 378 * \exp(-3.4^*t) + 80 * \exp(-0.08^*t) : \quad \text{for the nucleus}$$

where Y and t are intracellular B concentration and retention time, respectively. The good fit of the double exponential function on the experimental data indicates that there may be two separable processes involved in the elimination: the faster one may be responsible for elimination of the majority of intracellular B and the slower one for a small tightly bound portion. The majority of intracellular B was readily washed out within an hour after cells were moved into BSH free media, which could be a major difficulty in enhancing the tumor/blood concentration ratio, a critical parameter for the effectiveness of BNCT.

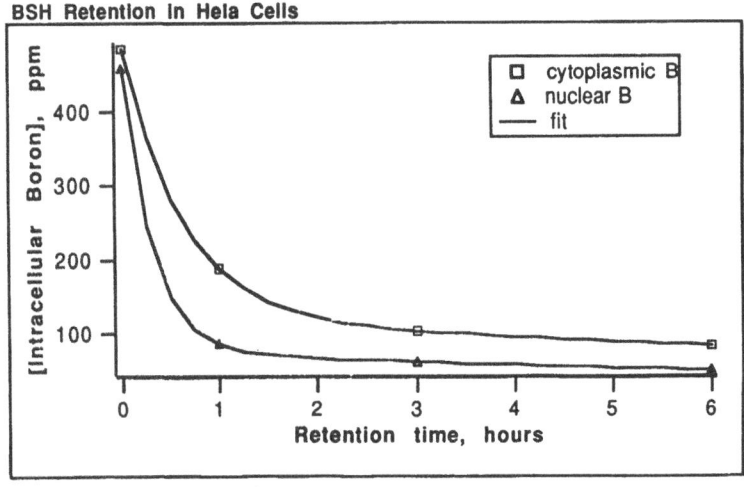

Figure 1. Elimination of BSH from Hela cells

We have developed a cell culture model system for the study of drug uptake into malignant melanoma. Use of the highly melanotic M-3 clonal strain[8] of mouse melanoma cells allows correlation of light microscopy and ion microscopy. We are able to match, area for area, pigment level (degree of melanization) to ion intensity from the photomicrographs and ion images. In a preliminary double label experiment, M-3 cells were treated with BPA (200 µg/mL) and deuterated tyrosine (L-tyrosine-(ring-D_4), 100 µg/mL) for one hour, freeze-fractured, freeze dried, photomicrographed, and analyzed with the ion microscope. The results are given Figure 2. The data show that the deuterium signal correlates to the amount of pigment, as would be expected for this melanin precursor. However, the boron signal does not correlate with pigmentation and has about the same intensity from cell to cell. This model system is now being used to elucidate the mechanism of BPA uptake and distribution utilizing specific transport and metabolic inhibitors.

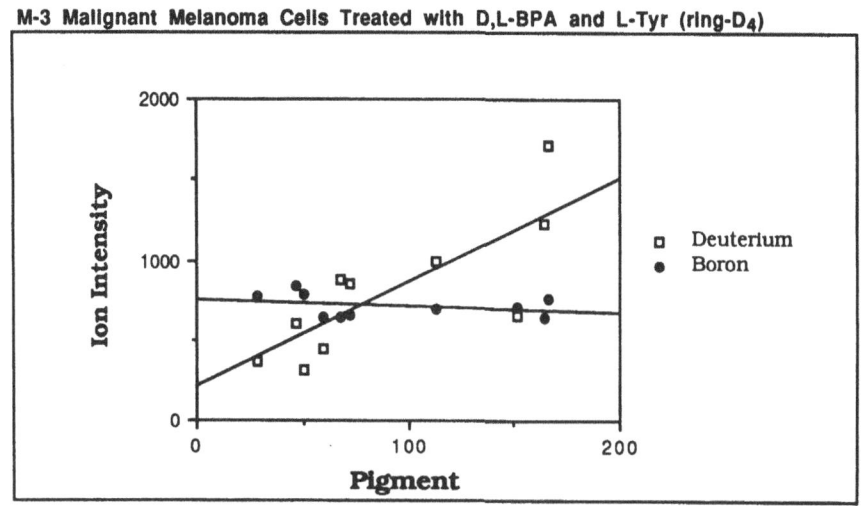

M-3 Malignant Melanoma Cells Treated with D,L-BPA and L-Tyr (ring-D_4)

Figure 2. Uptake of boron (from BPA) and deuterium (from D_4-Tyr) into M-3 malignant mouse melanoma. Note the positive correlation of deuterium with pigmentation ($R^2_{deuterium,pigment}$ = 0.62; $R^2_{boron,pigment}$ = 0.075, R^2 = coefficient of determination)).
Degree of pigmentation (melanization) was obtained by scanning the photomicrograph with Applescan and transferring the image into the "NIH Image" image processing program for pixel measurement. The values represent the average gray scale value from a region within a cell. The boron and deuterium intensities are the pixel counts integrated over a 5 minute acquisition for the corresponding area.

References

[1]Chandra, S. and Morrison, G. H. (1989) Methods Enzymol. 158, 157-179.

[2]Chandra, S., Morrison, G. H., and Wolcott, C. C..(1986) J. Microsc. (Oxford), 744, 15-37.

3Turner, L. K., Ling, Y-C., Bernius, M. T., and Morrison, G. H. (1987) Anal. Chem. 59, 2463-2468.

[4] Ling, Y-C., Bernius, M. T., and Morrison, G. H. (1987) J. Chem. Inf. Comput. Sci. 24, 86-95.

[5]Ausserer, W.A., Chandra, S., and Morrison, G. H.(1989) J. Microsc. (Oxford), 154, 39-57.

[6] Barth, R.F., Soloway, A.H., Alam, F., Clendenon, N. R., Blue, T.E., Mafune, N., Goodman, J.H., Gorden, W., Bapat,B., Adams, D.M., Staubus, A.E., Moeschberger, M.J., Gahbauer, R., Yates, A.J., Wang, C.K., Makroglou, G.E., Tzeng,J-J., and Fairchild, R.G. "Pre-clinical Studies on Boron Neutron Capture Therapy", Clinical Aspects of Neutron Capture Therapy, Ed. by R.G. Fairchild, V.P. Bond, and A.D. Woodhead, Plenum Press (1989), p. 95.

[7] Ausserer,W.A., Ling, Y-C., Chandra, S., and Morrison, G.H.,(1989) Anal. Chem., 61, 2690-2695.

[8] Yasumura, Y., Tashjian, A. H., and Sato, G. H., (1966) Science, 154, 1186-1189.

UPTAKE OF BORONATED MONOCLONAL ANTIBODIES BY MELANOMA CELLS VISUALISED

BY TRACK ETCH AUTORADIOGRAPHY AND ELECTRON ENERGY LOSS SPECTROSCOPY

D E Moore,[1] J R Stretch,[2] A L Dawes,[1] D J H Cockayne,[3]
B J Allen[4] and G Constantine[5]

[1]Department of Pharmacy, and [3]Electron Microscope Unit
  The University of Sydney, Sydney 2006 Australia
[2]Department of Plastic Surgery, Radcliffe Infirmary
  Oxford OX2 6HE England
[4]Biomedicine and Health Program, Australian Nuclear Science
  and Technology Organisation, Menai 2234 Australia
[5]AEA Technology, Harwell OX11 ORA England

The monoclonal antibody (MAb) NKI-C3 (Netherlands Cancer Institute) is a
murine IgG1 known to react with a formalin resistant antigen expressed by
more than 95% of human melanomas. In principle, it can be used in the
diagnosis of tissue sections for the presence of melanocytes, and with the
appropriate level of boron labelling, this antibody could also be used for
NCT of melanoma, provided its specificity is not impaired by the labelling
process. The present study involves the use of two imaging techniques:
first, α-track etch autoradiography to determine the specificity of the
MAb after boronation, and second, electron energy loss spectroscopy to
obtain information at the subcellular level concerning the localisation of
the boron label.

Boronated monoclonal antibody Modifying the approach of Alam [1] we used
a bifunctional reagent to link dodecaborane clusters to polyornithine as a
bridging macromolecule, which was then bound to the antibody by means of a
photoactivatable bifunctional reagent [2]. After separation by anionic
chromatography, the boron content of the antibody was determined by
inductively coupled plasma atomic emission spectrometry [3] to be 1150 B
atoms per antibody molecule. Polyornithine of average molecular weight 43
kD was chosen for the macromolecular bridge. This provides a large number
of amino groups necessary for the covalent linkage of the dodecaborane
clusters to the extent that only 4 or 5 boronated polyornithine bridges
(each carrying about 250 B atoms) are attached per antibody molecule. The
disadvantage of this product is that the molecular weight is increased
substantially, and its solubility reduced concommittantly. Nonetheless,
the boronated NKI-C3 antibody retained at least 90% of its specificity for
melanocytic lesions.

Neutron capture autoradiography Conventional histological techniques
were used to cut 6 μm thick tissue sections of a human melanoma onto CR-39
plastic. The melanoma sections were incubated with the boronated antibody
for 30 min at 20°C, thoroughly rinsed in tris-buffered saline and air
dried. The composite samples were positioned in the 6H filtered cold

neutron beam in the DIDO reactor at AEA Technology, Harwell. A one hour exposure at a flux of 3.5×10^8 neutrons cm^{-2} s^{-1} was adequate to generate sufficient tracks for demonstration of the MAb-tumour affinity reaction. The tracks were visualised by immersing the irradiated CR-39 sheet in a 6M KOH bath at 60°C for 3 hours. The damaged areas dissolve at an enhanced rate so that an etch pit forms around each track. These are individually visible under the microscope, but collectively give a frosted appearance to indicate the boron distribution image. The correlation of the boron neutron capture autoradiography with that produced by immunohistochemistry on an adjacent section was excellent as shown in Figure 1.

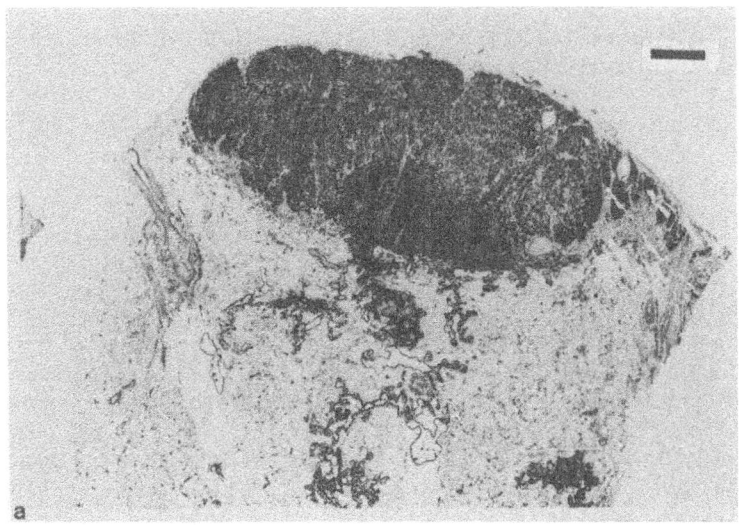

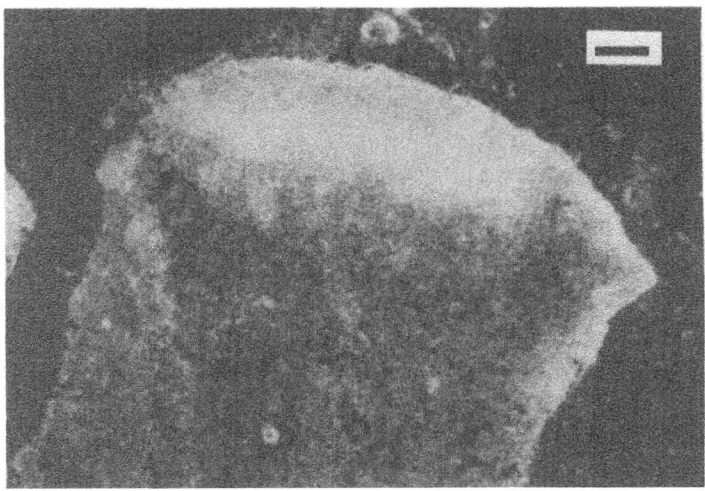

Figure 1. Melanoma section incubated with boronated antibody NKI-C3 and visualised by (a) α-track autoradiography and (b) immunohistochemistry. The scale bar indicates 1 mm.

Electron energy loss spectroscopic imaging Boron conjugation with MAb also provides a means whereby the time course and spatial distribution of B-MAb can be studied in detail by means of the technique of electron energy loss spectroscopy (EELS) in the electron microscope [4]. EELS is based on the detection of electrons which have lost a discrete amount of energy following interaction with specific atoms in the sample. The B label appears ideal since the EELS technique is particularly sensitive to low atomic number elements, and there is no B occurring naturally to create an interference.

EELS elemental mapping can be performed both in the scanning transmission analytical electron microscope (STEM), or in the energy-filtering transmission electron microscope (EFTEM). In EFTEM an energy filter is adjusted to select one energy loss at a time, so that the response due to one element in the sample can be collected very quickly at a resolution determined by the objective lens and chromatic aberration. In STEM the full spectrum is collected by the parallel detection system, so that several elements are determined concurrently, with the resolution limited by the minimum useful probe size and electron gun brightness. To develop a full elemental map, STEM is much slower than EFTEM, but has the ability to record a spectrum from an area where the elemental concentration may be too small to image.

Preliminary studies using parallel EELS in the STEM mode, have shown that spot analysis on various specimens containing B-MAb reveals a boron K-edge which varies in strength from position to position. The technique is yet to be developed to systematically scan an area of the sample such that an elemental map of one or more cells can be obtained. In elemental mapping of biological samples, the important criterion is the practical limit of detectability of the element being mapped. Among the factors influencing the limit are the sample thickness uniformity over the field of study.

If the thickness varies, the scattering of electrons varies and the sample image becomes less well defined. As a first step it was necessary to ascertain whether boron could be detected at the anticipated concentration levels, and whether the response could be quantified while accounting for variations in sample characteristics. Standard samples having uniform boron concentration were prepared by dissolution of known amounts of decaborane ($B_{10}H_{14}$) (Callery Chemicals) in Formvar solution in ethyl acetate. The film was cast to about 20 nm thick and collected on the

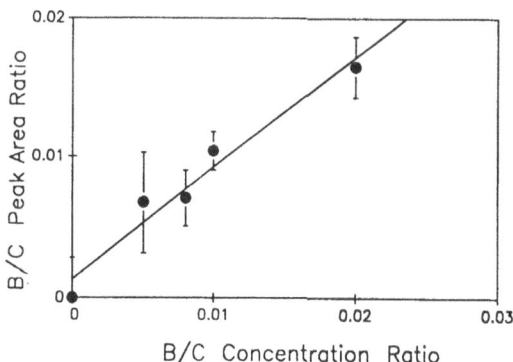

Figure 2. Standard curve for boron quantification by EELS.

sample grids. The films were viewed in a Philips EM430 transmission electron microscope operating at either 300 kV or 250 kV. Energy loss spectra were collected using a Gatan parallel spectrometer fitted beneath the microscope, and the spectra were processed using a TN 5500 MCA system. For each boron concentration, EELS spectra were taken at 20 different positions on the film for two separate grids, as an attempt to compensate for variation in thickness. From each spectrum, the signal areas due to boron and carbon after background subtraction were measured and averaged. The existing software enabled boron quantitation with reference to carbon as contained in the Formvar supporting film. A linear standard curve was obtained for the concentration range up to 2% boron, with the minimum detection level being 0.3% boron in the carbon film as shown in Figure 2.

For the B-MAb prepared as described here, the boron content achievable is 8% by weight, so that if the probe can successfully focus down to the resolution of one B-MAb molecule (about 10 nm) an accurate B map is possible. The next step is the development of the software to enable the systematic scanning of a sample to provide a map showing the distribution of boron in cellular systems. The boron elemental map then provides the marker of the MAb distribution in the cell.

ACKNOWLEDGEMENT

This project is supported by grants from the Leo & Jenny Leukemia and Cancer Foundation and the Australian Research Council.

REFERENCES

1. *F Alam, AH Soloway, RF Barth, N Mafune, DM Adams, WH Knoth.* Boron neutron capture therapy: Linkage of a boronated macromolecule to monoclonal antibodies directed against tumour-associated antigens. J. Med. Chem., *32*, 2326-2330, 1989.

2. *SR Tamat, DE Moore, A Patwardhan, P Hersey.* Boronated monoclonal antibody 225.28S for potential use in neutron capture therapy of malignant melanoma. Pigment Cell Res., *2*, 278-280, 1989.

3. *SR Tamat, DE Moore, BJ Allen.* Assay of boron in biological tissues by inductively coupled plasma atomic absorption spectrometry. Anal. Chem., *59*, 2161-2164, 1987.

4. *RD Leapman, RL Ornberg.* Quantitative electron energy loss spectroscopy in biology, Ultramicroscopy, *24*, 251-268, 1988.

INTERACTION BETWEEN BORON CONTAINING COMPOUNDS AND

SERUM ALBUMIN OBSERVED BY NUCLEAR MAGNETIC RESONANCE

W. F. Bauer,[1] K. M. Bradshaw,[1] and T. L. Richards[2]

[1]INEL BNCT Research Programs, Idaho National Engineering
Laboratory, P.O. Box 1625, Idaho Falls, ID   83415-3519
[2]Imaging Research Laboratory, University of Washington
Seattle, WA 98195

INTRODUCTION

The nature of the binding mechanism between the $B_{12}H_{12}SH^{-2}$ anion (BSH)
and serum albumin has long been a question.[1-3] Early experiments[1,2]
suggested that BSH may be bound covalently to the albumin molecule via a
disulfide bond, since the interaction of BSH to albumin was somewhat
stronger than that of $B_{12}H_{12}^{-2}$. One problem with many of the previous
experiments concerned with the binding of BSH to albumin was that a method
was not readily available with which to directly determine the nature of
the interaction without significant disruption of the system. Recently,
nuclear magnetic resonance (NMR) spectroscopy has been used to determine
that covalent bonding via the formation of disulfide bonding is not
significantly involved in the binding mechanism.[4]

More evidence as to the nature of BSH bonding to protein molecules
was discovered during experiments involving the development of a
noninvasive method for the *in-vivo* measurement of boron in tissue
utilizing [11]B magnetic resonance imaging (MRI).[5] It was noted that the
signal intensity and relaxation times for known boron concentrations and
boron in tissues varied as a function of temperature. Additional
experiments were performed on a GE Signa™ MRI system, where NMR measurements were obtained at temperatures ranging from 20-40 °C of solutions
containing BSH with either bovine, dog, or human serum albumin (BSA, DSA,
and HSA, respectively). The results indicated that as the temperature
increased, the NMR signal intensity more than doubled and the peak width
was reduced by almost a factor of 2.

Since the [11]B nucleus has a spin of $I=3/2$, it has a quadrupolar
moment (Q) and the primary modes of relaxation can be expected to be
associated with that moment.[6-8] The results obtained on the MRI system are
consistent with the behavior of quadrupolar nuclei (i.e., [35]Cl) in anions
associated with large proteins in aqueous solutions.[7,8] Anionic binding to
albumins is known and previous work has demonstrated that exchange
kinetics can play a significant role in relaxation at lower temperatures,[9]
and differences in the chemical nature of anions containing the same
nuclei can affect the nature of the interaction with the three-dimensional
protein structure; thus altering the relaxation mechanisms.[7,8]

EXPERIMENTS AND RESULTS

To confirm the observations from the experiments on the MRI system,
additional investigation was performed on a 7-Tesla, Bruker AC-300, high-
field, multinuclear NMR spectrometer equipped with a boron probe operating
at 96.2 Mhz for [11]B. Work on the high-field spectrometer also allowed the

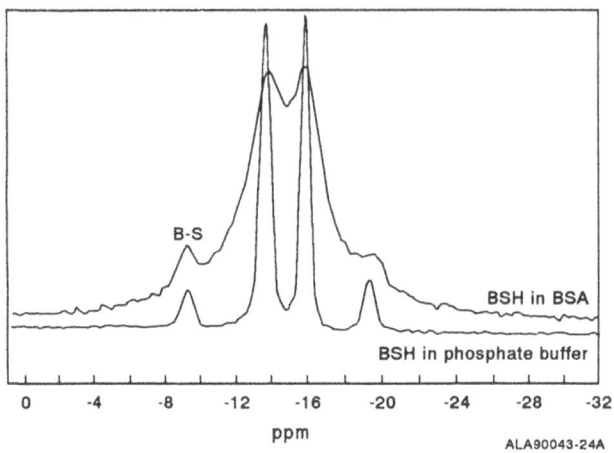

Figure 1. 100 µg boron/mL as BSH in phosphate buffer and BSA.

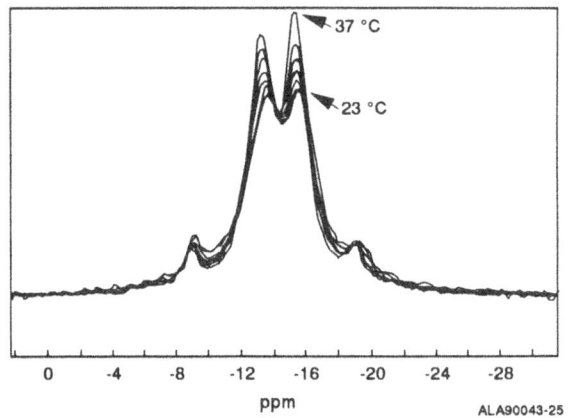

Figure 2. Temperature effects upon ^{11}B spectra of BSH in BSA.

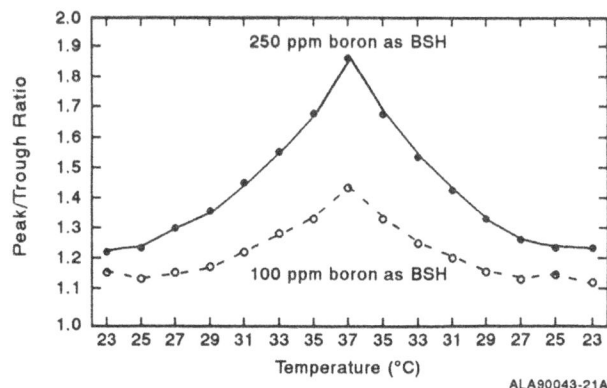

Figure 3. BSH binding with albumin, as observed by ^{11}B NMR.

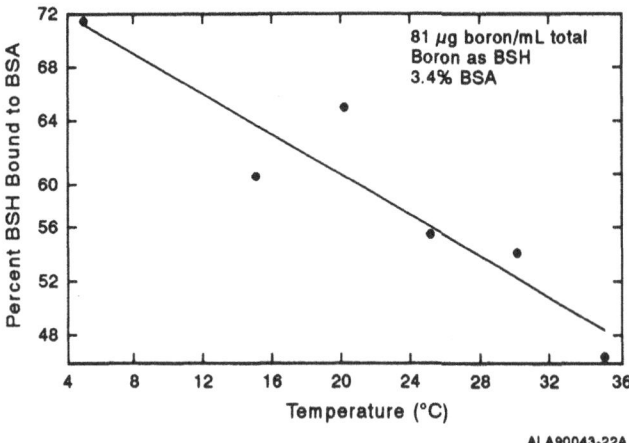

ALA90043-22A

Figure 4. Variation of percent BSH bound to
albumin with temperature.

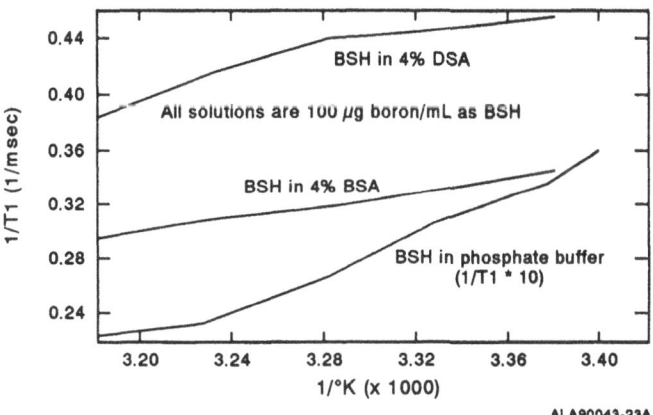

ALA90043-23A

Figure 5. Temperature effects on T1 at the
-15.5 ppm peak of BSH.

observation of each type of boron atom in BSH as the various parameters were changed. Experiments were conducted with BSH in both buffered (pH 7.4 phosphate buffer at 8.3 mM) and nonbuffered solutions and with and without approximately 4% (w/v) serum albumin (BSA, DSA, or HSA). Concentrations of 700-100 μg boron/Ml as BSH were selected, as this approximates the median serum levels observed in dogs that have been administered the BSH compound.[9]

The lack of any noticeable chemical shifts in the NMR spectra (as shown in Figure 1) once again indicate that the interaction between BSH and BSA is not via any significant covalent bonding. Similarly, no covalent type binding via the sulfhydryl group of BSH was noted when BSH was in solution with DSA or HSA. The extensive peak broadening and nearly an order of magnitude decrease in both the T_1 and T_2 values for all boron atoms does indicate a significant interaction with the protein; however, this interaction is more likely due to ionic or electrostatic interactions. The association of BSH with serum albumin causes the boron nuclei to become much more significantly influenced by the electric field gradients imposed by the large albumin molecule. This interaction causes an increases in the quadrupolar coupling, thus decreasing both T_1 and T_2.

The lack of covalent binding between BSH and serum albumin is also supported by the spectral data (Figures 2 and 3), obtained from a 100-μg boron/mL BSH in 4% BSA solution that was heated from 23-37 °C and then back to 23 °C. The increasing peak-to-trough ratio (~ δ -13.5/δ -14.4) and increasing net intensity in the spectra obtained at higher temperatures indicate that an exchange process is occurring that significantly changes as temperature increases. As the temperature increases, the molecular correlation time (τ_c) for the association of the boron cage compound with serum albumin decreases. Therefore, at higher temperature, more "free" BSH is present in the solution, and at temperatures as high as 50-60 °C, but before the protein begins to significantly denature, the spectrum begins to resemble that of a solution of BSH. IF the BSH was covalently bound to the albumin to any appreciable extent, very little change would be expected in the spectra over the temperature range studied, since the τ_c would only reflect a small change in the tumbling motion of a molecule as large as albumin.[7]

To support the hypothesis that BSH bonding to albumin is predominately ionic and the quantity of free BSH increases at high temperature, a separate study was performed to measure the bound and unbound BSH at temperatures in the range of approximately 5-36 °C. A stock solution containing 80 μg boron/mL as BSH and 3.4% BSA was prepared. Aliquots of this stock solution were inserted into an Amicon Centrifree™ Ultrafiltration unit with a molecular weight cutoff of 30,000 daltons. The ultrafiltration unit was placed into a refrigerated/heated centrifuge that had previously been quilibrated at the desired temperature. The samples were allowed to equilibrate at the desired temperature for at least 15 minutes and was spun at approximately 1000 x g for 20-25 minutes. The boron content of the filtrates and stock solution were determined by inductively coupled plasma-atomic emission spectroscopy (ICP-AES).[10] Bound boron was assumed to be the total boron minus the "free" boron found in the filtrate. Bound boron vs temperature is plotted in Figure 4 and clearly shows a trend indicating much more "free" boron (as BSH) at higher temperature. This result supports the NMR data that indicate no covalent bonding of BSH to albumin and more rapid exchange of bound and free BSH at higher temperatures.

Even though the NMR spectra for BSH solutions containing BSA, DSA, and HSA appear to be quite similar, the possibility exists that the "binding" sites may be in somewhat different microenvironments for each albumin. A limited set of inversion recovery experiments were performed and T_1 values were calculated for BSH from 22-37 °C in 8.3 Mm phosphate buffer, BSA, and DSA. The relationship between T_1 and temperature is consistent with that of quadrupolar relaxation mechanisms of ions in solution. The magnitude of T_1 shown in Figure 5 ($1/T_1$ vs $1/°K$) may indicate that the chemical microenvironments and strength of the binding could be quite different for BSH with each of the albumin species. The binding characteristics of BSH to HSA appear to be more closely related to that of DSA than BSA.[6] This effect is currently being studied in more detail.

CONCLUSIONS

The use of NMR spectroscopy can be a useful tool for the study of the interactions of boron-containing species with large biological molecules. Even though the relaxation mechanisms of quadrupolar nuclei, such as ^{11}B, are very complex, some qualitative information can be obtained

about the interactions. Examination of the spectra of BSH alone, and in a solution containing albumin, indicate that little, if any, covalent bonding between BSH and the protein occurs. The anionic sites involved in BSH binding appear to be different for each serum albumin studied. The ionic bonding and an exchange process between the BSH anion and the protein molecules is evident and future studies will involve determining such quantitative parameters as molecular correlation times, T_2 values, quadrupolar coupling constants, actual binding sites on the protein, and, possibly, exchange rate and binding constants.

REFERENCES

1. Soloway, A. H., H. Hatanaka, and M. A. Davis, "Penetration for Brain and Brain Tumor VII: Tumor-Binding Sulfhydryl Boron Compounds," J. Med. Chem. 10: 714 (1967).

2. Nakagawa and Nagai, "Interaction Between Serum Albumin and Mercapto-undecahydrododecaborate Ion (An Agent for Boron Neutron Capture Therapy of Brain Tumor)," Chem. Pharm. Bull. 24: 2934 (1976).

3. Soloway, A. H., F. Alam, R. F. Barth, and V. B. Bapat, "Boron Chemistry and Target Cell Affinity," Strahlenther. und Onkol. 165: (2/3) 118 (1989).

4. Samsel, E. G. and D. L. Miller, "High Resolution ^{10}B and ^{11}B Nuclear Magnetic Resonance (NMR) Spectroscopy of $Na_2B_{12}H_{11}SH$ Impurities and Metabolites," Strahlenther. und Onkol. 165: (2/3) 140 (1989).

5. Bradshaw, K. M., W. F. Bauer, and T. L. Richards, "Observations of the $Na_2B_{12}H_{11}SH$ Binding to Albumin Protein by NMR as a Function of Concentration, Temperature, and Albumin Species," presented at the Boron USA-II Workshop, Research Triangle Park, NC, June 7-9, 1990.

6. "Multinuclear NMR," J. Mason (ed), Plenum Press, NY (1987).

7. Reimarsson, P., T. Bull, and B. Lindman, "The ClO_4^- Ion as a Probe in NMR Studies of Protein Anion Binding Sites," FEBS Letters 59: (2) 158 (1975).

8. Norne, J., S. Hjalmarsson, B. Lindman, and M. Zeppezauer, "Anion Binding Properties of Human Serum Albumin from Halide Ion Quadrupole Relaxation," Biochemistry 14: 3401 (1975).

9. Kraft, S. L., P. R. Gavin, C. E. DeHaan, W. F. Bauer, and T. E. Ary, "The Biodistribution of Boron in Canine Spontaneous Intracranial Tumors Following Borocaptate Sodium Infusion," Proceedings of the Fourth International Symposium on Neutron Capture Therapy for Cancer, Sydney, New South Wales, Australia, December 4-7, 1990.

10. Bauer, W. F., D. A. Johnson, S. M. Steele, K. Messick, D. L. Miller, and W. A. Propp, "Gross Boron Determination in Biological Samples by Inductively Coupled Plasma-Atomic Emission Spectroscopy," Strahlenther. und Onkol. 165: (2/3) 176-179 (1989).

THE NECESSITY OF STOCHASTIC RADIOBIOLOGY IN BNCT
OR
WHAT IS THE RBE OF THE ^{10}B(n,α)^{7}Li REACTION

Detlef Gabel[1], Victor P. Bond[2], John Kalef-Ezra[3], Ralph G. Fairchild[2]

[1]Dept. of Chemistry, University of Bremen, Bremen, FR Germany
[2]Medical Department, Brookhaven National Laboratory, Upton, New York, USA
[3]Medical Physics Laboratory, Medical School, University of Ioannina, Greece

INTRODUCTION

In radiation biology and in radiotherapy, the details of the interaction of ionizing radiation with biological matter is of great importance. With the advent of high-LET, short range particles such as those utilized in BNCT, a more thorough and detailed knowledge of these interactions is of even greater importance. It would be desirable to predict the response of a biological system (e.g. an organ in an organism) from basic principles derived in simpler systems. This deductive approach would be highly satisfactory.

When dealing with different types of ionizing radiation (e.g. gamma rays, electron, protons, fast neutrons) it has become apparent quite soon that the physical description of the interaction with matter for these types of radiation does not translate directly to the observed response. Thus the same amount of energy deposited in a macroscopic volume element has been found to result in different types of radiation.

In order to reconcile the observed variation in biological effects of identical doses of different radiation, the concept of Relative Biological Effectiveness, RBE, has been created.

With this number, the radiotherapist has been put into position to choose for a given therapy modality, the dose level for the therapy of a given tumor at a given position, aiming at maximal tumor response and, even more important, minimal complications due to healthy tissue response.

As will be shown, for particles with high linear energy transfer (around 30 keV/μm and higher), RBE is not sufficient to describe the biological response. Two other parameters, the Hit Size Effectiveness Function (HSEF) and the Relative Local Efficiency (RLE), must be taken into account. With the high-LET particles in question, the appropriate Poisson statistics need also to be considered.

This paper summarizes the knowledge on these parameters, and draws conclusions for the clinical implication of BNCT.

A number of studies have been carried out on the radiobiological effect of the ^{10}B(n,α)^{7}Li reaction on cells and organs. The derived RBE value was found to be dependent on the chosen compound and end point.

For the radiation response of cells, it is important to realize in which geometrical environment they are irradiated.

HIT SIZE EFFECTIVENESS FUNCTIONS IN HIGH-LET RADIOTHERAPY

The amount of energy that is liberated in any of the ^{10}B(n,α)^{7}Li reactions is quite large. Thus, for an expected survival of 10 % (i.e. a dose of 1.7 Gy), only four events will occur within the volume of one cell. Clearly, at these low numbers, Poisson statistics will have to be taken into account. A considerable difference of energy deposition must be expected between different cells subjected to identical boron and neutron exposure. Gabel [1] has analyzed this situation.

When analyzing the radiation response of cells to low-LET radiation, it can be assumed, due to the large number of interactions necessary to damage the proliferative capabilities of cells, that all cells receive roughly the same amount of energy. Then the dose delivered to a macroscopic (e.g. 1 g) piece of matter will be a good indication of the energy deposited in the nuclei of the cells. This is not true for low-level exposure to low-LET radiation (usually resulting in mutations etc. rather than reproductive death). Therefore, it has been suggested by Bond [2] that the energy deposited in the nuclei of individual cells be called "hit size". For mutations, it was found that there is a strong dependence of the probability of response on the hit size. This dependence could be expressed in a "Hit Size Effectiveness Function", HSEF.

The analysis of cells exposed to the $^{10}B(n,\alpha)^{7}Li$ reaction, monitored for their proliferative potential, strongly suggests the existence of a HSEF also for high-LET radiation [1].

THE RELATIVE LOCAL EFFICIENCY OF HIGH-LET RADIATION

The geometrical arrangement of boron in and around the cells influences greatly both the average energy deposition in the nuclei, as well as their distribution pattern. This has been discussed for averaged hit sizes [e.g. 3] and for hit size distributions [e.g. 1].

In order to deliver lethal hits to every single target cell, enough boron (as well as thermal neutrons) must be present in this cell. If a cell does not take up boron, but is surrounded by boron-containing cells, a reduced hit size must be expected. This can be expressed numerically by the Relative Local Efficiency, RLE, and the Localization Factor, LF [1].

The geometrical arrangement of boron, together with the HSEF, will make it almost impossible to predict the biological response of cells to a BNCT treatment from the average boron concentration and the neutron fluence alone. In an intact organ, the response must, at present, still be determined empirically. As an example, if only the capillary cells of a tumor were to take up boron, damage to tumor cells would be greatly reduced. Vascular cells might make up a few percent (say 5 %) of the mass of a tumor. Therefore, an average boron concentration of 10 ppm in the tumor tissue could mean a concentration of 200 ppm in the vascular cells. The biological effect of extensive vascular damage upon neutron exposure is not known at present and would still have to be determined experimentally.

IMPLICATIONS FOR THERAPY

Tumor uptake versus tumor selectivity of boronated compounds

In the development of boronated tumor seekers, it is in principle possible to obtain compounds that are highly tumor specific (with uptake ratios of over 10 between healthy and tumor tissue), but with a low absolute concentration in the tumor. Other compounds are only moderately tumor specific (with uptake ratios of below 10 between healthy and tumor tissue), but with high absolute concentration in the tumor.

Whereas it might be tempting to assume that high specificity of tumor uptake might be of greater value than the absolute concentration that can be obtained, this is not so. Healthy tissue (as well as tumor tissue) will receive radiation dose contributions not only from the $^{10}B(n,\alpha)^{7}Li$ reaction, but also from other unavoidable sources. Therefore, less optimal tumor selectivity might be more than compensated for by high absolute uptake.

As an example, assume that in the absence of boron, a relative dose rate of 1 is found, but if the boron increases to 6 ppm, then a relative dose rate of 2 is observed. Then, for the tumor, a dose differential of 2 (i.e. a 100 % increase in dose) is found when 6 ppm are present in the tumor, and no boron in the healthy tissue (concentration ratio tumor/healthy tissue >> 10). If the same compound is present in the tumor in a concentration of 30 ppm, a dose differential of 2 would be obtained with 12 ppm boron in the healthy tissue (ratio = 2.5). For 60 ppm boron in the tumor, the same dose differential would be obtained with as much as 27 ppm boron in the healthy tissue (ratio = 2.2).

Treatment planning

In conventional beam radiotherapy, much emphasis is placed on treatment planning. With treatment planning one tries to maximize the dose to the tumor, while at the same time sparing healthy tissue.

In BNCT, treatment planning will not be possible to the same extent. This is due to the fact that a neutron beam, no matter how well collimated, will spread laterally once it enters the target. The contributions from the different dose components will change with depth. Tissue outside the beam, not exposed to neutrons, will still receive a substantial radiation dose from the long-ranging gammas generated by neutron capture in hydrogen.

However, more important than these factors is the considerable dose modification of the beam by the boron present in the target. The hit size to the individual cell depends on the amount of boron in and around this cell, as well as its subcellular distribution. Both of these parameters cannot be determined experimentally at present. A different subcellular localization can change the hit size to a cell by an order of magnitude and more.

The maximum dose of neutrons with a known amount of a given boron compound in BNCT will therefore be determined by the response of the healthy tissue. The treatment planning will be largely decided not by the shape and other parameters of the beam, but by the choice of compound.

Due to the importance of localization of boron, the maximally tolerated dose will be compound dependent. Thus, studies with one compound (e.g. BSH) will not yield much information for the treatment using a different boron compound (e.g. p-dihydroxyboryl phenylalanine). Equally, studies for one target organ (e.g. brain tissue) cannot, even for the same compound, be transferred easily to other treatment areas.

Fractionation

In radiotherapy, the presently available treatments are often carried out by administering repeated small fractions. For low-LET radiation, there is a marked increase in dose tolerance of healthy tissue with increasing fractionation. For high-LET radiation, this increase is reduced, but not always absent. A numerical value for RBE for the ^{10}B reaction in a practical therapy situation will have to take this into account. Also it is necessary to consider which organs are exposed to the beam, as the radiosensitivity of different healthy cells to both low-LET (i.e. reference radiation) and high-LET radiation varies considerably [4]. When boron is administered prior to each dose, retargeting to other cells must be expected, and might actually be beneficial.

CONCLUSION

It is highly uncertain that a defined RBE value can be assigned to the $^{10}B(n,\alpha)^{7}Li$ reaction in a tissue. The main uncertainty is the knowledge of the subcellular localization of boron. Different patterns of subcellular localization can result in differences of apparent RBE values of up to one order of magnitude and more. Furthermore, the heterogeneity of uptake found in tumors for all boron-containing tumor seekers would preclude that an effective dose can be defined for all tumor cells.

In the context of therapy, it will therefore be unlikely that a maximization of the dose to the tumor can be obtained. Instead, a minimization of the dose to the healthy tissue must be aimed for. The aim must be a reduction of the dose to healthy tissue below its tolerance level for serious side effects.

The response of the healthy tissue will, for the very same reasons, not be determined by simple multiplication of neutron fluence and gross boron concentration. Rather, it will also depend on the subcellular distribution of boron in all cells exposed. Because of the vastly different boron distribution patterns, it is unlikely that the cells determining the tolerance of the healthy tissue can be pointed at from previous knowledge. Therefore, any clinical trials with any boron compound must be preceded by a proper study of the response of healthy tissue to the proposed therapy.

It must be considered highly unethical to embark upon clinical trials with a new compound without having carried out the necessary and appropriate studies of the tolerance of healthy tissue to the proposed treatment. The results cannot be obtained deductively from other experiments. Even an exact determination of RBE values (which has aided radiotherapists in the past) for a given compound in a cell system will not yield the necessary information. Rather, an inductive approach to clinical trials in BNCT must be advocated.

ACKNOWLEDGMENTS
This work has been supported partly by the North Atlantic Treaty Organization.

REFERENCES

[1] Gabel, D., S. Foster, R.G. Fairchild (1987) Radiat. Res. 111, 14-25.
[2] Bond. V.P., L. Feinendegen, J. Booz (1988) Int. J. Radiat. Biol. 53, 1-12.
[3] Kobayashi, T., K. Kanda (1982) Radiat. Res. 91, 77-94.
[4] Geraci, J.P., P.D. Thrower, K.L. Jackson, G.M. Christensen, R.G. Parker, M.S. Fox (1974) Radiat. Res. 59, 496-503.

ENHANCEMENT OF THERMAL NEUTRON INDUCED KILLING EFFECT ON HeLa CELLS
CONTAINING BORON-10 NUCLEIC ACID DERIVATIVES

Y. Ujeno[1], M. Akaboshi[1], K. Akuta[1], T. Maki[1], K. Kawai[1], Y. Yamamoto[2]

[1] Research Reactor Institute, Kyoto University, Sennan-gun
Kumatori-cho, Osaka 590-04, Japan
[2] Department of Chemistry, Faculty of Sciences, Tohoku University
Sendai-shi, Aoba-ku, Miyagi 980, Japan

INTRODUCTION

The ^{10}B-compounds as the carriers of ^{10}B atoms are one of the keys to
make BNCT succeed. Recently, we synthesized some derivatives of nucleic
acids containing ^{10}B. The present study deals with the enhanced killing of
HeLa S3 cells containing these compounds in vitro by irradiation in the
thermal neutron beam of the Kyoto University Reactor (KUR). The
enhancement was measured with the changes in 4 radiobiological parameters.

MATERIALS AND METHODS

The ^{10}B-compounds used were 5-(1-hydroxymethyl)carboranyl-uridine
(5HMCBU), 5-carboranyl-2'-deoxyuridine(5CBdeoxyU),
5-carboranyluridine(5CBU) and 5-(para-deoxyborylphenyl)uridine (5BPU).
These compounds were initially dissolved in EtOH, then diluted with saline,
to dissolve in the culture medium of HeLa S3 cells. The final
concentration was 0.2, 1.0 or 2.0 μg ^{10}B/ml of MEM medium. The final
concentration of EtOH was less than 5%. The culture methods were reported
previously[1]. HeLa S3 cells were incubated for 2 hours at 0°C or 37°C in the
medium containing ^{10}B-compounds to allow uptake into cells before
irradiation. The irradiation was carried out at room temperature in the
biomedical radiation field of KUR. The irradiation methods were also
reported previously[1]. The cells were cultured in the medium without
^{10}B-compounds for 10 days to count the colony. The killing effect was
measured with a colony counting method.

The thermal neutron flux was measured with Au foils and γ-rays were
measured with TLD. The absorbed doses due to both radiations were
calculated from flux and exposure[1]. In this calculation, ^{10}B was assumed to
be extracellular.

The radiobiological parameters, α (Gy^{-1}), β (Gy^{-2}), the mean
inactivation dose $\bar{D}$(Gy), the surviving fraction at 2 Gy SF(2) which are
important to evaluate the effect of radiation in radiotherapy[2], and their
ratios relative to controls were calculated. These ratios show the
increase in absorbed dose in the cell nucleus but do not represent RBE
values[1]. The α ratios were taken to be ratios for irradiation with a ^{10}B
compound to irradiation without ^{10}B. The inverse was used for the $\bar{D}$ ratios,
namely the ratio for irradiation without ^{10}B to irradiation with ^{10}B.

Table 1. The radiobiological parameters of HeLa S3 cells incubated in the medium containing ^{10}B-5BPU and irradiated in the KUR thermal neutron beam.

incubation	α (ratios)	$\bar{D}$ (ratios)
0μg ^{10}B/g, 0°C, 120 min	1.135 (1.000)	0.792 (1.000)
2μg ^{10}B/g, 0°C, 120 min	2.611 (2.291)	0.383 (2.068)
2μg ^{10}B/g, 37°C, 30 min	2.405 (2.119)	0.416 (1.904)
2μg ^{10}B/g, 37°C, 60 min	2.766 (2.437)	0.362 (2.188)
2μg ^{10}B/g, 37°C, 120 min	3.011 (2.653)	0.322 (2.386)

Table 2. The effect of incubation temperature on the radiobiological parameters of HeLa S3 cells incubated in the medium containing four ^{10}B-compounds (0.2 μg ^{10}B/g) and irradiated in the KUR thermal neutron beam. Incubation time was 2 hours.

^{10}B-compounds	inc.temp.(°C)	α (ratios)	$\bar{D}$ (ratios)
	0	0.746 (1.000)	1.254 (1.000)
	37	0.740 (1.000)	0.977 (1.000)
5HMCBU	0	1.248 (1.673)	0.801 (1.566)
	37	1.931 (2.609)	0.518 (1.886)
5CBdeoxyU	0	0.333 (0.446)	0.774 (1.620)
	37	1.600 (2.162)	0.530 (1.843)
5CBU	0	3.473 (4.693)	0.288 (4.354)
	37	2.374 (3.172)	0.426 (2.293)
5BPU	0	1.341 (1.812)	0.746 (1.681)
	37	1.423 (1.923)	0.656 (1.489)

Table 3. The effect of incubation temperature on the radiobiological parameters of HeLa S3 cells incubated in the medium containing four ^{10}B-compounds (1.0 μg ^{10}B/g) and irradiated in the KUR thermal neutron beam. Incubation time was 2 hours.

^{10}B-compounds	inc.temp.(°C)	α (ratios)	$\bar{D}$ (ratios)
	0	0.490 (1.000)	1.492 (1.000)
	37	0.247 (1.000)	1.908 (1.000)
5HMCBU	0	0.964 (1.967)	1.037 (1.438)
	37	1.081 (4.377)	0.950 (2.008)
5CBdeoxyU	0	1.511 (3.084)	0.614 (2.430)
	37	1.077 (4.360)	0.804 (2.373)
5CBU	0	2.867 (5.851)	0.349 (4.275)
	37	2.964 (12.000)	0.410 (5.662)
5BPU	0	1.107 (2.259)	0.903 (1.652)
	37	0.602 (2.417)	1.661 (1.143)

The parameters in the experiments for four ^{10}B-compounds are listed in Tables 2 and 3. The enhanced killing effect of compounds was variable but largest for 5CBU. The ratios at 37°C incubation before irradiation, were always larger than those at 0°C incubation, except the data on $\bar{D}$ for compounds 5CBU and 5BPU. However, as the concentration of compounds increased from 0.2 μg ^{10}B/g to 1.0 μg ^{10}B/g, the ratios increased, except the data on $\bar{D}$ for 5BPU.

RESULTS

The α and $\bar{D}$ ratios increased with the prolongation of incubation time in the medium containing ^{10}B-5BPU(Table 1).

CONCLUSION

The ^{10}B-compounds used in the present experiment, contain one or ten ^{10}B atoms in one molecule. However, calculating the concentration of these compounds as the weight of ^{10}B, we can compare the data of the compounds. The compounds are derivatives of nucleic acids and are expected to be taken up into the cells or cell nuclei. The increase in α and $\bar{D}$ ratios with prolongation of incubation time at 37°C, suggests uptake into cells or cell nuclei. 5CBU appears to enhance the killing effect most effectively following 2 hours incubation. But ^{10}B-compounds outside of cells also showed enhanced killing effects, because the ratios of both parameters for incubation at 0°C were greater than 1.000. The parameters α and $\bar{D}$ show the radiosensitivity of cells in the comparatively low dose range. Increasing the ratios of both parameters, the present ^{10}B-compounds can increase the radiosensitivity of cells in the comparatively low dose range, but there are a few exceptions. This property is very valuable for BNCT.

REFERENCES

1. Ujeno, Y., Akaboshi, M., Maki,H. and Kawai, K., 1990, Mathematical analysis of the survival of HeLa S3 cells following neutron capture radiation: calculation of RBE by a linear-quadratic model, Annu.Rep.Res.Reactor Inst., Kyoto Univ., 23:91-96.

2. Fertil,B., Dertinger,H., Courdi,A. and Malaise,E.P.,1984, Mean inactivation doses: a useful concept for intercomparison of human cell survival curves, Radiat.Res.,99:73-84.

FURTHER IN VITRO RADIOBIOLOGICAL ANALYSIS ON ^{10}B-BPA BNCT OF MALIGNANT MELANOMA: CORRELATION OF DETERMINED ^{10}B-CONTENT AND CELL KILLING EFFECT

M. Ichihashi[1], M. Shiono[1], K. Yamamura[1], A. Komura[1],
Y. Mishima[1], K. Yoshino[2], T. Kobayashi[3], K. Kanda[3],
H. Fukuda[4] and Y. Hori[5]

[1]Depts. Derm., Special Inst. Cancer Neutron Capture
 Therapy, Kobe Univ. Sch. Med., Kobe 650,
[2]Dept. Chem., Fac. Sci., Shinshu Univ., Matsumoto 390,
[3]Kyoto Univ. Res Reactor Inst., Osaka 590-04,
[4]Natl. Inst. Radiol. Sci., Chiba 280,
[5]Shiseido Res. Cent., Yokohama 223, Japan

INTRODUCTION

The successful application of boron neutron capture therapy (BNCT) for melanoma depends on the following points, (1) high accumulation of ^{10}B in target melanoma cells (approximately 20 ppm) and (2) high tumor/normal tissue ^{10}B ratio, theoretically greater than 5.

We have already experimentally overcome both requirements and achieved successful treatment of several melanoma cases by BNCT using ^{10}B$_1$-paraboronophenylalanine (^{10}B$_1$-BPA)[1].

We are continuing further basic studies to enhance ^{10}B uptake by melanoma cells for the following reasons, (1) neutron radiation fluence could be reduced for safer application and (2) deep-seated melanomas (4-5cm from the skin surface) need to be treatable by BNCT.

Therefore, it is required to find out conditions which will enhance ^{10}B uptake by melanoma cells, and also to develop a method of measuring low ^{10}B levels (up to 0.1 ng/g tissue) using small samples, such as cultured melanoma cells (10^6 cells/dish). Such a method would serve to correlate ^{10}B-content in melanoma cells to its corresponding killing effect in BNCT and to measure increased selective accumulation of ^{10}B$_1$-BPA in melanoma cells as compared to normal cells.

MATERIALS AND METHODS

1.Determine number of cultured cells equivalent to one gram wet tissue
   Protein was extracted by the Schmidt-Thannhanser-Schneider method from 20mg of B-16 melanoma obtained from transplanted tumor mass, and its content (TP) per gram melanoma tissue was measured by the Lowry method[2]. Protein content (CP) of 4 x 10^6 cultured B-16 melanoma cells was also measured by the same method. Cell numbers (N) per gram were calculated as follows, assuming protein content of melanoma cells in vivo to be the same as in vitro.

$$N = \frac{TP}{CP} \times 4 \times 10^6$$

2. Measurement of Boron-10 of cultured cells by inductively coupled plasma-mass spectrometry (ICP-MS)

B-16 melanoma cells were grown in Falcon 3002 dish to semiconfluence and incubated with racemic $^{10}B_1$-BPA or $^{10}B_1$-L-BPA (0, 10, 50, 100, 200 μg/ml) in complete cell culture medium for 0-24 h at 37°C. Cells were washed 3 times with Ca-Mg free phosphate-buffered saline [BPS(-)], then trypsinized for cell count. For ^{10}B determination by ICP-MS, cells collected by rubber policeman were digested with 0.3 ml of 60% perchloric acid and 0.6 ml of 31% hydrogen peroxide, then decomposed for 1 h at 75°C. After membrane filtration (0.45 μm), ^{10}B content of sample solution was assayed by ICP-MS[2]. Yttrium was used as an internal standard.

3. Determination of accumulation characteristics of $^{10}B_1$-BPA in B-16 melanoma cells

$1.0-4.0 \times 10^6$ melanoma cells were incubated for 20 h with Eagle's MEM containing 200 μg $^{10}B_1$-BPA/ml, then the medium was changed with ^{10}B-free medium and continued culture for 0-24 h at 37°C in CO_2 incubator. At 0, 3, 6, 12 and 24 h after the medium change, cells were collected and processed for ^{10}B measurement by ICP-MS.

4. Evaluation of melanoma cell killing by BNCT using racemic and L-isomer $^{10}B_1$-BPA

B-16 melanoma cells incubated with medium containing $^{10}B_1$-D, L-BPA or $^{10}B_1$-L-BPA at various concentrations for 20 h were trypsinized, and 1.5×10^5 cells suspended in normal medium were kept in teflon tube. The teflon tubes were located at different distances from the bismuth surface to obtain various neutron fluences ($0.3-1.5 \times 10^{13} n/cm^2$)[3]. The total elapsed time from the beginning of removal of the cells from the incubation medium and the end of irradiation ranged from 5 1/2 to 6 1/2 hours.

After irradiation, cells were seeded in Falcon 3002 dish and cultured for 10 days. Cells were fixed and stained for colony counting. Either KUR or MITR were used as neutron source.

D_0 values were obtained from dose-survival curves.

RESULTS AND DISCUSSION

The cell number of cultured B-16 melanoma cells equivalent to 1 g wet weight was found to be 1.73×10^8, approximately 1/6 of 1×10^9 which has been widely used as the conversion value.

The ^{10}B concentration of cultured B-16 melanoma cells incubated with 50μg $^{10}B_1$-BPA/ml was 26.0 and 4.5 μg ^{10}B/g cells based on the former and newer calculation ratios respectively.

Melanoma cells incorporated $^{10}B_1$-BPA in a dose and time dependent manner. 1.5-2.0 times more $^{10}B_1$-L-BPA was uptaken by melanoma cells than was by racemic $^{10}B_1$-BPA (Fig. 1).

Further, $^{10}B_1$-L-BPA at the concentration of 200 μg/ml was not found to be cytotoxic and was incorporated as high as 21.4 μg/g cells measured by the new method. These results indicate that $^{10}B_1$-L-BPA is more suitable than racemic BPA for BNCT.

$^{10}B_1$-BPA incorporated into melanoma cells was released rather rapidly into the medium during the first 3 hours (50% remaining in the cells), then ^{10}B-content within the cells decreased gradually up to 24 h after medium change. The results suggest that melanoma cell killing by BNCT using $^{10}B_1$-BPA in vitro may be influenced by the time lag between trypsin treatment and thermal neutron radiation. D_0 values were obtained

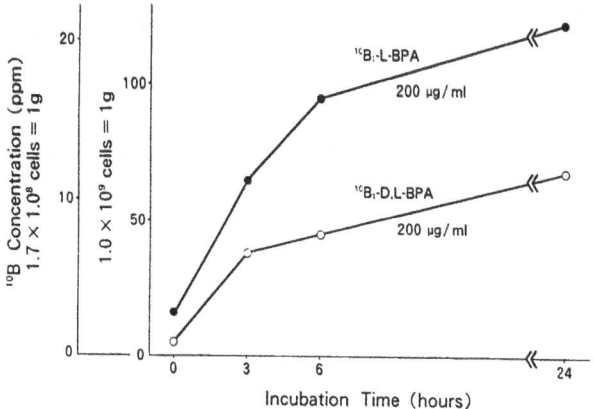

Fig. 1
^{10}B incorporated into B-16
melanoma cells pre-incubated
with $^{10}B_1$-L-BPA (●) or $^{10}B_1$-
D,L-BPA (○) was measured by
ICP-MS.

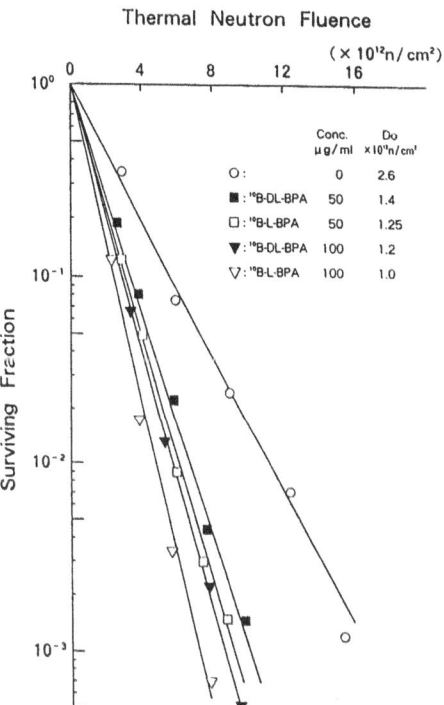

Fig. 2
Dose survival curves of B-16
Melanoma cells, exposed to thermal
neutron radiation after preincubation with various concentrations
of $^{10}B_1$-L-BPA or racemic $^{10}B_1$-BPA.
$^{10}B_1$-L-BPA shows more enhanced
killing of melanoma cells by BNCT
than racemic $^{10}B_1$-BPA.

from dose-survival curves of B-16 melanoma cells exposed to thermal neutron radiation after pre-incubation with $^{10}B_1$-D,L-BPA or $^{10}B_1$-L-BPA (Fig. 2). The D_0 value (1.25×10^{12} n/cm^2) of BNCT using 50 μg $^{10}B_1$-L-BPA/ml was significantly lower than that using racemic $^{10}B_1$-BPA (1.4×10^{12} n/cm^2). Similar results were obtained in other experiments in relevance to ^{10}B-BPA concentrations and isomer type.

Partial replacement of water with D_2O (10-30%) did not increase the uptake of $^{10}B_1$-BPA by cultured melanoma cells, however, an enhanced lethal effect of BNCT using $^{10}B_1$-BPA in D_2O occurred in a dose dependent manner. D_0 values at 0, 20 and 40% D_2O replacement were 1.4×10^{12}, 1.2×10^{12}, and 1.1×10^{12} n/cm^2, respectively.

CONCLUSIONS

1. ICP-MS is useful for measuring a low concentration of ^{10}B in samples.
2. $^{10}B_1$-L-BPA should be used for melanoma treatment by BNCT, since it was proved to be incorporated approximately 1.5-2.0 times more into melanoma cells than racemic $^{10}B_1$-BPA. Further, ^{10}B incorporated into melanoma cells after 24 h incubation with $^{10}B_1$-L-BPA was 21.4 μg/g cells, exceeding the level of ^{10}B content theoretically required for successful BNCT.
3. Partial replacement of normal water with D_2O could be effective in vivo to kill melanoma cells by BNCT.

REFERENCES

1. Mishima Y, Honda C, Ichihashi M, et al: Treatment of malignant melanoma by single thermal neutron capture therapy with melanoma-seeking ^{10}B-compound. Lancet 2:388, 1989.
2. Hori Y, Nakamura K, Matsuoka M et al: Determination of ^{10}B in biological samples by ICP-AES and IPC-MS. The 4th Japan-Australia International Workshop on Thermal Neutron Capture Therapy for Malignant Melanoma, Kobe, Feb. 13-17, 1989.
3. Ichihashi M, Sasase A, Hiramoto T, et al: RBE of thermal neutron capture therapy using $^{10}B_1$-paraboronophynelalanine for human and B-16 melanoma cells. Strahlen und Onkologie 165:198, 1989.

^{157}Gd-NEUTRON CAPTURE: POTENTIAL OF ^{157}Gd-LABELLED DNA LIGANDS FOR NEUTRON CAPTURE THERAPY

R.F. Martin, A. Haigh, C. Monger, M. Pardee
Peter MacCallum Cancer Institute, Melbourne

A.D. Whittaker, D.P. Kelly
Department of Chemistry, University of Melbourne

B.J. Allen
Australian Nuclear Science and Technology Organisation
Menai, NSW Australia

Introduction

The classical feature of BNCT is the limited range of the fission products of the ^{10}B-NC reaction. Although there are other nuclides with higher thermal neutron capture cross sections than that of ^{10}B, these have been considered of limited value for NCT because they are all n, gamma reactions. However, ^{157}Gd, which has the highest thermal neutron capture cross section (250,000 barns) has been re-evaluated in recent years [1,2]. We have been particularly interested in the possibility of exploiting the internal conversion and consequent Auger electron emission associated with the n-gamma reaction. Experiments with ^{157}Gd^{3+} and plasmid DNA demonstrated that DNA-associated ^{157}Gd-NC induces DNA double-strand breaks[1]. DNA-breakage was reduced by sequestering the Gd^{3+} from DNA by addition of EDTA, reflecting the limited range of Auger electrons, which is well-established[3] from experiments with Auger-emitting isotopes such as ^{125}I. These results demonstrate the potential of ^{157}Gd-DNA ligands for NCT, by analogy with the radiobiological effectiveness of ^{125}I decay in DNA[3].

In addition to the requirement that the ^{157}Gd-NC need be on DNA to exploit the Auger effect, there are also general advantages in locating NC events on DNA, from the NCT standpoint. Firstly, DNA is the critical radiobiological target, and the advantages of locating a BNC reaction in the cell nucleus has already been pointed out[4]. Secondly, DNA represents a substantial reservoir of binding sites for DNA ligands. The human genome[5] comprises 7 x 10^{+9}bp, so even at a modest binding ratio of one ligand per 100bp, this reservoir is considerably higher than that for say, cell surface receptors. For a thermal neutron fluence of 10^{13} n cm^{-2}, and one ^{10}B or ^{157}Gd atom per DNA ligand molecule, 7x10^{7} binding sites per genome corresponds to 3 or 180 NC-events per cell, for ^{10}B or ^{157}Gd respectively. However, the extent to which a ligand can occupy these sites without conferring toxicity is obviously critical. The fact that a ligand such as Hoechst 33342 can be used at saturating levels for fractionation of cells according to DNA content, without substantial loss in viability, is encouraging.

We have therefore undertaken the synthesis of ^{157}Gd- and ^{10}B-labelled DNA-binding bibenzimidazoles. The details of the synthesis are described elsewhere in these proceedings[6]. In this paper we report the results of preliminary DNA-binding and cellular uptake experiments with three such ligands.

Experimental

The three ligands tested were:-
-GdDTPA monoHoechst; the Gd chelate of the amide formed between diethylene triaminepentaacetic acid(DTPA) anhydride and an aminoethyl bibenzimidazole,
-GdDTPA bisHoechst; similar to the mono compound except the bisamide of the DTPA anhydride, and
-boroHoechst; the analogue of Hoechst 33342 in which the ethoxy group is replaced with a boronic acid.

All three ligands were purified by reverse-phase HPLC. DNA binding studies were done in 50mM Tris buffer (pH7.5), generally with the ligand at a concentration of 10uM. Calf thymus DNA was included to yield a ligand:DNA bp ratio of 0.1. UV-Vis spectra were recorded on a Varian DMS100 spectrophotometer. In some experiments the buffer also included 0.1M NaCl.

V79 monolayers were cultured as described[7], using 0.5ml chambers on microscope slides. A 20ul sample of the ligands in 20mM acetic acid in 50% methanol was added to give a final ligand concentration of 20uM. After 2 hours at 37°, the monolayers were rinsed in saline, and fixed in 4% formaldehyde in phosphate buffer. The slides were air dried, mounted with coverslips, and examined by fluorescence microscopy.

Results

In the spectrophotometric DNA-binding studies, all three ligands yielded a shift in the absorption maximum of the bibenzimidazole upon addition of DNA, indicative of DNA binding. The shifts for the Gd-monomer, Gd-dimer and boroHoechst were 3,10 and 14nm, respectively. As is the case for other minor-groove binding bibenzimidazoles, the shifts were maintained in 0.1M NaCl.

The fluorescence microscopy studies yielded variable results. For the GdDTPA monoHoechst, uptake was generally poor, with evidence of precipitation. The uptake was much better for the GdDTPA bisHoechst but there was little evidence of concentration in the nucleus, and fluorescence was sometimes apparently more intense on the cell membrane. In contrast, the boroHoechst yielded pictures very similar to those for Hoechst 33342; obvious concentration of the fluorescence in the nucleus and on chromosomes in mitotic figures.

358

Discussion

A major difference between the two Gd-labelled ligands is that for the monomer, the ligand has a net negative charge in the chelate moiety, whereas the dimer is neutral in this respect.

For the monomer, one of the five acetic acid groups is involved in an amide link and the remainder contribute four negative charges compared to the tripositive metal. The dimer has two amide links. This probably explains the poor cellular uptake of the monomer, but although the Gd-dimer is better, it is not ideal. We are hopeful that a smaller ligand, in which a single bibenzimidazole is conjugated to a chelating moiety that yields a neutral chelate with Gd^{3+}, will have improved uptake. However, both the present Gd-ligands will be useful for NC experiments with purified DNA.

The uptake experiments with boroHoechst are very encouraging, although it must be emphasised that the monitoring of fluorescence may grossly over-estimate the ratio of nuclear:cytoplasmic ligand concentrations. We now propose to proceed to NC experiments in V79 cells to monitor cell kill by clonogenic survival. Once a better Gd-labelled ligand is available we will be able to address the main objective of our research program: the relative effectiveness of ^{10}BNC vs $^{157}GdNC$ in DNA, with respect to cell kill. There seems little doubt that the former will be more effective, on a per event basis but it is the extent of the difference which is critical. In terms of therapeutic ratio, ^{157}Gd-DNA ligands will offer an overall advantage compared to ^{10}B-DNA ligands, only if the difference is substantially less than a factor of 60; the ratio capture cross-sections.

Acknowledgements: This project is supported by grants from the Anti-Cancer Counil of Victoria and the Australian Institute of Nuclear Science and Engineering.

References

1. Martin, R.F., D'Cunha, G., Pardee, M., and Allen, B.J. Induction of double-strand breaks following neutron capture by DNA-bound ^{157}Gd. Int. J. Radiat. Biol. 54: 205 (1988).
2. Brugger, R.M., and Shih, J.A., Evaluation of Gadolinium-157 as a neutron capture therapy agent. Strahlenther. Onkol. 165: 153 (1989).
3. Baverstock, K.F., and Charlton, D.E., "DNA Damage by Auger Emitters". Taylor and Francis (1988).
4. Kobayashi, T., and Kanda, K., Analytical calculations of boron dosage in cell nucleus for neutron capture therapy. Radiat. Res. 91: 77 (1982).
5. Alberts, B., Bray, D., Lewis, J., Raff, M., Roberts, K., and Watson, J.D., "Molecular Biology of the Cell", Garland (1983).

6.Whittaker, A., Kelly, D.P., Pardee, M., and Martin, R.F., Synthesis of ^{10}B- and ^{157}Gd-labelled DNA ligands for neutron capture therapy. These proceedings

7.Martin, R.F., Murray, V., D'Cunha, G., Pardee, M., Kampouris, E., Haigh, A., Kelly, D.P., and Hodgson, G.S., Radiation sensitisation by an iodine-labelled DNA ligand. Int. J. Radiat. Biol. 57: 939 (1990).

GADOLINIUM-NEUTRON CAPTURE REACTIONS: A RADIOBIOLOGICAL ASSAY

Y. Akine, N. Tokita, T. Matsumoto, H. Oyama
and O. Aizawa

Departments of Radiation Therapy and Neurosurgery,
The National Cancer Center, Tokyo, Japan and Atomic
Energy Research Laboratory, Musashi Institute of
Technology, Kawasaki, Japan

INTRODUCTION

Gadolinium neutron capture(GNC) therapy as proposed in 1936
by Gordon Locher[1] and recently by others[2,3,4,5,6] takes
advantage of its extraordinarily large cross section to thermal
neutrons. In GNC reactions, prompt high energy gamma rays, x
rays and electrons are released[3]. Because of the photons and
electrons, the intracellular presence of gadolinium is not
considered critical. This is an advantage over boron-neutron
capture therapy where the intracellular presence of boron is
required because of the short flight tracks of 2.4 MeV alpha
particles. In this study, the radiation effect of GNC reactions
was measured using Chinese hamster cells in an attempt to
evaluate the contributions of neutrons, gamma rays and electrons
on cell inactivation.

METHODS

Experiments were carried out using Chinese hamster
cells(V79) maintained as monolayered cultures in dishes
containing Eagle's MEM medium supplemented with 5% fetal bovine
serum in a humidified atmosphere containing 5% carbon dioxide.
Exponentially-growing cells in plastic dishes were trypsinized
and single cell suspensions were prepared. Teflon tubes(6 cm
long, 0.8 cm in outer diameter and 1 mm thick) were filled with
1.7 ml of cell suspensions(at a density of 0.4 million
cells/ml) with or without 5,000 ppm meglumine gadopentetate or
788 ppm Gd-157 (Schering AG, Berlin, Germany) and were exposed
to thermal neutrons generated by a TRIGA II reactor at the
Musashi Institute of Technology with an output of 100 kW[7] at
room temperature. A single teflon tube was used for each dose
point except for the 5 Gy dose point where two teflon tubes were
used to provide adequete numbers of cells for plating. After
exposure cells were plated onto 6 petri dishes for each and
colonies were counted after 7 days.   Two separate experiments
were carried out. Gamma rays produced in the sample and from the
reactor core were measured with (Mg2 SiO4;Tb) TLDs; and for
thermal neutrons, by gold foils. Doses from electrons were not
measured. Gamma dose rates measured for a teflon tube filled
with 1.7 ml of water, or 1.7 ml of cell samples containing 5,000

ppm gadolinium were 1.05 Gy/hr and 10.3 Gy/hr, respectively. There was a 35% depression of the thermal neutron fluence across the teflon tube as a result of absorption by the gadolinium-containing water. The fast neutron flux in the field was estimated to be 0.1% of the thermal neutron flux[7]. X-irradiation of cells was carried out in a similar manner using 250 kVp x-rays at a dose rate of 0.8 Gy/min at room temperature.

RESULTS AND DISCUSSION

A simple exponential survival curve was obtained for cells exposed to neutrons in the absence of gadolinium(Gd-), and the surviving fraction was expressed as S=EXP-[0.41N] where N= neutron fluence/10**12*cm**2. The survival curve for cells exposed in the presence of gadolinium(Gd+) exhibited a shoulder in the low neutron fluence region with the survival expressed as

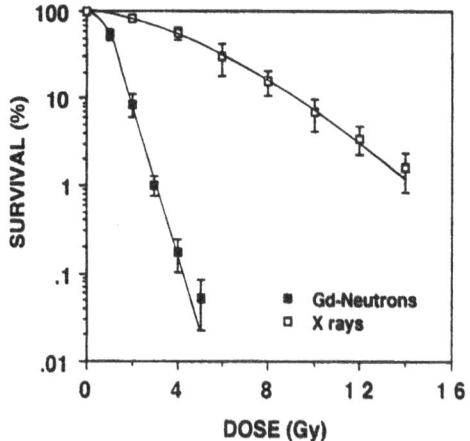

Fig. 1. Cell survival curves for Gd+ cells exposed to neutrons or x-irradiated cells plotted as a function of dose.

S=EXP-[0.87N+0.4N**2]. Comparison of the results at 10% survival levels shows that there was a 3.5-fold difference in neutron fluence (5.4*10**12 neutrons/cm**2 for GD- cells, and 1.55*10**12 neutrons/cm**2 for Gd+ cells). Gd+ cells required a considerably less number of neutrons and the cytocidal effect seemed to come largely from non-neutron radiations.

The same survival data were evaluated based on the available dosimetry data, which consisted of doses from neutrons, gamma rays from GNC reactions and from the core, but not from electrons. In Gd+ cells the contribution of neutrons was found to be small when compared to photons and electrons emitted from GNC reactions. There is a significant difference in the 10% survival doses between Gd+ cells(1.9 Gy) and X-irradiated cells(9.1 Gy)(Fig.1). The difference seems to result from the contribution of electrons and it is several-fold greater than that of gamma rays from GNC reactions. Although the RBE value of these electrons are not known at present, it appears that in GNC reactions a significant proportion of the radiation effect results from electrons.

This prediction, if comfirmed, will lead to a conclusion that the dose distribution within the treatment volume may be different from what has been expected with 7 MeV gamma rays. To verify the results, electrons dosimetry and estimation of RBE value are needed.

The Gd-157 concentration, in terms of the number of atoms per weight, used in this study was similar to that used in boron neutron capture therapy when taking into account the abundance ratio of 15.6% for Gd-157. Recently Gd-157 enriched to 90.96% abundunce has become commercially available and the use of the enriched form, presently being explored, will certainly result in a several-fold increase in the intensity of radiation released from GNC reactions for a given gadolinium concentration.

A physical disadvantage of thermal neutrons lies in the poor depth penetration in tissue. This has led to consider epithermal neutrons for therapy. Conde, et al. has proposed KeV neutrons produced in a spallation process by 72 MeV protons[8]. It is clinically far more desirable if slow neutrons are produced by an accelerator rather than by a reactor.

Successful therapy demands a higher Gd-157 concentration in tumors and a lower value in the normal tissue. One of our current efforts has been to deliver gadolinium to tumors by means of trascatheter arterial embolization (TAE) which results in prolonged retention of gadolinium in tumors as used in the treatment of liver tumors with iodine-containing oil. Another approach being explored is to develop and deliver Gd-157 deoxyuridine(GdUdR) through a feeding artery to be picked up by dividing tumor cells.

REFERENCES

1. Locher G L. Biological effects and therapeutic possibilities of neutrons. Amer J Roentgenol. 36:1,1936.
2. Martin R F, D'Cunha G, Pardee M and Allen B J. Induction of double-strand breaks following neutron capture by DNA-bound Gd-157. Int J Radia Biol. 54: 205, 1988.
3. Allen B J,McGregor B J and Martin R F. Neutron capture therapy with Gd-157. Strahlenther Onkol. 165: 156,1989.
4. Brugger R M and Shih J A. Evaluation of gadolinium-157 as a neutron capture therapy agent. Strahlenther Onkol. 165: 153,1989.
5. Ryabukhin Y S. Integrated approach in the planning of neutron capture therapy. Strahlenther Onkol. 165:158, 1989.
6. Akine Y, Tokita N,Matsumoto T, Oyama H, Egawa S, Aizawa O. Radiation effect of gadolinium-neutron capture reactions on the survival of Chinese hamster cells. Strahlenther Onkol. 166: 831, 1990.
7. Matsumoto T. Aizawa O, Nozaki T and Sato T.Present status of the medical irradiation facility at the Musashi reactor. Pigment Cell Res 2: 240, 1989.
8. Conde H, Crawford J F, Dahl B, Grussel E, Larsson B, Petterson C B, Reist H, Sjostrand N G, Sornsuntisook O and Thuresson L. The production by 72 MeV protons of keV neutrons for B-10 neutron capture therapy. Strahlenther Onkol. 165: 340,1989.

IN VITRO BIOLOGICAL EFFICACY OF BORONATED LOW DENSITY

LIPOPROTEINS FOR NCT

Stephen B. Kahl[1], David Pate[1], Brenda H. Laster[2], Edward A. Popenoe[2]
and Ralph G. Fairchild[2]
[1]Department of Pharmaceutical Chemistry
University of California, San Francisco
[2]Medical Department, Brookhaven National Laboratory

ABSTRACT

Low Density Lipoproteins (LDLs) are known to be internalized within the cell by receptor-mediated mechanisms. There is evidence that LDLs may be taken up avidly by tumor cells to provide cholesterol for the synthesis of cell membrane. Thus, the possibility exists that LDLs may provide an ideal vehicle for the transport of boron to tumor cells for Neutron Capture Therapy (NCT). A boronated analog of LDL has recently been synthesized for possible application in NCT. The analog was tested in cell culture for uptake and biological efficacy in the thermal neutron beam at the Brookhaven Medical Research Reactor (BMRR). It was found that boron concentrations ten times higher than that required for NCT were easily obtained, and that uptake data were constant with a receptor mediated binding mechanism. The measured intracellular concentration of ~240 μg ^{10}B/g cells is significantly higher than that obtained with any other boron compound previously evaluated for possible clinical application.

INTRODUCTION

The utilization of receptor-mediated uptake mechanisms (as are operational with low-density lipoproteins, or LDLs) presents the possibility of long-term binding, as well as internalization of the boron compounds. The metabolism of LDLs has recently been explored by Brown and Goldstein (1,2). As the major cholesterol transport agent from plasma to cells, LDL binds to specific, cell surface receptors, is internalized *via* endocytosis, and is processed by lysozomal action. It has been estimated that 90% or more of intracellular cholesterol is derived from receptor-mediated importation and less than 10% by *de novo* synthesis. Selective targeting of boron *via* boronated LDL is predicated on the assumption that LDL flux is inherently higher in cancer cells. This follows on the assumption that cholesterol requirements are greater due increased cell membrane synthesis as a consequence of high turnover and replication rates. While LDL metabolism is a relatively new field, with little overall knowledge of LDL receptor site densities in normal and transformed cells, there are a number of reports of significantly increased LDL flux in cancer cells (3,4).

MATERIALS AND METHODS

^{10}B-enriched elaidyl carborane carboxylate was synthesized from ^{10}B-enriched carborane carboxylic acid and elaidyl alcohol as described in reference 5. The ester was reconstituted into human low density lipoprotein as described in reference 6. Analysis of boronated LDL by prompt gamma ray spectrometry gave an average of ~12,000 boron atoms per LDL, equivalent to 20% boron per unit protein weight.

CHO and V-79 Chinese hamster cells in logarithmic growth were maintained in DME growth medium (Gibco) supplemented with 10% fetal bovine serum (Hyclone), 1% penn-strep-fungison (Gibco), and 2.0 mM L-glutamine. Detailed procedures are given in ref. (7).

Irradiations were carried out at the thermal neutron beam of the Brookhaven Medical Research Reactor (BMRR) in 1.5 cm Eppendorf microfuge tubes with the thermal neutron fluence rate being $2.8 \times 10^{11} n_{th}$ cm^{-2} min^{-1} at the center of the tube. Gamma irradiations were carried out using a 9000 Ci ^{137}Cs source at the Biology Department's Controlled Environmental Radiation Facility (CERF), at a dose rate of ~50 rads/min.

Survival was determined by colony assay; D_0 values were obtained by measuring the difference in irradiation time which reduced survival by a factor of $1/e$ on the linear portion of the curve. D_0 is expressed in units of time throughout this paper as the latter is the most basic parameter (8). Conversion to absorbed dose, biologically effective dose, fluence of thermal neutrons, etc. can be carried out directly using readily available BMRR beam data.

The biological efficacy of boronated LDLs was evaluated in terms of equivalent amounts of ^{10}B in the form of boric (H_3BO_3), or "boric acid equivalents"; the latter procedure is described in detail in ref. 7. This method of analysis is carried out in order to quantitate the results of an unknown boron distribution, in terms of a known quantity such as boric acid (H_3BO_3), where a uniform distribution inside and outside the cell is assumed. In order to obtain "boric acid equivalents", V-79 cells were grown in the presence of (H_3BO_3) in concentrations of 15 and 30 μg ^{10}B/g. If one uses the multi-hit formula $S = 1 - \{1 - exp(-D/D_0)\}^n$ and evaluates the slope of the survival curve in the linear portion when plotted on semi-log paper, the inverse of the slope is the dose in terms of time (or neutron fluence) that it takes to reduce survival by a factor of "e" (i.e., by 63%). The slope will be a linear function of ^{10}B content, so that if the negative slope is plotted vs ^{10}B content, a straight line is obtained, with its intercept on the abscissa equivalent to the slope produced by the adventitious or "background" radiations alone (7). Thus, if the negative inverse of D_0 for any experiment is evaluated from the calibration curve described above, the boron response in terms of equivalent concentration of ($H_3{}^{10}BO_3$) in μg ^{10}B/g can be obtained (boric acid equivalents), free of effects from contaminating radiations.

The growth medium in each experiment was analyzed for boron concentration in the prompt-γ-neutron activation analysis facility at the BMRR (8). For analysis of ^{10}B in cells, ~10^8 cells were grown in boronated growth medium, washed thoroughly, pelletized, and adjusted to 1 g with deionized water prior to activation.

RESULTS

Hamster V-79 and CHO cells were incubated for ~1 cell cycle (16 hours) at 37° in the presence of ~23 μg ^{10}B/ml of growth medium, washed thoroughly and then irradiated in the thermal neutron beam. Results are shown for CHO cells in Figure 1; similar results were obtained with V-79 cells. For comparison, survival curves obtained under similar conditions (30 μg ^{10}B/g) with $Na_2B_{12}H_{11}SH$ (BSH) and the boronated porphyrin BOPP. Calculated D_0's and the resulting boric acid equivalents for the above curves are summarized in Table 1. It is readily apparent that the biological efficacy of boronated LDL is ~10 times that of the boronated porphyrin in BOPP and ~100 times that of BSH.

Direct boron analysis (by neutron activation) of CHO cells incubated for 1 cell cycle in 19.5 μg ^{10}B/g of B-LDL and then washed 2 times prior to analysis, shows an absolute concentration of ~239 μg ^{10}B/g. Since the biological efficacy is equivalent to 100 μg ^{10}B/g of boric acid, one can assume that the boron location is predominantly intracellular. This follows since it is known that with V-79 cells, an extracellular location provide 10% of the effective nuclear dose from a uniform distribution, while cytoplasmic and nuclear location provide 45% each of the remaining dose (9). If, for example, the location of boron was extracellular, the absolute ^{10}B concentration would have had to have been ~1000 μg/g to obtain the observed response. Thus, these data are consistent only with a cytoplasmic (or intracellular) location of B-LDLs.

DISCUSSION

Our results clearly indicate that boronated LDL is recognized by the LDL receptor and is taken up by a process which is consistent with receptor-mediated endocytosis. Repeated washings of cells with boron-free medium did not result in wash-out of the boron, suggesting that once the LDL complex has been internalized the boronated contents of the hydrophobic core remain bound intracellularly. Cell survival experiments support the notion of a cytoplasmic locus for the [10]B since comparison with a compound having uniform distribution inside and outside the cell (H_3BO_3) shows an enhanced cell killing effect for the boronated LDL as predicted by Monte Carlo calculations (8).

When incubated with cells at boron concentrations similar to those used with other candidate NCT delivery agents, intracellular [10]B concentrations of ~240 μg [10]B/g are easily

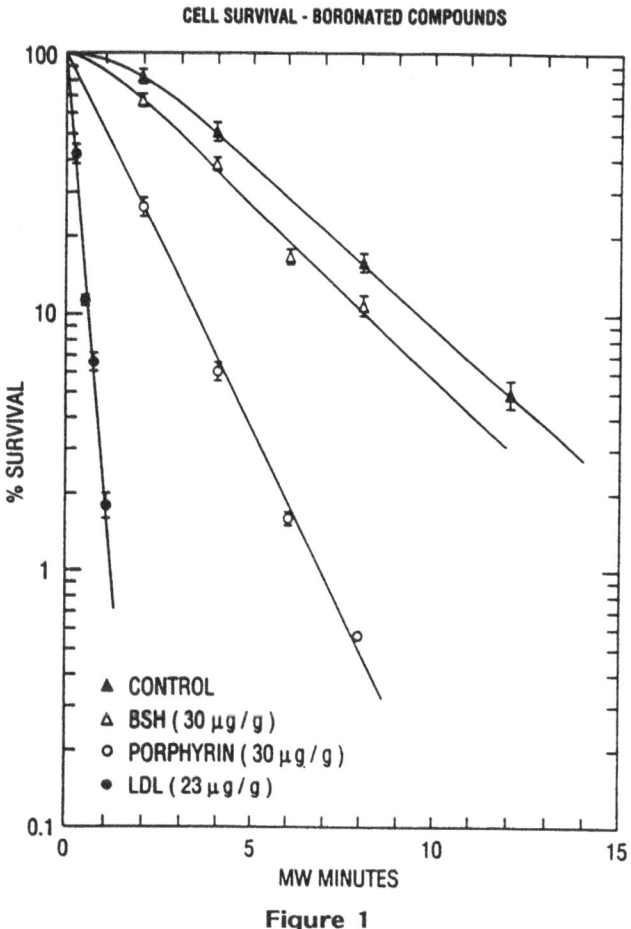

Figure 1

Comparative CHO cell survival curves for 16 hour incubation in the presence of various boron carriers. Following the boron pulse, cells were washed 3x with boron-free medium and irradiated at the thermal neutron beam port of the BMRR.

obtained. This value is an order of magnitude greater than the 20 μg/g generally regarded as necessary for BNCT. In fact, boronated LDL uptake, retention and biological efficacy *in vitro* are far greater than with any compound yet studied. If similar results are obtained *in vivo*, especially in the case of glioma where the normal blood brain barrier completely excludes low density lipoproteins, the possibility exists that boronated LDL may have major beneficial consequences for neutron capture therapy.

Table 1

Comparative D_0's and Boric Acid Equivalents from Figure 1

Compound	^{10}B conc. (µg/g)	D_0(min)	Boric Acid Equivalents (µg ^{10}B/g)
$Na_2B_{12}H_{11}SH$	30.0	3.3	0.5
BOPP	30.0	1.2	11.4
LDL	23.0	0.20	100.0
LDL	3.5	0.50	38.0

REFERENCES

1. Brown MS, Kovanen RT, and Goldstein JL, *Science* **212**:628 (1981).
2. Goldstein JL, Anderson RGW, and Brown MS. *Nature* **279**:679 (1979).
3. Gal D, Obashi M, McDonald PC, Bushbaum HJ, and Simpson E, *Gynecol.* **139**:877(1981).
4. Vitols SJ, Goldstein JL, Brown MS, Ralph JR, and Anderson RAW, *Proc. Natl. Acad. Sci. USA* **78**:5717 (1981).
5. Kahl SB, *Tetrahedron Lett.* **31**:1517 (1990).
6. Kahl SB and Callaway JC, *Strahlenther. Onkol.* 165:137 (1989).
7. Fairchild RG, Kahl SB, Laster BH, Kaelf-Ezra J, and Popenoe EA, *Cancer Res.* **50**:4860 (1990).
8. Fairchild RG, Gabel D, Laster BH, Greenberg D, Kiszenick W, and Micca PL, *Med. Phys.* **13**:50 (1986).
9. Gabel D, Foster S, and Fairchild RG. *Radiat. Res.* **111**:14 (1987).

IN VITRO INCORPORATION OF BORONOPHENYLALANINE BY AMELANOTIC AND MELANOTIC

MURINE AND HUMAN MALIGNANT MELANOMA CELL LINES

J.K. Brown[1], B.J. Allen[1], J.E. Chapman[1], M.H. Mountford[1], P.Parsons[2]

[1] Biomedicine and Health Program, Australian Nuclear Science and Technology Organisation PMB 1 Menai NSW 2234 Australia
[2] Queensland Institute of Medical Research, Herston, Queensland 4006, Australia

INTRODUCTION

In an earlier experiment[1], thermal neutron cell survival dose response curves were generated for early plateau phase cultures of three human malignant melanoma cell lines.

Pelleted cells were irradiated as previously described[1], following a 20 h incubation in RPM1 1640 medium, in the presence or absence of 10µg/ml D,L-paraboronophenylalanine hydrochloride ($^{10}B_1$-BPA.HCl). Thermal neutrons were derived from Moata, a 100-kW Argonaut-type light water reactor. The neutron flux was 2.6×10^9 $n/cm^2/s$, dose rate 3.7 Gy/h (n+γ) and the dose range 0.6 - 8.0 Gy. Cells were plated onto X-irradiated feeder layers in triplicate in $25cm^2$ Falcon flasks and colonies counted after 11-12 days. No differences in thermal neutron radiosensitivity were observed for two amelanotic cell lines (96E, 96L). A small but significant difference was observed for the melanotic cell line (418) grown in the presence or absence of BPA (D_0 values of 1.03 and 1.15 Gy respectively)[1].

Subsequent experiments showed that the uptake of boron was low in the B16 murine malignant melanoma cell line cultured in the presence of BPA. It was therefore necessary to investigate the boron uptake and incorporation in melanoma cells by increasing the BPA concentration, increasing melanisation using different variants of the B16 cell lines, and alternative methods of cell layer detachment.

METHOD

To improve uptake, the concentration of BPA was increased from 10 to 50 µg/ml and melanogenesis increased by the addition of 1mM theophylline to the RPMI medium. Cellular changes were observed in cells grown three days in theophylline medium: melanin was frequently seen as discrete polar bodies in swollen elliptical shaped cells in the population. These cells were easily ruptured, e.g. when harvested by scraping off the cell layer. Consequently, B16 cells for melanin and boron estimation were routinely harvested from two day cultures containing theophylline in which the cells did not show microscopic evidence of change.

About 40% of the boron incorporated by the CMc human malignant melanoma cell line, following incubation with a boronated monoclonal antibody, was lost when the cell layer was detached using trypsine-versene solution[2]. The possibility of boron loss from "melanised" B16 cells by trypsination was therefore investigated by comparing the boron content of two identical batches of B16 cells (and the supernatants after centrifugation of the cells) cultured two days in 1mM theopylline medium and 50 µg/ml BPA. Two methods were used for detaching the cells: trypsin-versene treatment (TV) or scraping off the cell layer (SO).

RESULTS

The results in Table 1 show that the boron content of the TV and SO supernatants was extremely low, similar in fact to the background level of boron in the reagent blank and cells cultured without boron. If confirmed, this suggests that the harvest of B16 cells by TV treatment does not elute boron incorporated intracellularly.

Table 1

Sample	No. of cells x 10^6	Boron uptake µg	Boron uptake µ g/10^9 cells
Cells TV (+B)	14.6	0.220	15.0
Cells SO (+B)	14.4	0.173	12.0
Supernatant TV	–	0.014	–
Supernatant SO	–	<0.013	–
Reagent blank	–	<0.013	–
Cell blank (-B)	22.1	<0.013	<0.6

The kinetics of melanin production and boron incorporation were examined in two subcultures of the Japanese B16 melanoma cell line received in Australia in June 1987 (designated B16) and in November 1988 (designated J-B16). The two subcultures differed in morphology and cellular properties when grown in Eagle's MEM or RPMI 1640 medium.

Table 2 lists data for several sets of measurement of plating efficiency (PE) and doubling time (DT). PE values were derived from five experiments with six petri dishes per experiment. Doubling times were calculated from serial cell counts of duplicate Falcon flasks harvested over the period 24 to 72h. Melanin was estimated[3] and boron determined by ICP analysis[4]. Melanin and boron were estimated simultaneously in two day theophylline medium for a terminal 20 h incubation and 50 µg/ml BPA.

Table 2

Cell Strain	Culture Medium	PE %	DT h	Melanin pg/cell +Th	Boron µg/10^9 cells +Th
B16	RPMI	75.5	18.7	14.7	8
B16	MEM	44.6	22.2	23.7	5
J-B16	RPMI	54.3	21.3	3.7	30
J-B16	MEM	29.1	28.3	4.1	11

The highest PE and shortest DT was observed for both B16 cell lines cultured in RPMI (medium used in Australia) and the lowest PE and longest DT in MEM (medium used in Japan) (Table 2). This is perhaps consistent with the higher concentrations and more varied ingredients in the RPMI medium formulation compared to MEM medium, although it is interesting to note that the latter medium contains higher concentrations of phenylalanine and tyrosine.

Striking differences in melanin content were observed between B16 and J-B16 cells in the different media (Table 2) containing 1mM theophylline (+Th) and 50 μg/ml BPA. The highest melanin content was detected in B16 cells cultured in MEM medium. These cells in ordinary medium (-Th) have a low melanin content such that the pellated cells show only a light buff colouration in contrast to the black pellets derived from cells grown two days in theophylline enriched medium. On average the melanin content of "melanised" B16 was about five times higher than J-B16 cells similarly treated.

Depending on cell type and medium the concentration of cellular boron varied widely with the highest uptake being recorded for J-B16 cells. Results to date, contrary to the finding of previous investigators, appear to show an inverse relationship between melanin content and boron uptake. However, the low number of cells processed in many samples for boron estimation in this group of samples casts doubt on the validity of the present results and indicates the need for confirmatory experiments.

CONCLUSIONS

The striking difference in cellular properties between the two strains of B16 cells in this study provides a clear indication of the importance of standardising cell cultures procedures for in vitro experimentation. The continuous culture of cells, especially if stressed, results in the selection of different cell types with altered phenotypic and genetic expression. To avoid such changes several criteria should be adopted: use of pure characterised cell lines, experimental use of cells for only 10-30 generations and the maintenance of a repository stock of the cell type to maintain consistency in vitro. Unless these precautions are exercised there is a good likelihood that the results of experiments on in vitro cell cultures will have little value scientifically relative to the in vivo situation.

REFERENCES

1.   K.J. Brown, M.H. Mountford, B.J. Allen, Y. Mishima, M. Ichihashi, and P. Parsons. Neutron irradiation of human melanoma cells. Pigment Cell Res. 2:319-374 (1989).

2.   S.R. Tamat. Boron Containing Pharmaceuticals for Neutron Capture Therapy of Malignant Melanoma, Thesis, University of Sydney, Australia, p.146-148 (1988).

3.   P.G. Parsons, and B.J. Allen. Accumulation of chloropromazine and thiouracil by human melanoma cells in culture. Aust. J. Exp. Med. Sci. 64:517-526 (1986).

4.   S.R. Tamat, D.E. Moore, and B.J. Allen. Boron assay in biological tissue by inductively coupled plasma atomic emission spectroscopy. Anal. Chem. 59, 2161-2164 (1987).

STUDIES ON THE UPTAKE OF PARA-BORONOPHENYLALANINE

IN MELANOMA CELLS

M. Papageorges,[1] C. A. Elstad,[2] G. G. Meadows,[2]
P. R. Gavin,[1] R. D. Sande,[1] and W. F. Bauer[3]

[1]College of Veterinary Medicine, Washington State University,
Pullman, WA   99164-6610
[2]College of Pharmacy, Washington State University, Pullman, WA
99164
[3]PBF/BNCT Research Programs, Idaho National Engineering
Laboratory, P.O. Box 1625, Idaho Falls, ID   83415-3519

INTRODUCTION

Cell-associated boron levels adequate for neutron capture therapy
(NCT) have been demonstrated *in-vitro* using cultured melanoma cells[1] and
in-vivo using xenografts in mice.[2-5] Preliminary *in-vivo* studies performed
by researchers at the College of Veterinary Medicine, Washington State
University (WSU), using a spontaneous canine melanoma model, showed
subtherapeutic tumor concentrations of para-boronophenylananine (p-BPA) in
a large proportion of dogs. Possible explanations include poor solubility
of p-BPA at physiological pH, physiological differences between transplanted and spontaneous tumors, and lack of metabolic incorporation at the
cellular level.[2-5]

Reports of *in-vitro* p-BPA uptake studies are few and contradic-
tory,[1,4] and the kinetics of boron uptake at the average p-BOA blood
concentration achieved in dogs (100 mg/L) is unknown. *In-vitro* and *in-
vivo* experiments were designed to study boron loading in melanoma cells
and to test the hypothesis that short-term tyrosine and phenylalanine
deprivation can increase the uptake of p-BPA.[1-3,5]

METHODS

Murine melanotic melanoma cells (B16-BL6) were grown *in-vitro* to
subconfluence and incubated with p-BPA (200 mg/L) in cell culture medium
for 0-12 hours at 37 °C. Cells were also incubated with p-BPA (100 mg/L)
for three hours at 0, 21, and 37 °C. Cells were washed three times with
Ca-Mg free Hanks' solution (CMF), detached with ethylene glycol tetra-
acetic acid (EGTA), counted by hemocytometer count, centrifuged, and
frozen. The boron content of the pellets was determined by inductively
coupled plasma-atomic emission spectroscopy (ICP-AES) analysis and
normalized for cell number. Cells were incubated with p-BPA before and
after being detached with EGTA, and the effect of EGTA and trypsin on
cell-associated boron was compared. Cells were incubated in a tyrosine-
phenylalanine deficient (88% decrease from normal levels[6]) cell culture
medium for 24 hours before incubation with p-BPA (100 mg/L).

Three nude mice, bearing canine melanoma xenografts, received p-BPA
by intraperitoneal injection (750 mg/kg) when tumors were larger than 1 cm
in diameter. Mice were sacrificed by cervical dislocation and boron
concentration in various tissues was determined by ICP-AES analysis.

Progress in Neutron Capture Therapy for Cancer
Edited by B.J. Allen *et al.*, Plenum Press, New York, 1992

RESULTS

The measured cell-associated boron was lower than that required for NCT (< 20 ppm) in all *in-vitro* assays. There was no increase in cell-associated boron uptake during longer incubation times. Preincubation in a tyrosine/phenylalanine deficient medium seemed to increase the amount of cell-associated boron (Figure 1). The analytical method, however, appeared to overestimate the amount of cell-associated boron for smaller samples (Figure 2) and the number of cells in the tyrosine/phenylalanine deficient group was 2-3 times lower. There was only minimal increase in cell-associated boron in cells incubated at 37 °C, compared to cells incubated at 0 and 21 °cells (Figure 3).

Detaching cells with EGTA before incubation with p-BPA reduced the amount of cell-associated boron compared to detaching the cells after p-BPA incubation, but a second incubation with EGTA did not reduce it further. Cell-associated boron was similar whether cells were detached with EGTA or trypsin after incubation with p-BPA (Figure 4). Boron concentration in the xenografts was higher than in all other tissues evaluated and higher than the *in-vitro* results (Figure 5).

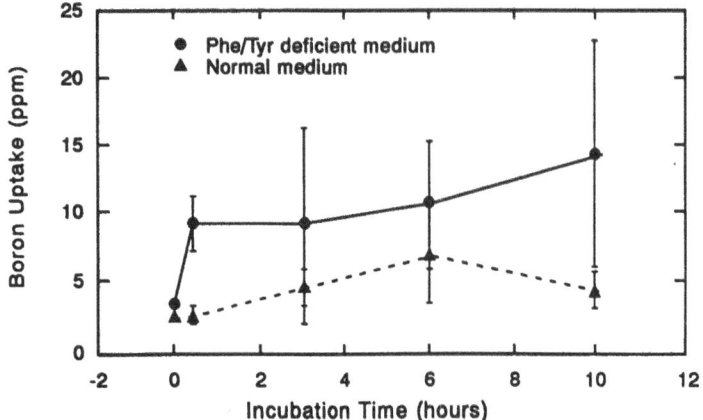

Figure 1.   Cell-associated boron measured by ICP-AES with p-BPA after in-vitro incubation.

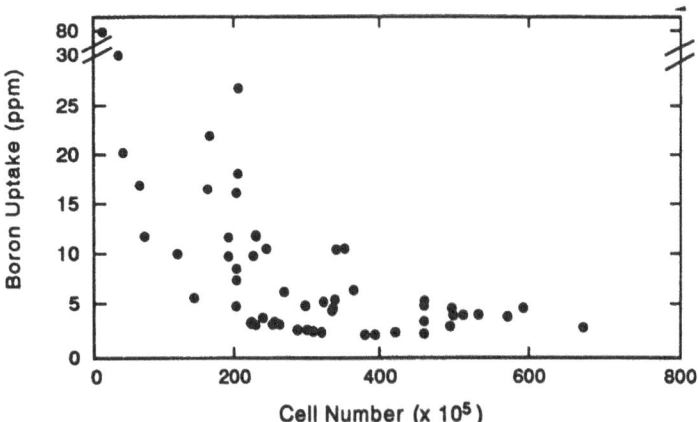

Figure 2.   Correlation between sample mass and cell-associated boron measured by ICP-AES.

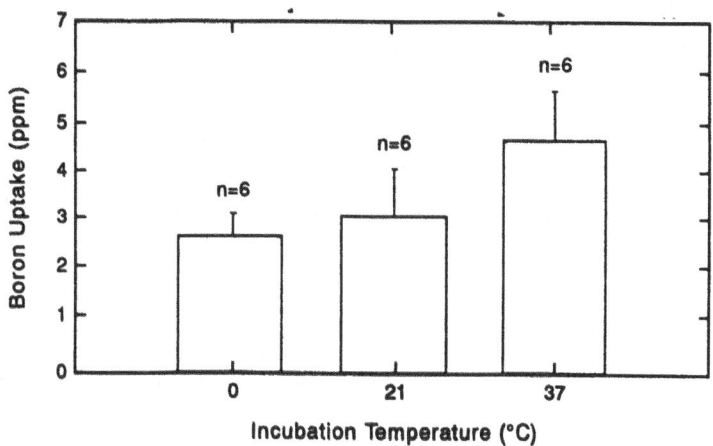

Figure 3. Effect of different temperature of incubation
on cell-associated boron measured by ICP-AES.

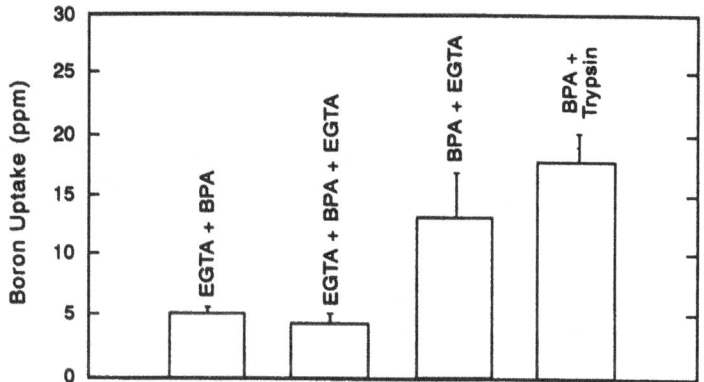

Figure 4. Effect of different methods of detaching cells
on cell-associated boron determination by ICP-AES.

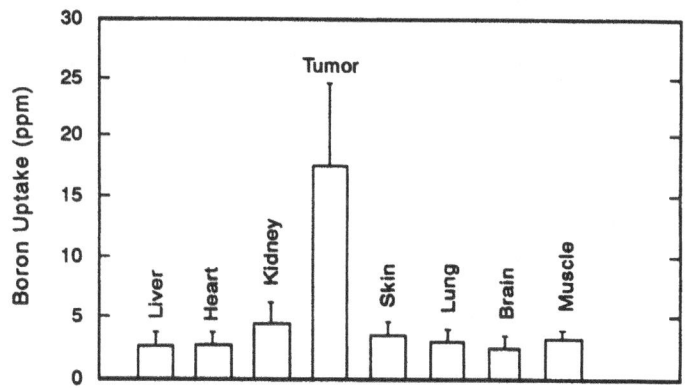

Figure 5. Biodistribution of boron in three nude mice.

DISCUSSION AND CONCLUSIONS

Cell-associated boron, as measured by ICP-AES, was insufficient for NCT when B16-BL6 cells were incubated *in-vitro* with p-BPA at a concentration of 100 mg/L (5 ppm of boron). Boron concentration in canine tumors transplanted in nude mice were higher and similar to those previously reported.[2,4,5] The reasons for the difference between *in-vitro* and *in-vivo* boron uptake and the difference between the murine and canine model are undetermined. Temporary higher blood p-BPA concentrations might be achieved in the mouse model, or there might be significant differences affecting boron uptake between transplanted and spontaneous tumors. Differences between *in-vitro* and *in-vivo* boron uptake should be studied using dose-response curves.

The absence of temperature-dependent uptake mechanisms and the fact that longer incubation did not significantly increase the amount of cell-associated boron suggest passive diffusion or binding to a cellular component without metabolic incorporation. These findings support those of others who found that continuous infusion of p-BPA did not increase boron concentration in melanomas transplanted in mice.[2] Whether boron is cleaved from the phenylalanine or the entire molecule is not incorporated is unknown. Preincubation of melanoma cells in a medium deficient in phenylalanine and tyrosine prior to incubation with p-BPA at a concentration of 100 mg/L (5 ppm of boron) might increase cell-associated boron levels, but levels suitable for NCT were not obtained.

Methods to detach cells and measure cell-associated boron should be compared to reduce the possibility of artifactitious boron determinations. Tumor-boron uptake, obtained with potential boron-delivery agents, should be studied using more than one model.

REFERENCES

1. Ichihashi, M., et al., "Specific Killing Effect of $^{10}B_1$-para-borono-phenylalanine in Thermal Neutron Capture of Malignant Melanoma: *In-Vitro* Radiobiological Evaluation," J. Invest. Dermatol. 78: 215-218 (1982).

2. Coderre, J. A., et al., "Selective Targeting of Boronophenylalanine in Melanoma in BALB/C Mice," Cancer Res. 47: 6377-6383 (1987).

3. Coderre, J. A., et al., "Boron Neutron Capture Therapy of a Murine Melanoma," Cancer Res. 48: 6313-6383 (1987).

4. Allen, B. J., et al., "*In-Vitro* and *In-Vivo* Studies of Boron Conjugated Melanoma Affined Biochemicals," Strahlen. & Onkol. 165: (2/3) 163-165 (1989).

5. Coderre, J. A., et al., "Selective Delivery of Boron by the Melanin Precursor Analogue p-boronophenylalanine to Tumors Other than Melanomas," Cancer Res. 50: 138-141 (1990).

6. Meadows, G. G., et al., "Dietary Influence of Tyrosine and Phenylalanine on the Response of B16 Melanoma to Carbidopa-Levodopa Methyl-Ester Chemotherapy," Cancer Res. 42: 3056-3063 (1982).

STUDIES TO USE FISSION NEUTRONS IN BNCT FOR DEEPER TUMOR LESION

Tsuyoshi Kadosawa[1], Munekazu Nakaichi[1], Tomihisa Kawasaki[1], Akira Takeuchi[1], Tetsuo Matsumoto[2], Hiroaki Wakabayashi[3]

1)Department of Veterinary Surgery, the University of Tokyo
2)Atomic Energy Research Laboratory, Musashi Institute of Technology
3)Nuclear Engineering Research Laboratory, the University of Tokyo

INTRODUCTION

When applying the selectivity of boron neutron capture therapy (BNCT) in the treatment of the tumors, the rapid attenuation of thermal neutrons in tissue presents serious limitations. Our basic idea was to irradiate a tumor in an acrylic block (30x 30x30cm^3) with fission neutrons and, in adjunct to the therapeutic effects of fast neutrons, to take advantage of thermalization of fast and epithermal neutrons within the acrylate or tissues for the BNCT of a deep neoplastic lesion[1].

The possibility of using fission neutrons for BNCT was studied by comparing the effects of the $^{10}B(n, \alpha)^7Li$ reaction and fast neutrons with the effects of γ-rays (^{137}Cs) on the colony forming ability of irradiated V-79 Chinese hamster cells. The depth to which the irradiated tumor might receive a higher dose than normal tissue was calculated.

MATERIALS AND METHODS
Cell culture

V-79 Chinese hamster cells were cultured in MEM medium containing 10% fetal calf serum and gentamicin (50μg/ml) and fungizone (1.5μg/ml), buffered with 5% CO_2 in air. Before irradiation, these cells were grown in 25cm^2 plastic flasks (Falcon) for 24 hours. Cells were incubated in medium containing 80μg^{10}B/ml (140μg$Na_2B_{12}H_{11}SH$/ml) for the latter 12 hours of the 24 hours' incubation. Just prior to irradiation, the medium was poured off and cells were washed twice with PBS. After irradiation, cells were detached from the flask by trypsinization (0.1% trypsin and 0.02% EDTA) and plated in 80mm petri dishes with 10ml medium (yielding between 50 and 100 colonies). For each dose, 4-8 dishes were used. After incubation for 7-10 days the colonies were fixed and stained with formaldehyde and crystal violet. Colonies in excess of 50 cells were counted manually.

Boron uptake by V-79 cells in culture

V-79 cells were grown in the medium containing 80μg^{10}B/ml for 12 hours. The cells were suspended by trypsinization and washed three times with PBS. Three specimens with approximately 3x10^{8}cells were analyzed for boron content by a colorimetric method[2].

Irradiation

Fission neutrons used in this study were from the reactor "YAYOI" of the University of Tokyo. YAYOI is a 2kW rated fast neutron source reactor ($\overline{En}$=0.9MeV)[3]. In this study, in order to scatter fast neutrons, an Al rod (ϕ5.2x20cm) was set in the center of the irradiation field. Fission neutrons were used to irradiate an acrylic block (30

x30x30cm^3, located 15 cm from the exit of 9x9cm^2 collimator) in which 25cm^2 culture
flasks were set at 4 cm from the surface. Fast neutron and γ-ray doses were measured
at the surface of the acryl block and the culture flask by paired ionization chambers
(gas flow type). Thermal neutron flux distributions were measured both axially and
laterally using Au foils with and without Cd cover and taking their difference.
Furthermore, In foils and TLD were used to check the fluence of fast neutron and
γ-ray dose when V-79 cells were irradiated. The fast neutron flux was calculated by
measuring 335 keV γ-rays from ^{115}In(n, n')^{115m}In.

Thermal neutrons were from the reactor at the Musashi Institute of Technology
(Musashi reactor, TRIGA-II, 100KW)[4]. Culture flasks were irradiated and the dose of
γ-rays was measured by TLD. The thermal neutron flux was measured by Au foils.
Irradiation with ^{137}Cs γ-rays was carried out at a dose rate of 1.6 Gy/min.

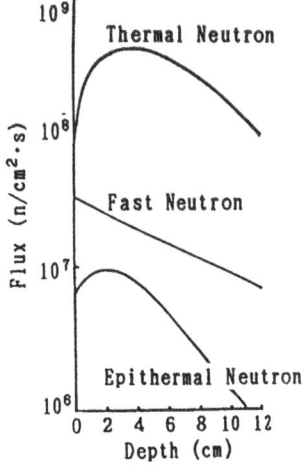

Fig.1 Axial Flux Distribution
in the Acryl Block at the
YAYOI beam with Al rod.

Table 1 Irradiation Dose to V-79
Chinese Hamster Cells.

Dose Rate (cGy/min)	Fission Neutrons (YAYOI)	Thermal Neutrons (MUSASHI)
γ-rays	5.4	1.9
Fast Neutron	6.9	0.25
^{14}N(n, p)^{14}C	0.15	1.6
^{10}B(n, α)^{7}Li	3.0	31.3

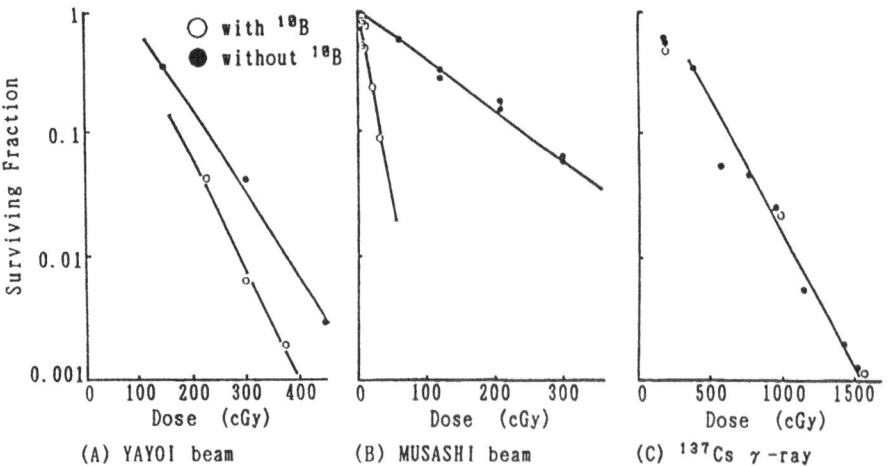

(A) YAYOI beam   (B) MUSASHI beam   (C) ^{137}Cs γ-ray

Fig.2 Dose-Survival Curves for Irradiation of V-79 Chinese Hamster Cells with (A)
YAYOI beam, (B) MUSASHI beam, and (C) ^{137}Cs γ-ray with (○) and without (●)
^{10}B. The mean of 4-8 dishes per data point is shown. The ^{10}B(n, α)^{7}Li reaction
is not included in the dose.

RESULTS

Figure 1 shows the axial flux distribution in the acrylic block ($30 \times 30 \times 30 \text{cm}^3$) of fast, epithermal and thermal neutrons for the YAYOI beam. The thermal neutron flux peaked several cm from the surface.

Table 1 shows the dose-rates of fast neutrons, γ-rays, $^{14}N(n,p)^{14}C$ and $^{10}B(n,\alpha)$ ^{7}Li reactions in a culture flask irradiated at the YAYOI and MUSASHI reactors. The ^{14}N $(n,p)^{14}C$ reaction was calculated from the thermal neutron flux and the nitrogen content of V-79 Chinese hamster cells (1.7% by weight in the wet cells[5]). The $^{10}B(n,\alpha)$ ^{7}Li reaction is calculated from the thermal flux and boron uptake by V-79 cells ($28.1 \pm 2.2 \mu g^{10}B/g$). The fast neutron dose rate at the Musashi reactor was estimated from the experiment by T.Matsumoto et al[4].

Figure 2 shows dose-survival curves for irradiation of V-79 Chinese hamster cells with (A) YAYOI beam, (B) MUSASHI beam and (C) ^{137}Cs γ-rays, with and without ^{10}B. In these figures, the dose of $^{10}B(n,\alpha)^{7}Li$ reaction is not included. The D_0 values for the YAYOI beam, the MUSASHI beam and ^{137}Cs γ-rays are 62, 98 and 202 cGy respectively (obtained from a straight line in each dose-survival curve). From these D_0 values, the gain factors of the YAYOI beam and the MUSASHI beam compared to ^{137}Cs γ-rays are 3.3 and 2.1 respectively.

DISCUSSION AND CONCLUSION

The YAYOI beam was passed through an acrylic block to thermalize the fast and epithermal neutrons. The thermal neutron flux increased for the first several cm and then formed a plateau-like peak, after which it gradually decreased. These results suggest that if a tumor at a depth of several cm in acrylic resin can be irradiated by fission neutrons, then the tumor will be in a uniform plateau-like thermal neutron field. This could make BNCT possible even for a thick tumor lesion.

In order to estimate the possibility of using such fission neutrons for BNCT, the effects of the $^{10}B(n,\alpha)^{7}Li$ reaction and fast neutrons on V-79 Chinese hamster cells were compared to the effects of ^{137}Cs γ-rays. The YAYOI beam and the MUSASHI beam are mixed beams composed of neutrons and γ-rays, and produce $^{14}N(n,p)^{14}C$ reaction in cells or tissues and $^{10}B(n,\alpha)^{7}Li$ reaction in the presence of ^{10}B. To evaluate gain factors of each radiation, it was necessary to assume that the survival rates of these radiations are logarithmically additive :

$S(N+\gamma+np+n\alpha)=S(N+\gamma+np) \cdot S(n\alpha)$, $S(\gamma)=S(^{137}Cs \ \gamma)$

where, $S(N+\gamma+np+n\alpha)$: Survival rate for the YAYOI beam with ^{10}B.

$\quad \quad S(N+\gamma+np)$: Survival rate for the YAYOI beam without ^{10}B.

$\quad \quad S(n\alpha)$: Survival rate for $^{10}B(n,\alpha)^{7}Li$ reaction.

$\quad \quad S(\gamma)$: Survival rate for the reactor γ-ray.

$\quad \quad S(^{137}Cs \ \gamma)$: Survival rate for the ^{137}Cs γ-ray.

Under this assumption the calculated gain factors of fast neutrons and $^{14}N(n,p)^{14}C$ are 5.0 and 2.9 respectively and the gain factor of $^{10}B(n,\alpha)^{7}Li$ is 3.7 in the YAYOI beam and 1.5 in the MUSASHI beam.

Assuming these gain factors are estimates of RBE values and using the results of dosimetry in acrylic resin, the distributions of total dose including ^{10}B were compared for irradiation with fission neutrons (the YAYOI beam) and with thermal neutrons (the MUSASHI beam). Figure 3 shows the expected axial total dose (total of each absorbed dose x each gain factor) for tumor tissue, under the following conditions.

*The YAYOI beam is passed through the Al rod and 4 cm acrylic resin to irradiate the normal or tumor tissues .

*The radiation field of the MUSASHI beam is $10 \times 10 \text{cm}^2$ [4].

*The normal tissue (skin) at the surface (0 cm) is not irradiated more than 18Gy.

*The nitrogen content of normal tissues is 4.6% by weight[6].

*The boron content of tumor tissue and normal tissue are $40 \mu g/g$, $0 \mu g/g$ respectively.

*The absorbed dose in tissue from $^{10}B(n,\alpha)^{7}Li$ reaction is twice that in monolayer cells[7].

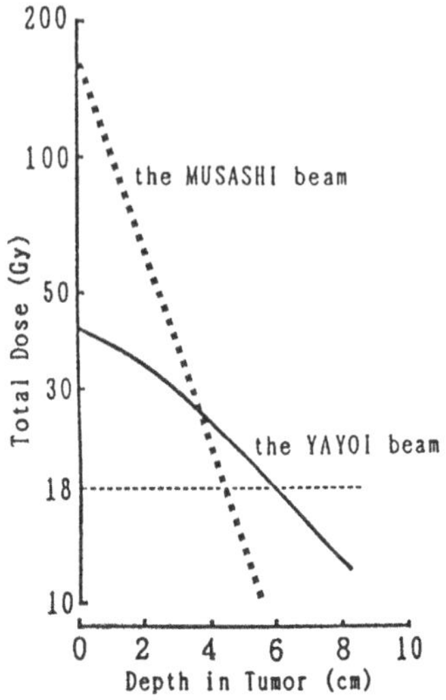

Fig. 3 Expected Axial Dose Distributions in Tumor Tissue Containing $40 \mu g^{10}B/g$ in Using the MUSASHI beam and the YAYOI beam.

Under these circumstances, within 4 cm of depth, the tumor containing $40 \mu g^{10}B/g$ could be damaged more selectively by using thermal neutrons (the MUSASHI beam) than using fission neutrons (the YAYOI beam). But thermal neutrons might be inferior to fission neutrons in attenuation of absorbed dose in tumor. With the same damage to the surface normal tissues, the depth to which the tumor is irradiated by more dose than normal tissue is about 4 cm and 6 cm in using the MUSASHI beam and the YAYOI beam respectively. The YAYOI neutron beam used in this study might still contain much fast neutron and γ-ray contamination, but even such a beam is superior to a thermal neutron beam for the BNCT of deeper tumor lesions. Though the spectrum of fission neutrons should be further improved by reducing the relative fast neutron flux, fission neutrons might be worth using for BNCT in treating malignant tumors at depth.

REFERENCES

1) T. Kadosawa, T. Kawasaki, R. Nishimura, F. Ohashi, A. Takeuchi, H. Wakabayashi, and I. Saito, 1986, Possible Use of Fast Neutrons in Boron Neutron Capture Therapy for Expanded or Deeply Located Tumor Lesions, in "Neutron Capture Therapy", H. Hatanaka, ed., Nishimura Co., Ltd., Niigata.
2) I. Ikeuchi, and T. Amano, 1978, A Colorimetric Determination of Boron in Biological Materials. Chem. Pharm. Bull., 26(9) : 2619-2623.
3) H. Wakabayashi, T. Yoshii, N. Sasuga, T. Inada, K. Kawachi, T. Kanai, and A. Ito, 1983, Dose Rate Characterization of the Biomedical Irradiation Facility of Fast Neutron Source Reactor YAYOI - Intercomperison of Independent Measurement of Dose Rates, Journal of the Faculuty of Engineering, the University of Tokyo(B), 37(2) : 241-251.
4) T. Matsumoto et al., 1986, Musashi institute of Technology Reactor as a Medical Facility with Reference to Dosimetry and in situ Boron Concentration Measurement, in "Boron Neutron Capture Therapy for Tumors", H. Hatanaka, ed., Nishimura Co., Ltd., Niigata.
5) D. Gabel, R. G. Fairchild, B. Larsson, and H. G. Borner, 1984, The Relative Biological Effectiveness in V79 Chinese Hamster Cells of the Neutron Capture Reactions in Boron and Nitrogen, Radat. Res., 98 : 307-316.
6) D. R. White, R. J. Martin and R. Parlison, 1977, Epoxy resin based tissue substitutes, British Journal of Radiology, 50 : 814-821.
7) M. A. Davis, J. B. Little, K. M. M. S. Ayyangar, and A. R. Reddy, 1970, Relative Biological Effectiveness of the $^{10}B(n, \alpha)^7Li$ Reaction in HeLa Cells, Radiat. Res., 43 : 534-553.

INTRACELLULAR DISTRIBUTION OF VARIOUS BORON COMPOUNDS

IN RAT 9L GLIOSARCOMA CELLS

T. Nguyen[1], B.A. Teicher[2], M. Miura[3], S.B. Kahl[4] and G.L. Brownell[1]

[1]Nuclear Engineering Department and Whitaker College, M.I.T., Cambridge, MA 02139 USA
[2]Dana-Farber Cancer Institute, Boston, MA 02115 USA
[3]Brookhaven National Laboratory, Upton, NY 11973 USA and
[4]Department of Pharmaceutical Chemistry, University of California at San Francisco, CA 94143 USA

The effect of neutron capture therapy depends on the selective localization of the ^{10}B atoms in target cells. It is generally preferred that the boron compound linked to the nuclear structure of the individual cancer cell, so that the neutron capture reaction occurs in the most sensitive part of the cell [1]. The currently used boron compound for clinical trials in Japan and for pre-clinical investigations in the USA is the monomeric sulfhydryl borane, BSH. Recently, interest has been shown to several new compounds: the dimeric sulfhydryl borane (BSSB), the boronophenylalanine (BPA), and the porphyrins such as BOPP and VCDP. This paper presents a parallel study of these compounds in terms of their cytotoxicity, uptake and subcellular distribution in 9L gliosarcoma cells.

METHOD

Cytotoxicity. Five boron compounds were investigated: the monomeric and dimeric sulfhydryl boranes (BSH and BSSB), D,L-P-Boronophenylalanine (BPA), and two carboranyl porphyrins (BOPP and VCDP). 9L gliosarcoma cells were maintained in culture in alpha medium supplemented with 10% fetal bovine serum and antibiotics. Cytotoxicity assays were performed by determining the survival fractions of colony-forming cells, describing elsewhere [2,3]. Briefly, cells were allowed to grow in the medium with the presence of the drug for one hour, then washed with phosphate buffered 0.9% saline (PBS) and reseeded in fresh medium. Surviving cells were allowed to grow colonies for one week. After staining with crystal violet, colonies of greater than 50 cells were counted and the results were expressed as surviving fractions of treated cells compared to the untreated cells. In the two porphyrin cases, the cells were kept in low light condition.

Uptake study. Five million cells were suspended in serum-free alpha medium before the drug was added to the medium. An iso-effective concentration that results in a surviving fraction of 0.70 of 9L cells by all five boron compounds was chosen for the uptake and subcellular studies. This iso-effective concentration for BOPP and VCDP was 25 µM, and for BSH, BSSB, and BPA was 500 µM. After preselected time periods (namely 60 min, 50, 40, 30, 20, 10, 5, 3, 2, 1 min, 30 sec, 15 sec and 0 sec), the drug-containing medium was separated from the cells by centrifugation, with the help of a layer of silicon oil. The medium and the silicon oil were then removed from the cells and the cells were lysed using a sonic demembrator. Lysed materials were injected to the atomic absorption spectrophotometer to measure boron levels. The 0 time point sample was used to obtain the background level.

Cellular Fractionation. For each timepoint (15 and 60 min), suspended cells were separated into one aliquot and the drug was added to one aliquot for 15 min and to the other for 60 min. The drug-containing medium was then removed, cells were washed 3 times with cold PBS, counted and lysed in distilled water by sonication on ice. The fractionation was performed at 4°C in distilled water, following Sharma and Edwards' procedure [4].

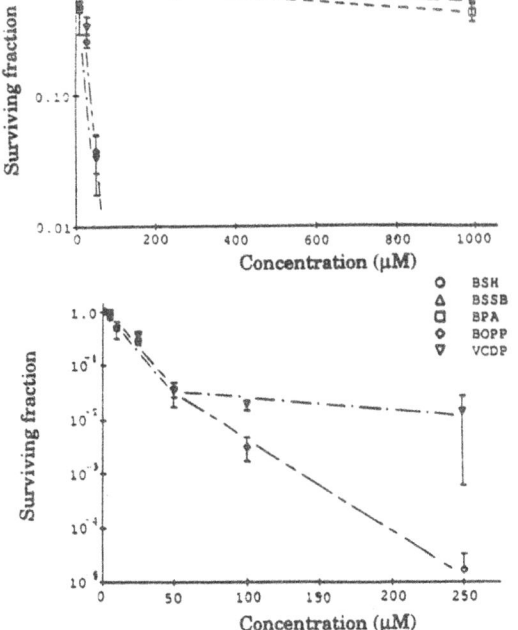

Fig. 1. Survival of 9L gliosarcoma cells exposed to various concentrations of each boton compound for one hour.

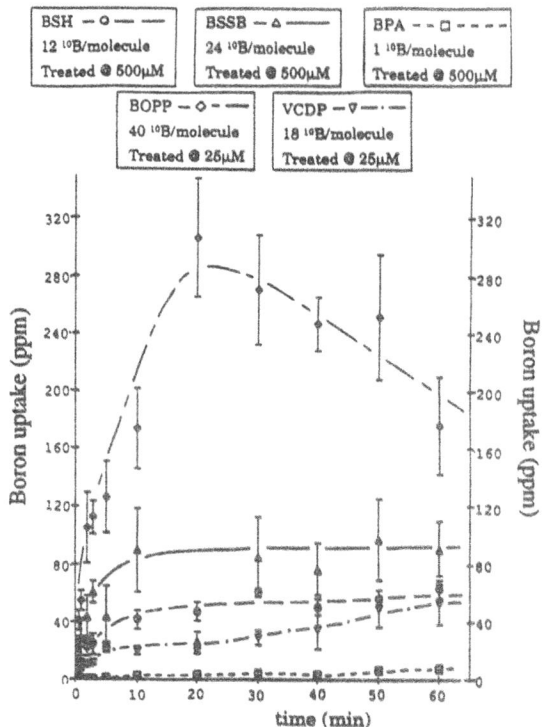

Fig. 2. Boron uptake by 9L cells, measured by boron atomic absorption. Points are the means of three separate experiments, error bars represent the SEM.

Figs. 3a - 3e. Drug content in various subcellular fractions of 9L gliosarcoma cells, measured by boron atomic absorption. Zero timepoint was the time of addition of drug to cell medium. The sixty minute timepoint was immediately after removal of drug. Points are the means of three separate experiments, error bars represent the SEM.

Drug concentration added to the medium of the cells:
BSH - 500μM, BSSB - 500μM, BPA - 500μM,
BOPP - 25μM, VCDP - 25μM.

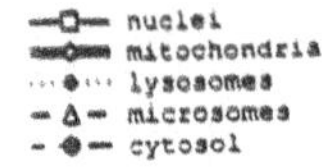

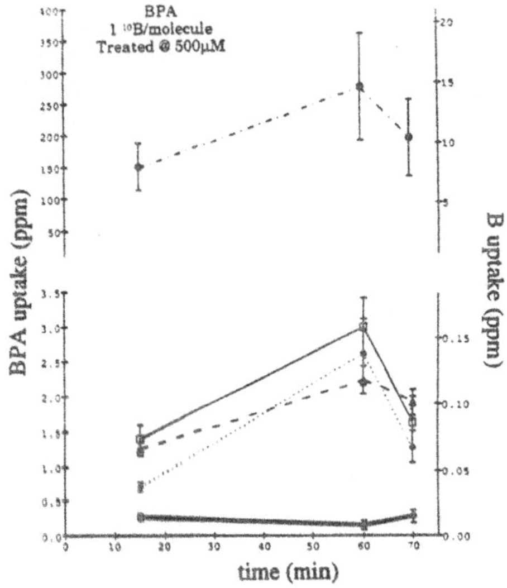

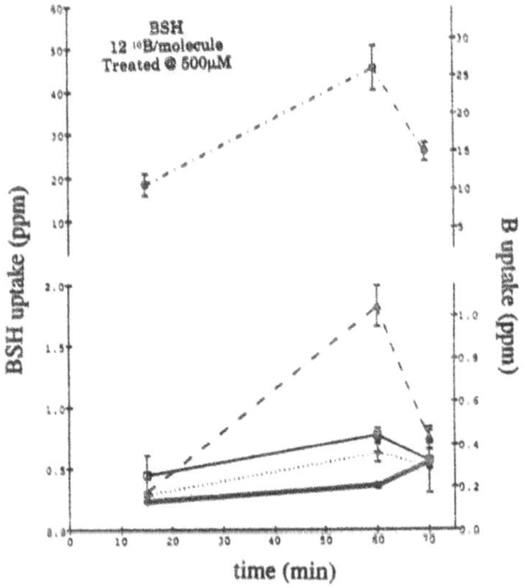

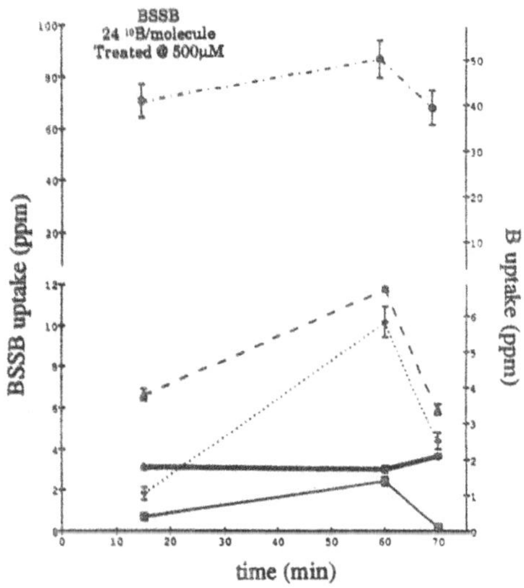

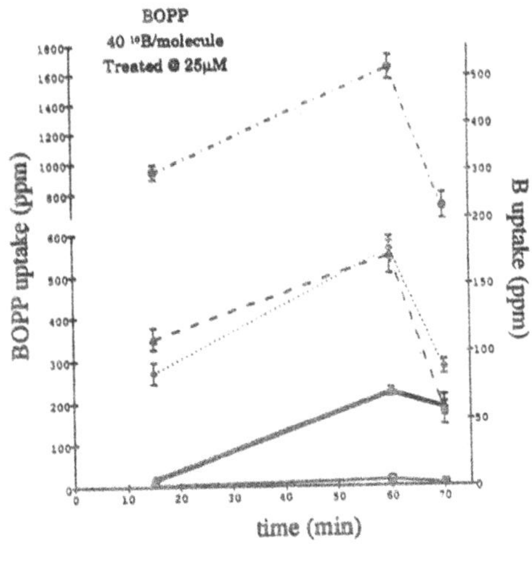

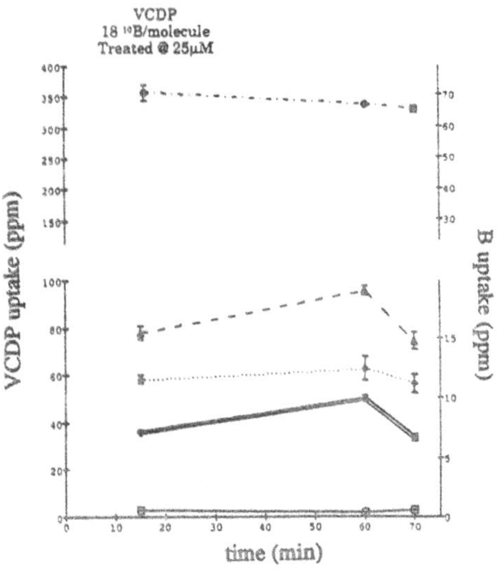

For the 70 min timepoint (10 min wash-off), the procedure was similar except that after the suspended cells were treated with drug for 60 min, they were removed from the drug-containing medium and allowed to grow in fresh medium for 10 min before being washed with cold PBS. The purpose of this part is to examine the wash-off of drug by the cell system after 10 min growing in the drug-free medium.

<u>Atomic Absorption Spectrophotometry</u>: Each collected pellet was lysed again in 30µl of distilled water using a sonic demembrator. Lyse materials were then injected to the atomic absorption spectrophotometer to measure the boron level. For each boron compound, a calibration curve was produced to calculate the efficiency of the atomic absorption spectrophotometer to that drug.

RESULTS AND DISCUSSION

The five boron compounds studied are among the most popular boron-containing compounds currently investigated for BNCT. Studies on these compounds have been done. Figure 1 shows the survival fractions of 9L cells after exposure to various concentrations of each compound for one hour. The two porphyrins are seen to be much more cytotoxic than the sulfhydryl boranes and the BPA. A 500µM concentration of a borane would leave about 70% survival cells while this survival fraction can be obtained only with roughly 25µM porphyrin. This iso-effective concentration was used in the uptake and subcellular distribution studies. At 25µM, one of the porphyrins, BOPP, shows the highest uptake of boron in 9L cells. It appears to reach the highest uptake at 20 min timepoint, and slightly fall off with time. At the same drug concentration, VCDP shows a lower uptake level, but slowly increases with time. Among the less toxic compounds, BSSB shows the highest uptake which seems to saturate after 60 min. BSH uptake in 9L cells also display a saturation after almost 60 min, but with a boron level about 70% lower than that of BSSB. BPA carries the least amount of boron into 9L cells. Figure 2 summarizes the uptake results, expressed in nanogram of boron in one million cells (ngB/10^6 cells, also denoted as ppm), after the drug was individually added to the growth medium of the cells at the concentration of 500µM for BSH, BSSB, BPA, and of 25µM for BOPP and VCDP. At a 20-fold lower concentration, BOPP still shows a higher boron uptake in 9L cells compared to the other compounds.

The subcellular distribution of each compound is shown in Fig. 3a to 3e. In each individual case, the cytosol shows the highest amount of boron in the cell, probably due to the largest volume of the cytoplasm compared to the volumes of other organelles. BPA, the smallest structure among the five compounds studied, can carry a relatively high percentage of intracellular boron into the nuclei of the cells. The mitochondria have the least amount of BPA. BSH also seems to be able to permeate the nuclear membrane partially, but the microsomes display the highest uptake rate of BSH among all the organelles. The mitochondria contain the least amount of BSH. BSSB, having a larger structure than BSH, appears to be unable to cross the nuclear membrane, showing the least percentage of BSSB in the nuclei of the cells. The microsomal pellet contains a relatively high amount of BSSB, while the lysosomes display the highest BSSB uptake rate. BOPP and VCDP, having the largest structures among the five investigated compounds, share the same result with BSSB in terms of their percentage uptake in the nuclear pellets. Similar to the case of BSSB, these 2 complexes seem to attach to the cell membrane structure (the microsomal pellets) more than any other cell organelle. BOPP, however, is found in the lysosomes at a higher percentage than VCDP.

The wash-off of these compounds by the cell system is also shown in Figs 3a - 3e (from timepoint 60 to timepoint 70). In general VCDP shows a smaller decrease compared to BOPP, suggesting a stronger bond in the cell structures. The mitochondrial pellets seem to gain some BSH and BSSB as the rest of the cell is losing the boron compounds during this wash-off period. In general, this study suggests that all five compounds seems to have loose bonds, if any, to the cell structure.

CONCLUSION

This study provides some data to compare the intracellular distribution of five different boron-containing compounds in 9L cells grown in culture. The initial limitation of a boron compound to be treated to these cells is clearly the cytotoxicity of each individual compound to this cell line. To allow the compound to permeate through the nuclear membrane, the size of these compounds appear to be important, unless a new compound will be found that will take advantage of the cellular physiological pathway to cross the nuclear membrane without hinder. The number of boron atoms per molecule is also an important factor. BOPP, having the highest number of boron atoms per molecule, apparently displays an advantage over the rest of the investigated compounds.

REFERENCES

1. D. Gabel, S. Foster and R. G. Fairchild. The Monte Carlo Simulation of the Biological Effect of the $^{10}B(n,\alpha)^{7}Li$ Reaction in Cells and Tissue and Its Implication for Boron Neutron Capture Therapy, Rad. Res., 111: 14 (1987).
2. V. S. Goldmacher, J. Anderson, W. A. Blattler, J. M. Lambert and P. D. Senter. Antibody-complement-mediated cytotoxicity is enhanced by ribosome-inactivating proteins, J. Immunol., 135:3648 (1985).
3. W. G. Thilly, J. G. DeLuca, H. Hoppe and B. W. Penman. Phenotypic lag and mutation to 6-thioguanine resistance in diploid human lymphoblasts, Mutat. Res., 50:137 (1978).
4. R. P. Sharma and I. R. Edwards. Cis-platinum: Subcellular distribution and binding to cytosolic glands, Biochem. Pharmac., 32:2665 (1983).

IN VITRO EVALUATION OF ^{10}B-BPA FOR MELANOMA AT MOATA - JOINT WORK BETWEEN JAPAN AND AUSTRALIA BNCT RESEARCH TEAMS

M. Ichihashi[1], H. Fukuda[2], J.K. Brown[3], M.H. Mountford[3], B.J. Allen[3], J.G. Wilson[3] and Y. Mishima[1]

[1]Department of Dermatology, Special Institute for Cancer Neutron Capture Therapy, Kobe University School of Medicine, Kobe 650, Japan
[2]National Institute of Radiological Science, Chiba 280, Japan
[3]Biomedicine and Health Program, ANSTO, NSW 2234, Australia

INTRODUCTION

A variety of conjugated compounds have been synthesized in Japan, the USA and Australia. Among these ^{10}B-compounds, ^{10}B$_1$-paraboronophenyl-alanine (^{10}B$_1$-BPA) has been widely tested in vitro and in vivo for boron neutron capture therapy of melanoma. We have shown that ^{10}B$_1$-BPA is selectively incorporated into melanoma cells in vitro[1] and in vivo[2]. Neutron capture therapy (NCT) using ^{10}B$_1$-BPA has been demonstrated not only to be highly lethal for melanoma cells in vitro[3] but also to be effective for suppressing melanoma growth in vivo.

As a result, NCT of malignant melanoma using ^{10}B$_1$-BPA entered its first clinical trial phase in Japan in 1987[4]. Six melanoma lesions have been successfully regressed by Mishima's group using ^{10}B$_1$-BPA for NCT.

Experimental data obtained by Japanese and Australian research groups on ^{10}B$_1$-BPA accumulation in melanoma cells and the lethal effect of NCT using ^{10}B$_1$-BPA, however, have varied significantly.

We therefore proposed to carry out a Japan-Australia joint work in vitro at ANSTO to investigate the cause for the varied results on the killing effect of NCT using ^{10}B$_1$-BPA in cultured melanoma cells. Four radiobiological experiments were undertaken using B-16 melanoma cells pre-incubated with ^{10}B$_1$-BPA by the method of Japanese group, and one radiobiological experiment was performed to evaluate gamma-ray dose in the mixed field of the 100 kW Moata reactor.

In addition to ^{10}B-BPA testing, toxicity and neutron capture experiments with ^{n}B-thiouracil[5] were performed. This compound contains 10 boron atoms[5] and on the average two of these atoms are boron-10. As such, incubation with ^{n}B-thiouracil should show a cell killing effect after neutron capture if uptake by melanoma cells occurs. These experiments were performed during Dec. 7-16, 1988, under the support of the Japanese and Australian governments.

MATERIAL AND METHODS

1. Determination of melanoma cell killing by neutron capture therapy using $^{10}B_1$-BPA and ^nB-thiouracil

$2-4 \times 10^6$ cells cultured in flask (Falcon 3024) were incubated with $^{10}B_1$-BPA (0-80 μg/ml medium) or with ^nB-thiouracil (0-10 μg/ml medium) for approximately 20 h at 37°C. 4-5 h before thermal neutron radiation $^{10}B_1$-BPA treated cells were trypsinized and $1-5 \times 10^5$ cells/ml were prepared in each teflon tube. The tubes were placed at different distances from the bismuth surface and irradiated at doses ranging from $0.3-10 \times 10^{13}$ n/cm^2 in the Moata field. 50-10,000 cells seeded on petri dish (Falcon 3002) were cultured for 7-9 days in CO$_2$ incubator, and then fixed and stained to count colonies.

2. Determination of radiobiological effect of capture gamma-ray on cell killing in comparison with ^{60}Co gamma-ray

A paraffin block of 4 cm thickness was located in front of the reactor's bismuth surface to generate a high flux of capture gamma-rays along with the 2.2MeV produced predominantly by $^1H(n, \gamma)^2H$ reaction. Cultured cells (1.5×10^5/ml medium) in teflon tubes were further loaded into ^6LiF shielded tubes to protect cells from thermal neutron radiation. The total gamma-ray dose (core + capture) was measured by TLDs (400 CAF$_2$ bulbs). After thermas neutron radiation, cells were seeded as also described in experimental procedure 1.

RESULTS AND DISCUSSION

^nB-thiouracil at the concentration of 100 μg/ml significantly suppressed B-16 melanoma cell growth, whereas 10 μg/ml ^nB-thiouracil inhibited cell growth only slightly (Fig. 1).

BNCT for B-16 melanoma cells using ^nB-thiouracil at the concentration between 1.0 μg/ml and 10 μg/ml did not enhance cell killing in comparison with thermal neutron radiation without boron-pretreatment. These results suggest that our ^nB-thiouracil may not be applicable for BNCT in vivo.

The cell killing effect of BNCT on B-16 melanoma cells using $^{10}B_1$-BPA pre-incubation at 40 or 80 μg/ml was slightly higher than that not treated with $^{10}B_1$-BPA (Fig. 2a), but much lower than that obtained previously by Japanese research group.

Measured total gamma-rays and γ/n ratio of the Moata field produced in the NCT experiment using cultured cells were significantly higher than those of MUSASHI reactor field (Fig. 3).

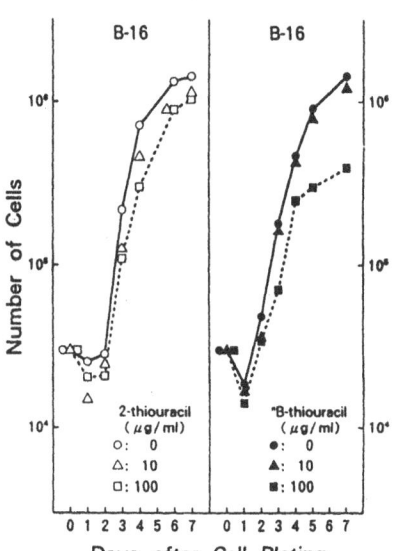

Toxic Effect of Thiouracil on Melanoma Cell Growth

Fig. 1

Since 240 and 280 cGy gamma-ray dose absorbed by the cells at the high neutron fluence locations (1.13 and 1.53×10^{13} n/cm^2 respectively) is much higher than the D_0 value of 154 cGy obtained from the dose-survival curve for B-16 melanoma cells exposed to ^{60}Co gamma-ray, the NCT effect needs to be evaluated after subtraction of the gamma-ray dose corresponding to the level of MUSASHI reactor field (181 cGy at 1.48×10^{13} n/cm^2, 155 cGy at 1.16×10^{13} n/cm^2).

D_0 values of the dose-survival curves for B-16 melanoma cells exposed to neutrons alone and NCT using $^{10}B_1$-BPA were significantly different when corrections for the killing effect of gamma-ray

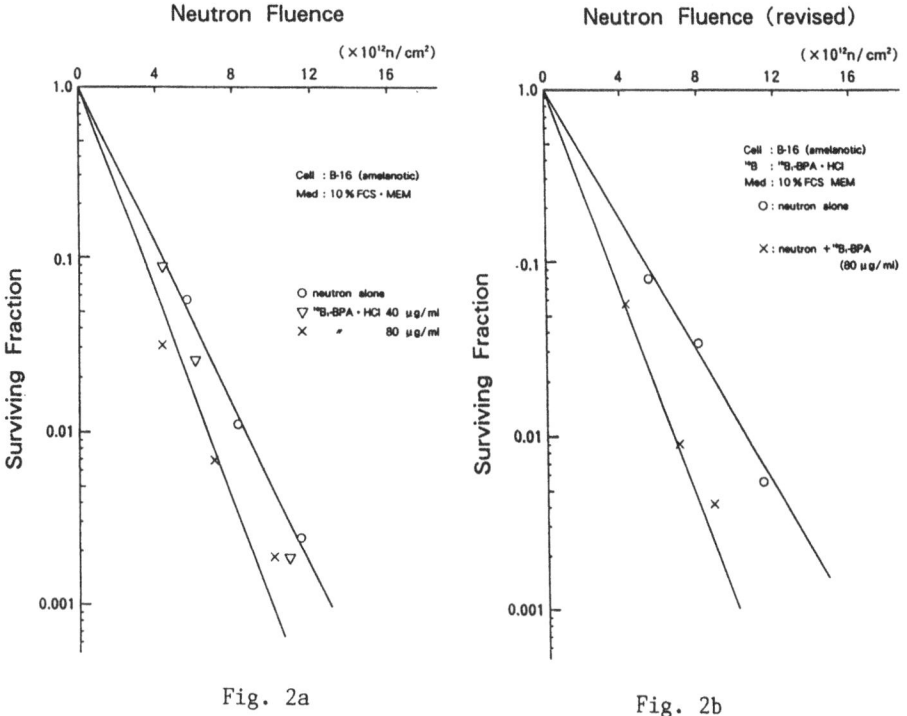

Fig. 2a   Fig. 2b

contamination are made to the same
level as that of MUSASHI reactor
field (Fig. 2b). In brief, the lethal
effect on B-16 cells induced by
contamination γ -rays, exceeding
that of the MUSASHI reactor field
experiment, was calculated from
the survival curve obtained by
[60]Co radiation and subtracted from
the survival curve of neutrons, and
NCT using [10]B$_1$-BPA for the Moata
reactor.

The total gamma ray component
of our experimental radiation in the
Moata field was much higher than that
of the MUSASHI reactor under similar
experimental conditions, and had
a similar killing effect to [60]Co
gamma-ray on melanoma cells (data
not shown). Further, the Do value
of neutrons alone after substraction
of contaminated gamma-ray to the level
of MUSASHI field was 2.7×10^{12} n/cm^2,
which was almost the same Do value of
the experiment done in MUSASHI field.
Therefore, we came to a conclusion
that an unexpectedly lower lethal

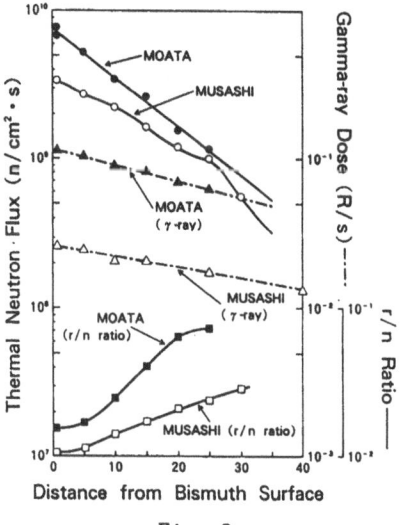

Fig. 3

effect of NCT using [10]B$_1$-BPA in Moata field compared to that of MUSASHI
field could be due to both the high γ/n ratio of Moata compared with
MUSASHI field and low uptake of [10]B$_1$-BPA by melanoma cells having scanty
melanogenic activity.

Table 1 Do values of NCT and BNCT using ^{10}B-BPA for
B-16 melanoma cells in the Moata reactor field.

	$Do \times 10^{12} n/cm^2$	
	N C T	B N C T
Moata reactor without substraction	1.8	1.2
Moata reactor with substraction	2.7	1.6

CONCLUSIONS

   To clarify the relation between ^{10}B content/g cultured melanoma
cells and killing effect of NCT in vitro, it is essential to develop a
method measuring ^{10}B at a low level of 1.0 ng/g sample.
   The gamma-ray dose in the Moata field should be reduced to the level
of MUSASHI reactor field for in vitro biological use.

RFERENCES

1)M.Ichihashi, M.Ueda, K.Hayashibe, S.Hatta, M.Tsuji, Y.Mishima, H.Fukuda,
  T.Kobayashi, K.Kanda: In vitro radiobiological evaluation of selective
  killing effects of ^{10}B$_1$-paraboronophenylalanine HCI in the thermal
  neutron capture therapy of malignant melanoma cells. KURRI-TR-260:23-31,
  1985.
2)C.Honda, Y.Mishima, M.Ichihashi, S.Hatta: In situ detection of cutaneous
  melanoma by prompt gamma-ray spectrometry using melanoma-seeking ^{10}B-
  dopa analogue. J. Dermatol. Sci., 1:23-32, 1990.
3)M.Ichihashi, Y.Mishima, M.Ueda, K.Hayashibe, S.Hatta, Y.Funasaka,
  H.Yoshino: Selective lethal effects of ^{10}B$_1$-para-boronophenylalanine on
  mouse and human melanoma cells in thermal neutron capture therapy by
  tyrosine and phenylalanine deficiency. Proc. of the Second International
  Symposium on Neutron Capture Therapy. "Neutron Capture Therapy",
  ed. H.Hatanaka, Niigata, Nishimura Co.Ltd., pp.237-246, 1986.
4)Y.Mishima, M.Ichihashi, S.Hatta, C.Honda, K.Yamamura, T.NaKagawa: New
  thermal neutron capture therapy for malignant melanoma: Melanogenesis-
  seeking ^{10}B molecule-melanoma cell interaction from in vitro to first
  clinical trial. Pigment Cell Res. 2:226-234, 1989.
5)J.G.Wilson: Synthatic approaches to a carboranyl thiouracil. Pigment
  Cell Res. 2:297-303, 1989.

THERMAL NEUTRON CAPTURE THERAPY (NCT) USING ^{10}B-CONJUGATED ANTIMELANOMA ANTIBODIES: QUANTIFICATION OF ^{10}B ON CULTURED HUMAN MELANOMA CELLS

A. Komura, T. Nakagawa, M. Ichihashi, and Y. Mishima

Department of Dermatology, Special Institute for Cancer
Neutron Capture Therapy, Kobe University School of Medicine
Kobe 650, Japan

INTRODUCTION

Since the success of human melanoma treatment by a single NCT application (Mishima et al., 1989) using ^{10}B-dopa analogue, ^{10}B$_1$-paraborono-phenylalanine, a metabolic substrate for melanin, we have been investigating other melanoma-seeking ^{10}B agents which could in principle be applicable to other cancers.

In order to accumulate a sufficient number of ^{10}B atoms on target cells, we first synthesized new ^{10}B-avidin compounds. These compounds can be effectively targeted on human melanoma cells by biotinated monoclonal antibodies (MoAbs) specific for the cells.

The precise quantification of ^{10}B atoms accumulated on a target cell has been successfully carried out using Inductively Coupled Plasma Mass Spectrometry (ICP-MS).

MATERIALS AND METHODS

1. Selection of the best combination of a cell line and an antibody human melanoma cell lines (Colo 38, SK-40, Seto 12, and Ihara) and mouse melanoma cell line (B16) were maintained in our laboratory. Other human melanoma cell lines (SK-Mel-26:P22 and MeWo:P39) were kindly supplied by Dr. M. Taniguchi, Chiba University, Chiba, Japan. Monoclonal mouse IgM antimelanoma antibody (M2590)(Wakabayashi et al., 1984), monoclonal mouse IgG1 antihuman melanoma antibody (763.74T) (Giacomini et al., 1984), and control mouse IgG1 monoclonal antibody (6A4)(Tokuhisa et al., 1982) were purified by ion-exchange chromatography using DEAE wet cellulose column. The cells were treated with biotinated antibodies (Komura et al., 1989) and avidin-fluorescein isothiocyanate (FITC) (Vector Laboratories, Inc., Burlingame, CA), then, fluorescence intensity on the cells was analyzed by a fluorescence-activated cell sorter (FACS-IV; B-D FACS Systems, Becton, Dickinson & Co., Sunnyvale, CA) (Fig.1). The best combination was P22 and 763.74T.

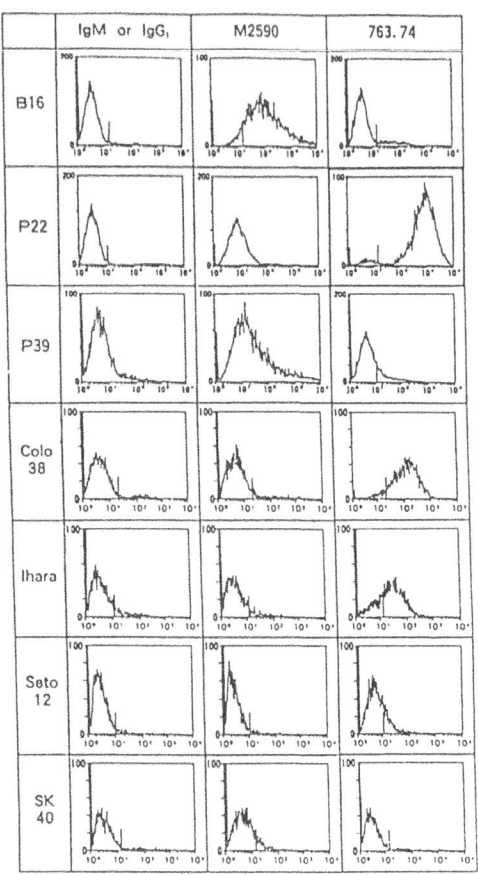

Fig. 1 FACS Profiles of Melanoma
        cells by MoAbs

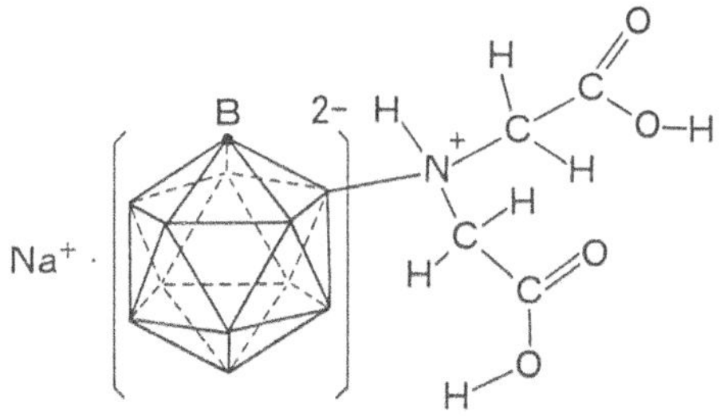

Fig. 2 Efficient $^{10}B_{12}$
        compound

2. Conjugation of $^{10}B_{12}$ compound to avidin

Sodium dodecahydrododecaborate ($Na_2B_{12}H_{12}$) was prepared from ^{10}B-enriched boric acid, the degree of enrichment being 92.4%. A new boron compound, $^{10}B_{12}$ compound, was synthesized from this material(Komura et al., 1989) (Fig.2).

3. Quantitative analysis of ^{10}B accumulated on P22 cells

^{10}B-avidin compounds were applied to biotinated 763.74T MoAb-treated P22 cells. First, 0.12 mg of biotin N-hydroxysuccinimide ester (Sigma B2643) in $120\,\mu l$ of dimethyl sulfoxide (DMSO) was added to 1.0 mg of purified antibodies at pH7.0 and incubated at room temperature (r.t.) for 4 hours.
    The mixtures were then extensively dialyzed against phosphate buffered saline of pH 7.5 (PBS).
    The boronation of avidin was done with $^{10}B_{12}$-compound in the presence of 1-ethyl-3-(3-dimethylaminopropyl)-carbodiimide under acidic conditions. After thorough dialyses, first against an NaCl solution of high concentration, then against distilled water, the boron concentration of the reaction mixture was determined by a conventional method (Ikeuchi and Amano, 1978). The result revealed, that about 3.5 molecules of the compound were conjugated to one avidin molecule.

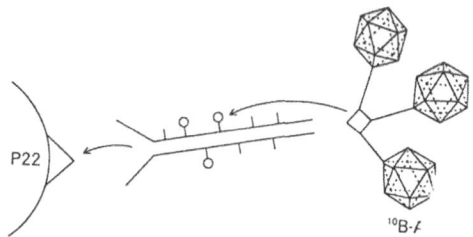

Fig. 3

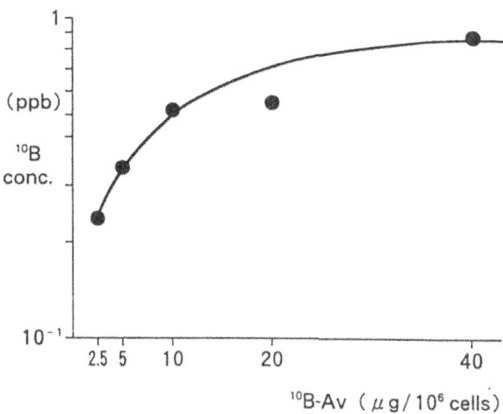

Fig. 4

5x10^5 of cells in 100 l of MEM medium (Nissui) containing 10 % fetal
calf serum (FCS:HyClone Laboratories) were reacted with 2.5 μg of the
biotin coupled 763.74 T for 1 hour at 4°C. These cells were washed 3
times with medium, then $^{10}B_{12}$-avidin was applied to the antibody treated
cells for 15 min at 4°C (Komura et al., 1989)(Fig.3). Then we estimated
the amount of ^{10}B on the cells using inductively coupled plasma-mass
spectrometry (ICP-MS:SPQ 6,500, Seiko Instruments Inc., Tokyo, Japan) by
the method of Hori et al. (Hori et al., 1989). Fig.4 shows the result.

RESULTS AND DISCUSSION

^{10}B concentration on 2x10^5/ml P22 melanoma cells treated with biotinated 763.74T MoAbs and ^{10}B-avidin compounds was 0.885 ng/ml, so the
weight of ^{10}B accumulated on one P22 cell was 0.885x10^{-9}/2x10^5(g)
(Fig.4). The weight of one ^{10}B atom is 10/6x10^{23} (g). Therefore, the
number of ^{10}B atoms accumulated on a P22 cell is about 2.6x10^8.
We have already estimated the necessary dose of ^{10}B atoms for
complete killing of malignant melanoma cells by neutron capture therapy.
20 μg of ^{10}B atoms are required to kill 1 g of melanoma. That is we need
1.2x10^9 ^{10}B atoms to kill a melanoma cell.
The number of ^{10}B atoms we could accumulate on a P22 cell was only
slightly smaller than the ideal number.
We have already irradiated P22 cells with thermal neutrons using this
system and estimated the cell survival by counting colonies (Fig.5).
Thermal neutrons did injure target cells boronated by MoAbs using our
system.

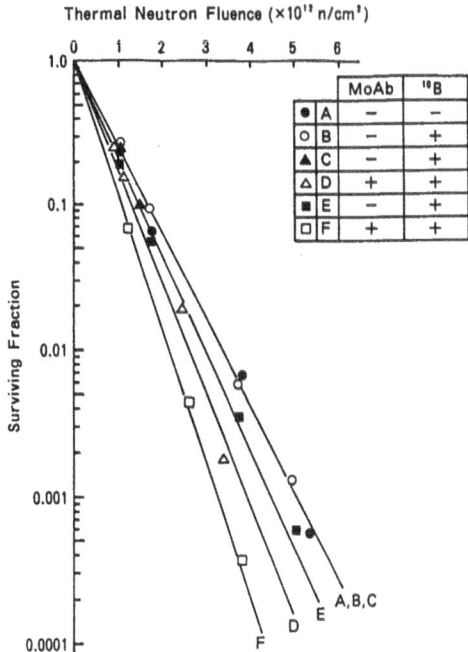

Fig. 5 Dose-survival curves of P22 irradiated with neutron

REFERENCES

1) Giacomini, P., F. Veglia, P. Cordiali Fei, T. Rehle, P.G. Natali, and
   S. Ferrone (1984) Level of a membrane-bound high-molecular-weight
   melanoma-associated antigen and a cytoplasmic melanoma-associated
   antigen in surgically removed tissues and in sera from patients with
   melanoma. Cancer Res., 44:1281-1287.
2) Hori, Y., K. Nakamura, M. Matsuoka (1989) Determination of ^{10}B in
   biological samples by ICP-AES and ICP-MS. The 4th Japan-Australia
   International Workshop on Thermal Neutron Capture Therapy for Malignant
   Melanoma, Kobe Feb., 13-17.
3) Komura, A., T. Tokuhisa, T. Nakagawa, A. Sasase, M. Ichihashi, S.
   Ferrone, and Y. Mishima (1989) Specific killing of human melanoma
   cells with an efficient ^{10}B-Compound on monoclonal antibodies. Pigment
   Cell Res., 2:259-263.
4) Mishima, Y., C. Honda, M. Ichihashi, H. Obara, J. Hiratsuka, H. Fukuda,
   H. Karashima, T. Kobayashi, K. Kanda and Y. Yoshino (1989) Treatment
   of malignant melanoma by single neutron capture therapy with melanoma-
   seeking ^{10}B-compound. Lancet 11:388-389(8659)
5) Tokuhisa, T., Y. Komatsu, Y. Uchida and M. Taniguchi (1982) Monoclonal
   alloantibodies specific for the constant region of the T cell antigen-
   receptors. J. Exp. Med., 156:888-897.
6) Wakabayashi, S., T. Saito, N. Shinohara, S. Okamoto, H. Tomioka, and
   M. Taniguchi (1984) Syngeneic monoclonal antibodies against melanoma
   antigens with species specificity and interspecies cross-reactivity.
   J. Invest. Dermatol., 83:128-133.

ULTRASTRUCTURAL CHANGES IN TUMOUR CELLS FOLLOWING BORON NEUTRON CAPTURE THERAPY

D.H. Barkla[1], J.K. Brown[2], H. Meriaty[2,] B.J. Allen[2]

[1] Department of Anatomy, Monash University, Clayton Vic 3168 Australia.
[2] Australian Nuclear Science & Technology Organisation PMB 1 Menai NSW 2234 Australia.

INTRODUCTION

In a previous study we reported on morphological changes in two human melanoma cell lines treated with ^{10}B-phenylalanine(BPA) and Boron Neutron Capture Therapy(BNCT)[1]. The present study describes morphological changes in melanoma and glioma cell lines treated with boron-tetraphenyl porphyrin(BTPP) and BNCT. Porphyrin compounds are selectively taken up by tumour cells and have been used clinically in phototherapy treatment of cancer patients[2]. Boronated porphyrins show good potential as therapeutic agents in BNCT treatment of human cancer patients and the structure of these compounds is described in detail elsewhere in this monograph.

MATERIALS AND METHODS

Two human melanoma cell lines, MM96 (non pigmented) and LiBr (moderately pigmented), and one glioma cell line U87MG, were maintained at 37°C in RPMI 1640 medium supplemented with 10% fetal calf serum, penicillin and streptomycin (both 50µg/ml). Some flasks were wrapped in aluminium foil (to exclude light) and then incubated with BTPP (15 µg/ml, courtesy of S. Kahl) for 15 hr. The cells were then washed with fresh medium and irradiated with thermal neutrons in the MOATA reactor (Dose 5.23 Gy, neutron fluence 1.2×10^3n cm^{-2}). Control flasks of cells were either (a) left untreated, (b) treated with BTPP but not irradiated, or (c) not treated with BTPP but irradiated (5.23 Gy) in the MOATA reactor. All cells were then harvested mechanically using a rubber cell-scraper, pelletted, fixed using 3% glutaraldehyde, post-fixed for 2 hr in 1% osmium tetroxide, followed by 1 hr in 1% uranyl acetate. Pellets were then dehydrated through graded alcohols, embedded in Epon-Araldite and sectioned for examination using light and electron microscopy. Thin sections were stained with lead citrate and uranyl acetate and examined in a Jeol 100S electron microscope at 60 k.V.

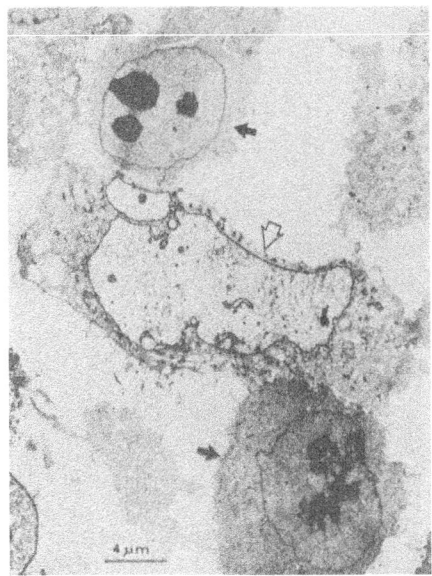

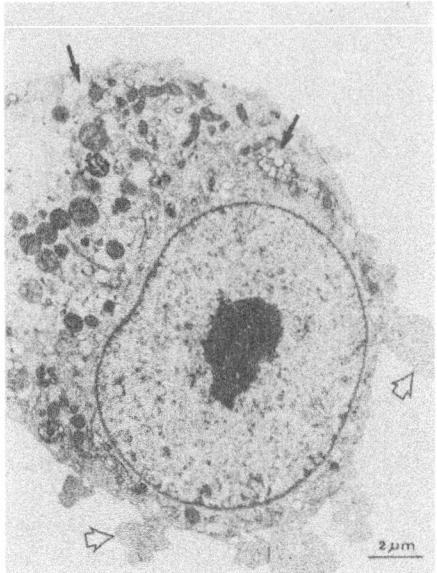

Fig.1. Electron micrograph of LiBr cells 24 hr after irradiation with thermal neutrons alone (MOATA reactor 5.25 Gy). These cells were not pretreated with BTPP. One cell (white arrow) shows morphological evidence of nuclear damage (dispersed chromatin). The other two adjacent cells (black arrows) lack morphological evidence of cell damage.

Fig.2. Electron micrograph of a U87-MG cell 12 hr after BNCT (5.25 Gy). The cells were pre-treated with BTPP (15 μg/ml for 15 hr in total darkness). Morphological changes include formation of surface blebs (white arrows) and cytoplasmic vacuoles (black arrows).

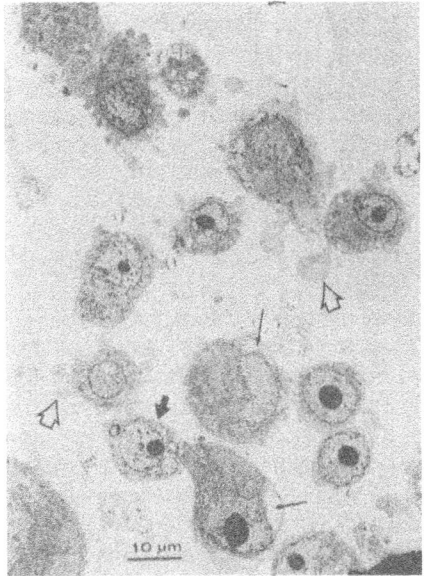

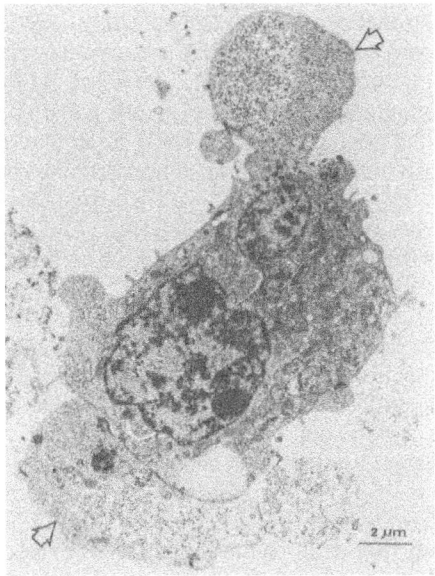

Fig.3. Low power electron micrograph of MM96 cells 24 hr after BNCT (5.25 Gy). The cells were pre-treated for 15 hr with BTPP (15 μg/ml for 15 hr in total darkness). Morphological changes include granulation of the cytoplasm (fine black arrows). Surface blebs (white arrows), and formation of "mini nuclei" in one cell (large black arrow).

Fig.4. Electron micrograph of a MM96 cell 48 hr after BNCT (5.25 Gy). This cell had been pretreated with BTPP (15 μg/ml for 15 hr in total darkness). Extensive loss of granular cytoplasmic material into baloon-like surface projections can be seen (white arrows).

396

RESULTS

Cytotoxicity

The ultrastructural morphology of cells treated with BTPP alone was unchanged from that of untreated cells indicating that BTPP was not cytotoxic at 15 μg/ml.

Cells treated with thermal neutrons alone

Morphological evidence of cell damage was seen in a minority of tumour cells after irradiation. At 12 and 24 hr, occasional nuclear profiles were enlarged and the nuclear chromatin was more dispersed (Fig. 1). Although at 48 and 72 hr, a few cells showed signs of advanced degenerative changes, the majority of cells retained the appearance of untreated cells.

Cells treated with BTPP and thermal neutrons

The response of each of the cell lines to this treatment was similar and the following description is common to all three cell lines: At 1 hr and 6 hr after irradiation, morphological changes were not apparent. At 12 hr after irradiation, many cells showed small surface blebs containing cytoplasmic material and membrane-bound vacuoles in the cytoplasm (Fig. 2). Changes in nuclear morphology were not apparent. At 24 hr after irradiation, formation of surface blebs continued (Fig. 3). Areas of granulation were seen in the cytoplasm of many cells (Fig. 3). Occasional cells showed formation of "mini-nuclei" where the profile of a single round nucleus was broken up into multiple small profiles containing euchromatin and heterochromatin (Fig. 3). At 48 hr after irradiation, many cells showed loss of cytoplasm into large balloon-shaped extensions of the plasmolemma (Fig. 4). Whilst many cells were necrotic and showed pyknotic nuclei, others showed only early signs of cell damage. At 72 hr after irradiation, the majority of cells were necrotic although occasional cells retained a normal appearance and a few mitotic figures were seen.

DISCUSSION

The results suggest that BTPP is taken up into the cytoplasm (but not the nucleus) of tumour cells and that the products of the neutron capture event physically disrupt structural components in cell membranes, especially the plasmolemma. The formation of mini-nuclei in [10]BPA/BNCT-treated cells has been described previously[1] and these can also be possibly explained by the temporary disruption of structural components in the nuclear membrane.

Changes in the appearance of nuclear euchromatin, heterochromatin and nucleolus were not a feature of BTPP/BNCT-treated cells although such changes are commonly seen in tumour cells irradiated with gamma rays (unpublished observation - DHB). The significance of this apparent difference in damage pattern between BNCT and gamma treatment is unclear.

Further morphological studies, using a new porphyrin compound (BOPP - Dr. S. Kahl, UCSF) are presently being conducted.

REFERENCES

1.   Barkla D.H., Allen B.J., Brown, J.K., Mountford, M., Mishima, Y. and Ichihashi, M. Morphological changes in human melanoma cells following irradiation with thermal neutrons. Pig. Cell Res. 2, 345-348, 1989.
2.   Morstyn G. and Kaye A.H. (Eds) Phototherapy of Cancer. Harwood Academic Press, Melbourne, 1990.

DOSE MODIFICATION BY NEUTRON CAPTURE IN CELL CULTURE USING A 1 MEV MEAN ENERGY FISSION NEUTRON BEAM

Wolfgang Sauerwein*, Heike Szypniewski*, Fred Pöller*, René Huiskamp**

*Dept. of Radiotherapy, University Hospital, Essen, Germany
** Radiobiology & Radioecology, Netherlands Energy Research Foundation
ECN, Petten, The Netherlands

INTRODUCTION

Experiments in a d(14)+Be fast neutron beam at the Essen Cyclotron demonstrate an enhancement of dose by neutron capture reactions which could be useful for clinical application (1,2). Based on these results, we underwent similar experiments using a different beam configuration. At the Low Flux Reactor in Petten, fast fission neutrons from a ^{235}U-converter with a mean energy of 1.0 MeV are available to irradiate animals or cells using the Biological Irradiation Facility BIBOP (3,4,5). This facility has been used to obtain more information about dose modification by neutron capture reactions in non (epi-)thermal neutron beams.

PHYSICAL ASPECTS

The exposure facility is optimized to obtain a neutron spectrum between 45 keV and 10 MeV (fig 1). The mean track average LET of the recoil protons in water is 57 keV/μm. The absorbed doses are given as neutron center line doses not including a nine percent gamma-ray contribution. The variation in dose over all irradiation positions is +/-2 percent. The fluence of thermalized neutrons at the center was measured by the gold activation method in Perspex phantoms of identical shape as the tubes used for cell irradiation. A fluence of 2.5×10^{14} thermal neutrons/m^2/s has been found. The fluence rate of thremalized neutrons in a larger volume has been stablished in a polystyrene phantom (22.5 cm x 22.5 cm x 20.0 cm). The depth distribution of the fluence rate is shown in fig 2.

CELL CULTURE EXPERIMENTS

A human melanoma cell line (MeWo) was grown in Eagle's Minimal Essential Medium supplemented with Earl's salts. Cells were irradiated in exponential growth as cell suspension in the BIBOP facility. Boric acid ($H_3{}^{10}BO_3$) was neutralized using 10-N-NaOH. This solution was then added to the medium to obtain a concentration of 0.5 mg

^{10}B/ml medium. 10 ml Falcon tubes containing 5.5 ml cell suspension with or without ^{10}B were placed in a 50 ml Falcon tube containing 15 ml H_2O for build-up of thermalized neutrons and proton-recoil reactions of the fission neutrons. Boron containing medium was given to the cells immediately before irradiation. After the irradiation, cells were incubated for colony formation. As a measure of the cytotoxic action of the treatment, the ability of cells to form a colony of more than 50 cells within two weeks was determined.

RESULTS AND CONCLUSIONS

The survival of MeWo cells after irradiation with fission neutrons in the presence or absence of ^{10}B is shown in fig 3. By using fission neutrons alone we observed a quadratic

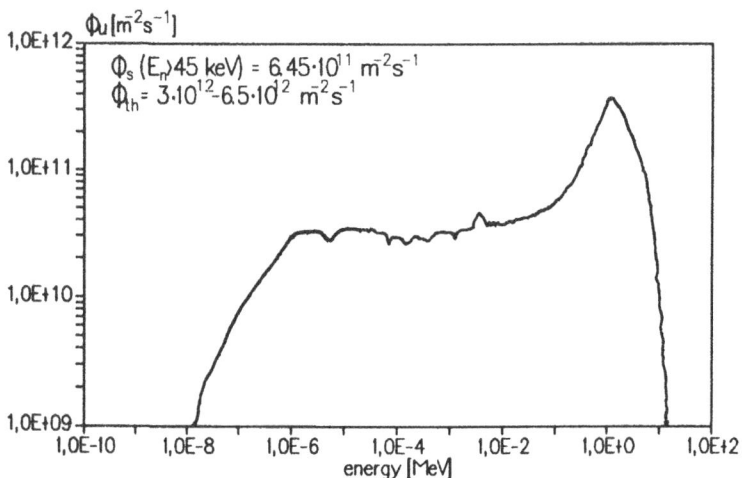

Fig 1. Neutron spectrum in BIBOP (5)

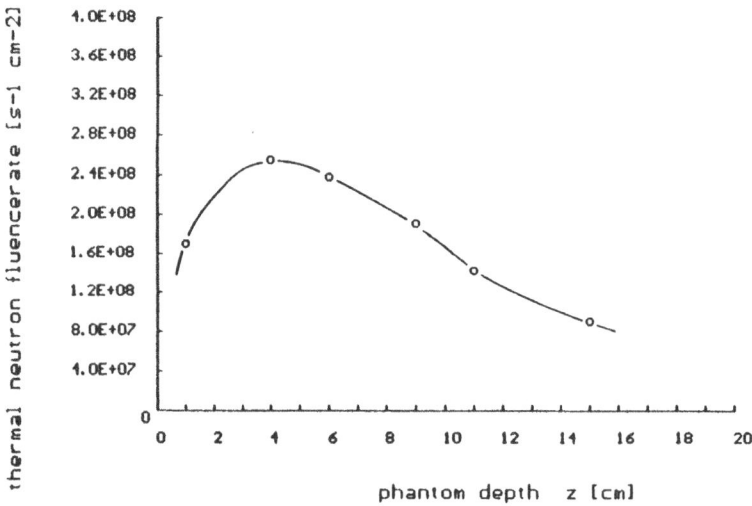

Fig 2. The depth distribution of thermalized neutrons in a polystyrene
phantom

400

component in the dose effect relationship whereas in presence of ^{10}B this quadratic component seems to disappear. At a neutron dose of 1 Gy we observed 15 percent survival without ^{10}B and 1.5 percent on the presence of 0.5mg/ml ^{10}B. A dose modification factor of about two could be derived from these curves. The considerable enhancement of cell kill due to the ^{10}B(n,α)^{7}Li reaction stress the possibility of a therapeutic gain using NCT in fast neutron therapy. To design an optimum configuration for such an application of NCT further experiments are necessary.

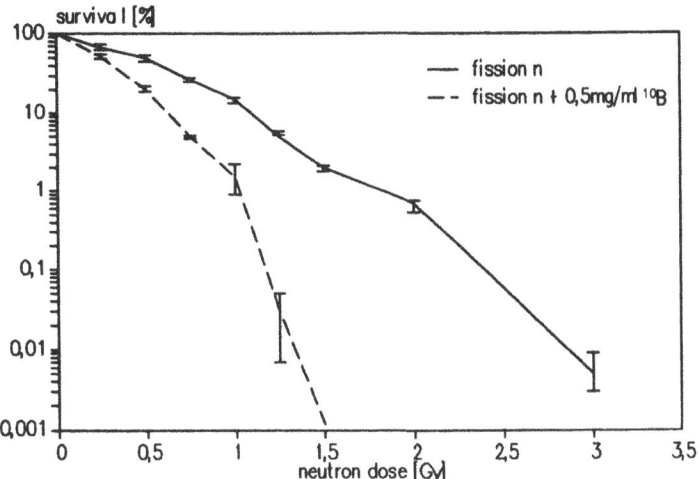

Fig 3. Survival of MeWo cells after irradiation with fission neutrons

LITERATURE

1. Sauerwein W., W. Ziegler, K. Olthoff, C. Streffer, J. Rassow, H. Sack: Neutron Capture therapy using a fast neutron beam: clinical considerations and physical aspects. Strahlenther. Oncol. 165 (1989), 208-210.
2. Sauerwein W., W. Ziegler, H. Szypniewski, C. Streffer: Boron neutron capture therapy (BCNT) using fast neutrons: effects in two human tumor cell lines. Strahlenther. Oncol. 166 (1990), 26-29.
3. Davids J., A. Mos, A. de Oude: Fast-neutron facility for biological exposures in an Argonaut reactor: design, tissue dosimetry and neutron spectrometry. Phys.Med.Biol. 14 (1969), 573-584.
4. Huiskamp R., J. Davids, O. Vos: Short and long term effects of whole body irradiation with fission neutrons or X-rays on the thymus in CBA mice. Radiat. Res. 95 (1983), 370-381.
5. Braak J.P., De Lage Flux Reactor te Petten. Stichting Energieonderzoek Centrum Nederland, ECN-87-172 (1987).

THERMAL NEUTRON INDUCED DECOMPOSITION AND INACTIVATION OF SEVERAL BIOMOLECULES

M. Akaboshi, K. Kawai, H. Maki, K.Akuta, Y. Ujeno

Research Reactor Institute, Kyoto University
Kumatori, Sennan, Oska-590, Japan

INTRODUCTION

Despite considerable work in the field of radiation effects of the $^{10}B(n,\alpha)^7Li$ reaction, the mechanisms of radiation damage to cells and biomolecules are not well understood. More knowledge of the generalities of comparative radiation effects of the other types of radiations, especially those relating to the $^{14}N(n,p)^{14}C$ reaction is needed. Irradiation by thermal neutrons of ^{10}B-containing biological materials inevitably involves exposure to radiations other than α- and Li-particles, namely those derived from the nuclear reactions $^{14}N(n,p)^{14}C$, $H(n,\gamma)D$, etc. Although ^{10}B has a larger cross-section for thermal neutron absorption (about 2000-fold larger than that, for example, of ^{14}N), the smaller abundance and lower accumulation of this nuclide in the usual biological samples make the additional contribution of other nuclear reactions to the total radiation effect inevitable. The initial purpose of this study is to quantitate the contribution of $^{14}N(n,p)^{14}C$ reaction to the total radiation effect when ^{10}B-containing biological materials are irradiated with thermal neutrons. The Tc-pneumatic irradiation facility (Tc-Pn) attached to KUR has a high thermal neutron flux (4×10^{11} n cm^{-2} sec^{-1}) as well as a high mixed γ-ray dose (2×10^3 Gy hr^{-1}). Hence it is useful for the analysis of the effect of $^{14}N(n,p)^{14}C$ reactions on biomolecules, such as amino acids, nucleotides, proteins and nucleic acids. The contribution of the $^{14}N(n,p)^{14}C$ reaction depends on the N-concentration of the samples. Our preliminary calculation for irradiation at the Tc-Pn indicated that when N-concentration is less than $10^{-2}M$, most of the radiation damage would arise via mixed γ-rays. But the contribution of the $^{14}N(n,p)^{14}C$ reaction comprises about 0.8 and 7.4% of total absorption dose when N-concentration of irradiated materials is 10^{-1} M and 10^0 M, respectively. It reaches nearly 50% when dry materials such as amino acids and proteins are irradiated at the Tc-Pn. In this investigation, an attempt was made to clarify the mechanism of the thermal neutron $^{14}N(n,p)^{14}C$ reaction on cells and bio-molecules by examining the inactivation of various enzymes in dry state.

MATERIALS AND METHODS

Crystalline samples of lysozyme, RNase and trypsin purchased from the Sigma Chemical Company were used without further purification. Thermal neutron irradiation was carried out using the Tc-Pn for 5 to 75 hours. For γ-ray irradiation, a 10000 Ci cobalt-60 source was employed with a dose rate of 4.8×10^4 Gy hr^{-1}. After irradiation and suitable dilution, the degree of denaturation of each protein was examined using High Performance Liquid Chromatography (HPLC). For this purpose, an exclusion column Shim-pack DIOL-300 was used. The enzyme activities of lysozyme, RNase and trypsin solutions were measured according to the methods of Smolelis[1], Dubos[2] and Kunitz[3], respectively.

Table 1. Contribution of the $^{14}N(n,p)^{14}C$ reaction to total absorbed dose versus N-concentration

Alanine	10^{-1} M	10^0 M	5×10^0 M	Dry
$^{14}N(n,p)^{14}C$ 10^3 Gy	0.016	0.16	0.80	1.79
mixed γ-ray 10^3 Gy	2	2	2	2
Contribution (%)	0.79	7.4	28.6	47.2

RESULTS AND DISCUSSIONS

Table 1 shows the absorbed dose and contribution of the nuclear reaction $^{14}N(n,p)^{14}C$ to the total absorbed dose when various concentrations of amino acid solutions were irradiated in the Tc-Pn irradiation facility for 1 hour. It can be seen that at our irradiation condition (dry state), the absorbed doses due to mixed γ-rays and the (n,p) reactions comprise about 50% each of the total absorbed energy.

Fig. 2 demonstrates the elution profile of γ-irradiated lysozyme. As shown, detection of the protein was made using the two monitors, absorbance at 210 nm and fluorescence measurement (OPA). From the figure, it can be seen that irradiation with 2.92×10^5 Gy of γ-rays results in a decrease of the areas of elution bands for both absorbance and fluorescence. The dose-response curves for the degradation of both γ-ray and thermal neutron irradiated lysozyme are shown in Fig. 2 together with those for enzyme inactivation. The enzyme is found to decrease exponentially with increasing dose of both the radiations. The slopes of the inactivation curves are somewhat steeper than those for degradation in both the radiations. This is a common tendency found in all the enzymes examined. From the slopes of the curves, the D_{37}s for enzyme inactivation of γ-ray and thermal neutron irradiated lysozyme, RNase and trypsin were obtained (Table 2). Here the RBEs of thermal neutrons were also determined to be 1.9, 2.8 and 2.4 for lysozyme, RNase and trypsin, respectively. In the calculation, the combined effect of thermal neutrons and mixed γ-rays was assumed to be additive. It should be noted that the RBE values obtained in the present experiment for enzyme inactivation are intermediate between those for cell survival of oxygenated (1.3) and hypoxic (3.6) Ehrlich ascites tumor cells[4].

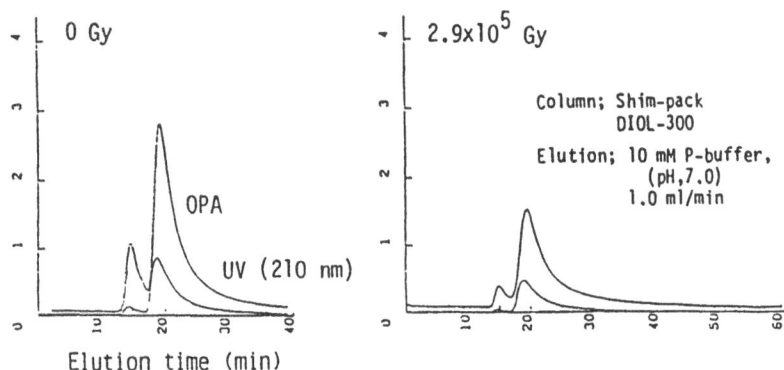

Fig. 1. HPLC-profile of γ-irradiated lysozyme (Chicken egg white)

404

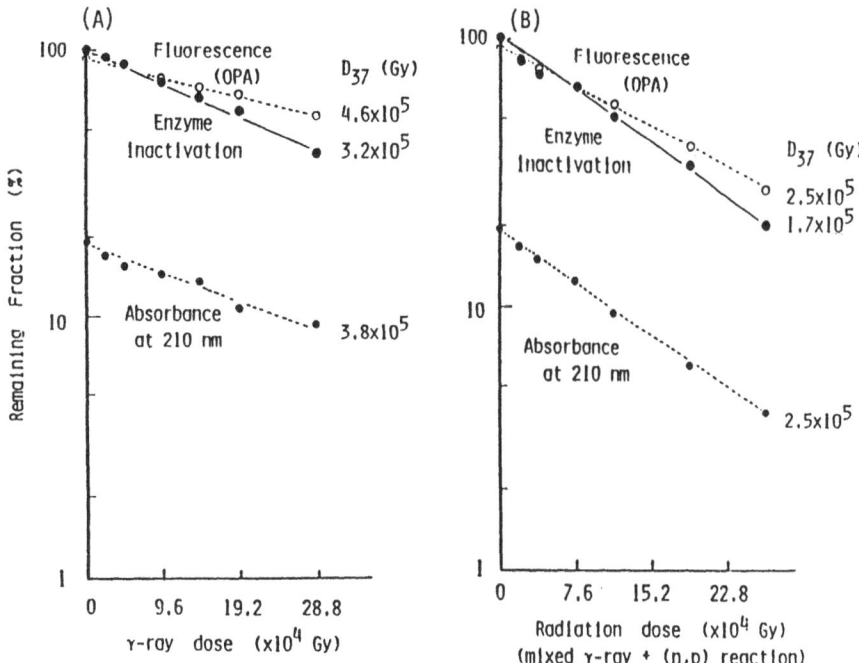

Fig 2. Dose-response curves of ^{60}Co-γ-ray (A) and thermal neutron (B) irradiated crystalline lysozyme. Values are means for three separate samples. In most cases, the standard deviations were less than 3% of means, and error bars did not exceed each point.

Table 2. D_{37}s and RBEs of irradiated enzymes

		D_{37} (γ)		D_{37} (n.th.)	
	M.W.	($\times 10^5$ Gy)	irrad.time	dose ($\times 10^5$ GY)	RBE
RNase A	1.37×10^4	7.77	70.1 hr	(n,p) : 1.26	2.8
				γ : 1.54	
Lysozyme	1.4×10^4	3.20	44.2 hr	(n,p) : 0.72	1.9
				γ : 0.88	
Trypsin	2.3×10^4	1.45	16.5 hr	(n,p) : 0.27	2.4
				γ : 0.33	

REFERENCES

1. A. M. Smolelis and S. E. Hartsell, The determination of lysozyme, J. Bact., 58:731-736 (1949).

2. R. J. Dubos and R. H. S. Thompson, The determination of yeast nucleic acid by a heat-resistant enzyme, J. Biol. Chem., 124:501-510 (1938).

3. M. Kunitz, Crystalline soybean trypsin inhibitor. II. General properties, J. Gen. Physiol., 30:291-310 (1947).

4. M. Akaboshi, K. Kawai and H. Maki, Lethal effect of thermal neutrons on hypoxic Ehrlich ascites tumor cells in vitro, J. Radiat. Res. 26:450-458 (1985).

KILLING EFFECTS OF GADOLINIUM NEUTRON CAPTURE REACTION ON BRAIN TUMORS

M. Takagaki[1], Y. Oda[1], S. Miyatake[1], H. Kikuchi[1],
T. Kobayashi[2], K. Kanda[2] and Y. Ujeno[2]
[1] Dept. Neurosurg., Sch. Med., Kyoto Univ., Kyoto Japan
[2] Research Reactor Institute of Kyoto Univ., Osaka Japan

INTRODUCTION

Boron Neutron Capture Therapy (B-NCT) has been successfuly reported during this quarter century (1).   In this therapy, boron accumulation into neoplastic tissue must be attained. Gadolinium has been proposed as an another potential nuclide of NCT (2,3,4).   Gd-157 has an approximately 64 times greater thermal neutron cross section, 255,000barns, than Boron-10, and the neutron capture reaction releases a total kinetic energy of 7.94MeV shared amongst prompt γ -rays, internal conversion electrons and Auger electrons (5).   The long range high energy γ -rays and electrons can deliver appreciable doses to infiltrating neoplastic satellite lesions of the tumor (3).   Also Gd-DTPA, which is an enhancement material for MR imaging, is clinically available as a tumor seeking agent(6).   In this study the tumorcidal effect of Gd-NCT was investigated using Gd-DTPA, and its killing effect was confirmed in in-vitro and in-vivo systems.

MATERIALS AND METHODS

The In Vitro Study

Human glioma cells, T98G, were suspended in Teflon tubes (10mm in diameter,30mm high) containing 1500μl of Dulbecco's modified Eagle's medium supplemented with 10% fetal bovine serum and Gd-DTPA, yielding 5,000ppm Gd (=780ppm Gd-157, corresponding to clinical standard of 50ppm B-10), and irradiated with thermal neutrons at the deuterium-thermal neutron facility of KUR.   After irradiation, cells were incubated in 6 cm diameter tissue culture dishes containing medium in a humidified atmosphere with 5% carbon dioxide at 37℃. Colonies were counted after 10 days incubation.

The In Vivo Study

Fisher-344 rats (7 weeks old female) bearing gliosarcoma brain tumor were prepared. Nitrosourea-induced gliosarcoma cells (9L, 10^6 cells in 10μl) were implanted into the right parietal region by stereotactic manoeuvres.   Mean survival of the 9L-rat was 16 days. Twelve days after implantation, at a nearly terminal stage, 9L-rats were exposed with thermal neutrons at the fluence rate of 3×10^9 cm^{-2} sec^{-1} for 1hr immediately after intravenous injection of 1mmol/kg Gd-DTPA.   Thermal neutrons were vertically directed onto

the parietal scalp surface under sedative condition.   During exposure, the body was
protected from neutron bombardment using ^{6}LiF holder.   Two weekes after irradiation, brains
were removed and submitted for pathological examination.   Tumor clearance of Gd-DTPA was
also measured by the prompt γ −ray spectrometry (7).

Human Brain Tumor Clearance of Gd-DTPA

Sixty four human brain tumor samples from 54 subjects were collected 5 to 100 minutes after
intravenous administration of 0. 1mmol/kg bw. Gd-DTPA during surgical manoeuvres.
Gd concentration was determined via ICP luminescence analysis.

RESULTS

The In Vitro Analysis

1% survival level was obtained at 3.75×10^{12} (n/cm^2) for Gd-loaded medium and 2.50×10^{13}
(n/cm^2) for Gd-free medium respectively; approximately a 6.7-fold difference (Fig-1L).
Similar tumorcidal effect on the cultur cell system of 9L was obtained (Fig.1R).

The In Vivo Analysis

9L-brain tumor cells were considerably destroyed by Gd-NCT, and almost no damage on normal
brain and vessels were observed.   But viable tumor cells were also identified.   9L-brain
tumor clearance of Gd-DTPA was measured.   About 60ppm Gd was detected immediately after
iv. injection of 0. 1mmol/kg Gd-DTPA.   When sacrifice was 5.5hrs after administration,
a slight difference of Gd concentration between tumor(3.5ppm) and blood(2.5ppm) was
detected (Fig.2).   Gd concentration in the opposite normal hemisphere was under the lower
detectable limit of about 1ppm.   Approximately 20 minutes after injection, Gd concentration
in tumor decreased to be half.

Human Tumor Clearance

All tumors contained from 0.06 to 25.01ppm of Gd, except one recurrent meningioma.
Concentration of Gd in tumors was calculated on subtraction of Gd in tumor vessels.
The lower detectable limit was 0.02ppm.   The maximum tumor/blood ratio of Gd was around 0.3
-0.6.   No correlations between Gd accumulation and tumor histological types were noted.

DISCUSSION

The Gd concentrations in brain tumors confirmed here after administration of 0. 1mmol/kg
Gd-DTPA were less than 100ppm, and it was measured to decrease in keeping equilibrium with
that in blood.   Gd-NCT, after high dose administration of 1mmol/kg Gd-DTPA, showed
tumorcidal effect on 9L-brain tumor without serious injury of normal brain and vessels after
thermal neutron exposure of 1.8×10^{13} (n/cm^2).   Using Gd-157 enriched DTPA, the concentration
of Gd-157 in tumor can be easily elevated 6-fold.   The linear dose relationship between the
Gd dose and the peak intravenous concentration of Gd was confirmed on our following
experiment for Gd-NCT.   Thus the muximum intravenous concentration of Gd is estimated to be
several thousnd ppm.   But the pulse infusions of Gd-DTPA during thermal neutron exposure is
necessary , becase the tumor clearance is too short.   Another potential use of Gd-DTPA,
intraventricular and/or intrathecal high dose injection can produce supplemental killing

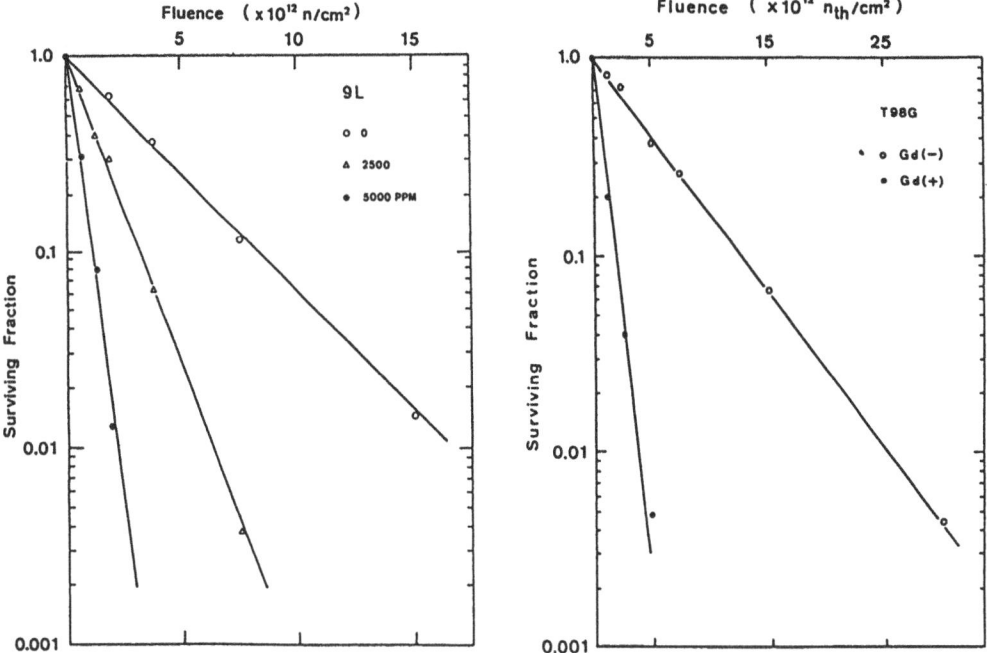

Fig. 1 Survival curve of Gd-NCT on malignant glioma cell (left) and nitrosourea indused gliosarcoma cell (right).

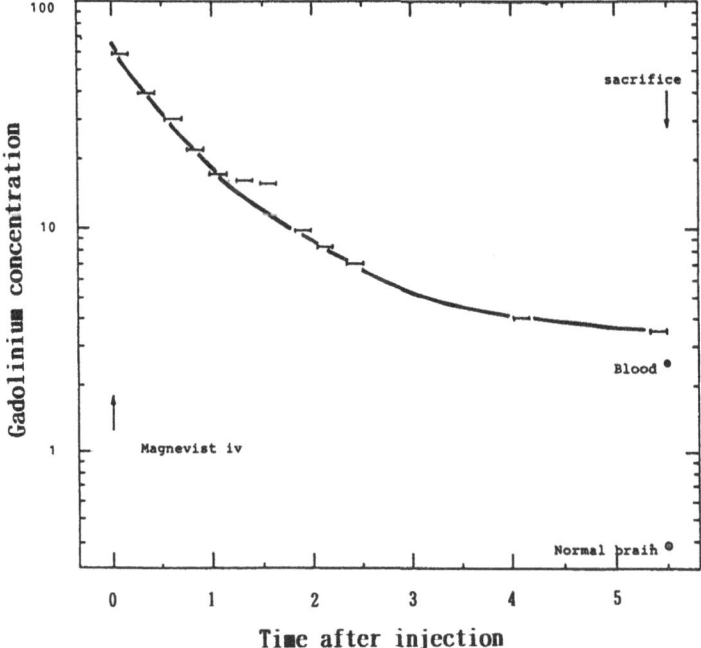

Fig. 2 Tumor clearance of Gd-DTPA after intravenous injection of 0.1mmol/kg analyzed by the prompt gamma ray spectroscopy. Half value of tumor clearance was about 20min.

effect on the cases of subependimal or intraventricular tumor disseminations by the simultaneously combined treatment with B-NCT. In Gd-NCT, dose distribution in tumor is not uniform. Theoreticaly in the case of spherical tumor with a radius of R, dose intensity: $\phi(r)$ caused by Gd(n, γ and/or e) reactions which uniformly occured in tumor is expressed as follows,

$$d^2\phi(r)/d^2 r + 2d\phi(r)/rdr + B^2\phi(r) = 0$$
$$\phi(r) = (A/r)\sin(\pi r/R)$$
$$A = \pi\phi(0)/R = \pi N\sigma\Phi/R$$

where, r:distance from tumor center, N: ^{157}Gd concentration, σ:255,000barns, Φ:thermal neutron fluence and B:constant depending on diameter of spheroid. The total absorbed dose distribution is estimated as follows,

$$\gamma * + {}^{157}Gd(n, \gamma \text{ and/or e}) {}^{158}Gd + {}^{14}N(n, p){}^{14}C$$
$$= \gamma * + \{N(Gd)\sigma(Gd)RBE(\gamma \text{ and/or e}) + N(N)\sigma(N)RBE(p)\}\Phi$$

where, $\gamma *$: caused by reactor core, structural materials and hydrogen atoms in tissue, RBE:relative biological effectiveness, N:concentration of ^{157}Gd and/or ^{14}N in tissue. Dose distribution onto tumor surrounding tissue caused by high energy γ-rays and electrons might be useful for infiltrating tumors. The gamma dose and proton dose caused by nitrogen and hydrogen atoms in tissue and also core gamma are inevitably exposed, and strongly restrict the irradiation period. This tantalizing situation can be lessened by Gd+B-NCT.

Acknowledgements-This work was supported by a Grant-in Aid for Cancer Research from the Ministry of Education, Science and Culture, Japan.

REFERENCES

1. Neutron Capture Therapy for Brain Tumors. H. Hatanaka ed. Niigata, Nishimura Co., Ltd., 1986
2. R. F. Martin, G. D'cunha, M. Pardee and B. J. Allen.:Induction of double-strand breaks following neutron capture by DNA-bound ^{157}Gd., Int. J. RADIAT. BIOL., 54(2), 205-208, 1988
3. R. M. Brugger, J. A. Shih.:Evaluation of Gadolinium-157 as a neutron capture therapy agent .,Strahlenther. Onkol., 165(2/3), 153-156, 1989
4. Akine Y., Tokita N., Matsumoto T., Oyama H., Egawa S. and Aizawa O.:Radiation effect of gadolinium neutron capture reaction and survival of chinese hamster cells., Strahlenther Onkol., 166(Nr.12), 831-833, 1990
5. R. C. Greenwood.:Collective and two-quasiparticle states in Gd-158 observed through study of radiative neutron capture in Gd-157., Nuclear Physiol., A304, 327-428, 1978
6. Oda Y., Takagaki M., Miyatake S., Kikuchi H.:Basic study of gadolinium neutron capture therapy for malignant brain tumors. Neurosurgery Letters, 1(5), 11-16, 1991
7. Kobayashi T. and Kanda K.:Microanalysis system of ppm-order B-10 concentratrion in tissue for neutron capture therapy by prompt gamma-ray spectrometry. Nucl. Instr. Meth., 204:525-531, 1983

SPONTANEOUS CANINE ORAL MELANOMA: A LARGE ANIMAL MODEL FOR BNCT

P.R. Gavin,[1] S.L. Kraft,[1] C.E. DeHaan,[1] R.D. Sande,[1]
M. Papageorges,[1] W.F. Bauer[2]

[1]Veterinary Clinical Medicine & Surgery, Washington State
University, Pullman, WA
[2]Idaho National Engineering Laboratory, Idaho Falls, ID

INTRODUCTION

Spontaneous tumors, in comparison to transplantable tumors, in animals offer several advantages for investigating new therapeutic modalities prior to human clinical trials. The main advantages are "typical" tumor vasculature, normal anatomical sites, slow growth rates and long cell-cycle times, and a nonimmunogenic nature.

Oral melanomas in dogs are the most common malignant neoplasm of the oral cavity. Prevalence has been recorded at 127 per 100,000 dogs/year. There is a predilection for the gingiva of male dogs with heavy pigmentation. The tumors are resistant to treatment with conventional radiation and chemotherapy. The tumors are very aggressive and have generally metastasized to the regional lymph nodes at the time of initial diagnosis. Distant metastases occur in approximately 85% of patients. Metastatic sites include lungs, kidneys, liver, brain, skeleton, and gastrointestinal (GI) tract.

METHODS

Fifteen (15) dogs with oral lesions biopsied and diagnosed as malignant melanoma were entered in the study. A thorough diagnostic regimen was performed in an attempt to detect the regional spread and distant metastases of the tumor. The protocol included computed tomography (CT) of: 1) the head, lungs, and liver, 2) thoracic radiographs, and 3) hepatic ultrasonography. Patients with distant metastases were entered into an acute terminal pharmacokinetic study using p-boronophenylalanine (p-BPA). Patients without detectable metastasis were administered the same compound and had radical surgery in an attempt to control the disease and provide sufficient tissue for boron analysis. Blood samples were taken before, during, and after p-BPA administration. Tissues for boron analysis were obtained at necropsy or at surgery 6 to 48 hours following administration of the compound. Following surgery, the dogs were returned to their owners for routine care and were re-examined at 6-month intervals for potential recurrence or metastasis. Those dogs that developed metastases following surgery were entered into the terminal pharmacokinetic study when their health deteriorated. Table I lists the dogs and the basic nature of the pharmacokinetic study. The p-BPA was administered subcutaneously in physiologic saline, 800 ml total volume, or orally in water (11 mg/kg body weight).

Table I. Canine Melanoma Pharmacokinetic Summary of Patient Data for the D,L p-BPA Study.

Animal #	Boron Dose	Form of p-BPA	Administration Route	Collection Length	Surgery or Euthanasia
001	50 mg/kg	D,L,HCl	Orally	6 hrs	Euthanasia
002	50 mg/kg	D,L,HCl	Orally	6 hrs	Euthanasia
003	50 mg/kg	D,L,HCl	Orally	6 hrs	Euthanasia
004	200 mg/kg	D,L	SQ,QID	36 hrs	Euthanasia
005	200 mg/kg	D,L	SQ,QID	48 hrs	Surgery
006	200 mg/kg	D,L	SQ,QID	48 hrs	Surgery
007	200 mg/kg	D,L	SQ,QID	48 hrs	Surgery
007-2(repeat)	500 mg/kg	D,L	Orally	6 hrs	Euthanasia
008	203 mg/kg	D,L	SQ,QID	48 hrs	Surgery
009	250 mg/kg	D,L	SQ,QID	12 hrs	Euthanasia
010	750 mg/kg	D,L	SQ,QID	48 hrs	Euthanasia
011	400 mg/kg	D,L	SQ,QID	48 hrs	Surgery
012	491 mg/kg	D,L	Orally,QID	48 hrs	Euthanasia
013	750 mg/kg	D,L	Orally	6 hrs	Euthanasia
015	250 mg/kg	D,L	Orally	6.5 hrs	Surgery

SQ = subcutaneously; QID four times per day

RESULTS

Nine of the 15 dogs had regional and distant metastases at the time of original diagnosis. The sites of metastases included the lungs, kidneys, liver, adrenals, lymph nodes, and brain.

Four of the 6 dogs that had radical surgery have developed metastases to date. The p-BPA was suspended in water for oral administration. The p-BPA was dissolved in saline for subcutaneous administration. The serum boron peaked at the end of subcutaneous administration and maintained the level for approximately 12 to 18 hours before declining. Oral administration of p-BPA resulted in a serum peak at about 1 hour, lasting for the 6 hours studied. There was a direct relationship between dose of compound administered and the serum boron concentration with a high degree of variability (Figures 1 and 2). The serum boron in the dogs varied from <1 - 7.3 ppm. Eight dogs had complete tissue sampling and analysis. Tissues with high boron concentrations ($\geq$ blood-boron concentration) were the kidneys, liver, lungs, oral mucosa, and brain (Figures 3 and 4). The tumors also all had boron concentrations in excess of the blood concentration. The tumor-to-blood ratio varied from 3 to 32. None of the variables was found to correlate to the most favorable ratios. This variability was also seen in the metastases and these often had boron concentrations in excess of the tumor. The tumors of three dogs had boron concentrations judged sufficient for BNCT (>20 ppm). The three dogs do not represent a clear indication of factors to exploit (Table II).

DISCUSSION

Dogs with spontaneous oral melanoma are a common and available source for experimental therapies. The 15 dogs were admitted to the protocol within one year. Most dogs have distant metastases at the time the primary tumor is diagnosed. This provides numerous sites in

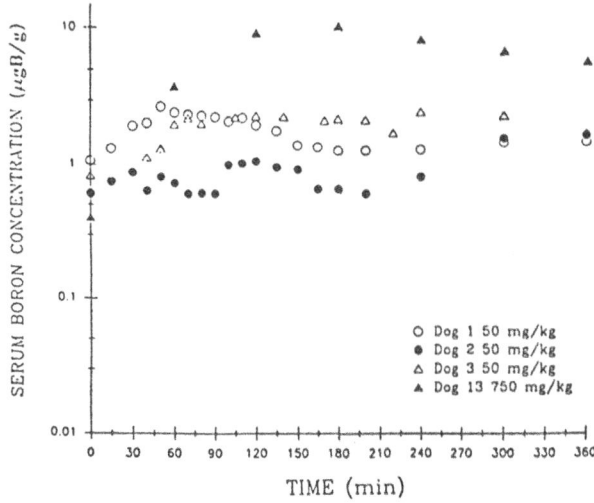

Figure 1. Serum Boron Concentration: Melanoma dogs 1, 2, 3, 13 - Oral p-Boronophenylalanine.

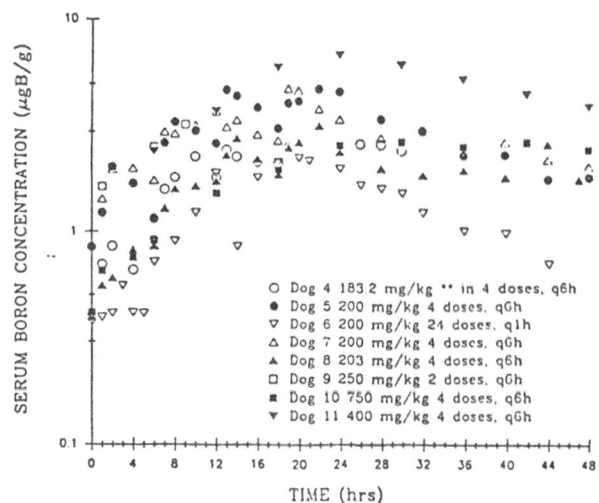

Figure 2. Serum Boron Concentration: Melanoma dogs 4-11 - p-Boronophenylalanine, given subcutaneously.

Table II. Canine Melanomas with Boron Concentration >20 ppm.

Dog #	Blood Boron Concentration	Tumor:Blood	p-BPA Dose (mg/kg)	Route of Administration	Time From End of Administration to Collection
007-2	7.2	n=22 x=3.2 σ=11.1	500	Oral Q6h x 4	6 hours
009	2.1	n=2 x=9.2	250	Subcutaneous Q6h x 2	12 hours
012	0.7	n=4 x=32.8 σ=13.8	500	Oral Q6h x 4	24 hours

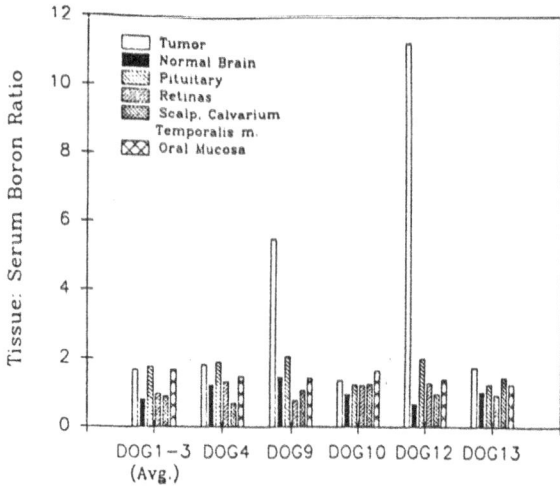

Figure 3. Tissue: Serum Boron Concentration, Melanoma
Dogs 1-3 (avg.), 4,9,10,12,13 - Given
p-Boronophenylalanine, sampled at various times.

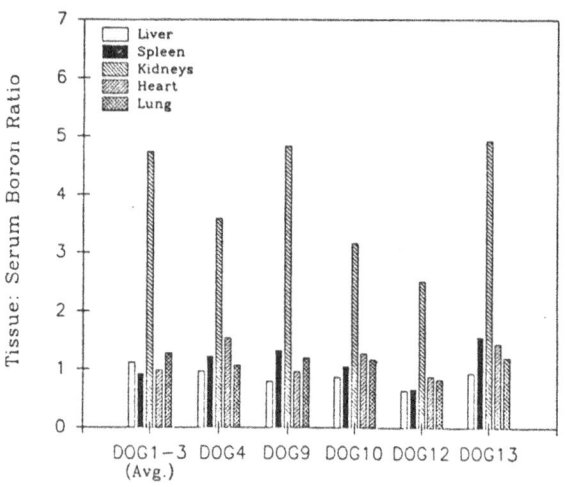

Figure 4. Tissue: Serum Boron Concentration, Melanoma
Dogs 1-3 (avg.), 4,9,10,12,13 - Given
p-Boronophenylalanine, sampled at various times.

multiple tissues for boron analysis in acute studies. The metastatic sites correspond to those of human melanoma patients; therefore, tolerance studies of the appropriate organ systems could be performed. Preliminary pharmacokinetic data reflects the variation in dose delivery during oral administration when administered subcutaneously. The amount of fluid needed to administer p-BPA subcutaneously may have prevented total absorption during the time studied. Future work will involve complexing the compound to materials to increase solubility at body pH and allow intravenous administration.

This preliminary study demonstrated therapeutic boron concentrations could be obtained in some dogs with spontaneous melanoma despite the limitations encountered. The boron concentration in tumors and other pigmented tissues did not increase with longer postadministration periods, which may indicate that boron is not metabolically incorporated. The boron concentration in the brain was often greater than the blood concentration, indicating p-BPA may not be the compound of choice to treat metastases of melanoma to the brain.

DOSE-RESPONSE ANALYSIS FOR BORON NEUTRON CAPTURE THERAPY OF THE B16

MURINE MELANOMA USING p-BORONOPHENYLALANINE

J.A. Coderre, P.L. Micca, D.N. Slatkin, and M.S. Makar

Medical Department, Brookhaven National Laboratory, Upton,
NY, 11973, USA.

Boron Neutron Capture Therapy (BNCT) of a well-pigmented B16 melanoma implanted subcutaneously in the mouse thigh has been carried out at the Brookhaven Medical Research Reactor (BMRR) using the synthetic amino acid p-boronophenylalanine (BPA) as the boron delivery agent. The response of the B16 melanoma to BNCT was compared with the response to 250 kVp x-rays using both tumor growth delay and an *in vivo/in vitro* assay that measures clonogenic survival. These experiments allow a comparison of tumor growth delay, log cell kill and damage to normal tissues produced by BNCT or photon irradiation.

METHODS

Mice (C57Bl/6) were dosed with intragastric (ig) slurries of 15 mg of the L-enantiomer of BPA in 0.5 ml water. First-passage tumors were initiated sc from $\approx 2 \times 10^5$ cells of a melanoma subclone (G3.12; Stackpole, 1985). Thigh tumors for irradiation (≈ 10-100 mg) grew from ≈ 1 mm^3 fragments of ≈ 200-300 mg first-passage tumors in 12 to 14 days. The outcome of a BNCT (Coderre, 1988) or an x-irradiation (Joel, 1990) procedure was measured by either the time to a spontaneous, tumor-related death or the time for the tumor to grow to a volume ($ab^2/2$, a>b; where a and b are perpendicular diameters) of 500 mm^3. Clonogenic survival was assayed in tumors removed <5 min post-treatment, which were then minced, trypsinized, cell-counted in suspension, and plated for colony-forming assay.

RESULTS AND DISCUSSION

^{10}B concentrations of ≈ 20 μg/g were obtained in the tumor 5 hours after one ig dose of BPA, that yielded tumor-to-blood-and tumor-to-muscle ratios of 8:1 and 6:1, respectively. Two ig doses given 5 hours apart resulted in ≈ 40 μg ^{10}B/g tumor (3 hours after the second dose); the tumor-to-blood-and tumor-to-muscle concentration ratios of 8:1 and 6:1 remained unchanged.

The fast-neutron dose from BNCT was 0.23 Gy/MW-min. The gamma dose from the reactor core and from activation of the collimator material was 0.08 Gy/MW-min. The dose from the ^{14}N(n,p)^{14}C reaction was 0.13 Gy/MW-min, based on 2.6% N (w/w) in tissues. A dose of 0.04 Gy/MW-min resulted from ^{1}H(n,γ)^{2}H reactions. The tumor dose resulting from 6 MW-min and 20 or 40 μg ^{10}B/g was 7.3 or 12.8 Gy, respectively; 10 MW-min with 20 μg ^{10}B/g resulted in a tumor dose of 12.1 Gy. The dose from BNCT irradiations is expressed as gray-equivalent (Gy-Eq), calculated by summation of physical doses (Gy) of the component radiations multiplied by appropriate relative biological effectiveness (RBE) factors. RBE values of 2.3 and 2.0 have been assumed for the ionizing particles from the ^{10}B(n,α)^{7}Li and ^{14}N(n,p)^{14}C reactions, respectively, and 2.0 has been assumed for fast neutrons.

Figure 1 (top panel) shows the response of the B16 melanoma to irradiations at the thermal neutron port of the BMRR with or without BPA. Tumor growth rates were inversely related to BNCT radiation doses. Median survivals were extended from 12 days for untreated tumor-bearing mice to 47, 51 or 115 days for mice that received BNCT doses of 21.5 Gy-Eq (n=17), 34.1 Gy-Eq (n=5) or 36.4 Gy-Eq (n=6), respectively. One tumor in each of the two latter groups regressed completely. At the two highest BNCT doses, reversible erythema and edema occurred in the foot distal to the irradiated tumor. The bottom panel in Figure 1 shows the response of the B16 melanoma to increasing doses of 250 kVp x-rays. X-ray doses of 5, 10, 15 or 20 Gy produced median survivals of 19, 27, 28 or 43 days, respectively, compared to 12 days for unirradiated controls. Normal tissue in the treatment field sustained severe damage (moist desquamation, muscle necrosis) from x-ray doses of ≥ 30 Gy. Damage (edema and atrophy) also occurred in the foot distal to the irradiated tumor. Although tumor growth was controlled by x-ray doses of 30 or 45 Gy, these mice had to be euthanized because of leg damage that was not observed to the same degree in any of the BNCT-treated mice.

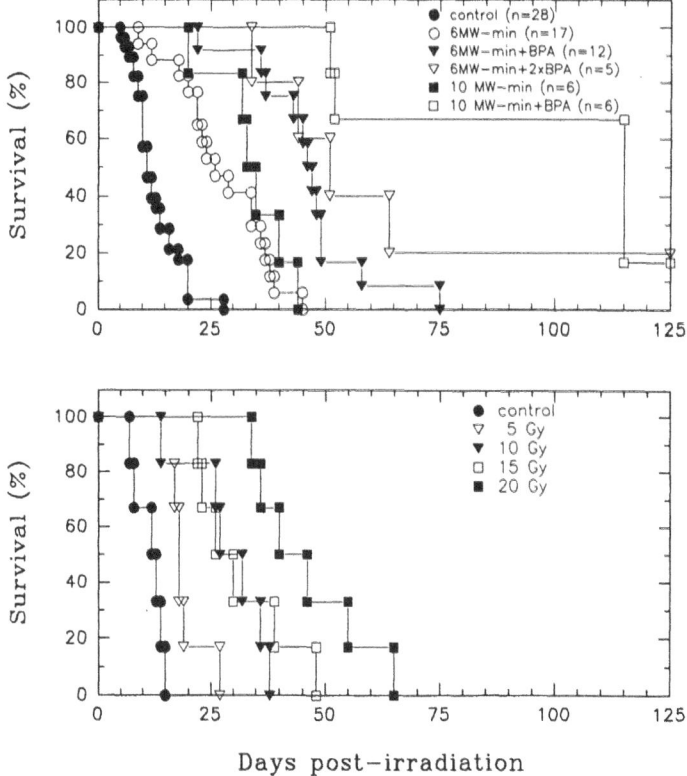

Fig. 1. (Top panel) Mouse survival data following irradiation of thigh tumors with thermal neutrons at the BMRR in the presence or absence of BPA. The control group was untreated. Thermal neutron fluences of $4.9 \times 10^{12} n_{th} cm^{-2} sec^{-1}$ (6 MW-min) and $8.0 \times 10^{12} n_{th} cm^{-2} sec^{-1}$ (10 MW-min) were used. The 6 MW-min group received reactor irradiation only (tumor dose = 4.7 Gy-Eq); the 6 MW-min+BPA group received one dose of BPA (20 μg ^{10}B/g tumor, tumor dose = 21.5 Gy-Eq); the 6 MW-min+2xBPA group received two doses of BPA (40 μg ^{10}B/g tumor, tumor dose = 34.1 Gy-Eq). The 10 MW-min group received reactor irradiation only (tumor dose = 8.6 Gy-Eq); the 10 MW-min+BPA group received a single dose of BPA (20 μg ^{10}B/g tumor, tumor dose = 36.4 Gy-Eq). (Bottom panel) Mouse survival following irradiation of thigh tumors with 250 kVp x-rays.

Figure 2 shows the fraction of surviving cells in irradiated tumors immediately after treatment. If the BNCT cell survival curve is extended by log-linear extrapolation to the doses used in these therapy irradiations, the log cell kill is on the order of $\approx 10^{-8}$ to 10^{-7}. This contrasts sharply with the degree of cell kill produced by 250 kVp x-rays, which is $\approx 10^4$-fold less than that produced by similar doses from BNCT. Tumor growth delays were similar from 20 Gy of x-rays and from 21.5 Gy-Eq of BNCT (Fig.1), yet the corresponding log cell kills apparently differed by $\approx 10^4$-fold.

Interestingly, BNCT did not produce permanent or long-term regression of tumor (Fig.1, top panel) until doses were used that apparently (Fig.2) yielded survival fractions of the order of 10^{-7}. Similar doses of x-rays, however, destroyed the leg as well as the tumor but allowed up to 1% of the cells in the tumor to survive the irradiation (Fig.2).

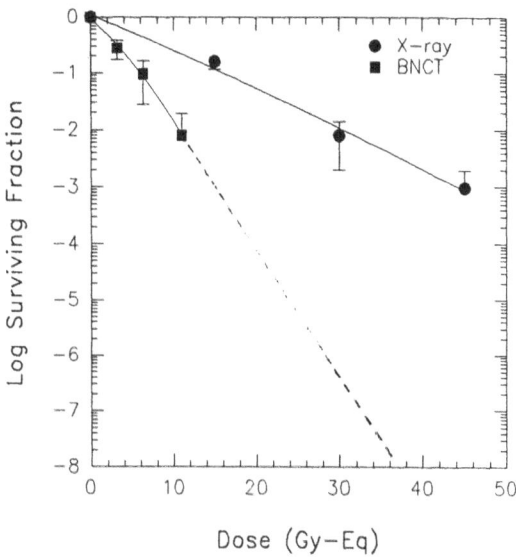

Fig. 2. Clonogenic survival in solid tumors determined by colony forming assay < 5 min after either BNCT or x-ray irradiation. Each point is the mean (± SD) of 4 - 6 tumors; 3 different dilutions were plated per tumor with 5 replicate plates per dilution.

ACKNOWLEDGEMENTS

The research described in the report involved animals maintained in animal care facilities fully accredited by the American Association for Accreditation of Laboratory Animal Care. This research was supported in part by the US Department of Energy under contract DE-AC02-76CH00016, and by Grant No. CA42446 (JAC) from the NIH.

REFERENCES

Coderre, J. A., J. A. Kalef-Ezra, R. G. Fairchild, P. L. Micca, L. E. Reinstein, and J. D. Glass, Boron neutron capture therapy of a murine melanoma. *Cancer Res.* **48**, 6313-6316 (1988).

Joel, D. D., R. G. Fairchild, J. A. Laissue, S. K. Saraf, J. A. Kalef-Ezra, and D. N. Slatkin, Boron neutron capture therapy of intracerebral rat gliosarcomas. *Proc. Natl. Acad. Sci., USA* (1990) in press.

Stackpole, C. W., A. L. Alterman, and D. M. Fornabaio, Growth characteristics of clonal cell populations constituting a B16 melanoma metastasis model. *Invasion Metastasis* **5**, 125-143 (1985).

INCREASED SELECTIVE ^{10}B-UPTAKE BY MALIGNANT MELANOMA USING SYSTEMIC ADMINISTRATION OF ^{10}B$_1$-BPA·FRUCTOSE COMPLEX

C. Honda[1], M. Shiono[1], N. Wadabayashi[1], M. Ichihashi[1],
Y. Mishima[1], T. Kobayashi[2], K. Kanda[2], Y. Hori[3], and
K. Yoshino[4]

[1]Department of Dermatology, Special Institute Cancer Neutron
Capture Therapy, Kobe University School of Medicine, Kobe
650, Japan.
[2]Kyoto University Research Reactor Institute, Osaka 590-04,
Japan.
[3]Shiseido Toxicological & Analytical Research Center,
Yokohama 223, Japan.
[4]Department of Chemistry, Shinshu University, Matsumoto 390,
Japan.

INTRODUCTION

^{10}B$_1$-para-Boronophenylalanine (^{10}B$_1$-BPA) has selective affinity for malignant melanoma. In our first human case, we succeeded in obtaining complete regression of a metastatic subcutaneous melanoma lesion by neutron capture therapy (NCT) using distant perilesional injections of ^{10}B$_1$-BPA hydrochloride.

Furthermore, we have cured primary cutaneous melanoma lesions of various types(1) in 5 additional patients by single or once repeated NCT using a combination of oral administration, subcutaneous and distant perilesional injections of ^{10}B$_1$-BPA·fructose complex at around pH 7.4(2). We have been pursuing NCT using increased systemic administration of ^{10}B$_1$-BPA, which can lead to cure of multiple (widely-distributed) melanoma lesions.

In this study, we analyzed boron dynamics in melanoma, skin and blood in tumor-bearing hamsters and a human patient after intravenous (i.v.) or subcutaneous (s.c.) injection of ^{10}B$_1$-BPA·fructose complex.

MATERIALS AND METHODS

^{10}B$_1$-BPA solution (pH 7.4) was prepared by complex formation with fructose. ^{10}B$_1$-BPA and fructose concentrations were 30 mg/ml (3%) and 66 mg/ml (6.6%), respectively.

In experiments using female Syrian golden hamsters bearing Greene's melanoma in subcutis, we analyzed tissue boron concentrations: i)by prompt gamma-ray spectrometry(3) at Kyoto Univ. Reactor, in order to follow ^{10}B dynamics in melanoma and normal skin without resection; or ii) by inductively coupled plasma atomic emission spectrometry (ICP-AES) at Shiseido Res. Center; after i.v. or s.c. injection of ^{10}B$_1$-BPA·fructose complex.

In a 63-year-old male patient with right thigh, multiple metastatic melanoma lesions of amelanotic type which were to be surgically removed in two operations, $^{10}B_1$-BPA fructose complex was administered by drip i.v. infusion in the first operation, and by s.c. left buttock injection in the second. Collected tissue samples were submitted for ICP-AES boron assay.

RESULTS AND DISCUSSION

I. Intravenous Administration

In Fig. 1, ICP-AES assay showed that after a single i.v. injection of $^{10}B_1$-BPA, the boron concentration in melanoma was maintained at about 14 ppm for at least 2 hours, while the concentrations in skin and blood decreased rapidly. These results further support a selective incorporation of $^{10}B_1$-BPA into melanoma cells.

In human melanoma patients using drip i.v. infusion of $^{10}B_1$-BPA·fructose complex, no side effects or complications were noted, and promising results for drip i.v. infusion of $^{10}B_1$-BPA in NCT were observed, as described elsewhere(4).

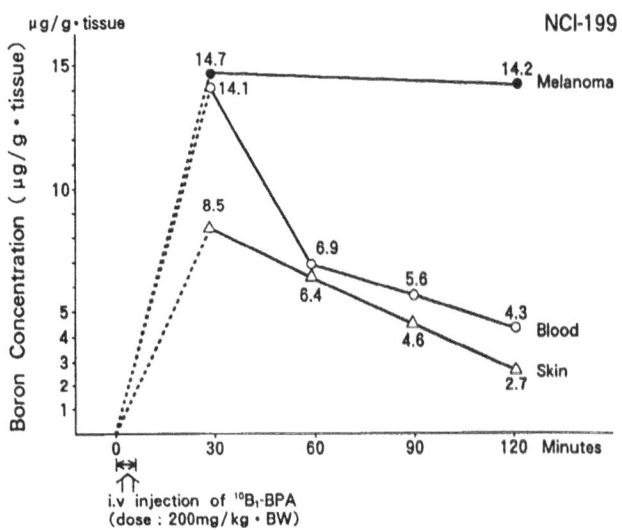

Fig.1. Time course of boron concentrations analyzed by ICP-AES in blood (O), skin (△) and Greene's melanoma (●) after intravenous injection of $^{10}B_1$-BPA·fructose complex to melanoma-bearing hamsters.

II. Subcutaneous Injection

We have found that boron concentrations in blood, melanoma, and skin collected 3 hours after s.c. injection increased almost linearly in proportion to the administered dose, as long as the dose was within 500 mg/kg·BW(4).

In Fig.2, in situ assay by prompt gamma-ray spectrometry of ^{10}B in a hamster shows a linearly increasing ^{10}B concentration in the melanoma for about 3 hours following a single s.c. injection (dose of $^{10}B_1$-BPA: 250 mg/kg·BW). On the other hand, as shown in Fig.3, by administering the same total $^{10}B_1$-BPA of 250 mg/kg·BW in 5 divided doses at 3 hour intervals melanoma can accumulate increasing amounts of ^{10}B, while ^{10}B concentration in normal skin shows relatively small increases in response to repeated

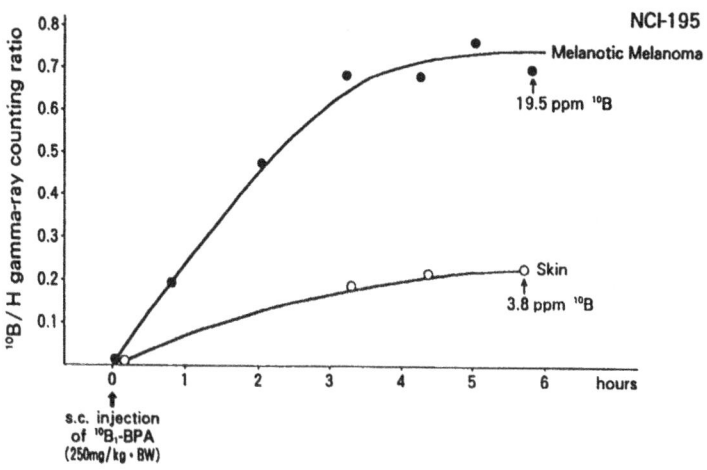

Fig.2. In vivo ^{10}B dynamics determined by prompt gamma-ray spectrometry in melanotic melanoma (●), and normal skin (○) after a single s.c. injection of $^{10}B_1$-BPA・fructose complex ($^{10}B_1$-BPA : 250mg/kg・BW) into a melanoma-bearing hamster.

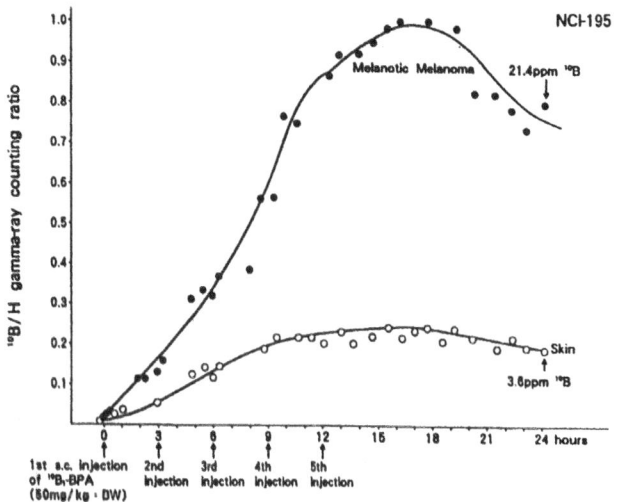

Fig.3. In vivo ^{10}B dynamics determined by prompt gamma-ray spectrometry in melanotic melanoma (●), and normal skin (○) after multiple s.c. injections of $^{10}B_1$-BPA・fructose complex ($^{10}B_1$-BPA : 50mg/kg・BW × 5) into a melanoma-bearing hamster.

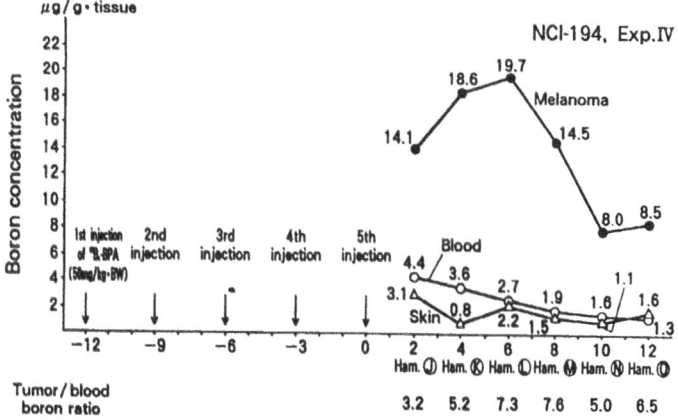

Fig.4. Time course of boron concentrations deter-mined by ICP-AES in blood (○), skin (△) and Greene's melanotic melanoma (●) after multiple s.c. injections of $^{10}B_1$-BPA・fructose complex ($^{10}B_1$-BPA : 50mg/kg・BW × 5) into melanoma-bearing hamsters.

injections. It is suggested that such divided s.c. injections of $^{10}B_1$-BPA may be more advantageous than single s.c. injection of the same total dose because boron concentrations in skin can be reduced. In Fig.4, assay by ICP-AES for B in hamsters revealed that at 6 hours after the last injection, the boron concentration reached approximately 20 ppm in melanoma, while both that in blood and skin were lower than 3 ppm.

In response to divided s.c. injections, a human melanoma patient, who displayed multiple metastatic lesions again several months after the first operation, showed that the boron concentrations in normal skin may decrease below 3 ppm after a longer time than did the hamster, as shown in Fig.5.

These experiments indicate that the most suitable method of systemic administration of $^{10}B_1$-BPA·fructose complex for optimal NCT can be established in the near future.

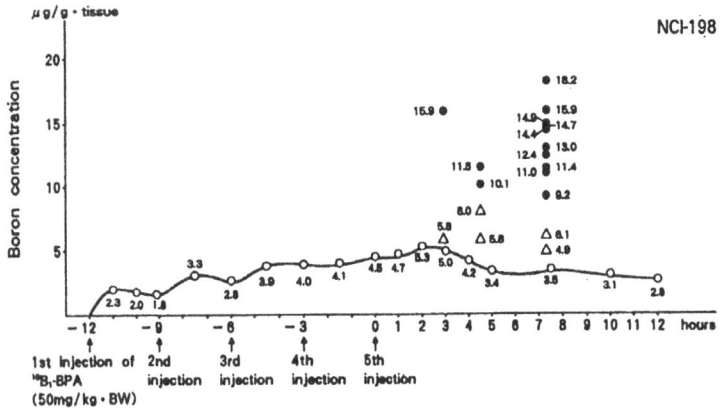

Fig.5. Time course of boron concentrations determined by ICP-AES in blood (○), skin (△) and amelanotic melanoma (●) by multiple s.c. injections of $^{10}B_1$-BPA·fructose complex ($^{10}B_1$-BPA : 50mg/kg·BW × 5) to a 63-y-o male melanoma patient bearing multiple subcutaneous metastatic tumors on his right thigh.

REFERENCES

1. Y.Mishima, C.Honda, M.Ichihashi, et al, Treatment of malignant melanoma by single thermal neutron capture therapy with melanoma-seeking ^{10}B-compound.
   Lancet 2:388 (1989).
2. K.Yoshino, A.Suzuki, Y. Mori, et al, Improvement of solubility of p-boronophenylalanine by complex formation with monosaccharides.
   Strahlenther. Onkol. 165:127 (1989).
3. C.Honda, Y.Mishima, M.Ichihashi, et al, In situ detection of cutaneous melanoma by prompt gamma-ray spectrometry using melanoma-seeking ^{10}B-dopa analogue. J. Dermatological Science 1:23 (1990).
4. Y.Mishima, M.Ichihashi, C.Honda, et al, Advances in the cure of human primary and metastatic melanoma by thermal neutron capture therapy.
   in: "Proc. 4th Int. Symp. Neutron Capture Therapy", (1991).

LOCAL CONTROL OF MURINE MELANOMA XENOGRAFTS IN NUDE MICE BY NEUTRON CAPTURE

THERAPY

B.J. Allen[1], S. Corderoy-Buck[1], D.E. Moore[2], Y. Mishima[3], M Ichihashi[3]

[1] Biomedicine and Health Program, Australian Nuclear Science and Technology Organisation PMB 1 Menai NSW 2234 Australia
[2] Department of Pharmacy University of Sydney NSW Australia
[3] Department of Dermatology University of Kobe, Kobe Japan

INTRODUCTION

In recent years considerable progress has been made in the development and implementation of neutron capture therapy (NCT) for the treatment of cancer. In particular, the boron analogue of the melanin precursor phenylalanine, ie DL-p-boronophenylalanine (BPA), has been used to demonstrate the regression and cure of Harding-Passey (HP) melanoma in syngeneic mice[1]. However, 18 to 25% cures were obtained for neutron irradiations without boron, suggesting that the neutron dose alone plays an important role. Neutron capture therapy of B-16 melanoma xenografts in nude mice[2] showed substantial tumour regression over 35 days, but the survival rate of NCT treated mice after 7 weeks was only 40-60%.

In this paper we demonstrate the equivalence of the nude mouse model with a syngeneic model, using the same Harding-Passey murine melanoma line, and delineate the conditions required for maximum differential response between neutron irradiation with and without BPA administration, with complete local control as the end point.

MATERIALS AND METHODS

The Harding Passey murine melanoma cell line (supplied by B Laster BNL) is a highly melanotic and reproducible cell line. Cells were batch cloned and held in liquid nitrogen. The ampoules were then thawed following standard reconstitution procedures and allowed to achieve normal growth rates over 2-3 weeks. Between 1.5 and 1.75 million cells were then implanted subcutaneously on the outer surface of the thigh, and tumours invariably grew to a few millimetres diameter within two weeks.

Athymic nude mice are bred at our laboratory and are derived from BALB/c Nu/Nu inbred/outbred stock. The mice are maintained in biohazard cabinets under specific pathogen free (spf) conditions. The mice used in this experiment were generally 14 weeks old and in excellent health.

The DL-p-boronophenylalanine.HCl was dissolved in physiological saline at a concentration of 24 mg/ml (ph = 1.5) prior to a 0.5 ml intraperitoneal (ip) injection of a glycol mixture.

For the biodistribution studies, mice were sacrificed at time intervals up to 24 h post-injection by cervical dislocation. Tissue samples were dissected out and prepared for analysis by the ICP method[3].

All mice are anaesthetised before loading into the irradiation capsule, using Ketamine (1 mg/kg), Zylazine (0.3 mg/kg) in 0.11 ml ip injection. This is well tolerated by the mice which show complete recovery within 90 minutes.

Throughout the experiment, spf conditions are maintained by loading the anaesthetised mice into sterile neutron shield tubes of ^{6}LiF epoxy, which are then placed inside a perspex box. One rear leg is pulled through a side aperture and exposed to the incident neutron flux. The neutron fluence inside the shield tube is reduced to a few percent of the value incident on the tube.

The mice were divided up into three groups of eight. In the control group of untreated mice, the tumours were allowed to grow to about 0.5 ml volume, and the mice subsequently sacrificed. The second group of mice were irradiated with 1.1×10^{13} n cm^{-2}, while the third group received 12 mg BPA.HCl 4 hours before the same neutron exposure. Irradiations occurred at $T_0 = 5,7,11,13$ days post-inoculation, for tumour sizes from 2 to 10 mm diameter.

The NCT facility is located in the graphite column of the 100 kW Moata Argonaut reactor. Within the NCT cavity, immediately behind the 20 cm thick bismuth shield, the neutron flux is 10^{10} n cm^{-2} s^{-1} and the concomitant gamma dose rate is 4.8 Gy/h at 100 kW full power. The mice were irradiated at 100 kW for 22 minutes for an incident neutron fluence at the perspex box of 1.8×10^{13} n cm^{-2} and reactor gamma dose of 1.8 Gy. The fluence at the mouse thigh, located in the aperture of the shield tube, is typically 1.1×10^{13} n cm^{-2}. The measured and calculated radiation dose components are given in Table 1, assuming 28.5 ppm ^{10}B in the tumour and 2 ppm ^{10}B in the skin.

Table 1. Radiation dose components in NCT experiment

Radiation Measured	Reactor gamma	Capture gamma	Fast neutron	Whole body	thermal neutron
absorbed dose (Gy)	1.8	0.2	–	2.0	2.4
dose component calculated	^{10}B 2 ppm	skin dose	^{10}B 28.5 ppm	Tumour dose	TG
absorbed dose (Gy)	1.7	6.1	27.7	32.1	5.3

RESULTS AND DISCUSSION

The growth pattern of the Harding Passey melanoma in the nude mouse model is initially lateral and then vertical for larger tumours. The normalised growth rates are therefore calculated as the ratio of tumour area at post-irradiation times to the area at the time of irradiation, as shown in fig.1 Results are shown for relative area growth normalised at 5, 7, 11 and 13 days post-inoculation.

The therapeutic gain (TG) is the ratio of tumour dose and maximum normal tissue dose. For this experiment, TG=5.3 for the ratio of absorbed doses. Thus the tumour receives over 5 times the radiation dose to the overlying skin, and the boron dose component to the tumour is 90% of the total radiation dose.

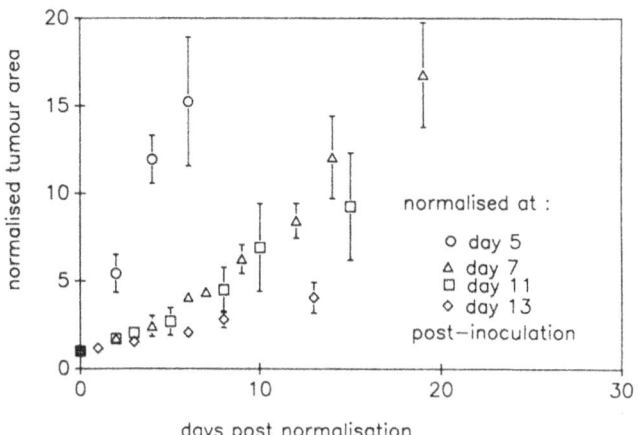

Fig. 1. Harding Passey melanoma relative area growth rates, normalised at 5
to 13 days post inoculation

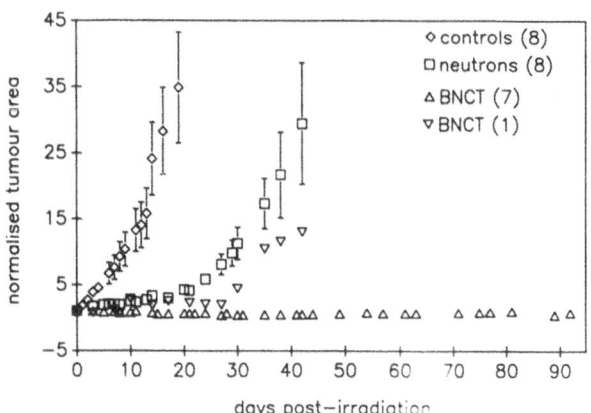

Fig. 2. Growth rates, growth delay and cure of Harding-Passey melanoma in the
nude mouse model by neutron capture therapy. One case of recurrance
(∇) was observed in 8 NCT treatments. Error bars are within data
points for surviving BNCT mice.

The growth rates, normalised to the area (product of orthogonal diameters) at the time of irradiation are shown in fig 2. for neutron only irradiations, and for neutron exposures following ip administration of enriched $^{10}BPA.HCl$. The same neutron fluence was applied in both cases. The control data are selected to have the same T_0 values as those found in the irradiated groups of mice. A growth delay of about 23 days is apparent for the neutrons only data, but not one case of complete local tumour control was observed.

Complete tumour regression was achieved for 7 of 8 NCT exposures following BPA administration and an estimated tumour dose of 32 Gy. Most NCT mice have survived to more than 200 days, and a second recurrence was observed at 250 days. However, in this case the tumour increased in thickness but the area did not change. In some cases the tumour completely disappeared, but more often the well delineated black mass gave way to a grey mass with ill-defined borders which slowly reduced in thickness. Erythema, or dry desquamation in the longer term, was not observed.

ACKNOWLEDGEMENTS

The assistance of I Delaney and M Bilek is much appreciated. The Australia-Japan collaboration has been sponsored by the Department of Industry, Technology and Commerce in Australia and Monbusho in Japan. The support of the Government Employees Assistance to Medical Research Fund has been critical to the success of this work.

REFERENCES

1. J.A. Coderre, J.A. Kalef-Ezra, R.J. Fairchild, P.L. Micca, L.E. Reinstein, J.D. Glass (1988). Boron neutron capture therapy of a murine melanoma, Cancer Res 48: 6313-6316

2. N. Tamaoki, M. Ueda, S. Tamauchi, K. Yamamoto, Y. Mishima (1989). Use of nude mice in experimental neutron capture therapy with ^{10}B-BPA, Pigment Cell Res 2: 343-344.

3. S.R. Tamat, D.E. Moore, B.J. Allen (1987). Determination of boron in biological tissues by inductively coupled plasma atomic emission spectrometry, Anal Chem 59: 1261-2164.

A RAT MODEL FOR THE TREATMENT OF MELANOMA METASTATIC TO THE BRAIN BY MEANS OF NEUTRON CAPTURE THERAPY

Khalid Z. Matalka, Michael Q. Bailey, Rolf F. Barth, Alfred E. Staubus, Dianne M. Adams
Albert H. Soloway, Steven M. James, and Joseph H. Goodman
The Ohio State University, Columbus, Ohio 43210, U.S.A.

Jeffrey A. Coderre and Ralph G. Fairchild
Brookhaven National Laboratory, Upton, New York 11973, U.S.A.

Einar K. Rofstad
Norwegian Radium Hospital, Oslo Norway

Introduction

Melanoma metastatic to the brain is a serious clinical problem for which there currently is no satisfactory treatment[1,2]. Boron neutron capture therapy (BNCT) has been shown by Mishima et al. to be clinically effective in the treatment of cutaneous melanoma using ^{10}B-enriched boronophenylalaine (BPA) as the capture agent[3]. Similarly, Coderre et al. have demonstrated efficacy of BNCT in the treatment of the Harding-Passey melanoma in BALB/c mice[4]. Our previous experience in the treatment of a rat glioma by means of BNCT[5] has lead us to develop a rat model for the treatment of melanoma metastatic to the brain. We have employed a human melanoma cell line, MRA 27, which when implanted intracerebrally into immunologically deficient nude rats, grows progressively and ultimately kills the host. Survival time is dependent upon the size of the initial tumor inoculum, and death occurs as a result of the expanding intracranial mass. Although human melanoma metastatic to the brain may be multicentric[6], the biological behavior of intracerebrally implanted MRA 27 simulates it in a number of ways, and therefore provides a good model for the human tumor. The purpose of the present study was to evaluate the efficacy of BNCT for the treatment of intracerebrally implanted MRA 27 using BPA as the capture agent and to compare its efficacy with external beam gamma irradiation.

Methods

Animals and cell line. The human melanoma cell line MRA 27 was derived from a 60 year old Norwegian male and has been propagated both in vitro and in vivo in nude mice and rats. Six to eight week old athymic female nude rats of NIH-rnu strain were purchased from the Animal Production Branch, National Cancer Institute, Frederick, MD. The rats were maintained under specific pathogen-free conditions and fed sterilized food and water.

Implantation. A stereotactic implantation procedure, previously used by us for studies on BNCT of a rat glioma, was employed[5]. Briefly, nude rats were sedated with a 1.2/1 mixture of ketamine/xylazine and a plastic screw was embedded in the skull. MRA 27 cells were injected into the right caudate nucleus at a concentration of 2×10^5 or $10^6/10$ μl of serum-free McCoy's 5A medium containing 1% agarose at a gelling temperature of $<30°C$. The implantation procedure employed a relatively slow injection time, rapid filling of the screw hole with bone wax following withdrawal of the needle, and flushing of the operative field with betadiene before closing the scalp incision with a single sterilized clip.

Pharmacokinetics. A solution of ^{10}B-enriched D,L-BPA, generously provided by Callery Chemical Co. (Callery, PA), was converted to a fructose complex by mixing 1:1 molar ratio of BPA and fructose to yield a final concentration of 120 mg of BPA/2 ml of water at pH 8.8. Two ml of the complex were administered i.p. to rats 37 days following intracerebral implantation of 10^6 tumor cells. Animals were killed 1, 3, 6, 9, 12, and 18 hours later and samples of blood, brain, tumor skin, liver, kidneys, muscle, eyes, and skull were obtained. Boron concentrations were determined by means of direct current plasma atomic emission spectroscopy, as described in detail elsewhere[7].

Irradiation studies. For photon irradiation rats were implanted with 2×10^5 MRA 27 cells and 31 days later they were divided into three groups of 5-6 animals each. Group 1a received a single 12 Gy dose of gamma photons and group 2a received 9 fractions of 2 Gy each, delivered over an eleven day period using a Picker ^{137}Cs Teletherapy machine, which had a dose rate of 1 Gy/min when a 2 cm (OD) cone was used, and group 3a consisted of untreated controls.

BNCT was initiated 35 days following implantation of 2×10^5 MRA 27 cells, unless indicated otherwise. Rats were divided into five groups of 3-7 animals each. Groups 1b and 2b were irradiated at either 6 hrs or 12 hrs post i.p. administration of 120 mg of ^{10}B-enriched L-BPA. Group 3b received two i.p. doses of 120 mg each of L-BPA, administered 9 and 6 hrs prior to irradiation. Group 4b received radiation only and group 5b were untreated controls. All irradiations were carried out at the Brookhaven Medical Research Reactor (BMRR), which has a thermal neutron flux density of 2.8×10^{11} n cm^{-2} min^{-1} at 1 megawatt (MW) power. All of the treated rats received 6 MW-minutes of irradiation or 2.73 Gy. Animals were weighed at 2 day intervals following irradiation, survival times were recorded, and Kaplan-Meier plots and mean and median survival times were determined.

Results and Discussion

Pharmacokinetic studies. Distribution of BPA in nude rats that had been implanted intracerebrally with MRA 27 melanoma are summarized below (Table 1).

Since the boron concentration of the blood and brain determine tissue tolerance, the optimum time for irradiation was chosen on the basis of maximum tumor/brain (T/Br) and tumor/blood (T/Bl) ratios. Blood levels of BPA exhibited biexponential decay ($t_{\frac{1}{2}\alpha} = 1.1$ hrs, $t_{\frac{1}{2}\beta} = 5.6$ hrs) and tumor levels of BPA exhibited monoexponential decay ($t_{1/2} = 5.39$ hrs) with the terminal time points (6-18 hrs) in an apparent distribution equilibrium with BPA levels observed in blood. The best

Table 1. Distribution of BPA following i.p. administration to nude rats carrying i.c. melanoma.

Tissue	Tissue boron concentrations (μg/g) at varying times post injection (hours)*				
	1	3	6	9	12
Brain	2.3	4.3	5.4	5.2	2.4
Blood	54.9	27.0	5.7	3.8	2.3
Tumor	27.6	19.4	13.7	9.2	8.7
Liver	36.1	11.1	7.1	4.2	2.6
T/Bl ratio	0.5	0.7	2.4	2.4	3.8
T/Br ratio	12.0	4.5	2.5	1.8	3.6

*average of four rats

Table 2. Survival of nude rats carrying i.c. implants of MRA 27 melanoma.

Group	Treatment	n[a]	Dose	MeST	MST $\pm$ S.D.	%ILS(Me)[b]	%ILS(M)[c]
Gp 1a	Gamma	6	12 Gy	86	83 $\pm$ 20	83	81
Gp 2a	Gamma	6	2 Gy x 9	79	78 $\pm$ 10	67	69
Gp 3a	None	5		47	46 $\pm$ 5	-	-
Gp 1b	BNCT	4	5.51 Gy[d]	159	>159 $\pm$ 60	261	>273
Gp 2b	BNCT	5	4.49 Gy[d]	93	93 $\pm$ 23	111	119
Gp 3b	BNCT	3	5.33 Gy[d]	221	>171 $\pm$ 94	402	>302
Gp 4b	Neutrons	5	2.73 Gy[d]	62	79 $\pm$ 48	41	86
Gp 5b	None	7		44	43 $\pm$ 4	-	-

a = number of animals per group
b = percent increased life span determined from median survival time (MeST)
c = percent increased life span determined from mean survival time (MST)
d = dose based on previous determination of ^{10}B tumor concentrations

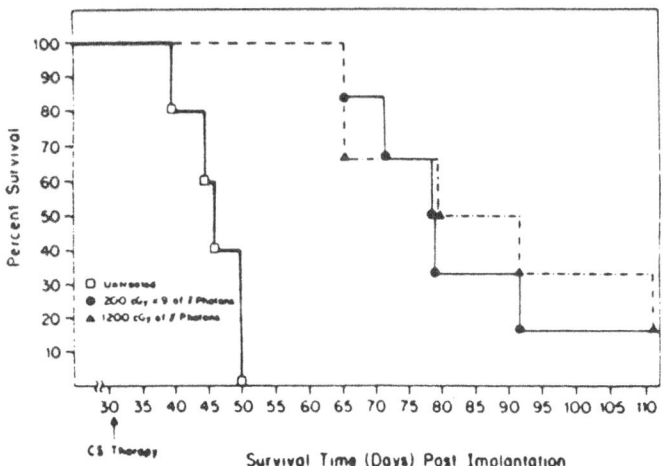

Figure 1

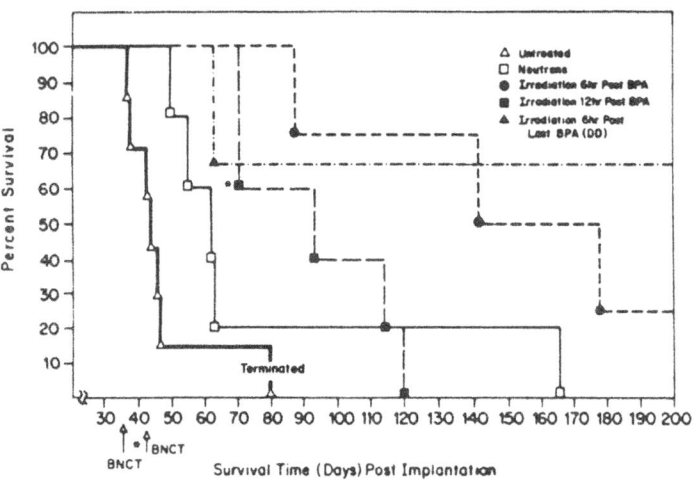

Figure 2

composite T/Br and T/Bl ratios were observed 6 hrs following BPA administration at which time the boron concentration in the tumor was 13.7 μg/g and T/Bl and T/Br ratios were 2.4 and 2.5 respectively, while the corresponding normal brain levels of boron ranged from 1.1-5.4 μg/g.

Irradiation studies. Kaplan-Meier plots for rats implanted intracerebrally with MRA 27 melanoma and then treated 31 d later with gamma photons are shown in Fig. 1. The median survival times (MeST) of rats treated with 12 Gy and 2 Gy x 9 were 86 d and 79 d respectively, compared to 47 d for the untreated animals. The mean survival times (MST) were 83 d and 78 d respectively compared to 46 d for the untreated rats. The percent increase in life span (%ILS) were 83% and 67% (determined from MeST) for the 12 Gy and 2 Gy x 9 groups respectively (Table 2).

Kaplan-Meier plots for BNCT treated animals are shown in Fig. 2. The MeST of neutron irradiated animals (gp 4b) was 62 d compared to 44 d for untreated controls (gp 5b). The MST were 79 d and 43 d respectively. The MeST of BNCT rats irradiated at 6 hrs (gp 1b) and at 12 hrs (gp 2b) after receiving BPA were 159 d and 93 d respectively. Those animals that received a double dose of BPA (gp 3b) had a MeST of 221 d. As determined from MeST, %ILS of the BNCT groups were 2.6-9.8 x > irradiated controls (gp 4b). Furthermore, as determined from MeST, the %ILS for BNCT rats irradiated 6 hrs post administration of BPA (gp 1b) was 2.4 x > those irradiated 12 hrs post BPA administration (gp 2b). There are at least two possible explanations for this enhanced survival. First, the boron concentrations in the tumors of gp 1b were greater than those of gp 2b (13.7 v.s. 8.7 μg/g). Second, the time at which BNCT was initiated for gp 1b was seven days earlier than gp 2b suggesting that earlier treatment may have been more effective than later treatment. Although the % ILS of the BNCT treated animals were 1.3 - 4.8 x > 12 Gy photon irradiated rats, the comparison of the effects of BNCT and gamma irradiation cannot be determined from this study. However, a more definitive study, which is in progress, will compare the two arms based on iso-effect tumor analysis.

In the present pilot study we have observed a significant prolongation in survival time of nude rats bearing intracerebral implants of the human melanoma cell line MRA 27 following administration of BPA and neutron irradiation. These findings suggest therapeutic efficacy, but tumor control studies which have been planned will define the parameters of BNCT that are important for future BNCT experiments.

Acknowledgments

This work was supported by grant 5 R01 CA 41288 and CA 53896 from the National Cancer Institute and grant DE-FG02-90ER60972 and contract DE-AC02-76CH00616 from the Department of Energy, and The Ohio State University Office of Research and Graduate Studies.

References

1. M.S. Mitchell: Relapse in the central nervous system in melanoma patients successfully treated with Biomodulators. Journal of Clinical Oncology 7, 1701-1709 (1989).
2. S. Madajewicz, C. Karakousis, C. West, J. Caracandas, A. Avellanosa: Malignant melanoma brain metastases. Cancer 53, 2550-2552 (1984).

3. Y. Mishima, M. Ichihashi, S. Hatta, C. Honda, K. Yamamura, T. Nakagawa: New thermal neutron capture therapy for malignant melanoma: melanogenesis-seeking ^{10}B molecule-melanoma cell interaction from in vitro to first clinical trial. Pigment Cell Research 2, 226-234 (1990).

4. J.A. Coderre, J.A. Kalaf-Ezra, R.G. Fairchild, P.L. Micca, L.E. Reinstein, J.D. Glass: Boron neutron capture therapy of a murine melanoma. Cancer Research 48, 6313-6316 (1988).

5. N.R. Clendenon, R.F. Barth, W.A. Gordon et al: Boron neutron capture therapy of a rat glioma. Neurosurgery 26, 47-55, (1990).

6. S.M. de la Monte, G.W. Moore, G.M. Hutchins: Patterned distribution of metastases from malignant melanoma in humans. Cancer Research 43, 3427-3433 (1983).

7. R.F. Barth, D.M. Adams, A.H. Soloway, E.B. Mechetner, F. Alam, A.K.M. Anisuzzaman: Determination of boron in tissues and cells using direct-current plasma atomic emission spectroscopy. Analytical Chemistry 63, 890-893 (1991).

RADIOBIOLOGY OF BORON NEUTRON CAPTURE THERAPY: PROBLEMS WITH THE CONCEPT OF RELATIVE BIOLOGICAL EFFECTIVENESS

J.A. Coderre and M.S. Makar

Medical Department, Brookhaven National Laboratory, Upton, NY, 11973, USA.

The radiation dose delivered to cells *in vitro* or *in vivo* during boron neutron capture therapy (BNCT) is a mixture of photons, fast neutrons and heavy charged particles from the interaction of neutrons with nitrogen and boron. The concept of relative biological effectiveness (RBE) has been developed to allow comparison of the effects of these radiations with the effects of standard photon treatments such as 250 kVp x-rays or ^{60}Co gamma rays. The RBE value for all of these high linear energy transfer radiations can vary considerably depending upon the experimental conditions and endpoint utilized (c.f. Fukuda, 1989). The short range of the particles from the $^{10}B(n,\alpha)^{7}Li$ reaction make the precise subcellular location of the ^{10}B atom of critical importance. The microscopic distribution of the ^{10}B has a decided effect on the dosimetry. Monte Carlo simulations have shown that, at the cellular level, there is a profound difference in the probability of cell kill depending on the location of the ^{10}B relative to the nucleus (Gabel, 1987). Convenient analytical techniques for the detection of boron at the cellular and subcellular level remain to be developed. Different boron-delivery agents will almost certainly have different distribution patterns at the subcellular level. For equivalent ^{10}B concentrations at the macroscopic level (e.g. μg ^{10}B/gram wet tissue), different boron-delivery agents may have vastly different cytotoxic effects. The application of a single RBE value for the $^{10}B(n,\alpha)^{7}Li$ reaction to different boron-delivery agents without some experimentally determined compensatory factor for subcellular localization could lead to gross under- (or over-) estimates of the actual absorbed dose.

The effect of BNCT with the amino acid *p*-boronophenylalanine (BPA) was compared with the effect of 250 kVp x-rays on a pigmented B16 melanoma subclone, both *in vitro* and *in vivo*. Generally accepted RBE values were applied to the relevant components of the Brookhaven Medical Research Reactor (BMRR) thermal neutron beam, however, there were still discrepancies when the resulting dose response curves were compared with the response to 250 kVp x-rays.

METHODS

B16 melanoma (subclone G3.12; Stackpole, 1985) cells were maintained in DMEM to which 5% (v/v) fetal bovine serum, 1% (v/v) antibiotics (penicillin, 100 IU/ml, amphotericin-B, 0.25 μg/ml and streptomycin 100 μg/ml) and 1% (v/v) L-glutamine (200 mM) were added. Solid tumors were initiated in C57B1/6 mice by s.c. injection of 2 x 10^5 cells in 0.1 ml of growth medium. Tumors were utilized after $\approx$ 12-14 days of growth when they weighed $\approx$ 50-100 mg. Irradiations at the BMRR have been previously described for *in vitro* (Gabel, 1984) and *in vivo* (Coderre, 1988) conditions. Clonogenic survival was assayed in tumors removed <5 min post-treatment, which were then minced, trypsinized, cell-counted in suspension, and plated for colony-forming assay. BPA (35 μg ^{10}B/ml) was added to the cell growth medium 24 hours prior to irradiation and was present in the medium during reactor irradiation. Mice were dosed with intragastric (ig) slurries of 15 mg of the L-enantiomer of BPA in 0.5 ml water. Two ig doses given 5 hours apart resulted in $\approx$ 40 μg ^{10}B/g tumor at the time of irradiation (3 hours after the second dose).

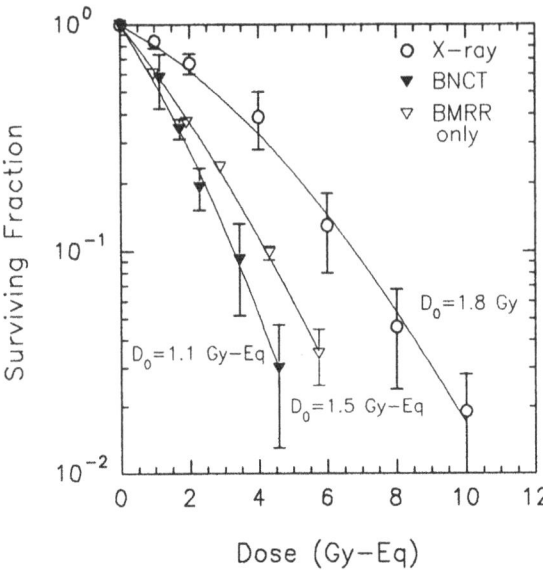

Figure 1. Survival of B16 melanoma cells exposed *in vitro* to x rays, BNCT or reactor irradiation only (no BPA). Each point is the mean of 3-5 experiments, 3 dilutions per point with 5 replicate plates per dilution.

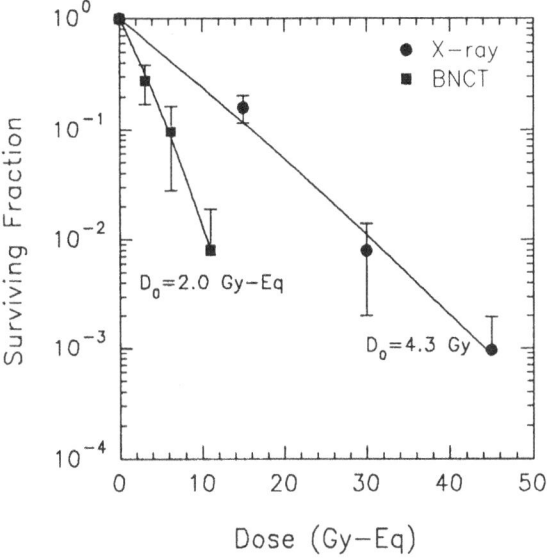

Figure 2. Clonogenic survival in solid tumors determined by colony forming assays <5 min after either BNCT or x-ray irradiation. Each point is the mean (± SD) of 4-6 tumors; 3 different dilutions were plated per tumor with 5 replicate plates per dilution.

RESULTS AND DISCUSSION

Dosimetry. The dose from BNCT irradiations is expressed as gray-equivalent (Gy-Eq), calculated by summation of physical doses (Gy) of the component radiations multiplied by appropriate relative biological effectiveness (RBE) factors. RBE values of 2.3 and 2.0 have been assumed for the ionizing particles from the $^{10}B(n,\alpha)^7Li$ and $^{14}N(n,p)^{14}C$ reactions, respectively, and 2.0 has been assumed for fast neutrons. BNCT *in vivo* resulted in the following dose rates to the tumor (at 1 MW reactor power) for the various beam components: fast neutrons, 0.23 Gy/min; gamma, 0.12 Gy/min; $^{14}N(n,p)^{14}C$ reaction, 0.13 Gy/min; and $^{10}B(n,\alpha)^7Li$ with 40 μg $^{10}B/g$ tumor, 2.13 Gy/min. BNCT *in vitro* produced the following dose rates: fast neutrons, 0.15 Gy/min; gamma, 0.07 Gy/min; $^{14}N(n,p)^{14}C$ reaction, 0.05 Gy/min; and $^{10}B(n,\alpha)^7Li$ with 35 μg $^{10}B/ml$ (ambient), 1.0 Gy/min.

In vitro irradiations. Figure 1 shows cell survival *versus* dose (Gy-Eq) following irradiation *in vitro* with either x-rays (D_0 = 1.8 Gy), BNCT (D_0 = 1.1 Gy-Eq) or with the BMRR thermal neutron beam in the absence of BPA (D_0 = 1.5 Gy-Eq). In theory, all three survival curves should superimpose if all of the RBE assumptions are accurate and if RBE correction alone is sufficient. It is possible that cells exposed to BPA in culture accumulated ^{10}B to levels higher than in the surrounding medium, resulting in an underestimate of the dose.

In vitro irradiations. Figure 2 shows clonogenic cell survival in tumors irradiated *in vivo* with either x-rays (D_0 = 4.3 Gy) or BNCT (D_0 = 2.0 Gy-Eq). The presence of hypoxic cells could account for the lower cell kill by x-rays *in vivo*. Interestingly, the cell kill produced by BNCT *in vivo* (D_0 = 2.0 Gy-Eq) is close to that produced by x-rays *in vitro* (D_0 = 1.8 Gy; Fig. 1).

The different response of the B16 melanoma cells to irradiation with 250 kVp x-rays *in vitro* (D_0 = 1.8 Gy; Fig. 1) or *in vivo* (D_0 = 4.3 Gy; Fig. 2) is most likely due to the resistance of hypoxic cells *in vivo* to photon irradiation; the magnitude of the oxygen enhancement ratio for cells in culture versus air-breathing mice was 2.4 (ratio of D_0 values). The different response of the B16 melanoma cells to BNCT *in vitro* (D_0 = 1.1 Gy-Eq; Fig. 1) or *in vivo* (D_0 = 2.0 Gy-Eq; Fig. 2) is unlikely to be due to an oxygen effect; the gamma component of the total tumor dose was only $\approx$ 5%. It is possible that non-uniform distribution of ^{10}B within the tumor resulted in a fraction of the cells receiving a lower dose.

ACKNOWLEDGEMENTS

The research described in the report involved animals maintained in animal care facilities fully accredited by the American Association for Accreditation of Laboratory Animal Care. This research was supported in part by the US Department of Energy under contract DE-AC02-76CH00016, and by Grant No. CA42446 (JAC) from the NIH.

REFERENCES

Coderre, J.A., J.A. Kalef-Ezra, R.G. Fairchild, P.L. Micca, L.E. Reinstein, and J.D. Glass, Boron neutron capture therapy of a murine melanoma. *Cancer Res.* 48, 6313-6316 (1988).

Fukuda, H., Ichihashi, M., Kobayashi, T., Matsugawa, D., Kanda, K., and Nishima, Y. Review: Biological Effectiveness of Thermal Neutrons and $^{10}B(n,\alpha)^7Li$ Reaction on Cultured Cells. *Pigment Cell Research* 2, 333-336 (1989).

Gabel, D., R.G. Fairchild, B. Larsson, and H. Börner, The relative biological effectiveness in V79 Chinese hamster cells of the neutron capture reactions in boron and nitrogen. *Rad. Res.* 98, 307-316 (1984).

Gabel, D., S. Foster, and R.G. Fairchild, The Monte Carlo simulation of the biological effect of the $^{10}B(n,\alpha)^7Li$ reaction in cells and tissue and its implication for boron neutron capture therapy. *Radiat. Res.* 111, 14-25 (1987).

Stackpole, C.W., A.L. Alterman, and D.M. Fornabaio, Growth characteristics of clonal cell population constituting a B16 melanoma metastasis model. *Invasion Metastasis* 5, 125-143 (1985).

IN VIVO CELLULAR PHARMACOLOGY ON THE SELECTIVE AFFINITY OF $^{10}B_1$-BPA FOR MALIGNANT MELANOMA

M. Shiono[1], T. Shibata[1], C. Honda[1], N. Wadabayashi[1], M. Ichihashi[1], Y. Hori[2], K. Yoshino[3] and Y. Mishima[1],

[1]Department of Dermatology, Special Institute of Cancer Neutron Capture Therapy, Kobe University School of Medicine, Kobe 650, Japan.
[2]Analytical Research Group, Shiseido Toxicological & Analytical Research Center, Yokohama 223, Japan.
[3]Department of Chemistry, Faculty of Science, Shinshu University, Matsumoto 390, Japan.

INTRODUCTION

We have previously shown that $^{10}B_1$-paraboronophenylalanine ($^{10}B_1$-BPA) has selective affinity for both melanotic and amelanotic melanomas in vitro and in vivo[1]. We have also shown complete suppression of implanted melanoma in hamster by thermal neutron capture therapy (NCT) using $^{10}B_1$-BPA[1]. Further, we have already treated succesfully six human melanoma cases by NCT using $^{10}B_1$-BPA[1,2].

For safer and more successful application of NCT using $^{10}B_1$-BPA for human melanoma eradication, it is important to understand the mechanism of $^{10}B_1$-BPA accumulation in melanoma cells. Therefore, we examined the intracellular distribution of $^{10}B_1$ BPA in melanoma cells.

MATERIALS & METHODS

Four Syrian (golden) hamsters were implanted subcutaneously in the dorsal region with four separate pieces of Greene's melanotic melanoma (about 30 mm^3).

On day 14, the implanted tumors became thumb sized and about 8 grams, and then the hamsters were treated with 1.3 ml intraperitoneal injection of $^{10}B_1$-BPA·fructose complex (total 200 mg $^{10}B_1$-BPA/kg·body weight). The hamsters were sacrificed 5 hours after injection.
^{10}B concentration in melanogenic compartments of melanoma cells, especially premelanosome, melanosome, and coated vesicles were compared with that of non-melanogenic compartment, mitochondrial fraction.

The subcellular fractions were obtained by the method of Mishima et al[3] (Fig.1). Briefly, the tumor mass of 15-20 gram net weight was cut into pieces, washed 3 times with MES-buffer[2-(N-morpholino)ethane-sulfonic acid](pH6.5) and homogenized in ice bath, then centrifuged at 1,000 G for 10 minutes. The supernatant was isolated and then re-centrifuged two more times. The pellet contained intact cells, nuclei, connective tissue and red blood cells.

The supernatant was then twice centrifuged at 12,000 G for 60 minutes and separated into two parts, pellet or large granule fraction (LGF), and

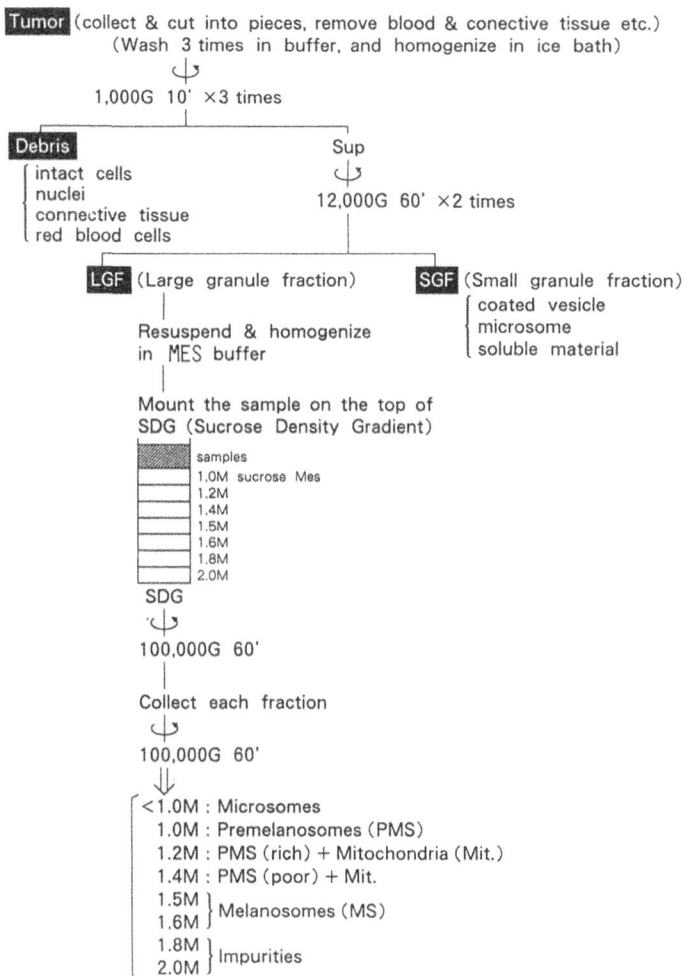

Figure 1. The method of fractionation of melanogenic compartments in pigments cells.

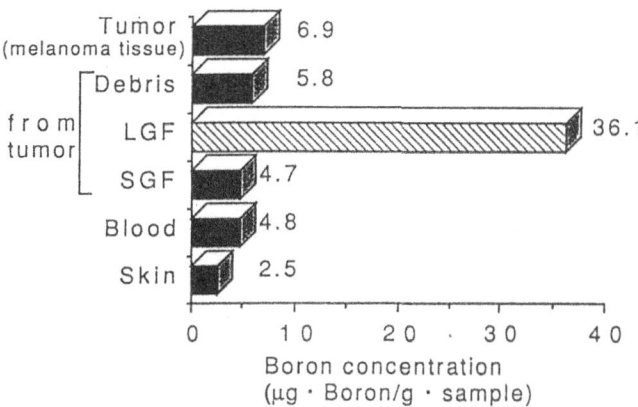

Figure 3. The boron concentration in LGF subfractions

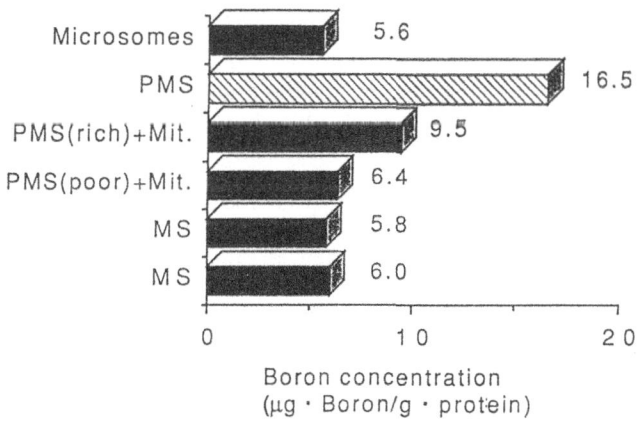

Figure 2. The boron concentration of subcellular fractions of
melanoma cells in comparison with that of melenoma tissue,
blood and skin.

supernatant or small granule fraction (SGF). LGF contained microsomes, mitochondria (Mit), premelanosomes (PMS) and melanosomes (MS). SGF contained coated vesicles, microsomes and soluble materials.

LGF was resuspended, homogenized in MES-buffer and mounted on the top of a sucrose density gradient and centrifuged at 100,000 G for 60 minutes. Each fraction was collected individually, washed in MES-buffer and re-centrifuged at 100,000 G for 60 minutes. The subcellular fractions contained in each sucrose density are summarized in Fig. 1.

After acid digestion with H_2O_2 and $HClO_4$, the concentration of ^{10}B atom was measured by inductively coupled plasma-mass spectrometry (ICP-MS, Seiko Instruments Inc., Model:SPQ 6500).

RESULTS AND DISCUSSION

Selective accumulation of $^{10}B_1$-BPA in melanotic and amelanotic melanoma tissue in vivo has been reported by Tsuji et al[4] and Honda et al[5]. These authors showed an active uptake and accumulation of $^{10}B_1$-BPA by melanin synthesizing melanoma cells.

In the present study, in order to explain the selective accumulation of $^{10}B_1$-BPA in melanoma cells in comparison with other normal tissue and blood, we demonstrated high concentration of ^{10}B in the melanogenic compartment of melanoma cells. In LGF with MS and PMS, ^{10}B concentration was much higher than that of SGF without MS and PMS (Fig.2). In the finaly separated LGF, ^{10}B concentration of PMS subfraction is higher than that of other subfractions (Fig.3).

Our present results suggest that $^{10}B_1$-BPA may accumulate in melanoma tissue due to high localization in PMS, a subcellular melanogenic compartment where specific melanin polymer formation proceeds.

REFERENCE

1. Mishima, Y., M. Ichihashi, S. Hatta, C. Honda, K. Yamamura, and T. Nakagawa (1989) New thermal neutron capture therapy for malignant melanoma: melanogenesis-seeking ^{10}B molecule-melanoma cell interaction from in vitro to first clinical trial. Pigment Cell Res., 2:226-234
2. Mishima, Y., C. Honda, M. Ichihashi, H. Obara, J. Hiratsuka, H. Fukuda, H. Karashima, T. Kobayashi, K. Kanda and K. Yoshino (1989) Treatment of malignant melanoma by single thermal neutron capture therapy with melanoma-seeking ^{10}B-compound. Lancet II:388-389 (8659)
3. Hamada, T., and Y. Mishima (1972) Intracellular localization of tyrosinase inhibitor in amelanotic and melanic malignant melanoma. Brit. J. Dermatol., 86:385-394
4. Tsuji, M., M. Ichihashi, and Y. Mishima (1983) Selective affinity of ^{10}B-para-boronophenylalanine·HCl to malignant melanoma for thermal neutron capture therapy. Jpn. J. Dermatol., 93:773-778
5. Honda, C., Y. Mishima, M. Ichihashi, and S. Hatta (1990) In situ detection of cutaneous melanoma by prompt gamma-ray spectrometry using melanoma-seeking ^{10}B-dopa analogue. J. Dermatol. Science 1:23-31

COMPARATIVE PHARMACOKINETICS AND DISTRIBUTION STUDIES OF BORIC ACID, L-BPA AND BSH IN TWO MURINE TUMOUR MODELS

V.G. Gregoire[*], R. Huiskamp[**], R. Verrijk[*] and A.C. Begg[*]

[*]Department of Experimental Therapy, The Netherlands Cancer Institute, Amsterdam, The Netherlands
[**]Radiobiology and Radioecology, Netherlands Energy Research Foundation ECN, Petten, The Netherlands

INTRODUCTION

One of the requirements of Boron Neutron Capture Therapy (BNCT) is that the boronated compounds be selectively incorporated and retained in the tumour cells while remaining at a low level in irradiated normal tissues. To achieve this, different boronated compounds have been synthesized and tested, among them boron-phenyl-alanine (BPA) and borocaptate sodium (BSH). Despite clinical application in melanoma and grade IV glioma respectively, there are few data on the tumour selectivity of these different boronated compounds. Pharmacological studies with these compounds have therefore been initiated in two murine tumour models as part of the European BNCT project.

MATERIALS AND METHODS

Two murine tumour models were used in this investigation. The RIF-1 (radiation induced fibrosarcoma) in C3H/km mice was used as a reference tumour. The B16 melanotic melanoma tumour in C57Bl mice was chosen as a relevant model for BNCT experiments. For both models, 10^5 cells were implanted subcutaneously on the flank of the animals which were used when the tumours reached 7-9 mm diameter.

A saline solution of 3 mg B/ml were prepared for boric acid (Merck Chemical) and BSH (Centronic limited), while for L-BPA (Callery Chemical Company) the powder was dissolved in a 0.3 M fructose solution at a pH of 8.2 to a final concentration of 1.42 mg B/ml. All three compounds were injected ip at a boron dose of 50 µg B/g mouse (BSH and boric acid) or 12.5 µg B/g mouse (L-BPA). A lower dose was used for the latter because of limited supply.

The mice (4-5 mice per experimental point) were sacrificed at different time after injection ranging from 5 minutes to 21 hours and boron concentrations were measured in blood, plasma, tumour, brain, liver muscle and kidneys using inductively coupled plasma atomic emission spectroscopy (ICP-AES, Jobin Yvon JY70 plus). All samples, including blood and plasma, were digested with an acid mixture composed of 90% (w/w) of nitric acid (HNO3; 65%), 5% (w/w) of perchloric acid (HCl04; 68%) and 5% (w/w) of hydrofluoric acid (HF; 48%). The samples (maximum 1.3 g of tissue) were digested for 15 minutes in a pressure controlled microwave oven (CEM MDS-81D) at a power of 630 watts. For the ICP-AES, the 249.773 nm emission line was chosen to measure boron. Zinc at a concentration of 10 ppm was used as a internal standard to correct for the variation in the nebulization between each measurement. For a 4 ml sample, the detection limit defined as the mean value of the background + 3 standard deviation, was between 0.001 and 0.015 ppm. This allowed the detection of between 0.04 and 0.6 ppm of boron in a 0.1 g sample (plasma, blood), between 0.013 and 0.2 ppm in a 0.3 g of tissue (tumour, brain, muscle) and between 0.004 and 0.06 ppm in a 1 g sample (liver). All the measurements were done in triplicate with a coefficient of variation less than 2%. The recovery was in the 95% range.

For all tumour/compound combinations, the tumour and plasma concentration versus time curves were fitted according to standard pharmacokinetic models (PCNONLIN programme). A one compartment with first order output model was used for boric acid and L-BPA, while the BSH data were fitted with a two compartment model with first order output.

Table 1 summarizes the pharmacokinetic parameters for the RIF-1 and B16 tumours. After boric acid and BSH injection, an adequate boron concentration (>20-25 ppm) could be achieved, with no significant differences being observed between tumour types for boric acid and BSH, although L-BPA showed a greater uptake in the melanoma, as expected. Maximum concentrations were higher after boric acid than after BSH. For L-BPA, in both models, the maximum boron concentration didn't reach, but was close to, the target concentration of 20-25 ppm. This could be explained by the lower injected boron dose. It is worthwhile to note that maximum tumour concentrations were 1.4-2.0 times higher for BSH than for L-BPA, although four times more boron as BSH was administered. This indicates that boron was concentrated in tumours to a higher extent for L-BPA even in the non-melanoma (RIF-1). The same trend was observed between boric acid and L-BPA, i.e. greater relative tumour concentration with L-BPA.

It is also apparent from table 1 that retention of boron was longer after L-BPA administration, where according to the pharmacokinetics model 67% and 42% of the maximum boron concentration was retained in the tumour 5 hours post injection for B16 and RIF-1 respectively. Tumour retention after BSH injection was no better than after boric acid injection; i.e. not more than 20% of the maximal boron concentration was detectable in either tumour 5 hours after BSH injection, compared with 27% (B16) and 12% (RIF-1) for boric acid.

The changes in the tumour-plasma ratio as a function of time post injection are presented in figure 1 for the three compounds. The points were derived directly from the ratio of the measured concentration in tumour and plasma at each time, while the lines were calculated from the fitted pharmacokinetic profiles. Tumour-plasma ratios above unity were observed for the B16 melanoma after both boric acid and L-BPA, although only for L-BPA did the ratio remain advantageous for up to 18 hours. For BSH, the tumour-plasma ratio was unity or less for all times tested, except at 13 hours.

Concerning the normal tissues, maximum boron concentration were below 4 ppm in brain and 12 ppm in muscle after BSH and L-BPA injection, with no significant difference between the two models (mouse strains). After BSH injection, there was an large accumulation in the liver, however.

TABLE 1

Summary of pharmacokinetic parameters for the RIF-1 and
B16 tumours after ip boric acid, L-BPA and BSH.

Pharmacokinetic parameters	RIF-1 tumour	B16 melanoma tumour
Boric acid: 50 μg B/g		
C_{max} (μg/g tissue)	44.40 ± 1.76	43.22 ± 2.17[*]
T½ elimination (h)	1.42 ± 0.25	2.17 ± 0.35
L-BPA: 12.5 μg B/g		
C_{max} (μg/g tissue)	15.41 ± 0.86	20.62 ± 2.21
T½ elimination (h)	3.84 ± 0.34	7.51 ± 2.06
BSH: 50 μg B/g		
C_{max} (μg/g tissue)	31.13 ± 2.40	28.07 ± 4.86
T½ α elimination (h)	0.82 ± 0.12	0.26 ± 0.08
T½ β elimination (h)	6.53 ± 1.64	10.14 ± 2.44

[*] standard error

444

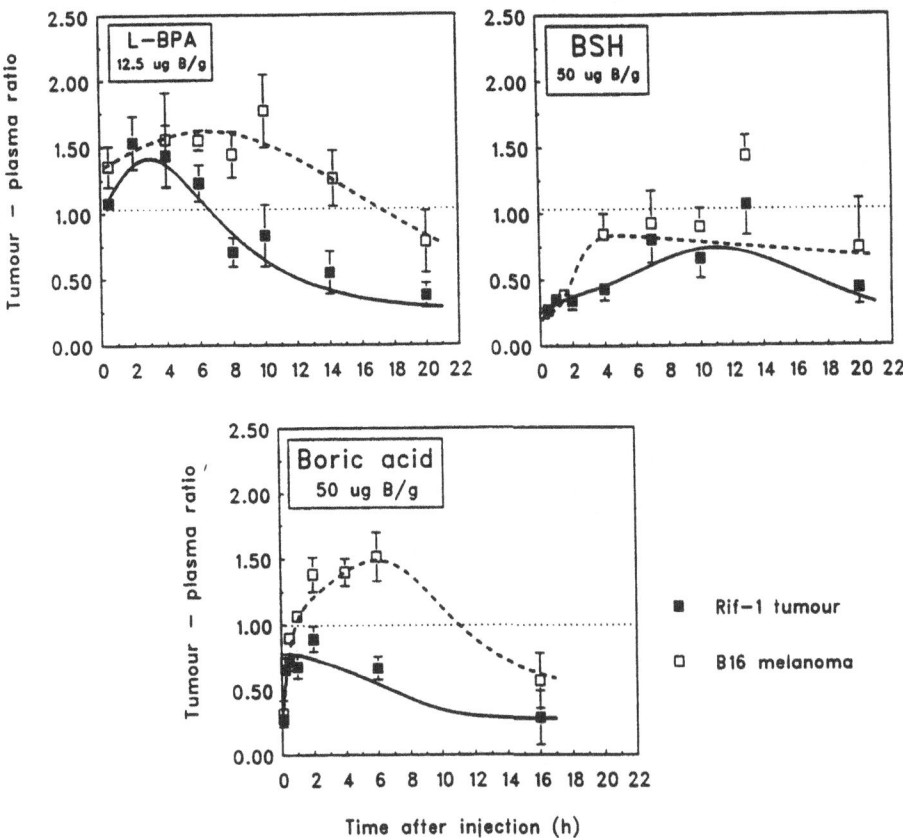

Figure 1. Tumour-plasma ratios as a function of time post injection for RIF-1 and B16 melanoma
models after L-BPA (upper left), BSH (upper right) and boric acid (lower)
administration.

In conclusion, these data show that adequate tumour boron concentration can be achieved, depending
on the injected dose, without prohibitively high boron concentrations in relevant normal tissues such
as brain and muscle. L-BPA appeared to show a slight preference for the melanoma model, although
the difference in uptake compared with the other tumour model was not great. The other two
compounds, boric acid and BSH, showed no tumour specificity. Higher injected L-BPA doses are being
tested and the studies are also being extended to a include a glioblastoma model.

ACKNOWLEDGMENTS

This work is supported by the Dutch Cancer Foundation (project NKI90-10). Dr.V.G.Gregoire benefited
from a grant from the Catholic University of Louvain, Belgium. We thank Prof.Dr.D.Gabel and
Dr.W.Sauerwein for providing us with BSH and L-BPA respectively, J. Bonouvrie for technical
assistance and D.Borger (ECN, Petten) for the running of the ICP-AES.

EVALUATION OF RESPONSE OF HEPATOCYTES(IN VIVO) TO THERMAL NEUTRON

IRRADIATION BY MICRONUCLEUS ASSAY

Keizo Akuta[1], Koji Ono[2], Tooru Kobayashi[1],
Mitsuhiko Akaboshi[1], Yowri Ujeno[1] and Mitsuyuki Abe[2]

1:Research Reactor Institute, Kyoto University, Kumatori-cho,
  Sennan-gun, Osaka 590-04, Japan.
2:Dept. of Radiology, Faculty of Medicine, Kyoto University,
  Sakyo-ku, Kyoto 606, Japan.

INTRODUCTION

In order to apply neutron capture therapy to malignant liver tumors,
it is necessary to know the effects of thermal neutron irradiation on the
normal liver precisely. In this study, we have investigated the response
of the hepatocytes in vivo to thermal neutron irradiation by micronucleus
assay[1,2].

METHODS AND MATERIALS

C3H/He mice weighing approximately 25 g were used for the studies.
Each mouse was held in a plastic case and was irradiated with thermal
neutrons generated by Kyoto University Reactor. Thermal neutrons were
collimated with LiF tile so that the upper abdomen including the liver
could be irradiated from the right side. To induce ^{10}B-thermal neutron
capture reaction in the liver, ^{10}B-enriched H_3BO_3 dissolved in saline was
administered intra-venously 5 min before irradiation. Six mice were used
in each treatment condition.

Since the hepatocytes are in the G_o phase of the cell cycle, irradiation alone to the liver can not produce the micronucleus effectively.
Therefore, partial hepatectomy was performed immediately after irradiation
in order to promote the cell cycling of hepatocytes in resting phase. Five
days after the treatment, a laparotomy was done and a polyethylene tube was
inserted into the portal vein. Through the tube, 2 ml of mixture of 0.05 %
trypsin and 0.02 % EDTA was perfused slowly, then the regenerating liver
was removed. Since the thermal neutrons attenuate steeply in the body, the
extracted liver was divided into right lateral and medial portions and
then, each part of the liver was minced in PBS respectively. The mixture
of liver fragments and PBS was filtered through fine nylon mesh. To get a
good single hepatocyte suspension, the filtrate was centrifuged at 500 rpm
for 40 sec and the pellet of the hepatocytes was resuspended in PBS. This
procedure was repeated two times. The cell suspension was centrifuged
again and the pellet was fixed with 70 % ethanol for several hours. Then
the fixative was changed to Carnoy's fluid (ethanol:acetic acid=3:1). 30
μl of this suspension was dropped onto microslide glass and dried.

Micronuclei in the hepatocytes were observed by fluorescence microscope after staining with ethidium bromide. About 500 hepatocytes were examined, and the frequency was defined as a ratio of total number of micronuclei and number of hepatocytes scored.

To estimate the absorbed dose of the hepatocytes irradiated with thermal neutrons, the thermal neutron fluence in the liver was measured with a phantom and the time course of ^{10}B concentration in the liver was

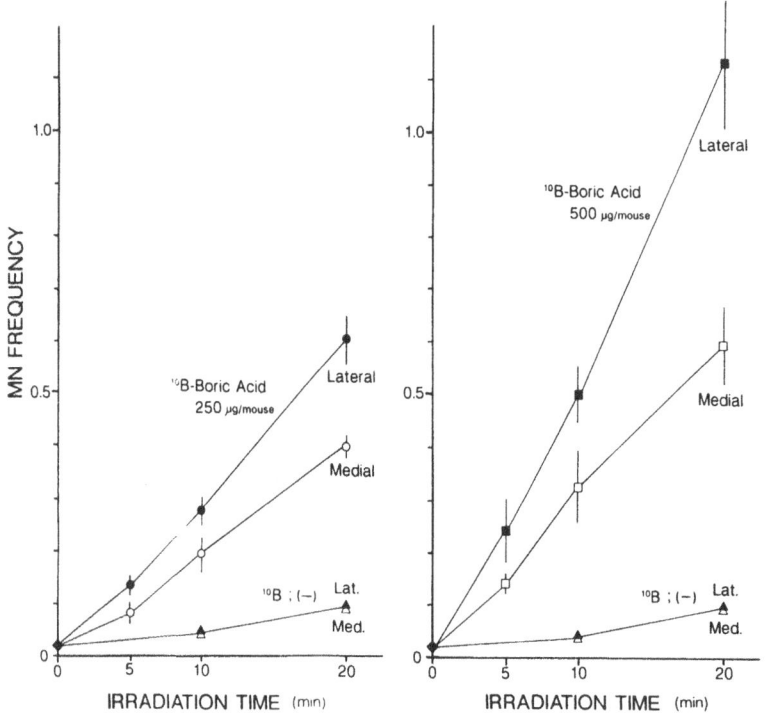

Fig. 1. Frequency of micronuclei in hepatocytes according to the irradiation time with thermal neutrons.
(Vertical lines represent standard deviations.)

also measured in vivo by prompt gamma-ray spectrometry[3]. Gamma-ray contamination from the reactor was also measured with TLD powder.

RESULTS AND DISCUSSION

Fig. 1 shows the micronucleus (MN) frequency according to the irradiation time. The frequency of MN increased as the irradiation time increased. MN frequency was markedly increased by the administration of the ^{10}B-boric acid. Further, MN were more frequently observed in the right lateral portion of the liver than in the medial portion when ^{10}B-boric acid was injected. This seems to reflect the attenuation of thermal neutron fluence in the liver according to the depth from the surface.

The phantom experiment showed that the average neutron flux measured was 2.6×10^9 and 1.6×10^9 n/cm$^2 \cdot$ sec in the lateral and medial portions, respectively.

To obtain the relative biological effectiveness (RBE) for boron neutron capture reaction, the MN frequency for thermal neutrons with boron neutron capture reaction in hepatocytes is compared with that following X-ray irradiation[2]. In the present study, the absorbed dose was estimated assuming that the energy was mainly delivered by ^{10}B(n,α)^{7}Li reaction and gamma-ray contamination. The energy from the ^{10}B(n,α)^{7}Li reaction was

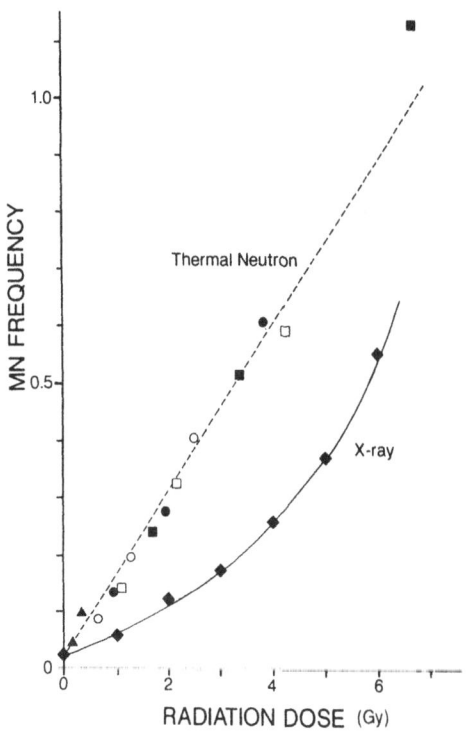

Fig. 2. Frequency of micronuclei as a function of
absorbed dose for BNCT and X-rays.
(Symbols in Fig. 1. are commonly used.)

calculated from the thermal neutron fluence and ^{10}B concentration of the liver. Average ^{10}B concentration in the liver during the irradiation (5-25 min after injection) was 20 and 11 µg/g tissue when 500 and 250 µg/mouse boric acid was administered, respectively. The gamma-ray contamination was 1.6 cGy/min. In Fig. 2, the MN frequencies with the thermal neutron irradiation and X-rays are plotted according to the estimated absorbed dose. The dose response curve following thermal neutron irradiation with boron was linear as compared with that of X-ray irradiation which was upward bending. The RBE was obtained from these data, and for thermal neutrons on hepatocytes in vivo was around 2.0(1.6-3.3). This value is similar to that observed with various normal or tumor cells in vitro and in vivo[4].

REFERENCES

1. I. Cliet, E. Fournier, C. Melcion, and A. Cordier, In vivo micronucleus test using mouse hepatocytes, Mutation Research, 216:321(1989).
2. K. Ono, Y. Nagata, K. Akuta, M. Abe, K. Ando, and S. Koike, Micronucleus frequency in hepatocytes following X-ray and fast neutron irradiation -An analysis by linear quadratic model-, Radiation Research, 123:345(1990).
3. T. Kobayashi and K. Kanda, Microanalysis system of ppm-order ^{10}B concentrations in tissue for neutron capture therapy by prompt gamma-ray spectrometry, Nuclear Instruments and Methods, 204:525(1983).
4. Y. Ujeno, Physical modification of thermal neutron-induced biological effects, in: Modification of Radiosensitivity in Cancer Treatment, T. Sugahara ed., Academic Press, Tokyo (1984).

LIPOSOMES AS CARRIERS OF BORONATED THIOURACILS FOR NCT OF MELANOMA

Douglas E Moore,[+] Alana K Chandler,[+] Sue Corderoy-Buck,[*]
J Gerald Wilson,[*] and Barry J Allen [*]

[+]Department of Pharmacy, The University of Sydney, Sydney 2006
Australia
[*]Biomedicine and Health Program, Australian Nuclear Science and
Technology Organisation, Menai 2234 Australia

Boronated Thiouracils

5-(3-(1,2-decaboronyl)propyl)-6-methyl-thiouracil, DBTU-1, and
5-(1,2-decaboronyl-methyl)-6-methyl-thiouracil, DBTU-2, are boron
derivatives of thiouracil, which is reported to localise in melanoma as
a false precursor in the synthesis of melanin.[1,2] The chemical
structures of DBTU-1 and DBTU-2 are given in Figure 1. Their
preparation and characterisation is to be found elsewhere.[3]

Experiments carried out *in vitro* showed that DBTU-1 accumulated in
melanoma cells in culture at least 11 times more effectively (based on B
content) than a mono-boronated thiouracil.[4] These studies, however, do
not distinguish between incorporation of the compound within the cell
and adsorption to the exterior of the cellular membranes.

Biodistribution studies with nude mice bearing melanoma xenografts of
both murine and human origin revealed only a slow uptake of boron by the
various tumours 48-72 hours after *intra peritoneal* injection of DBTU-1
dissolved in a small volume of dimethyl-sulfoxide (Table 1). The
relatively slow absorption has been related to the very low aqueous
solubility of these compounds. The solubility problem can be overcome by
either modifying chemically the molecule, or by the design of an
alternative drug delivery system to enhance the solubility. In this
report, liposomes are examined as an example of the second approach.

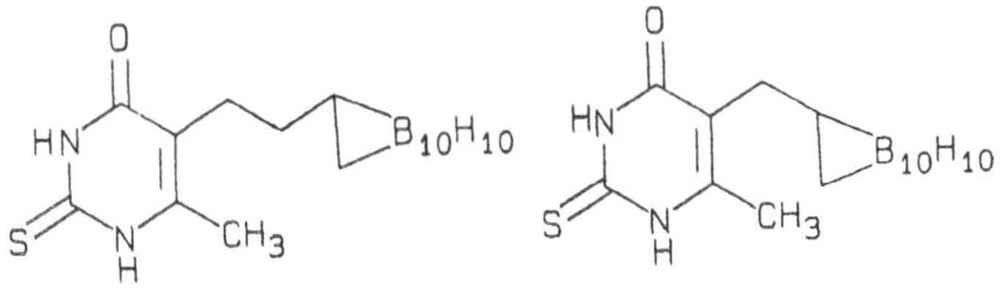

Figure 1. Structures of decaborono-thiouracils, DBTU-1 & 2.

Table 1. Uptake of boron by mice with various tumour xenografts
following administration of 300 µg B as DBTU-1 in 0.1 mL DMSO.

	B16	MM96	LiBr	MM418
No of mice	2	2	2	2
Time to peak B h	72	8	36	48
Peak B conc ppm	7.8	3.5	3.7	4.9
Tumour/blood ratio	4.4	2.5	3.7	4.9
Tumour/liver ratio	3.2	2.7	2.3	2.0

Liposomes as Drug Delivery Vehicles

Liposomes are single or multi-lamellar structures formed by the self
association of surface-active molecules which have a lipophilic
hydrocarbon chain coupled to a hydrophilic group which may carry an
anionic or cationic charge. Within the structure it is possible to
incorporate other compounds which have an affinity for that specific
environment. The use of phospholipids (naturally occurring membrane
constituents) enables the preparation of non-toxic liposomes. The
formulation used in these experiments consists of 7.5 mg (20 µmole) of
DBTU-1 or -2, L-α-phosphatidylcholine (120 µmole) and cholesterol (36
µmole) with either dicetyl phosphate or stearylamine (36 µmole) as the
component which determines the electrostatic charge to be negative or
positive, respectively. The liposome components were sonicated in 3.5 mL
of phosphate buffered saline and passed through a 0.45 µm membrane
filter before administration (0.5 mL per mouse).

The quality of the preparation was established by examination in the
electron microscope. A uniform size distribution with a mean diameter
about 100 nm is desirable to avoid trapping by the liver and spleen on
administration. The presence of boron within the liposomes was
confirmed by the observation of the electron energy loss spectroscopic
signal corresponding to boron. In this preparation the DBTU compounds
are expected to be localised in the lipophilic regions of the liposomes

Biodistribution of Boronated Thiouracils using Liposomes

Nude mice bearing human or murine melanoma xenografts were used for
biodistribution studies following *ip* injection of the drug-liposome

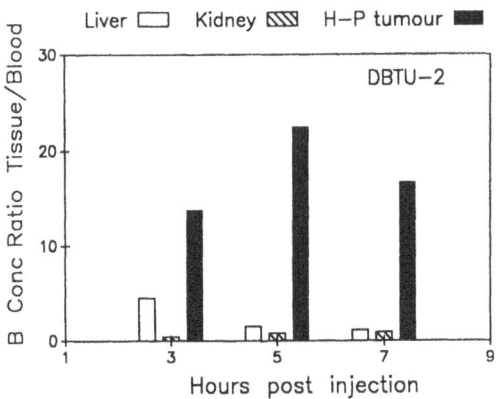

Figure 2. Biodistribution of DBTU-2 (negative liposome formulation) in
mice bearing Harding-Passey melanoma xenografts. Each data point is the
average from 3 mice; 300 µg B administered per mouse.

preparation. The boron content of dissected tissue samples was determined, after perchloric acid/hydrogen peroxide digestion, by inductively coupled plasma atomic emission spectrometry (ICP-AES).[5]

Wide variation between different cell lines was observed with respect to accumulation of boron in the tumour, but the liposome vehicle showed a significant advantage for delivery of the insoluble DBTU-1 in the amelanotic MM418 tumour and for DBTU-2 in the highly melanised Harding-Passey tumour (Figure 2). Although there was measurable accumulation in the liver, kidney and spleen, these results suggest that a therapeutic advantage can be achieved by liposome delivery.

Comparison with a Non-specific Compound

Liposomes have been promoted as having an inherent tumour targetting capability, so that the molecules carried may not require their own specific affinity for the tumour. Decaborane is also water insoluble but

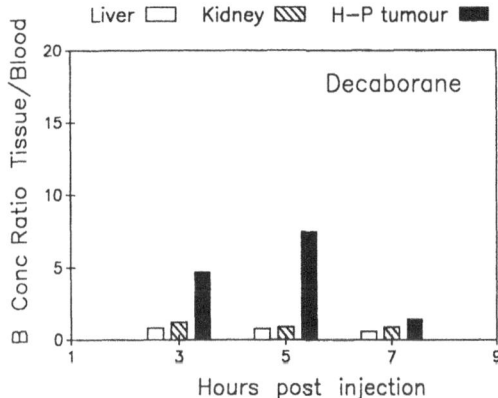

Figure 3. Biodistribution of Decaborane (negative liposome formulation) in mice bearing Harding-Passey melanoma xenografts. Details as in Fig 2.

has not been reported to bind to melanin, although it is relatively reactive. It was used as a marker of possible uptake by tumours by virtue of their altered vascular permeability.

When decaborane was administered in the liposome vehicle, there was an enhanced boron concentration in the tumour, as shown in Figure 3 for the negative liposome formulation in Harding-Passey tumours. Different cell lines, which have quite different growth rates, showed a variability in rate and extent of uptake of the decaborane. This reflects the differing blood perfusion of the tumours, and differences in affinity between cell membranes and the influence of liposome charge characteristics. Liposomal vehicles have therefore demonstrated the capacity to deliver non specific boron compounds to the tumour site for NCT. The retention of the decaborane within the tumour may be a manifestation of the ability of this molecule to react with amino groups.

Work supported in part by grants from the NSW Cancer Council and the Government Employees Medical Research Fund.

REFERENCES

1. *RG Fairchild, S Packer, D Greenberg, P Som, AB Brill, I Fand and WP McNally*, Thiouracil distribution in mice carrying transplantable melanoma. <u>Cancer Res</u>., <u>42</u>, 5126-5132, 1982.

2. *K Yamada, BS Larsson, A Roberto, L Dencker and S Ullberg*, Selective incorporation of thiouracil into murine metastatic melanomas. <u>J. Invest. Dermatol</u>., <u>90</u>, 873-876, 1988.

3. *JG Wilson*, Synthetic approaches to a carboranyl thiouracil. <u>Pigment Cell Res</u>., <u>2</u>, 297-305, 1989.

4. *S Corderoy-Buck, BJ Allen, JG Wilson, JK Brown, M Mountford, W Tjarks, D Gabel, D Barkla, A Patwardhan, AK Chandler and DE Moore*, Investigation of boron conjugated thiouracil derivatives for NCT of melanoma. <u>Proc. Sixth Int. Conf. Radiopharmacol</u>., Sydney, 1989, pp 114-127.

5. *SR Tamat, DE Moore, BJ Allen*. Assay of boron in biological tissues by inductively coupled plasma atomic absorption spectrometry. <u>Anal. Chem</u>., <u>59</u>, 2161-2164, 1987.

BIODISTRIBUTION, TOXICITY AND EFFICACY OF A BORONATED

PORPHYRIN FOR BORON NEUTRON CAPTURE THERAPY

Michiko Miura, Peggy Micca, Detlef Gabel*,
Ralph Fairchild and Daniel Slatkin

Brookhaven National Laboratory, Medical Department, Upton, New York
11973, USA. *Department of Chemistry, University of Bremen,
Box 330 440, D-2800 Bremen 33, Germany

Boron-containing porphyrins may be useful for boron neutron capture therapy (BNCT) in the treatment of brain tumors. Porphyrins have been shown to accumulate in tumor tissue and to be essentially excluded from normal brain. However, problems of toxicity may prevent some boron-containing porphyrins from being considered for BNCT.

We have synthesized the boronated porphyrin 2,4-bis-vinyl-o-nidocarboranyl-deuteroporphyrin IX (VCDP), shown in Figure 1 [1]. Preliminary studies in tumor-bearing mice showed considerable uptake of boron at a total dose of 150 μg/gbw with low mortality [2]. We now report that a total dose to mice of ≈275 μg VCDP/gbw administered in multiple intraperitoneal (ip) injections can provide 40-50 μg B per gram of tumor with acceptable toxicity. Toxicity experiments and a preliminary trial of BNCT in mice given such doses are also reported.

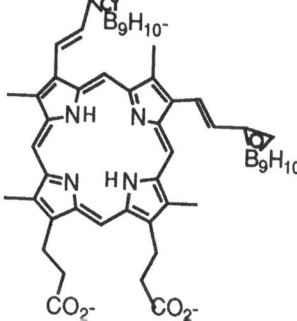

Figure 1. Structure of VCDP

Materials

Drugs. VCDP was prepared from hemin and vinyl carborane as described[1]. Solutions of VCDP were dissolved in isotonic phosphate-buffered saline (PBS) at pH 7.0 and kept shielded from ambient light and refrigerated for <3d before use.

Animals. Female 10-16 week-old BALB/c and C57Bl/6 mice were used. KHJJ mammary carcinomas [3] and B16 (G3.12) melanomas [4] were implanted subcutaneously in BALB/c mice and in C57Bl/6 mice, respectively. Right ventricular blood was collected for chemical analyses and for boron analysis by prompt-gamma spectrometry [5]. Tumor, liver, kidney, spleen, lung, skeletal muscle and brain tissues were also removed for boron analysis.

Results and Discussion

VCDP was administered to KHJJ tumor-bearing mice (275 μg VCDP/gbw), in which biodistribution and pharmacokinetics were evaluated after 18h, 2d, 4d or 6d clearance periods. Figure 2 shows 40-50 μg B/g of tumor 18h to 4d after the last injection. These are well above the minimum boron concentration, ≈15μg/g, recommended for therapy [6]. The boron concentrations of liver, spleen and kidney, which are higher than those of tumor, decrease with time. Tumor boron also decreases, but this is mainly attributable to tumor growth. The absolute amount of boron in tumor is actually higher at 6d than 4d but it does not match the increase in tumor weight. Most significant is that the brain boron concentration is negligible. The blood boron concentration dropped from ≈30 μg/g at 18h to ≈10 μg/g at

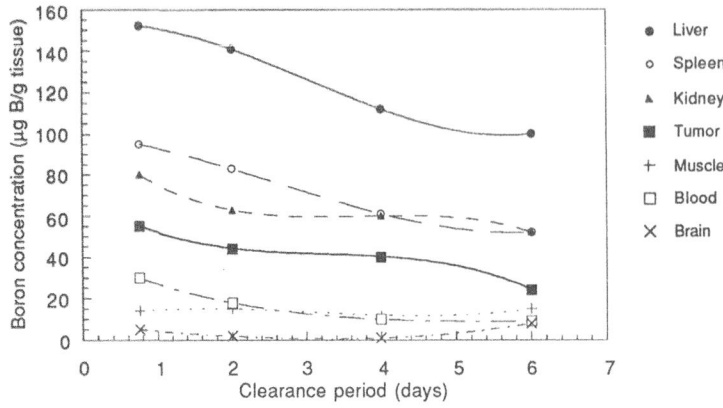

Figure 2. Boron distribution is tissues after various clearance times in KHJJ tumor-bearing mice given 275 μg VCDP/gbw in multiple ip injections (3/day for 4 days). Boron concentrations were determined using prompt-gamma spectrometry [5].

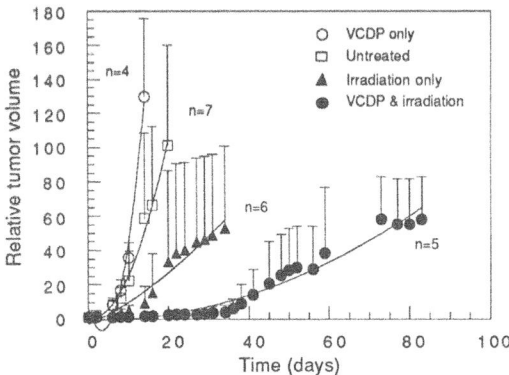

Figure 3. BNCT experiment on B16 melanoma-bearing C57Bl/6 mice treated with 232 μg [10]B-enriched VCDP/gbw and 6 MW-min (Group 4) in a comparison with three control groups: 1. No drug, no irradiation, 2. Drug only (232 μg VCDP/gbw), 3. Reactor irradiation only (BMRR thermal neutron port; 6 MW-min).

4d, yielding a 4:1 tumor:blood ratio. Tissue distribution ratios are similar to those for Photofrin II, the porphyrin mixture used in photodynamic therapy [7].

We also carried out a biodistribution study with VCDP in C57Bl/6 mice bearing the Stackpole B16 (G3.12 subclone) melanoma, which has been used in experimental BNCT [8]. After a dose of 232 μg VCDP/gbw and a 4d clearance period, tumor boron was ≈30 μg/g and the tumor:blood ratio was 2:1.

The results of our preliminary BNCT experiment with [10]B-enriched VCDP in mice with the same melanoma implanted subcutaneously in the thigh are shown in Figure 3. There is no significant difference between groups 1 (untreated) and 2 (VCDP only). Group 3 (irradiation only) showed a ≈20d growth delay and Group 4 (BNCT with VCDP) showed a ≈50d growth delay.

There appears to be reversible toxicity associated with VCDP at the 275 μg VCDP/gbw dose level in KHJJ tumor-bearing mice. Table I shows that blood platelets had decreased significantly at the 18h time point. At 4d, however, platelet counts had returned to within normal limits. Thrombocytopenia has also been observed with another boronated porphyrin [9]. Blood leukocytes increased with time in tumor-bearing mice given VCDP. This could be attributable in part to the tumor itself, since a comparison of groups I and J indicates that VCDP alone does not induce significant leukocytosis.

Table I. Hematologic parameters. Tabulated values are median and range (in parentheses). Group A comprises normal mice given the same volume of PBS as were groups B and C. Mice in groups B-H had transplanted KHJJ tumors. Group B was given TPPS (210 µg/gbw) at a rate of 30µg/gbw per injection. Group C was given VCDP at the same total dose and dose rate. Group D was given the same volume of PBS as were groups E-H, and euthanized 6d post-injection. Groups E-H were given VCDP (265 µg/gbw) at a rate of 22 µg/gbw per injection, and euthanized after the clearance periods indicated. Groups I and J are normal mice given PBS and 275 µg VCDP/gbw, respectively, and euthanized 4d post-injection.

Group	Clear. time	Number of mice	Dose (µg/gbw)	Tumor (yes/no)	Leukocytes ($10^3/mm^3$)	Platelets ($10^3/mm^3$)	Blood urea nitrogen (mg/dl)
A	3h	11	(PBS only)	n	3.5 (1.5-4.4)	1005 (547-1217)	28 (21-37)
B	3h	11	210 (TPPS)	y	4.2 (2.1-9.7)	652 (216-906)[a]	27 (20-32)
C	3h	16	210 (VCDP)	y	6.6 (2.6-13)	528 (103-796)[a]	24 (14-60)
D	6d	6	(PBS only)	y	12.7 (8.1-14.2)[a]	979 (840-1182)	23 (20-25)[e]
E	18h	6	265 (VCDP)	y	8.7 (4.7-10)[a]	137 (78-398)[a]	60 (22-140)[e]
F	2d	5	265 (VCDP)	y	12.4 (6.7-19.5)[a]	762 (635-798)[e]	18 (16-19)[a]
G	4d	5	265 (VCDP)	y	10.8 (7.1-15.1)[a]	819 (735-952)	17 (14-33)
H	6d	3	265 (VCDP)	y	25.4 (18.8-34.2)[a]	905 (796-965)	22 (19-30)
I	4d	6	(PBS only)	n	4.4 (3.2-4.8)	1141 (1040-1396)	27 (22-37)
J	4d	4	275 (VCDP)	n	6.0 (3.5-9.7)	828 (788-1050)	20 (17-24)

[a-e] The Wilcoxon non-parametric two sample test shows these values to differ from normal mice (Group A) with the following uncertainties: [a]$P<0.001$, [b]$P<0.002$, [c]$P<0.005$, [d]$P<0.01$, [e]$P<0.05$

Erythrocyte tests (hemoglobin, hematocrit, cell count, mean cell volume, mean cell hemoglobin and mean cell hemoglobin concentration) showed no differences among groups A-J.

In summary, doses of ≈275 µg VCDP/gbw in mice can yield ≈40-50 µg B/g in tumor, with a 4:1 tumor:blood ratio and negligible boron in brain. Toxicity experiments indicate a reversible thrombocytopenia and BNCT delayed growth of a subcutaneously implanted B16 mouse melanoma at these doses. VCDP, among other boronated porphyrins, should be considered as a potential boron-carrier for BNCT of brain tumors.

References

1. Miura, M., Gabel, D., Oenbrink, G., Fairchild, R., Syntheses of boronated porphyrins for boron neutron capture therapy, *Tetrahedron Let.*, 31:2247-2250, 1990.
2. Miura, M., Gabel, D., Warkentien, L.S., Laster, B.H., Fairchild, R.G. Synthesis and *in-vivo* properties of a carboranyl porphyrin. *Strahlenther. Onkol.*, 165:131-134, 1989.
3. Rockwell, S.C., Kallman, R.F., Fajardo, L.F., Characteristics of a serially transplanted mouse mammary tumor and its tissue-culture adapted derivative. *J. Nat. Cancer Inst.* 49:735-747, 1972.
4. Stackpole, C.W., Alterman, A.L., Fornabaio, D.M., Growth characteristics of clonal cell populations constituting a B16 melanoma metastasis model. *Invasion Metastasis*, 5:125-143, 1985.
5. Fairchild, R.G., Gabel, D., Laster, B.H., Greenberg, D., Kiszenick, W., Micca, P.L., Microanalytical techniques for boron analysis using the $^{10}B(n,\alpha)^7Li$ reaction. *Med. Phys.*, 13:50-56, 1986.
6. Fairchild, R.G., Bond, V.P., Current status of ^{10}B-neutron capture therapy: Enhancement of tumor dose via beam filtration and dose rate, and the effects of these parameters on minimum boron content: A theoretical evaluation. *Int. J. Radiation Oncology Biol. Phys.*, 11: 831-840, 1985.
7. Bellnier, D.A., Ho, Y.-K., Pandey, R.K., Missert, J.R., Dougherty, T.H., Distribution and elimination of photofrin II in mice. *Photochem. Photobiol.*, 50:221-228, 1989.
8. Coderre, J.A., Slatkin, D.N., Micca, P.L., Makar, M.S., Dose-response analysis for BNCT of the B16 murine melanoma using p-boronophenylalanine. Fourth International Symposium on Neutron Capture Therapy, Plenum Press, in press.
9. Kahl, S.B., Joel, D.D., Nawrocky, M.M., Micca, P.L., Tran, K.P., Finkel, G.C., Slatkin, D.N., Uptake of a nidocarboranyl porphyrin by human glioma xenografts in athymic nude mice and by syngeneic ovarian carcinomas in immunocompetent mice. *Proc. Natl. Acad. Sci. USA*, 87:7265-7269, 1990.

BASIC STUDIES IN BNCT —TOLERANCE TO HEAVY WATER

Tsuyoshi Kadosawa[1], Munekazu Nakaichi[1], Akira Takeuchi[1], Hiroshi Hatanaka[2]

1) Department of Veterinary Surgery, the University of Tokyo
2) Department of Neurosurgery, Teikyo University

INTRODUCTION

Advantages in application of heavy water (D_2O) to BNCT are to increase the penetration of thermal neutrons and enhance radiation produced by the $^{10}B(n, \alpha)^7Li$ reaction at depth in tissue[1]. Furthermore, D_2O decreases the capture γ-ray dose due to the $^1H(n, \gamma)^2H$ reaction[1]. In this paper, substitution of H_2O with D_2O and the physiological effects of oral and intraperitoneal administration of D_2O were studied in rats.

MATERIALS and METHODS

D_2O (>99.8%) was given orally (D_2O approximately 20ml/day) and intraperitoneally (lactated Ringer's solution made of D_2O, 20ml×2/day) to 15 and 18 Wistar rats (235±6 g, ♂, 7-8weeks) respectively and its physiological effects were compared with H_2O. To measure the substitution of H_2O with D_2O in tissues, three rats per day were euthanized on 1st, 2nd, 3rd, 5th and 7th day in oral administration, and on 1st, 2nd, 3rd and 5th day in intraperitoneal administration. Distilled water from blood and tissues was analysed for D_2O content by gas chromatography[2]. Furthermore, 3 rats were observed for 2 weeks after 2 days intraperitoneal administration of D_2O and another 3 rats after 3 days intraperitoneal administration of D_2O.

RESULTS

Table 1 shows D_2O content of water in blood and various tissues in oral administration of D_2O. There was little difference in D_2O substitution among organs. The same result was gained in intraperitoneal administration of D_2O.

Table 1 D_2O Content of Water in Blood and Various Tissues in Oral Administration of D_2O

Duration (day)	D_2O content of water in blood and tissues (%)					
	Blood	Brain	Liver	Kidney	Intestine	Muscle
1	9.43±1.08	9.45±1.11	9.30±1.02	9.32±0.92	9.55±1.24	9.39±1.07
2	15.74±3.13	15.73±3.15	15.59±3.45	15.78±3.08	15.28±3.26	15.67±3.23
3	17.52±0.03	17.51±0.02	17.52±0.01	17.53±0.01	17.52±0.01	17.52±0.01

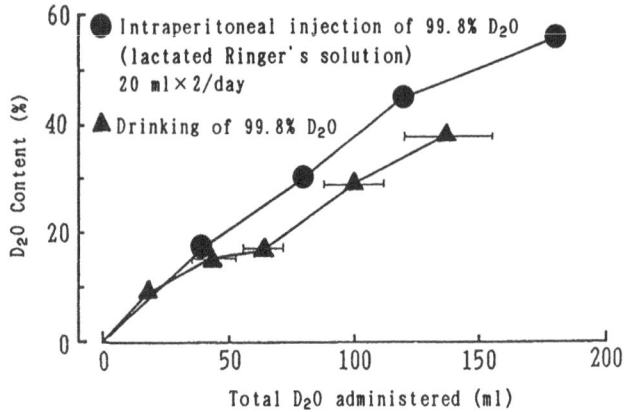

Fig.1 Total D_2O Administered and D_2O Content of Water in Blood

The relationship between the administered dose of D_2O and D_2O content in blood is shown in Figure 1. Intraperitoneal D_2O deuterated rats more efficiently than oral D_2O, but in each administration, D_2O substitution increased in proportion to the increase in total D_2O dosage.

Figure 2 shows changes of D_2O content of blood, body weight and physical condition in oral administration. Open circles indicate body weight in oral administration of H_2O. In oral administration of D_2O, depression of activity and decrease in body weight were observed on the 2nd day and the 3rd day, respectively. All rats showed hyperirritability on the 7th day, however not one of the rats died or showed anorexia.

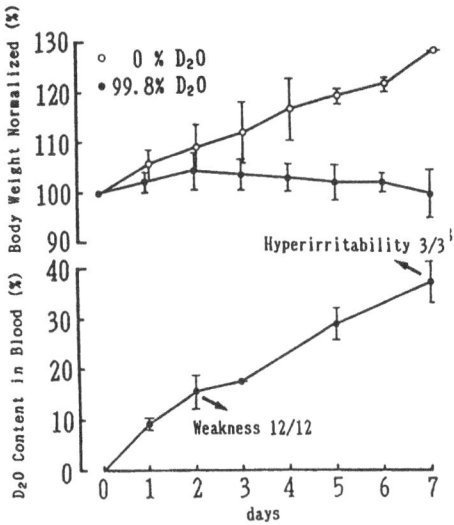

Fig.2 Physical Changes during D_2O Administration
[Oral]

Figure 3 shows changes of D_2O content of blood, body weight and physical conditions in intraperitoneal administration. Open circles show body weight in intraperitoneal injection of lactated Ringer's solution made of H_2O. In intraperitoneal injection of D_2O, depression of activity and decrease in body weight were observed on the 2nd day. On the 3rd day, one of nine rats showed hyperirritability. On the 4th day, two of three rats showed the above symptom and all of three rats showed immobility and anorexia. On the 5th day D_2O was administered intraperitoneally once only. All of three rats administered D_2O for 2 days and one of three rats administered D_2O for 3 days survived.

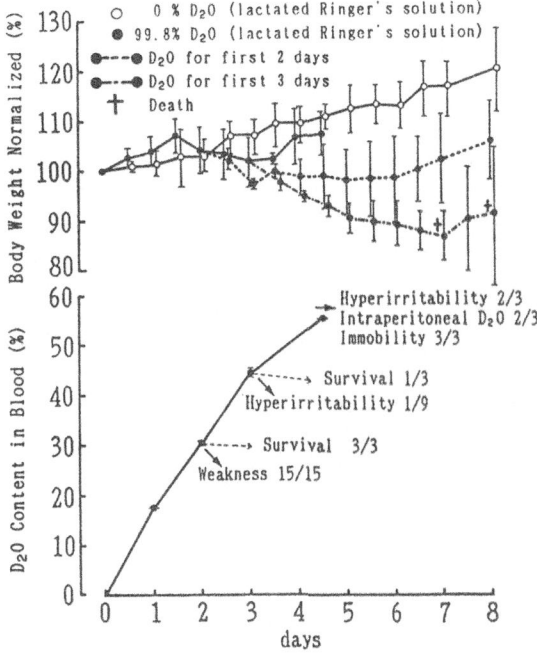

Fig 3 Physical Changes during D_2O Administration
[Intraperitoneal]

DISCUSSION and CONCLUSION

The Volume of D_2O substitution for H_2O in blood could be increased in proportion to the increase in D_2O administered, either orally or intraperitoneally. There was little difference in D_2O content between blood and other tissues. Because D_2O diffused rapidly from blood to other tissues, it would be possible to monitor D_2O substitution in those tissues by monitoring that in blood.

Daily administration of D_2O caused physiological effects, such as depression of activity, hyperirritability, immobility and death. All rats administered D_2O for 2 days, with 30% D_2O substituted for H_2O, survived. Two of three rats administered D_2O for 3 days, with 45% D_2O substituted for H_2O, died. It was found that deuteration to a level over 30% by daily administration of D_2O was dangerous. Though deuterium is an isotope of hydrogen, deuterium differs from hydrogen in both its thermodynamic and kinetic properties[3]. The change in reaction rate occasioned by the replacement of deuterium for hydrogen in the tissues could cause such physiological effects. In our study, D_2O substitution rate for H_2O was analyzed from distilled water in each tissue, that is from the body water. The replacement rate of deuterium for hydrogen (for instance : -C-H → -C-D) was not detected by analysis of water from the combustion[4] of each tissue. Oral administration of D_2O caused hyperirritability in rats at a lower D_2O concentration (all rats with 40% D_2O substituted showed hyperirritability) than intraperitoneal administration of D_2O (one of nine rats with 45% D_2O substituted and two of three rats with 55% D_2O showed the same symptom). These results might indicate that deuterium replaced hydrogen slowly in the tissues. Therefore, rapid substitution with D_2O followed by rapid restoring with H_2O might be able to reduce the disturbance of biological systems.

Deuteration of body water is advantageous to BNCT, although some toxicity is observed. Rats were able to tolerate approximately 30% D_2O substitution for body water by daily administration of D_2O. Transient or partial deuteration might be achievable safely with more than 30% D_2O substitution in the tissues applied to BNCT.

REFERENCES

1) D. N. Slatkin, M. M. Levine and A. Aronson, 1983, The Use of Heavy Water in Boron Neutron Capture Therapy in Brain Tumours. Phys. Med. Biol., 28 (12) : 1447-1451.

2) M. Mochizuki, S. Noda and T. Morishita, 1987, A Simple Method for Determination of Heavy Water by Combined Use of Gas Chromatography and Platinum Catalyst. Radioisotopes, 36 : 163-168.

3) J. J. Katz, H. L. Crespi, R. J. Hasterlik, J. F. Thomson and A. J. Finkel, 1957, Some Observations on Biological Effects of Deuterium, with Special Reference to Effects on Neoplastic Processes. J. Natl. Cancer Inst., 18 (5) : 641-659.

4) J. J. Katz, H. L. Crespi, D. M. Czajka and A. J. Finkel, 1962, Course of Deuteriation and Some Physiological Effects of Deuterium in Mice. Am. J. Physiol., 203 (5) : 907-913.

BORON NEUTRON CAPTURE THERAPY OF OCULAR MELANOMA AND INTRACRANIAL

GLIOMA USING p-BORONOPHENYLALANINE

J.A. Coderre, S. Packer[1], D. Greenberg, P.L. Micca, D.D. Joel and S. Saraf

Medical Department, Brookhaven National Laboratory, Upton, NY 11973, USA
[1]Department of Ophthalmology, North Shore University Hospital, Manhasset, NY 11030, USA

INTRODUCTION

During conventional radiation therapy, the dose that can be delivered to the tumor is limited by the tolerance of the surrounding normal tissue within the treatment volume. Boron neutron capture therapy (BNCT) represents a promising modality for selective irradiation of tumor tissue. The key to effective BNCT is the selective localization of ^{10}B in the tumor. The ratio of the ^{10}B concentration in the tumor to that in the normal tissues within the treatment volume will largely determine the therapeutic gain that can be achieved in any subsequent irradiation.

We have shown that intragastric (i.g.) administration of the synthetic amino acid p-boronophenylalanine (BPA) as an aqueous slurry at neutral pH is an effective method of drug administration (Coderre, 1988). BPA is non-toxic even at very high doses, is rapidly solubilized in the acidic environment of the stomach and is absorbed in the gastrointestinal tract. The time-course of tumor uptake and clearance of boron following i.g. doses was similar to that observed following i.p. doses of BPA. BPA is an analogue of the melanin precursor tyrosine and as such was originally intended as an agent for BNCT of melanoma. Subsequent studies with BPA have shown that this amino acid analogue is capable of selectively delivering boron to tumors other than melanoma; a murine mammary carcinoma and a rat gliosarcoma (Coderre, 1990). These results indicate that systemically administered BPA may have a general utility as a boron delivery agent for BNCT.

Our therapy experiments have progressed from irradiation of s.c. murine thigh tumors (Coderre, 1988) to the use of more sophisticated tumor models in order to demonstrate the ability of BNCT to effectively treat a tumor in the presence of radiosensitive normal tissues. Thermal neutron irradiations have been carried out at the Brookhaven Medical Research Reactor (BMRR), following i.g. administration of BPA, using the non-pigmented Greene melanoma carried in the anterior chamber of the rabbit eye and the GS-9L gliosarcoma implanted in the rat brain.

METHODS

BPA (as the free amino acid) was administered i.g. by transesophageal intubation with a feeding tube, as an aqueous slurry at neutral pH. Animals received a dose of approximately 750 mg BPA per kg body weight; rats received either 150 mg of L-BPA or 300 mg of D,L-BPA per dose in 3 ml of water, rabbits received up to 2.0 g of D,L-BPA in 15 ml of water. ^{10}B analysis was performed by the prompt gamma spectroscopic technique.

The rabbit ocular melanoma model. The Greene melanoma forms an amelanotic tumor when transplanted into the anterior or posterior chamber of the rabbit eye. During surgical procedures, rabbits were anesthetized with intramuscular ketamine hydrochloride (35mg/kg)/xylazine (5mg/kg). Iris melanomas were initiated in New Zealand White rabbits by implantation of approximately 1 mm^3 fragments of tumor tissue into the anterior chamber through an incision in the sclera at the limbus. Tumor size was measured with a hand-held caliper; 2 perpendicular dimensions were recorded. Tumors grew to about 200 mg in 2-3 weeks.

The rat glioma model. Subcutaneous (s.c.) tumors were initiated in F-344 rats by the injection of 5×10^6 cultured GS-9L gliosarcoma cells in 0.1 ml of growth medium. Tumors were palpable 4-5 days after inoculation and had a volume-doubling time of approximately two days. For initiation of brain tumors, 10^4 cultured cells in 1 μl of medium were injected, at a depth of 3-4 mm, into the left frontal lobe (Joel, 1990). This technique produced a locally expanding tumor with no evidence of blood-borne metastasis or seeding to ventricular or leptomeningeal surfaces. Rats survived an average of 22 ± 4 (SD) days after implantation.

RESULTS AND DISCUSSION

BPA distribution studies in the rabbit. Figure 1 shows the boron concentrations in the anterior chamber melanoma, blood and lens following a single i.g. dose of BPA. At 20 hrs post-administration there was ≈ 20 μg ^{10}B/g tumor with a tumor-to-blood concentration ratio of $\approx 4:1$. ^{10}B concentrations

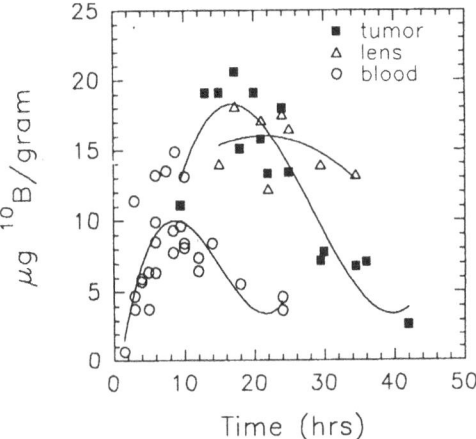

Figure 1. ^{10}B concentrations in anterior chamber Greene melanoma, blood, and lens *versus* time following one i.g. dose of BPA in the rabbit. Individual data points are shown.

in liver and muscle (not shown) were similar to those observed in the blood. Quantitative neutron capture radiography of tumor-bearing eyes following BPA administration indicated that the ^{10}B concentration in normal eye tissues was on the order of 3-5 μg/g with the exception of the lens, which showed higher levels of ^{10}B (10-15 μg/g) at the periphery. BNCT irradiations were carried out 20 hours after a single i.g. dose of BPA.

BPA distribution studies in the rat. The time course of ^{10}B accumulation and washout in the tumor as well as the maximum concentration of ^{10}B attained in the tumor were not significantly different when BPA was given as either the purified L-enantiomer (150 mg) or as the racemic mixture (300 mg). Evidently the D-enantiomer is not absorbed efficiently from the gastrointestinal tract and contributes little to the levels of ^{10}B in normal tissues.

Figure 2 shows the concentration of ^{10}B in tumor and normal tissues following i.g. administration of BPA (300 mg D,L-BPA per dose). The slow rate of accumulation of boron in the tumor following a single i.g. dose of BPA (Fig. 2) suggested that a second i.g. dose might produce an additive effect. This was confirmed by comparison of the time courses of boron uptake and clearance from tumor, blood and normal tissues in intracerebral GS-9L rat gliomas following a single i.g. dose of BPA and following two i.g. doses of BPA given 3 hours apart (Fig. 2). The second dose in the sequence substantially increased the maximum concentration of ^{10}B in the tumor, from 24 to 39 μg ^{10}B/g. Blood ^{10}B was also increased, but a tumor/blood ^{10}B concentration ratio of $\approx$3.3:1 was maintained. BNCT irradiations were carried out eight hours after the first of two i.g. doses given three hours apart.

Dosimetry. The dose from BNCT irradiations is expressed as gray-equivalent (Gy-Eq), calculated by summation of physical doses (Gy) of the component radiations multiplied by appropriate relative biological effectiveness (RBE) factors. RBE values of 2.3 and 2.0 have been assumed for the ionizing particles from the ^{10}B(n,α)^{7}Li and ^{14}N(n,p)^{14}C reactions, respectively, and 2.0 has been assumed for fast neutrons.

Tumor-bearing rabbits were irradiated for 6 minutes at 1 megawatt reactor power (6MW-min) using a collimator with a 1.55 cm diameter aperture. The thermal neutron fluence at the tumor position was 5.3 x 10^{12}n$_{th}$cm^{-2}. The contributions from the beam components to the total dose within the treatment volume for the 6 MW-min eye irradiation were as follows: fast neutrons, 1.56 Gy; photons from the reactor and the collimator, 0.80 Gy; products of the ^{14}N(n,p)^{14}C reaction, 1.03 Gy; and particles from the ^{10}B(n,α)^{7}Li reaction, 0.46 Gy per μg of ^{10}B present per gram wet tissue. In the BPA-BNCT group, the ^{10}B concentration in tumor and normal tissue at the time of irradiation was 20 and 3 μg/g, respectively. The total radiation dose was calculated to be 12.62 Gy (29.05 Gy-Eq) to the tumor and 4.77 Gy (9.44 Gy-Eq) to the normal eye tissues (cornea, retina). These data imply an average therapeutic gain of approximately 3. The ^{10}B distribution within the lens was non-uniform, as determined by neutron capture radiography; a local ^{10}B concentration of 15 μg ^{10}B/g would result in a dose of 10.3 Gy (21.9 Gy-Eq).

Tumor-bearing rats were irradiated for 4 minutes at a reactor power of 1.25 megawatts (5 MW-min) using a collimator with a 1.1 cm diameter aperture. The thermal neutron fluence at the tumor center was 2.0 x 10^{12} n$_{th}$cm^{-2}. The contributions from dosimetrically significant beam components to the total dose within the treatment volume for a 5 MW-min brain irradiation were as follows: fast neutrons, 1.35 Gy; photons from the reactor and the collimator, 0.55 Gy; products of the ^{14}N(n,p)^{14}C reaction, 0.38 Gy; and particles from the ^{10}B(n,α)^{7}Li reaction, 0.17 Gy per μg of ^{10}B present per gram wet tissue. In the BPA-BNCT group, boron concentrations in the tumor, normal brain, and the blood at the time of irradiation were estimated to be 39, 12 and 10 μg ^{10}B/g, respectively. The total radiation dose was

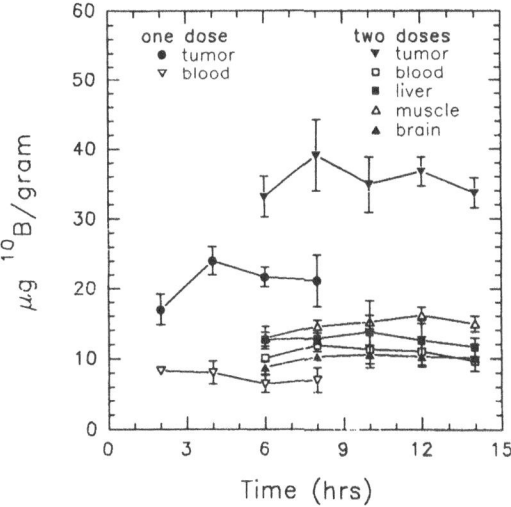

Figure 2. ^{10}B concentration in intracranial GS-9L gliosarcomas and normal tissues *versus* time following either one i.g. dose of BPA at t=0 hrs or two i.g. doses of BPA at t=0 and t=3 hours. The experiment was carried out 18 days after tumor initiation. Each point represents 4 or 5 rats, mean ± 1 SD.

calculated to be 8.9 Gy (19.3 Gy-Eq) to the tumor, 4.3 Gy (8.7 Gy-Eq) to the blood, 4.0 Gy (7.9 Gy-Eq) to the brain, and 4.1 Gy (8.2 Gy-Eq) to the capilary endothelium. The dose to the capillary endothelial cell was calculated as 1/3 of the dose to the blood plus 2/3 of the dose to the normal brain. These data imply average therapeutic gains of 2.2 - 2.4.

BNCT of ocular melanoma. A total of 31 rabbits with anterior chamber melanomas were divided into three groups. Figure 3 shows the tumor growth *versus* time in the groups that received no treatment (Fig.3A), reactor irradiation only (Fig.3B), or BPA-based BNCT (Fig.3C). Three of 13 BNCT-treated tumors grew (Fig.3C); the remaining tumors were monitored for various periods of time. Rabbits with controlled tumors were euthanized at increasing time intervals and the eyes examined histologically. At approximately 3 to 6 months post-irradiation cataract formation was observed in treated eyes as well as a mild to moderate keratitis; the vasculature in the treated eyes appeared normal. All 9 tumors in the reactor-irradiation-only group (Fig.3B) as well as all 9 control tumors (Fig.3A) grew at roughly the same rate.

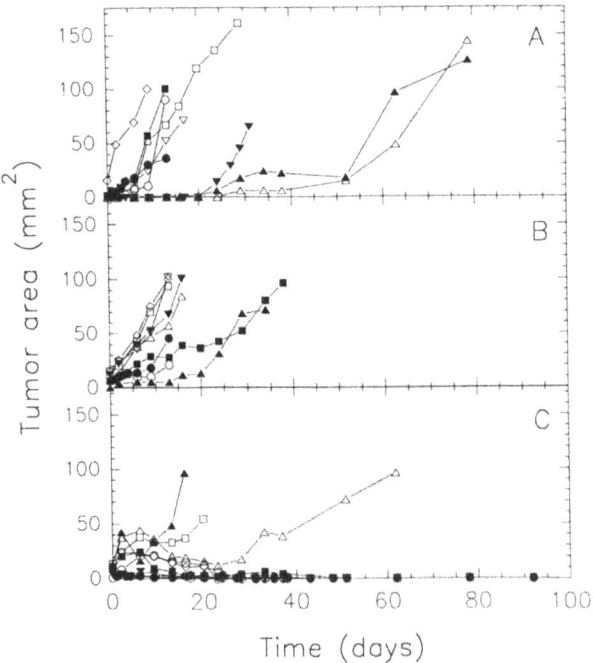

Figure 3.   Growth of the Greene melanoma in the anterior chamber of the rabbit eye (tumor area *versus* time) following (A) no treatment (n=9); (B) reactor irradiation only (n=9) and (C) BPA-based BNCT (n=13).

BNCT of intracranial glioma. A total of 44 rats bearing intracerebral tumors were divided into three treatment groups; 1) no treatment (n=13); 2) reactor irradiation alone (n=15); and 3) reactor irradiation after two i.g. doses of BPA (n=16). Reactor irradiations alone caused a transient weight loss. There was no evidence of radiation-induced nasopharyngitis. No post-irradiation supportive therapy was given. Figure 4 shows survival versus time following tumor initiation. The median survival of untreated rats with implanted gliosarcomas was 22 ± 4 (SD) days. Reactor irradiation was performed on day 14 after tumor initiation. Rats receiving reactor irradiations alone had a median survival of 25 days. There were no survivors in group 1 or group 2. The median survival of rats in group 3 was 80 days. Seven of the 16 animals in group 3 are long-term survivors; 4 are alive 13 months post-irradiation and 3 are alive 10 months post-irradiation. All of the seven long-term surviving rats developed cataracts in the left eye 3 to 6 months after BNCT; 4 developed cataracts in the right eye 6-9 months after irradiation.

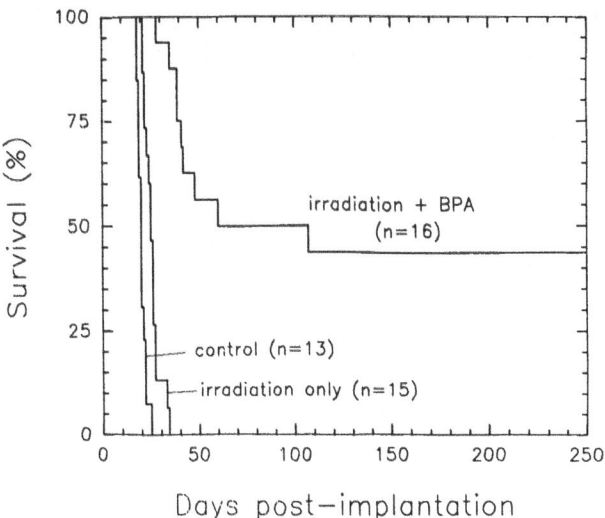

Figure 4. Survival of control and BNCT-treated rats bearing intracerebral GS-9L gliosarcomas *versus* time. Control rats (n=13) received no treatment. All reactor irradiations were performed 14 days following tumor initiation. Fifteen rats received reactor irradiation only. Sixteen tumor-bearing rats received 2 i.g. doses of BPA (300 mg D,L-BPA each) given 3 hours apart; the rats were irradiated 5 hours after the second dose.

Table 1. BNCT of the Intracerebral GS-9L Gliosarcoma: Comparison of BPA with the Sulfhydryl Borane Dimer.

	BNCT Treatment Conditions		
	Dimer 5MW-min[1]	BPA 5MW-min[2]	Dimer 7.5 MW-min[3]
Tumor Dose (Gy-Eq)	14.2	19.3	25.6
Endothelial Cell Dose (Gy-Eq)	8.8	8.2	15.2
Long-Term Survivors	2/12	7/16	6/10

[1] At the time of irradiation, ^{10}B concentrations in tumor, blood and brain were 26, 35, and 1.4 μg ^{10}B/gram, respectively (Joel, 1990).

[2] At the time of irradiation, ^{10}B concentrations in tumor, blood and brain were 39, 12, and 10 μg ^{10}B/gram, respectively.

[3] At the time of irradiation, ^{10}B concentrations in tumor, blood and brain were 35, 45, and 1.4 μg ^{10}B/gram, respectively (Joel, 1990).

Joel et al. (1990) have recently reported the results of successful BNCT trials in the GS-9L rat gliosarcoma using the dimer form of the sulfhydryl borane ($Na_4B_{24}H_{22}S_2$). There are differences in the distributions of ^{10}B in blood and normal brain between BPA and dimer which may have radiobiological implications *in vivo*. Table 1 shows, for BPA and the two dimer experiments reported by Joel *et al.* (1990), radiation doses to critical tissues based on comparable tumor ^{10}B concentrations and the corresponding fractions of long-term survivors. These data suggest a dose-response relationship with a 50% tumor control dose of roughly 23 Gy-Eq. Barker et al. (1979) reported a long-term survival of only 1 of 20 rats bearing the intracerebral GS-9L gliosarcoma following 20 Gy of x-rays to the whole head. Joel et al. (1990) also reported long-term survival fractions of 1/10 and 4/16 following x-ray doses of 15.0 and 22.5 Gy, respectively. X-ray doses in the 20 Gy range may be effective in controlling tumor growth in a small percentage of animals but have also been reported to cause delayed brain damage up to two years later (van der Kogel, 1983).

The radiation dose to the vascular endothelium in the brain is more significant, in terms of delayed damage, than similar doses to brain parenchyma (Hopewell, 1989). The lower ^{10}B concentrations in blood following BPA administration compared to the concentrations in blood following dimer infusion and the resulting lower radiation doses to the vascular endothelium may be advantageous in the prevention of delayed damage to the vasculature.

ACKNOWLEDGEMENTS

The research described in the report involved animals maintained in animal care facilities fully accredited by the American Association for Accreditation of Laboratory Animal Care. This research was supported in part by the US Department of Energy under contract DE-AC02-76CH00016, and by Grant No. CA42446 (JAC) from the NIH.

REFERENCES

Barker, M., D.F. Deen, and D.G. Baker, BCNU and x-ray therapy of intracerebral 9L rat tumors. *Int. J. Rad. Oncol. Biol. Phys.* 5:1581-1583 (1979).

Coderre, J.A., J.A. Kalef-Ezra, R.G. Fairchild, P.L. Micca, L.E. Reinstein, and J.D. Glass, Boron neutron capture therapy of a murine melanoma. *Cancer Res.* 48:6313-6316 (1988).

Coderre, J.A., J.D. Glass, R.G. Fairchild, P.L. Micca, I. Fand, and D.D. Joel, Affinity of the melanin precursor analog p-boronophenylalanine for tumors other than melanoma. *Cancer Res.* 50:138-141 (1990).

Hopewell, J.W., W. Calvo, D. Campling, H.S. Reinhold, M. Rezvani, and T.K. Yeung, Effects of Radiation on the microvasculature: Implications for Normal-Tissue Damage. In *Radiation Tolerance of Normal Tissues. Frontiers of Radiation Therapy and Oncology* Vol. 23:85-95 (1989).

Joel, D.D., R.G. Fairchild, J.A. Laissue, S.K. Saraf, J.A. Kalef-Ezra, and D.N. Slatkin, Boron Neutron Capture Therapy of Intracerebral Rat Gliosarcomas. *Proc. Natl. Acad. Sci., USA* (1990) in press.

van der Kogel, A.J., The cellular basis of radiation-induced damage in the central nervous system. In: *Cytotoxic Insult to Tissue; Effects on Cell Lineages* (C.S. Potten, and J.H. Hendry, eds) pp. 329-352, Churchill Livingstone, New York, 1983.

A QUANTITATIVE STUDY ON PHARMACOKINETICS AND BIODISTRIBUTION OF BSH

IN A RAT GLIOMA MODEL

Raphael J.B. Hemler*, Crister P. Ceberg**, Arne Brun***,
Detlef Gabel+, Börje Larsson++, Bertil R.R. Persson**
and Leif G. Salford*

*Dept of Neurosurgery, **Dept of Radiation Physics,
***Dept of Pathology, Lund University Hospital, Lund, Sweden
+Dept of Chemistry, University of Bremen, Germany
++Dept of Radiation Sciences, Uppsala, Sweden

INTRODUCTION

Less than 3 adult patients out of 1000 with astrocytoma grade III-IV survive more than 10 years (1). New therapeutic tools are required to improve this situation, and Boron Neutron Capture Therapy (BNCT) provides an attractive concept.

The ^{10}B carrier $Na_2{}^{10}B_{12}H_{11}SH$ (BSH) to be used in combination with a source for epithermal neutron irradiation in Petten, Holland, constitutes the basis for the European Collaboration on BNCT, supported by the Commission of the European Communities.

In parallel with this clinical feasibility study, we are collecting detailed information on biodistribution and pharmacokinetics of BSH in a rat glioma model in order to find the optimal time interval between BSH administration and neutron irradiation. Preliminary results are presented here.

MATERIAL AND METHODS

BSH in a dose equivalent to $175\mu g{}^{10}B/g$ body weight, was given i.v. to 19 Fischer 344 rats with RG2 glioma cells inoculated in the caudate nucleus 18 days earlier.

All animals were used for a comparison of histopathology and ^{10}B distribution and received their BSH 3-72 hours before sacrifice. Five animals were whole-body freeze-sectioned. In 3 cases the brains were removed to be separately fixed in formaldehyde-gas. In another 11 cases the brains were dissected and removed before freeze-sectioning. Eight out of these 11 animals were also used for studies of pharmacokinetics and received BSH 3 hrs (3), 6 hrs (3), 12 hrs (1) and at 24 hrs (1) before sacrifice.

Immediately thereafter, the brain including the tumor, and specimens from skin, muscle, dura, lung, liver, spleen and kidney were frozen in isopentane containing dry ice (-70°C). Blood samples were taken at 5, 15 minutes and 1, 3, 6, 12 and 24 hours after the BSH infusion when feasible. The blood samples were treated with EDTA, frozen and stored in tissue glue (OCT) at -22°C.

The ^{10}B content was evaluated with quantitative neutron capture radiography (QNCR) as documented by Gabel et al (2). The specimens were exposed to heavy-water moderated thermal neutrons ($10^{13}cm^{-2}$) at the R2-0 reactor facility in Studsvik, Sweden.

In the present work a new method for film evaluation has been developed (3). A macro-lens equipped CCD-camera (MTI), connected to a PC386-based imaging system (MIS), provided grey-scale transmission images of the film. The grey-scale was calibrated against known ^{10}B concentrations in standard samples. In such images, large enough to cover e.g. a rat brain, any region of interest can be evaluated for its ^{10}B content and compared to the histopathology of parallel stained adjacent sections.

RESULTS

In all of the 19 animals, gliomas had developed with sizes ranging from 3 to 8 mm diameter.

Comparison of histopathology and ^{10}B-distribution

In whole body slices from five animals, alpha-particle tracks were seen corresponding to the major blood containing vessels. Tracks were also seen in the skin and in organs such as the liver and the spleen. A concentration of tracks in the brain tumors could also be seen.

The difference in ^{10}B uptake between tumor tissue and surrounding brain was best demonstrated in the 3 formaldehyde-gas fixed brains, where the freezing artifacts were omitted. Extensive ^{10}B uptake was demonstrated in the tumors, while only a few scattered points of uptake could be seen in the surrounding histopathologically normal brain tissue. It was even possible to demonstrate a higher concentration of tracks in the peripheral portion of the tumors under the microscope.

For the 11 cases where the brains were dissected and removed before freeze-sectioning, ^{10}B distribution images and corresponding histological preparations were documented as shown in figures 1 and 2 respectively. Figure 1 shows the boron distribution in a slice through the tumor in a rat brain, 6 hours after the BSH administration. In figure 2, the histological preparation of the directly adjacent slice is shown. Some brains displayed a very close correlation between the histological tumor cell distribution and the boron uptake, while other cases demonstrated some boron uptake far outside the tumor mass. Higher magnification of the histological preparation, revealed that these areas contain small clusters of tumor cells spread in the otherwise normal brain tissue surrounding the tumor. Arrow A indicates such an area.

In the case shown in figures 1 and 2, even in the contralateral side, a small (0.2x0.5mm) cluster of tumor cells showed a corresponding boron uptake (arrow B).

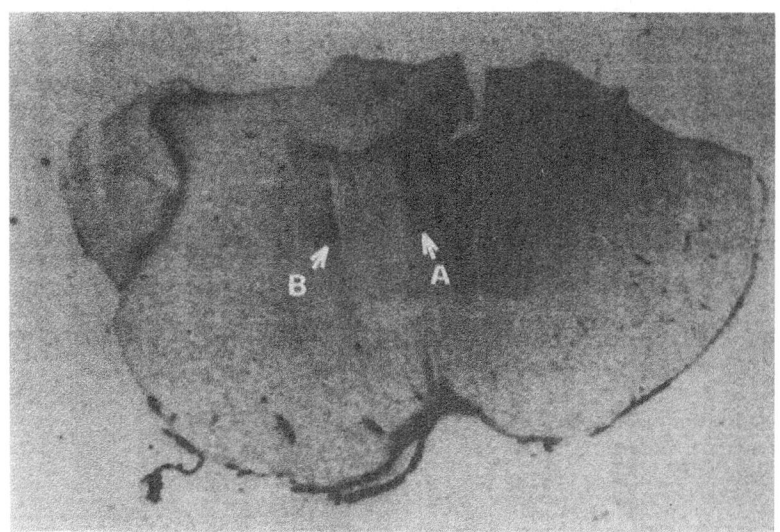

Figure 1. Transmission image of a nuclear track detector film, showing the boron distribution in a slice through the tumor in a rat brain 6 hours after the BSH administration.

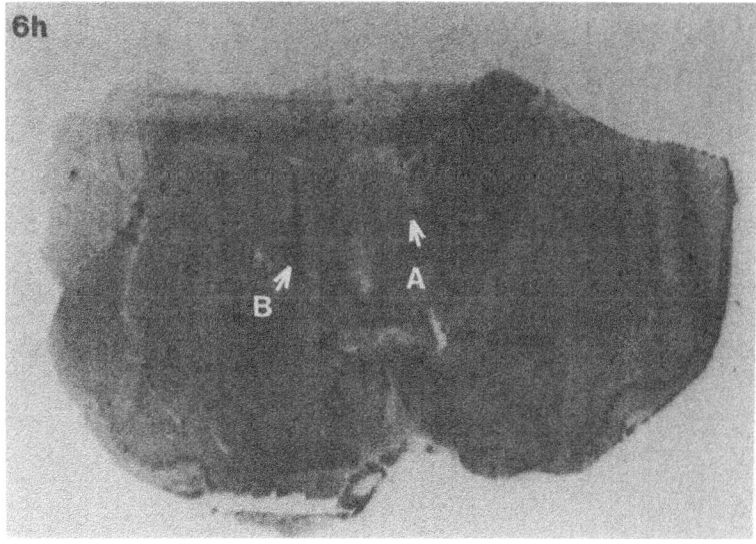

Figure 2. Digital image showing the histological preparation of the slice directly adjacent to the one in figure 1.

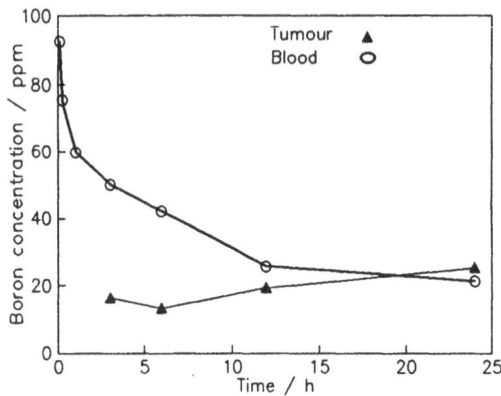

Figure 3. The ^{10}B concentration in blood and tumor. The blood concentration falls in a biphasic pattern, and the build-up of tumor concentration seems to approach the blood value at around 20 hours in this rat model.

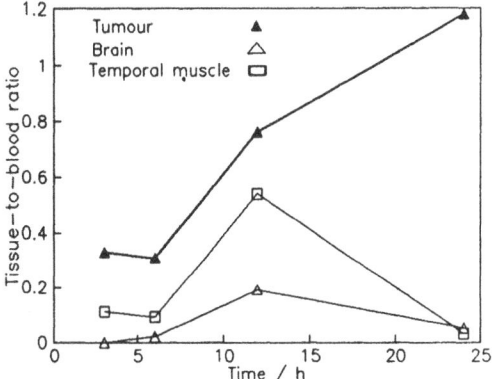

Figure 4. The tumor-to-blood ratio builds up continuously whereas other tissue-to-blood ratios decrease after about 12 hours.

Boron pharmacokinetics and biodistribution

For the 8 animals that were used for studies of the pharmacokinetics, the boron concentrations in blood, brain tumor and muscle tissue are shown in figures 3 and 4.

DISCUSSION

Following some modifications, our RG2 rat glioma model now mimics the human astrocytoma, and sends migrating "guerilla" glioma cells into the surrounding brain. There they might hide behind an intact blood-brain barrier, which shelters from therapeutic attacks. This is a crucial point for the future success of BNCT. Hitherto it has just been proven that BSH reaches the major portion of the tumor, where the blood-brain barrier is broken down. We have shown that boron can be revealed in minute clusters of tumor cells (Fig. 1) located far away from the bulk of the tumor in a region where there is a good reason to believe that the blood-brain barrier is still intact. This finding supports the potential of BNCT to *cure* astrocytomas.

In our continued research we have started parallel studies where the leakage of albumin, indicating blood-brain barrier breakdown, is measured around the tumor and in the vicinity of minor tumor cell clusters by the use of mouse anti-rat albumin antibodies. These investigations will be used in our efforts to clarify whether or not boron can be brought to and accumulated in the "guerilla" cells, in spite of an intact blood-brain barrier.

The pharmacokinetics of boron in this rat model points to an improving tumor-to-blood ratio during the first 24 hours. This is not directly applicable to the human situation, because of the higher metabolic rate of the rat as compared to the human. It should also be noted that these preliminary results only include single rats at the 12h and 24h time points.

REFERENCES

1. Salford LG, Brun A and Nirfalk S: **Ten year survival among patients with supratentorial astrocytoma grade III and IV.** *J. Neurosurg. 69:506-509, 1988.*

2. Gabel D, Holstein H, Larsson B et al.: **QNCR for studying the biodistribution of tumor-seeking Boron containing compounds.** *Cancer Res. 47:5451-5454, 1987.*

3. Ceberg C, Hemler RJB, Persson BRR and Salford LG: **Neutron Capture Imaging of ^{10}B distribution in tissue specimens.** *Manuscript in preparation.*

BIODISTRIBUTION AND PHARMACOKINETICS OF p-BORONOPHENYLALANINE IN C57BL/6 MICE WITH GL261 INTRACEREBRAL TUMORS, AND SURVIVAL FOLLOWING NEUTRON CAPTURE THERAPY

G. Solares[1], R. Zamenhof[2], S. Saris[2], D. Wazer[2], S. Kerley[2], M. Joyce[2], H. Madoc-Jones[2], L. Adelman[2], O. Harling[1]

[1]Nuclear Reactor Laboratory, Massachusetts Institute of Technology, 138 Albany Street, Cambridge, MA 01239, USA
[2]Tufts University School of Medicine and New England Medical Center Hospitals, Boston, MA 02111, USA

INTRODUCTION

Because much of the theoretical rationale for NCT rests on the availability of agents capable of selectively transporting ^{10}B to tumor cells, the ability to quantify differential ^{10}B distributions in tissue exposed to such agents is clearly of major importance. Also, since the precise intracellular location of ^{10}B can strongly influence the biological effect of the alpha particle and ^{7}Li recoil radiation following thermal neutron capture by ^{10}B[1], an analytic technique with a resolution of 2-3 μm is of obvious value. We have implemented a modified version of an autoradiography technique, originally developed in our laboratory at MIT[2] and added a computer-aided analytic capability based on a Macintosh-II computer with a CCD TV camera and Image Analyst software (Automatix Corp., Billerica, Massachusetts)[3-4]. We will briefly describe our implementation of this technique and present results from a p-boronophenylalanine (BPA) biodistribution and pharmacokinetic study in an intracerebral mouse glioma and a survival study to evaluate the efficacy of NCT in this tumor model.

HIGH RESOLUTION α-TRACK AUTORADIOGRAPHY

The autoradiographic technique we employ is diagrammatically summarized in Fig.1 A description of the current experimental technique has been published elsewhere[4]

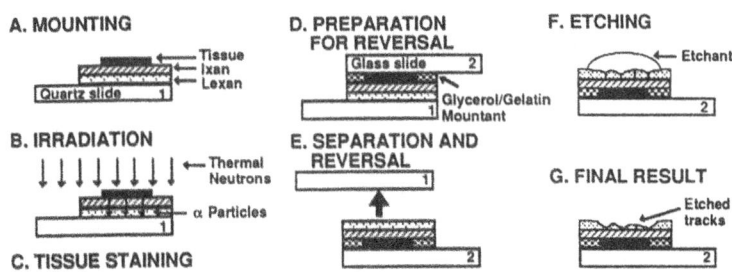

Fig. 1. Diagrammatic representation of procedure for performing high resolution alpha-track autoradiography.

Fig. 2 shows a 2-μm thick brain tumor section of a mouse after administration of 40 mg of ^{10}B/kg body weight of racemic BPA in which the tracks are visible simultaneously with the stained tissue. The left side of the figure shows the alpha tracks as circular black dots, the nuclei as dark gray objects, and the cytoplasm as the lighter gray area surrounding the nuclei (no cell boundaries have been defined). The white regions represent extracellular space including blood vessels, sectioning artifacts, etc. The right side of the figure shows the same section after image processing using a modified blurred mask subtraction technique. The processed image contains a more uniform background in which the tracks can be identified by thresholding. The tracks are then automatically counted using an edge gradient detection algorithm. The ^{10}B concentrations are calculated from a calibration curve of track density versus ^{10}B concentration derived from a set of tissue standards containing known ^{10}B concentrations. These standards were calibrated using the prompt gamma technique which, in turn, was cross-calibrated with the BNL prompt gamma facility.

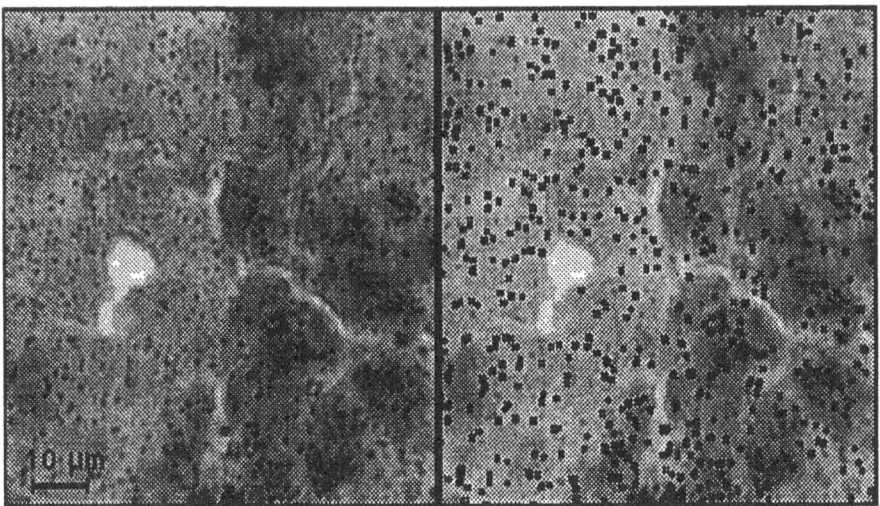

Fig. 2   High-resolution autoradiogram of a brain tissue section of a glioma-bearing mouse. The left side shows the original image in which tracks and tissue are visible simultaneously, while the right side shows the same image after computer processing where the tracks have been automatically separated from the original image, enhanced, and superimposed back onto the original image.

BIODISTRIBUTION AND PHARMACOKINETICS

Using this technique a BPA biodistribution and pharmacokinetic study was carried out on the GL261 glioma-bearing C57BL/6 mouse model. Although the biodistribution data is strictly that for ^{10}B, it will be loosely referred to as being that for BPA. Mice received oral doses of BPA ranging from 30 to 100 mg of ^{10}B/kg body weight.The animals were bled at time intervals ranging from 1 to 24 hours after which they were killed. Blood, brain, and tumor ^{10}B concentrations were measured by alpha-autoradiography as described earlier. Fig. 3 shows the boron concentration in the GL261 tumors, normal brain, and blood as a function of time following administration of BPA. It is evident that the boron concentration in tumor is markedly higher than in normal brain and blood. The tumor uptake of BPA reaches a maximum 3 h after BPA administration. The tumor-to-brain boron concentration ratio from 1 to 9 hours is maintained in the range of 3:1, peaking to 3.75:1 at approximately 7 h. The ^{10}B concentrations in tumor after 3 h are approximately 25% of the administered doses. Tumor-to-blood ratios at 3 h are 11:1. These distribution characteristics were maintained approximately constant over a 10-fold range in administered BPA dose. Macroscopic (LR115 track detector) BPA biodistribution data using an intracranial rat GS9L glioma model have been reported by Coderre[6]

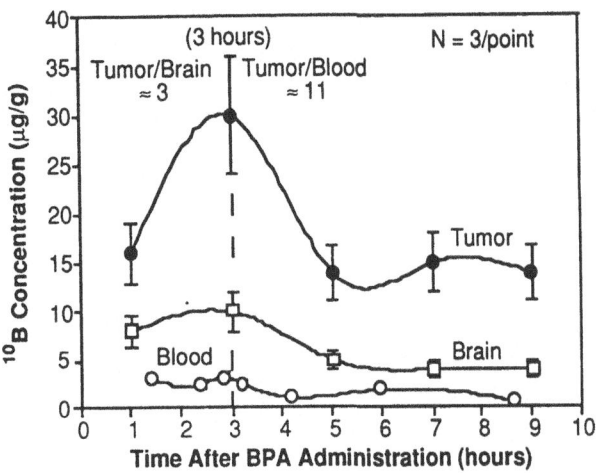

Fig. 3 ^{10}B concentrations in GL261 tumor., normal brain tissue, and blood. Each point is the average of 3 mice (mean ± SD). Each mouse received from 30 to 100 mg of ^{10}B/kg body weight of BPA orally. Highest tumor ^{10}B concentrations occurred after 3 hours following BPA administration with a tumor-to-normal brain ratio of 3:1. Highest tumor to normal brain ratio 3.75:1 occurred after 7 hours. Tumor-to-blood ratios at 3 h were 11:1.

NCT SURVIVAL STUDIES

An NCT survival study using the mouse/tumor model described above was carried out. This tumor has demonstrated infiltrative characteristics and aggressive growth similar to that of human glioblastoma multiforme. Four groups of control animals and one group of NCT treatment animals, each containing 6 animals were prepared The implanted tumors were allowed to grow for 3 to 4 days after which anesthetized animals were administered 95% ^{10}B-enriched racemic BPA through an orogastric stent with doses ranging from 50 to 200 mg of ^{10}B/kg body weight. Irradiations were carried out at the medical thermal beam facility of the Massachusetts Institute of Technology Research Reactor, MITR-II, 3 hours after BPA administration. The experimental details will be published elsewhere.

Fig. 4 summarizes median survival post irradiation for the NCT treated mice and controls. The two lower dose levels showed no statistically significant difference between treated and untreated mice. The median survival for the untreated and X-ray treated mice was 19.5 ± 5 days. For the two higher dose levels a statistically significant increase in the median survival for the treated mice was observed. The RBE's assumed in this paper were based on recommendations in ref (7), and were: 2.3 for the ^{10}B dose, 1.6 for all neutron doses, and 1.0 for all gamma doses. The median survival for the 4300 RBE cGy treated group was 63 days: a three-fold increase with respect to the untreated controls (p < 0.02). It also can be observed that the median survival for the X-ray treated mice at these higher dose levels is only 8 days, indicating radiation toxicity which does not appear in the NCT treated mice.

BIODISTRIBUTION IN HUMANS

NEMC/MIT, Boston University Medical Center, Brookhaven National Laboratory, Stonybrook Medical Center, North Shore Hospital (Long Island), and Ohio State University Medical Center are collaborating in a human biodistribution study to examine the potential suitability of BPA for clinical trials of NCT. Currently, approximately 15 ocular and cutaneous melanoma and glioblastoma patients have been studied. Tumor, normal brain, and skin boron distributions have been analyzed by high resolution alpha-track autoradiography, while the blood

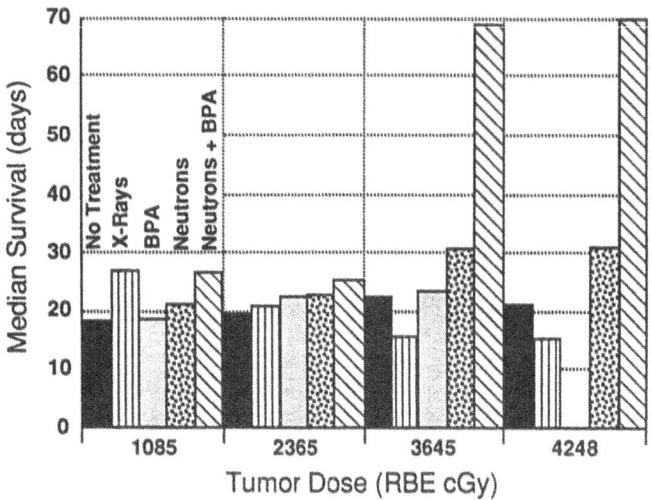

Fig. 4   Median survival for GL261 tumor-bearing mice after BNCT. Each group represents approximately 6 mice. ^{10}B-enriched racemic BPA was given orally 3 hours before irradiation.

and urine samples have been analyzed by prompt-gamma. Initial results indicate tumor/normal ^{10}B ratios slightly better than in Fig. 3, and tumor/blood ratios slightly worse.

ACKNOWLEDGMENTS

Funding for these studies have been partially provided by the U.S. Department of Energy under Grant No.DE-FG02-87ER-6060, by the Chairmans' Fund of the NEMC Department of Radiation Oncology and Neurosurgery, and by funding from the U.S. Department of Energy Reactor Sharing Program awarded to the MIT Nuclear Reactor Laboratory.

REFERENCES

1.   D. Gabel, S. Foster, R. Fairchild, "The Monte Carlo Simulation of the Biological Effect of the ^{10}B(n,α)^{7}Li Reaction in Cells and Tissue and Its Implication for Boron Neutron Capture Therapy," Radiation Res., 111:14, (1987).
2.   J. Kirsch, "Neutron-induced Track Etch Autoradiography: Studies in Track Detection and Neutron Capture Therapy," Ph.D. Thesis, MIT Department of Nuclear Engineering, February (1984).
3.   R. Zamenhof, S. Clement, K. Lin, C. Lui, D. Ziegelmiller, O. Harling, "Monte Carlo Treatment Planning and High-Resolution Alpha-Track Autoradiography for Neutron Capture Therapy," Strahlenther. Onk., 165:90, (1989).
4.   G. Solares, "High Resolution Alpha Track Autoradiography and Biological Studies of Boron Neutron Capture Therapy," Ph.D. Thesis, MIT Department of Nuclear Engineering, May (1991).
5.   O. Harling, R. Zamenhof, J. Yanch, R. Choi, G. Solares, R. Rogus, D. Moulin, L. Johnson, I. Olmez, S. Wirzek, J. Bernard, C. Nwanguma, D. Wazer, S. Saris, C. Sledge, H. Madoc-Jones,"Boron Neutron Capture and Radiation Synovectomy Research at the MIT Research Reactor," Nucl. Sci. Eng.(in press)
6.   J. Coderre, J. Glass, R. Fairchild, P Micca, I. Fand, D. Joel,"Selective Delivery of Boron by the Melanin Precursor Analogue p-Boronophenylalanine to Tumors Other Than Melanoma," Cancer Res., 50:138, (1990).
7.   O. K. Harling, J. Bernard, R. G. Zamenhof, eds., Neutron Beam Design, Development, and Performance for Neutron Capture Therapy, Plenum Press, New York (1990).

A LARGE ANIMAL MODEL FOR BORON NEUTRON CAPTURE THERAPY

P.R. Gavin,[1] S.L. Kraft,[1] C.E. DeHaan,[1]
M.L. Griebenow,[2] M.P. Moore[1]

[1]Veterinary Clinical Medicine & Surgery, Washington State
University, Pullman WA 99164
[2]EG&G Idaho, Inc., Idaho Falls ID 83415

ABSTRACT

An epithermal neutron beam is needed to treat relatively deep
seated tumors. The scattering characteristics of neutrons in this
energy range dictate that in vivo experiments be conducted in a large
animal to prevent unacceptable total body irradiation. The canine
species has proven an excellent model to evaluate the various problems
of boron neutron capture utilizing an epithermal neutron beam. This
paper discusses three major components of our study: I) the
pharmacokinetics of borocaptate sodium ($NA_2B_{12}H_{11}SH$ or BSH)
in dogs with spontaneously occurring brain tumors, II) the radiation
tolerance of normal tissues in the dog using an epithermal beam alone
and in combination with borocaptate sodium, and III) initial treatment
of dogs with spontaneously occurring brain tumors utilizing borocaptate
sodium and an epithermal neutron beam.

INTRODUCTION

Several in vitro and in vivo systems have documented the potential
advantages of boron neutron capture for the treatment of malignant
disease. The studies to date have, by necessity, used a thermal neutron
beam. The thermal neutron can be equally well used in tissue culture
studies and in various transplantable tumor models in rodents. The
unnatural growth characteristics, immunogenicity, and abnormal anatomic
sites of these models cast some doubt on their clinical utility.
However, positive results in these initial studies stimulated further
investigation with more realistic models. The control of experimental
variables using a relatively large number of animals with homogeneous
breeding provided statistical evidence of the positive benefits of boron
neutron capture therapy.

Spontaneous malignant diseases targeted by boron neutron capture
will require more penetration than is available from a thermal beam.
The present filtered beam at the Brookhaven Medical Research Reactor
provides the physical characteristics needed to perform canine studies.
Difficulties encountered in large animal studies, including accrual of a

relatively small number of animals with high variability, and the expensive nature of these studies, are recognized. However, information obtained from this study is imperative to allow continued development towards eventual safe clinical trials in human patients.

I. PHARMACOKINETICS

Materials and Methods

Dogs with spontaneously occurring brain tumors were obtained via a referral network. The dogs were administered intravenously borocaptate sodium at a dosage of 50 mg B/kg body weight. Serum was sampled at numerous time intervals prior to, during, and after boron infusion.[1] The animals were euthanized with an overdose of barbiturates 2, 6, and 12 hours post-compound administration.[2] All serum, urine samples, and tissue samples were analyzed using inductively coupled plasma-atomic emission spectroscopy (ICP-AES) for boron level determination.

Results

The boron concentration peaked at the end of infusion and underwent distribution over the next 1 to 2 hours with a $T_{1/2}$ of 110 minutes for that phase. Following distribution, most of the compound was excreted in the urine. This excretory phase had a $T_{1/2}$ of 274 minutes. Ultra-filtration studies of the serum revealed that approximately 80% of the detectable boron was associated with serum protein. Serum protein levels did not change significantly over the time periods studied.

Very little boron was detected within the blood-fibrin clot which remains after serum removal. Therefore, blood concentration is estimated to be roughly half that of serum concentration. Liver, spleen, lung, and kidneys (highly vascular tissues, and other tissues associated with elimination pathway) had boron concentrations significantly greater than blood. A few tissues had roughly the same boron concentration as blood. These tissues included skin and oral mucous membranes. Some tissues, including the brain and cerebrospinal fluid, had virtually no boron. Finally, there were tissues with boron concentrations between blood and brain concentrations. Such tissues included skeletal muscle and bone. The vascular compartment of most tissues is in the range of 3 to 10% of volume. Therefore, given equal tissue and blood-boron concentrations, 90 to 97% of tissue boron measurements would be extravascular.

All tissues appeared to lose boron at the same rate (Fig. 1). Tumor concentration varied markedly between animals. Variation was not as marked in multiple samples of the same tumor. Tumor to blood ratios generally varied in the range of 0.5 to 1.0 and remained constant while tumor to normal brain ratios varied in the range of 6 to 14 and decreased with time (Figure 1). The degree of contrast enhancement quantitated on computed tomography was directly related to the boron level detected in the tumor.[1]

Discussion

The pharmacokinetics of the BSH compound appear to be best described by the two-compartment model with the majority of the boron in the central compartment. This was especially true when sampling was confined to the 12 hour period post-boron administration. There did appear to be a tailing of the curve at later time periods indicating

480

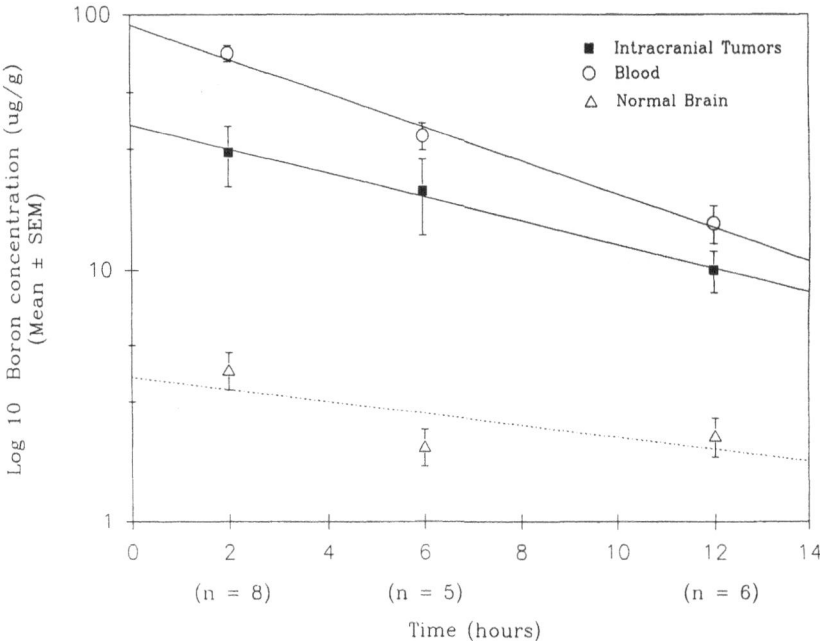

Fig. 1. Tissue boron concentration at 3 time
intervals post BSH administration

longer half-lives may be found at later periods. This was not
intensively investigated due to the low boron concentrations at those
times. The decision was made to concentrate on the earlier times with
higher blood-boron concentrations.

Higher blood-boron concentrations are needed for sufficient tumor
boron concentration. The tumors rarely had a higher boron concentration
than the blood. Boron concentration of the tumor tissue was of similar
magnitude as the skin and oral mucosa of the head. Peritumor brain
tissue had highly variable levels of boron, from the extremely low
normal brain boron concentrations to levels approaching that of the
blood. The normal tissues had remarkably constant boron concentrations
compared to the blood in all dogs studied. Therefore, it appears that
the macroscopic gross boron concentrations of the normal tissues can be
readily predicted from serum boron concentration. The ability to
predict the tissue concentration from serum measurement will be highly
useful in the clinical setting. It must be stressed that the boron
concentrations measured in this study are gross measurements.
Microscopic tissue and cellular distribution remain unknown. These
distributions could have a marked effect on the eventual outcome of
boron neutron capture therapy.

II. NORMAL TISSUE TOLERANCE STUDY

Materials and Methods

An initial dose range study placed 13 dogs in 5 dose groups from 0
to 60 Gy. These dogs were given 95% enriched ^{10}B BSH compound
intravenously at the dosage described previously (BSH dogs). Dogs were
irradiated with the epithermal beam from the BMRR reactor with a
projected mean blood-boron concentration of 50 µg/gm.[2]

A second group of 12 dogs was irradiated with the epithermal beam alone (EPI dogs). Two dogs served as sham irradiated controls. Five dogs were in the 10 Gy dosage group and 5 in the 15 Gy group. All radiation doses are described as the peak physical radiation dose.

Results

Acute Effects. Acute reactions were limited to the superficial tissues of the head. The initial reactions were moist desquamation, and epilation that peaked 3 to 4 weeks following irradiation. These changes occurred in dogs BSH receiving 27 Gy and higher. Only one animal receiving 27 Gy total peak physical dose developed significant moist desquamation. All EPI dogs (except controls) receiving only epithermal neutron radiations had considerable moist desquamation and epilation.

Three to four weeks following irradiation the areas of desquamation reepithelialized. In many of the dogs, the lesions continued to heal, leaving an area of partial epilation and a relatively normal, thin epithelial covering. In the two BSH dogs receiving 60 Gy and the five 15 Gy EPI dogs, the transient healing response was followed by dermal necrosis at approximately 12 weeks post-irradiation. Numerous surgical attempts to control the area of dermal necrosis failed in the two BSH dogs. The EPI dogs were euthanized following dermal necrosis by an overdose of intravenous barbiturates.

Late Effects. All animals remained neurologically normal for the first 4 months post-irradiation. In the BSH dogs, all dogs receiving total peak physical doses of 39 Gy or more had neurologic complications. These changes were seen at 18 to 22 weeks post-irradiation. The neurologic abnormality was initiated with a mild ataxia of the hind limbs followed by recumbency and inability to rise within 24 to 48 hours. This phase was accompanied by seizures that were not readily controlled with standard anticonvulsant therapy. The animals were given as thorough a workup as possible in the 24 to 48 hours following the onset of clinical signs and before euthanasia.

In the animals exhibiting neurologic abnormalities, magnetic resonance imaging revealed areas of contrast enhancement in the white matter of the cerebrum. This contrast enhancement was indicative of a break in the blood-brain barrier compatible with vascular necrosis. The changes were most prominent in the right side in the periventricular region but extended across midline to the left side. Post-mortem examination revealed areas of hemorrhage in the sites seen on magnetic resonance imaging and in additional areas as well. Histopathologic examination of these areas revealed a hemorrhagic necrosis compatible with vascular damage. These areas were associated with local demyelination.

Discussion

In the BSH dogs, dermal necrosis occurred at a dose significantly higher (60 Gy) than that associated with brain necrosis at a later time (39 Gy). Dogs irradiated with the epithermal neutron beam alone had dermal necrosis at a dose presumably lower (15 Gy) than that probably required for brain necrosis. The five dogs in the 15 Gy EPI group all had dermal necrosis; however, none of the dogs in the 10 Gy EPI group had brain changes similar to that seen in the BSH dogs. Subsequent experiments will add a dosage group between these two (12.5 Gy).

The doses reported are peak physical doses to blood. Peak dose in both cases is approximately 2 to 3 cm beneath the surface. The composition of the dose varies markedly between the two groups. The radiation consists of a mixture of neutron capture (boron in some dogs and nitrogen-hydrogen capture in all dogs) resulting in alpha particles, protons, and gamma photons. In addition, there are incident gamma photons and fast neutrons in the beam. The dogs containing 50 μg/gm boron in the blood would have 80% of the total peak physical dose associated with boron capture. The fast neutron dose at the peak would be proportionately smaller. In the EPI dogs, the fast neutron dose is proportionately larger in the absence of the boron capture dose. The resultant change in tissue tolerance obtained in these two groups at 50 and 0 μg/gm boron indicate the need for further studies to better define the normal tissue tolerance. Additional BSH dogs need to be done at levels above and below 50 μg/gm to better understand the change in tolerance with the change in the proportion of boron capture dose. Apparently, there is normal tissue sparing from the boron capture dose in normal brain and skin. In normal brain, geometric and other dosimetric considerations may spare the cerebral vasculature. The high boron tissue concentrations in normal skin suggest that the tissue or cellular distribution of the boron again results in a large sparing effect.

It was anticipated that the boron concentration in the normal brain would lead to reactions centered around the vasculature. Previous radiation studies of the brain with photons result in global irradiation to both the cerebral endothelium and glial cells. Considerable debate has arisen over the relative importance of these cellular types in the tolerance of the brain to radiation. The extremely low concentration of boron in the normal brain suggests that glial cells are spared from the boron capture dose. Therefore, this model yields an excellent way to separate vascular dose from glial dose. This lack of glial cell irradiation may have yielded a greater tolerance of the central nervous system tissues to neutron capture therapy.

III. SPONTANEOUS TUMOR DOG TREATMENT

The details of this portion are presented in detail in another paper.[3] Essentially nine dogs with spontaneous brain tumors underwent BNCT using the epithermal neutron beam at Brookhaven National Laboratory. The projected peak physical blood dose was 19 Gy with an anticipated boron concentration of 25 ppm following standard BSH administration.

DISCUSSION

It is interesting to note that two of the dogs treated with peak physical doses of as low as 20 Gy had delayed CNS change similar to that seen in the dose tolerance dogs at 27 Gy. The dose tolerance dogs had a mean blood-boron concentration of 50 ppm compared to the tumor dogs of 25 ppm. This is a further indication of a change in tolerance as the proportion of boron capture dose changes. This change in tolerance of the normal tissue in all of the tolerance dogs and treated dogs has been summarized (Fig. 2). Subsequent treatment dogs will be performed at higher blood-boron concentrations to document this difference.

OVERALL SUMMARY

An epithermal neutron beam will be needed to further the use of Boron Neutron Capture Therapy in human patients. This canine model

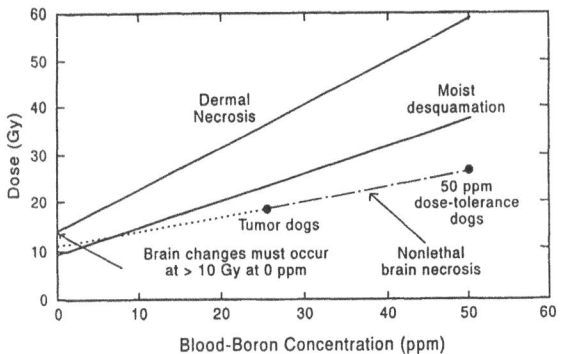

Fig. 2. Healthy tissue complications
in dogs vs blood-boron and dose

provided valuable information concerning the use of an epithermal beam and the readily available compound borocaptate sodium. Dosimetric models used to predict the dose rely on blood-boron concentration. Therefore, any other compounds screened in this model could derive boron concentrations for the blood in various tissues. Subsequent tissue tolerance data will be readily extrapolated to other compounds using a computational model.

Vascular sparing has been predicted previously. The direct relationship between normal tissue tolerance and blood-boron concentration verifies this occurrence. Change in blood-boron concentration and resultant tumor boron concentrations would indicate that the best time for brain tumor treatment would be early, following the distribution of the BSH compound. At an early time, one can maximize the tumor to normal brain concentration. Subsequent tumor treatments will utilize these facts in an attempt to verify this finding.

REFERENCES

1. S. L. Kraft, P. R. Gavin, C. E. DeHaan, C. W. Leathers, W. F. Bauer, and R. V. Dorn III, "The biodistribution of boron in canine spontaneous intracranial tumors following borocaptate sodium infusion," Abstract and Presentation, Fourth International Symposium on Neutron Capture Therapy for Cancer, Sydney, Australia, December 1990.

2. C. E. DeHaan, P. R. Gavin, S. L. Kraft, F. J. Wheeler, and C. A. Atkinson, "Acute and late reactions following epithermal-neutron irradiation of the normal canine brain," Abstract and Presentation, Fourth International Symposium on Neutron Capture Therapy for Cancer, Sydney, Australia, December 1990.

3. P. R. Gavin, C. E. DeHaan, S. L. Kraft, M. P. Moore, L. R. Wendling, and R. V. Dorn III, "Acute and late reactions following boron neutron capture epithermal-neutron therapy in dogs with spontaneous brain tumors," Abstract and Presentation, Fourth International Symposium on Neutron Capture Therapy for Cancer, Sydney, Australia, December 1990.

RADIOBIOLOGY STUDIES AT PETTEN: STATUS ON CELL CULTURE, MICE AND DOG

EXPERIMENTS

R. Huiskamp[1], A.C. Begg[2], V.G.A. Gregoire[2], R. Verrijk[2], D.Gabel[3], A.Siefert[4], and R.L. Moss[4]

[1]Radiobiology and Radioecology, Netherlands Energy Research
 Foundation ECN, Petten, The Netherlands.
[2]Department of Experimental Therapy, The Netherlands Cancer Institute,
 Amsterdam, The Netherlands.
[3]Department of Chemistry, University of Bremen, Germany.
[4]Commission of the European Communities, Joint Research Centre (JRC)
 Petten, The Netherlands.

INTRODUCTION

Boron neutron capture therapy (BNCT) with epithermal neutrons (1 eV to 10 keV) will achieve the necessary deep penetration for treating brain tumours. Epithermal neutrons will be moderated by the tissue mass between skin and tumour to produce the thermal neutrons necessary for the $^{10}B(n,\alpha)^7Li$ reaction in the target tissue. Beams of epithermal neutrons with sufficient fluence rate can be produced by filtration of spectrum fission neutrons obtained from the High Flux Reactor (HFR) of the Joint Research Centre (JRC) Petten, The Netherlands. During the Summer of 1990, an optimized neutron filter was installed in the HB-11 beam hole of the HFR for BNCT applications. Due to inevitable incomplete filtration, the beam will contain a fast neutron component, i.e. neutrons with energies $\geq$ 10 keV, and a γ-photon component originating from the reactor and produced in structural and filter materials.

In order to initiate a clinical trial with BNCT at Petten, an extensive programme of beam characterization, dosimetry and radiobiology is required. The physical characterization measurements of the HB-11 beam commenced in Autumn 1990. For the biological dosimetry and radiobiology, a programme has been designed which can be divided into two areas of interest: 1. preclinical "biological" characterization of the epithermal patient beam (HB-11), including normal tissue studies, and 2. biological studies to find and assess suitable boron compounds for BNCT, including measurement and mechanisms of therapeutic gain.

PRECLINICAL BIOLOGICAL CHARACTERIZATION OF HB-11

In vitro characterization

In order to verify and corroborate physical dosimetry and calculations of an epithermal neutron beam irradiating a realistic target, V79 Chinese hamster cells in suspension will be irradiated free-in-air and in a tissue-equivalent phantom in the presence of different amounts of boric acid and assayed for clonogenic survival. From a physical and mathematical point of view, a phantom with a rotational symmetry (cylinder or sphere) has been preferred. Cylinders are less ideal for dosimetry but small plastic vials containing cells in suspensions can be inserted more easily. Polyethylene cylinders, with or without a hemispherical end, have therefore been made by the University of Bremen, Germany, which will be filled with tissue-equivalent fluid. These phantoms are fitted with in depth adjustable crossed vial holder bars which will enable us to obtain the lateral dose distribution at different depths within the phantom.

Instrumentation for the phantom dosimetry will consist of activation foils (neutrons) and thermoluminescent dosemeters (γ-photons). The dimensions of these phantoms, i.e. 16.6 cm diameter; 23.0 cm length, are similar to those used for the characterization of the Brookhaven Medical Research Reactor (BMRR) beam. This would allow the direct comparison of an isotropic beam (BMRR) with an almost parallel beam (HB-11). With parallel beams, the thermal fluence at depth per incident neutron will increase whereas the maximum of thermal fluence will occur further down in the target.

The geometrical environment of cells (monolayer or suspension) is of considerable influence on the radiation response of cells after high linear energy transfer (LET) α-particle irradiation (Gabel et al, 1984). This will be investigated using a rapid multi-well survival assay using the DNA specific fluorescent dye Hoechst 33258 (Begg & Mooren, 1989).

In vivo characterization of HB-11

With respect to the treatment of patients with malignant glioma, preclinical studies on healthy tissue tolerance in dogs (Gavin et al., 1989) and the dose-depth profile of the BMRR epithermal beam in a phantom (Fairchild et al., 1990) have indicated that the tissue at risk is not the skin but normal brain. Healthy tissue tolerance will therefore be studied in dogs given different quantities of $Na_2B_{12}H_{11}SH$ (BSH) and irradiated with graded doses of epithermal neutrons form HB-11 (Table I). The biological endpoint in these studies will be non-lethal vascular damage to the central nervous system as measured by gadolinium-DTPA contrast enhanced magnetic resonance imaging (MRI) detectable brain lesions. MRI will be performed before irradiation and on days 1, 14, 180 and 360 post-irradiation or when neurological signs are observed. Besides MRI, other parameters will be investigated such as skin reactions, cellular blood count, blood chemistry, cerebrospinal fluid analysis, urine analysis and a total necropsy including histology will be performed at the end of the experiment. These studies will be performed in close collaboration with Washington State University (WSU), Idaho National Enginering Laboratory (INEL) and Brookhaven. The beam characteristics of HB-11 will be implemented in the INEL computer dosimetry system (Nigg et al., 1991) to estimate the expected normal tissue damage for HB-11. The modelling will be validated by the experiments described earlier.

In addition, split-dose studies will be carried out to evaluate the effect of low LET repair. The lower ^{10}B dose was chosen (Table I) because it likely that the first clinical trials will start off with low BSH concentration and fractionation. The interval between the two fractions will be 24 hrs since low LET repair is completed within 24 hrs. The second fraction will be given 3 hrs after the second BSH administration. The administered second BSH dose will depend on the blood level observed prior to the second fraction to get an the same peak blood level as with the first fraction. Special attention has to be given to the function of the blood brain barrier during these split-dose experiments.

TABLE I

Experimental setup for the healthy tissue tolerance studies in dogs

Single fraction		
peak ^{10}B dose (ppm)[*]	peak dose to blood (Gy; 3cm depth)[**]	number of dogs
25	15	5
	18	5
	23	5
50	24	5
	27	5
	30	5

Two fractions		
25	15	5
	18	5
	23	5

[*]Peak ^{10}B dose in blood measured with ICP-AES or prompt gamma.
[**]Total physical peak dose (Gy) to blood 3 cm below surface without modification by relative biological effectiveness (RBE) factors.

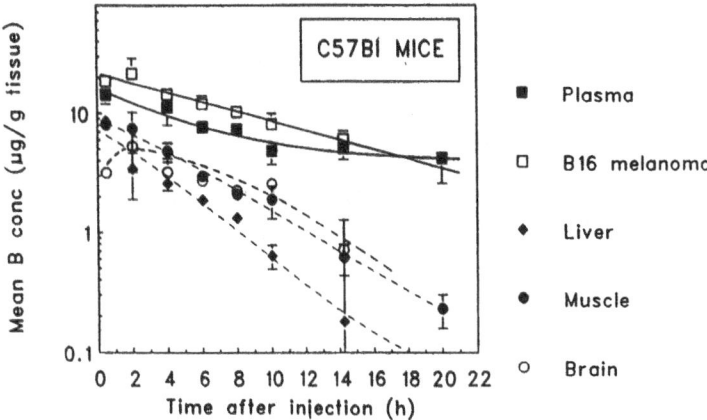

Biodistribution of L–BPA

Fig. 1. Biodistribution of L-BPA in C57Bl mice carrying s.c. the B16 melanoma. 12.5 μg B/g bw (257 μg/g bw) L-BPA was administered i.p. in 0.3 M fructose. Solid lines for plasma and tumour concentration (mean $\pm$ sem) are nonlinear least squares regression lines obtained with a pharmacokinetics programme (PCNONLIN). Dashed lines are graphical fits through the experimental points.

BIOLOGICAL STUDIES

In order to investigate the therapeutic gain of BNCT in experimental models, the uptake specificity of boronated compounds in different tumour types was studied. Pharmacokinetics and biodistribution studies were carried out in two murine tumour models in vivo. The compounds used in this investigation were two compounds considered for clinical use, BSH and L-BPA and boric acid as reference. The tumour models used were the B16 melanoma in C57Bl mice and the RIF-1 sarcoma model in C3H mice. The B16 model was chosen as a compound-related model and the RIF-1 model as a compound-unrelated model. The method of boron determination used for these studies was Inductively Coupled Atomic Emission Spectroscopy (ICP-AES). Sample preparation involved digestion of tissue with a mixture of HNO_3, $HClO_4$ and HF with a CEM MDS 81 D pressure controlled microwave system. Boron levels were measured with ICP-AES at the boron wave length 249.773 nm and corrected for Fe interference. As an example of these studies, the biodistribution of L-BPA in B16 carrying C57Bl mice is shown in Fig. 1. The B concentration in the tumour remained higher than the plasma concentration until 18 hrs after i.p. administration with a maximal tumour to plasma ratio of about 1.6 at 6 hrs after administration. However, plasma concentrations remained relatively high. A detailed description of these preliminary studies on pharmacokinetics of boronated compounds in the different tumour models will be reported by Gregoire et al. (This volume).

These studies will be extended using other modes of compound administration. Furtermore a more clinically relevant U87 glioma xenograft model will be used to investigate the preference of BSH or BPA for brain tumours. In addition, the pharmacokinetics and biodistribution of other boronated compounds such as BSSB, BTU and porphyrins will be investigated. The therapeutic gain of these compounds in these models will be studied using the thermal neutron beam of the Low Flux Reactor at Petten.

ACKNOWLEDGEMENTS

Part of this investigation was supported by the Netherlands Cancer Foundation (Koningin Wilhelmina Fonds, project NKI90-10). The work of the European Collaboration on Boron Neutron Capture Therapy is supported by the Commission of the European Communities.

REFERENCES

Begg, A.C. and Mooren, E., 1989, Rapid fluorescence-based assay for radiosensitivity and chemosensitivity testing in mammalian cells in vitro, Cancer Res. 49:565.

Gabel, D., Fairchild, R.G., Larsson, B. and Börner, H.G., 1984, The relative biological effectiveness in V79 Chinese Hamster cells of the neutron capture reactions in boron and nitrogen, Radiat. Res. 98:307.

Fairchild, R.G., Kalef-Ezra, J., Saraf, S.K, Fiarman, S., Ramsay, E., Wielpolski, L., Laster, B. and Wheeler, F., 1990, Installation and testing of an optimized epithermal neutron beam at Brookhaven Medical Research Reactor (BMRR), in: Neutron beam design, development, and performance for neutron capture therapy, Plenum Press, New York, in press.

Gavin, P.R., DeHaan, C.E., Kraft, S.L., Moore, M.P., Wheeler, F.J. and Miller, D.L., 1990, Dosimetric considerations: radiation tolerance of the normal canine brain following boron neutron capture, Abstract 38th Annual Meeting Radiation Research Society, New Orleans, April 7-12, 1990.

Gregoire, V.G.A., Huiskamp, R., Verrijk, R., and Begg, A.C., Comparative pharmacokinetics and distribution studies of boric acid, BPA and BSH in two murine tumour models, This volume.

Nigg, D.W., Randolph, P.D. and Wheeler, F.J., 1991, Demonstration of three-dimensional deterministic radiation transport theory dose distribution analysis for boron neutron capture therapy, Med. Phys. 18:43

THE BIODISTRIBUTION OF BORON IN NORMAL CANINE TISSUES FOLLOWING BOROCAPTATE SODIUM ADMINISTRATION AND THE EFFECT OF PLASMA EXCHANGE

S. L. Kraft, P. R. Gavin, C. E. DeHaan,[1] W. F. Bauer,[2] and T. E. Ary[3]

[1]College of Veterinary Medicine and Surgery, Washington State University, Pullman, WA   99164-6610
[2]INEL/BNCT Research Program, Idaho National Engineering Laboratory, Idaho Falls, ID   83415-3519
[3]Present Address: North Dakota State University, Fargo, ND

INTRODUCTION

Normal tissue tolerance establishes the dose limitations for any form of radiation therapy. The complexity of the mixed form of radiation from Boron Neutron Capture Therapy (BNCT) makes it difficult to predict normal tissue tolerance. A premise for BNCT is that the ideal boron compound should result in minimal boron concentrations in normal tissues and blood and high concentrations in tumor tissue.[1]

Borocaptate sodium ($Na_2B_{12}H_{11}SH$ or BSH) was administered to a set of dogs with naturally-occurring, intracranial tumors to evaluate the relative boron distribution in neoplastic and normal tissue. Data on the biodistribution of boron to these normal tissues is presented here in context of normal tissue tolerance. Since boron from BSH binds significantly to plasma proteins, plasma exchange following BSH infusion in a set of normal laboratory dogs was performed to evaluate the effect on blood and tissue concentrations as a potential means to increase normal tissue tolerance.

MATERIALS AND METHODS

Twenty-seven (27) dogs with naturally-occurring, intracranial lesions (ages ranging from 3 to 13, either sex, multiple breeds) were administered BSH intravenously at a natural isotopic ratio[1] at 55 mg boron/kg body weight (1 mg/kg-min^{-1}). The natural isotopic ratio was used to simulate the distribution of the more expensive, 95% ^{10}B-enriched compound. Serial blood and urine samples were obtained during and after infusion. Euthanasia was performed 2, 6, or 12 hours after end of infusion. At necropsy, samples of normal tissues were obtained, in addition to tumor and peritumor tissues.

For plasma exchange studies, 20 normal Beagle dogs (aged 2-5 years, either sex) were divided into experimental groups (Table I). BSH was administered intravenously at 33 mg boron/kg body weight. Plasma

---

[1] Callery Chemical Company, Pittsburgh, PA

[2] Autopheresis-C, Fenwal Division, Baxter Healthcare Corporation, Deerfield, IL

Table I. Experimental Groups Receiving Plasma Exchange[a]

| | Exchange at 6 Hrs Post-BSH | | Exchange at 6 Hrs Post-BSH with a 6-Hr Delay | |
	Controls (n=6)	Plasma, Boron Free (n=6)	Controls (n=3)	Plasma, Boron Free (n=5)
% Reduction Bld Boron Concentration	-1.75 (5.1)	-31.5 (7.1)	8.0 (7.8)	-23.9 (3.7)
Mean TBR[b] Cerebral Cortex	0.09 (0.04)	0.12 (0.04)	0.05 (0.01)	0.16 (0.04)
Mean TBR[b] Pituitary	0.74 (0.09)	0.81 (0.22)	1.33 (0.46)	0.99 (0.42)
Mean TBR[b] Liver	2.65 (0.32)	3.27 (0.56)	2.22 (0.19)	2.92 (0.32)
Mean TBR[b] Kidneys	1.36 (0.09)	1.65 (0.31)	1.68 (0.20)	1.56 (0.21)
Mean TBR[b] Scalp	1.07 (0.16)	1.28 (0.17)	1.25 (0.25)	1.30 (0.2)

[a] All values reported as mean (standard error of the mean).
[b] TBR = tissue to blood-boron concentration ratio

extraction (40 mls/kg body weight) was performed six hours later with an automated donor plasmapheresis unit.[2] Previously banked (boron-free) plasma was simultaneously infused at the same rate as plasma extraction. The (boronated) plasma being extracted was immediately returned at a similar rate in control dogs. Additional studies exchanging plasma at an earlier postinfusion time period and studies exchanging plasma with physiologic saline have been performed, but results are not yet available and are not reported here. Serial blood (for serum) and urine samples were obtained during and after BSH infusion and during plasma exchange. Euthanasia was performed at the end of plasma exchange with the exception of one set of dogs, where a six-hour postexchange delay was used to evaluate for a possible lag effect on tissue boron concentrations. Samples of normal tissues were obtained. Boron analysis of fluid and tissue samples was performed with inductively coupled plasma-atomic emission spectroscopy (ICP-AES).

RESULTS

Normal Tissue Concentrations in Dogs with Intracranial Lesions: Mean blood-boron concentrations were higher than the boron concentration of any tissue of the head (Figure 1). Skin had boron concentrations of similar magnitude to blood. Pituitary had mean boron concentrations of similar magnitude to mean tumor-boron concentrations. Normal brain consistently had the lowest mean boron concentrations. Liver, lung, and kidney mean boron concentrations exceeded that of blood (Figure 2).

Normal Laboratory Dogs Receiving Plasma Exchange: Blood-boron concentration declined rapidly in correspondence with plasma exchange (Table I). Blood-boron concentrations were reduced by approximately 25% relative to predicted (nonexchange) levels. Mean TBRs were similar for control and experimental groups (Table I).

DISCUSSION

Normal tissue-boron concentrations and TBRs are useful in under-standing observed tissue reactions in BNCT radiation tolerance studies. Measured blood concentrations are used in conjunction with derived TBRs to estimate physical tissue doses. Normal tissue boron concentration is

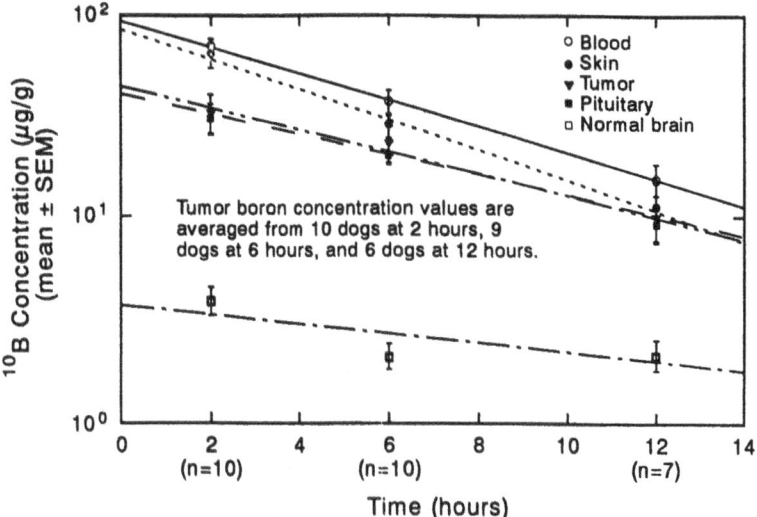

Figure 1. Boron concentrations in blood and selected tissues of the head in dogs with intracranial tumors at 2, 6, and 12 hours following BSH infusion.

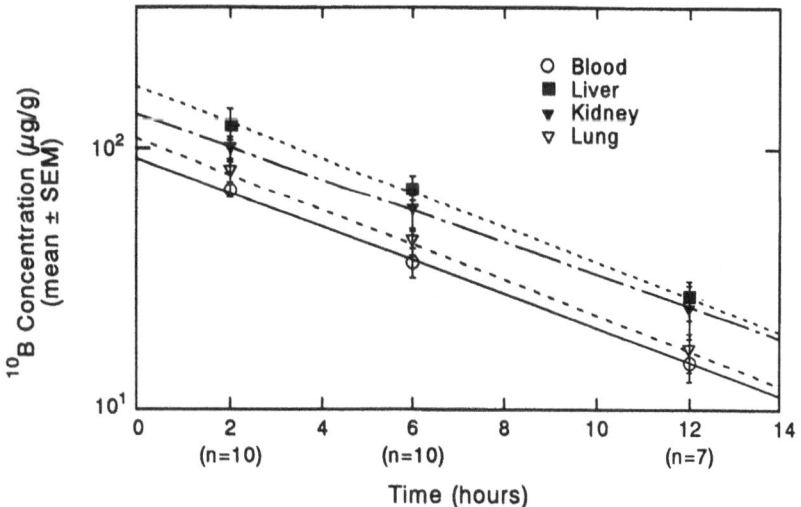

Figure 2. Boron concentrations in blood and selected systemic tissues in dogs with intracranial tumors at 2, 6, and 12 hours following BSH infusion.

crucial to BNCT tolerance, but this issue is complex. The macroscopic (intravascular vs extracellular) and microscopic distribution of ^{10}B critically determines radiation dose to parenchymal cells and, ultimately, tissue tolerance.[2] The low boron concentration of normal brain is compatible with confinement of boron with the intravascular space because of the blood-brain-barrier made up by vascular endothelium. This nonuniform distribution of boron within normal brain should lead to a dose-sparing effect of brain parenchyma. The low boron concentration of tissues, such as muscle and bone, likewise suggest little extravascular leakage of boron and a similar sparing effect may be expected.

In contrast, high boron concentrations in skin, pituitary, liver, lung, and kidney indicate the presence of extravascular boron. Upon initial evaluation, adverse radiation effects might be anticipated in such tissues within the primary beam. However, empirical results from animal tolerance studies and human BNCT trials show high tolerance of tissues of the head.[3,4] This leads to the supposition that microscopic nonuniformity in boron distribution may exist for many of these tissues with high boron concentration, leading to a high degree of dose sparing.

Blood-boron concentration will ultimately determine normal brain tolerance through effects on brain vascular endothelium. Blood-boron levels were high relative to tissues and tumor. A substantial decrease in blood-boron concentration was caused by single volume plasma exchange in the normal laboratory dogs, but the lack of substantial difference in mean TBRs between experimental groups suggests that extraction of blood boron was paralleled by a similar loss at the tissue level. In tumor-bearing dogs, mean tumor-boron concentrations declined at a rate similar to normal tissue and blood-boron concentrations, suggesting the absence of significant binding of boron to tumor tissue. Therefore, decline in tumor-boron concentration would be expected if plasma exchange were performed using banked (boron-free) plasma. However, plasma extraction could provide a significant therapeutic gain by allowing an increase in total administered dose, if tumor boron could be spared. Possibly, the use of saline as the infusate may lessen the extraction of boron from tissues, and may produce more selective reduction in blood boron while sparing tumor-boron concentration.

REFERENCES

1. Barth, R. F., A. H. Soloway, and R. G. Fairchild, "Boron Neutron Capture Therapy of Cancer," Cancer Research 50: 1061-1070 (1990).

2. Gabel, D., S. Foster, and R. G. Fairchild, "The Monte Carlo Simulation of the Biological Effect of the $^{10}B(n,\alpha)^{7}Li$ Reaction in Cells and Tissue and Its Implication for Boron Neutron Capture Therapy," Radiation Research 111: 14-25 (1987).

3. Goodman, J. H., J. M. McGregor, N. R. Clendenon, R. A. Gahbauer, R. F. Barth, A. H. Soloway, and R. G. Fairchild, "Ultrastructural Microvascular Response to Boron Neutron Capture Therapy in an Experimental Model," Neurosurg. 24: 701-708 (1989).

4. Hatanaka, H. and Y. Urano, "Eighteen Autopsy Cases of Malignant Brain Tumors Treated by Boron Neutron Capture Therapy Between 1968 and 1985," in BNCT for Tumors (H. Hatanaka, ed) Nishimura Co. Ltd., Japan, 381-417 (1986).

COPYRIGHT

DISTRIBUTION OF A BORONATED PORPHYRIN (BTPP) IN OSTEOSARCOMA BEARING NUDE MICE

Akira Takeuchi, N.Ojima, T.Kadosawa

Dept. of Veterinary Surgery, Faculty of Agriculture, Univ. of Tokyo, Tokyo

H. Hatanaka

Dept. of Neurosurgery, Teikyo University, Tokyo, Japan

Introduction

Osteosarcoma is known as one of the malignant tumor which is highly resistant to the ordinary irradiation therapy, and amputation of the affected limb at an early stage has been a treatment of choice for long years. Our final goal in this study is to find out a possibility to treat the osteosarcoma conserving the affected limb by irradiating high dose to the tumor specifically using the characteristics of boron-neutron capture thetapy (BNCT). For the success of this study, the development of the boron carrier with specific affinity to tumor or osteosarcoma is essential. In this paper, a recently developed boronated derivative, boronotetraphenylporphyrin (BTPP)[1] was studied for its distribution in osteosarcoma bearing nude mice by means of whole body alfa-track autoradiography[2]

Materials and Methods

Osteosarcoma bearing nude mice was produced by subcutaneus injection of cultured cells of canine osteosarcoma (5×10^6 cells) in female BALB/C nude mice, 7 to 10 weeks of age. The tumor has developed at the site of injection very rapidly and uniformly, and reached the size as large as approximately 2cm in diameter 8 weeks after inoculation.

Alfa-track autoradiography was studied by sacrificing the osteosarcoma bearing nude mice (8 weeks after inoculation) 6, 24, 48, and 72 hours after 100 mg/kg BW (25 mg Boron/kg) of BTPP was administered. The whole body was frozen in aceton with dry ice, and the sagital section 40 μ m as thick was prepared by cryomicrotome and was mounted on cellulose nitrate films (CN 85 KODAK). Following these preparation processes, approximately 10^{13} n/cm^2 of the thermal neutron was irradiated and was treated with etching with 10% NaOH for 3 min. at 60°C. By means of microscopic counting of thus produced alfa-tracks, the boron concentrations of tumor and other tissues were calculated using the calibration curve between number of alfa-tracks and boron concentration.

Table 1 BORON CONCENTRATION FOLLOWING I. P.
ADMINISTRATION OF BTPP.

Tissue	6hours	24hours	48hours	72hours
Tumor	42±26	63±29	92±36	11±12
Blood	138±21	119±24	86±20	16±9
Skin	63±34	83±24	92±10	16±13
Bone Marrow	118±29	106±25	136±30	15±10
Bone	18±10	19±9	20±7	3±3
Muscle	6±5	15±11	26±12	-2±1

(μg Boron/cm^3 Tissue)

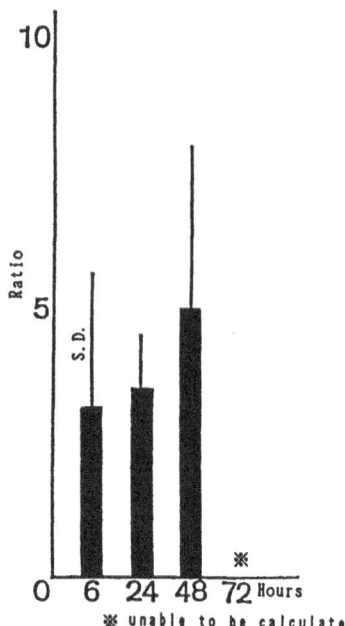

※ unable to be calculated

Fig. 1 TUMOR:BONE RATIOS
OF BORON CONCENTRATION

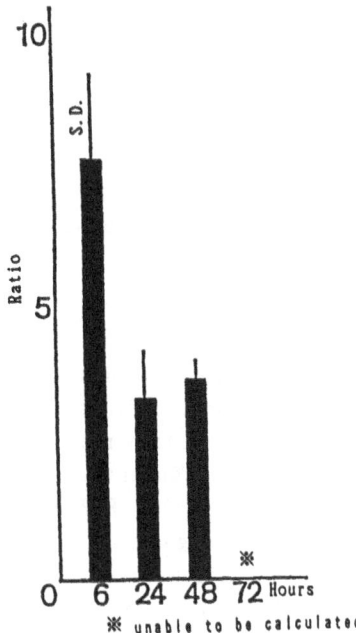

Fig. 2   TUMOR:MUSCLE RATIOS
         OF BORON CONCENTRATION

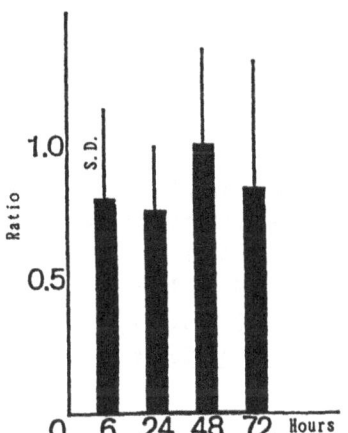

Fig. 3   TUMOR:SKIN RATIOS
         OF BORON CONCENTRATION

Results

The boron concentration in the tumor, the blood, the skin, the bone marrow, the bone and the muscle 6, 24, 48, and 72 hours after administration of BTPP respectively are summarized in Table 1. The peak value, as high as 92 μ g/cm^3 was gained in the tumor 48 hours after BTPP administration, however, boron concentration in the blood, the skin, and the bone marrow were also high as well. While, boron concentration in the bone and muscle are extensively low and kept less than 26 μ g/cm^3 throughout the experiment period.

The tumor:blood, tumor:skin, tumor:bone marrow, tumor:bone, and tumor:muscle ratios were also studied (Fig. 1, 2, 3). Although tumor:blood, tumor:skin, and tumor:bone marrow ratios were not significantly high, tumor:bone and tumor:muscle ratios were as high as 5 at 48 hours after administration of BTPP.

Discussion and Conclusion

It became clear that the significantly high boron concentration in osteosarcoma was able to be obtained by the intraperitoneal administration of BTPP in the nude mice. It was also clarified that boron concentration in normal bone and muscle is considerably low instead of high concentration in blood and skin. This may suggest us to be a big advantage for BTPP to be used as a boron carrier for BNCT of osteosarcoma, since, in general, many osteosarcomas of the limb are surrounded by bone and muscle, which have to be irradiated by thermal neutron at the time of BNCT. Therefore, if only the skin covering the tumor is peeled off, it might be possible to give the significantly high dose of irradiation specifically to osteosarcoma by BNCT whithout giving serious damages to the normal bone and muscle close to tumor.

Meanwhile, in order to consider the clinical use of BTPP in BNCT of osteosarcoma, the study on toxicity of BTPP is essential. The purpose of this paper is only to know the specific distribution of BTPP, and a certain dosage was selected to be used without major concern to its toxicity. If certain dose of BTPP with high concentration in the tumor with less toxicity can be established, then BTPP could be used in successful BNCT for osteosarcoma.

References

1) S. B. Kahl, D. D. Joel, M. M. Nawrocky, P. L. Micca, K. P. Tran, G. C. Finkel, and D. N. Slatkin, 1990, Uptake of a nide-carboranylporphyrin by human glioma xenografts in athymic nude mice and by syngeneic ovarian carcinomas in immunocompetent mice, Proc. Natl. Acad. Sci., 87 : 7265 - 7269.
2) O. Matsuoka, H. Hatanaka, and M. Miyamoto, 1977, Neutron capture whole body autoradiography of [10]B compounds, Acta Pharmacol. Toxicol., 41 : 56.

FEASIBILITY STUDY OF BORON NEUTRON CAPTURE THERAPY FOR INOPERABLE LIVER CANCERS

D. Chiaraviglio[1], A. Zonta[1], G. Rescigno[1], C. Cuzzoni[1], L. Calamita[1], A. Clerici[1], T. Pinelli[2], F. Fossati[2], S. Altieri[2], A. Perotti[3], C. Minoia[4], E. Capelli[5], H. Rief[6], R. Ricchenna[6], G. Bottiroli[7], A.C. Croce[7]

[1]   Dept Surgery, University of Pavia, P. Botta 10, 27100 Pavia, Italy.
[2]   Dept Nuclear Theoretical Physics and INFN, Univ Pavia
[3]   Dept General Chemistry, University of Pavia
[4]   Lab Industrial Hygiene, Foundation 'Clinica del Lavoro', Pavia
[5]   Dept Genetics & Microbiology University of Pavia
[6]   JRC Ispra, Commission European Communities
[7]   Centre for Study of Histochemistry, CNR, Pavia

AIM AND NATURE OF THE PROJECT

Presently only about 6% of liver cancers are curable, namely those most delimited and surgically resectable. The aim of our project is to investigate the possibility of curing patients with unresectable liver-only cancers, either primary or secondary to a resectable primary malignancy, consisting mainly of hepatocellular carcinoma and liver metastases from colonic carcinoma. The curability of liver cancers would increase by nearly 30% (1,2) and in Italy about 3400 patients per year could be saved (3). To reach this goal a specifically targeted treatment on both organ and neoplastic tissue should be realized. In fact conventional therapies (systemic chemotherapy, external radiotherapy) are only palliative, because of their hepatic or systemic toxicity. Also more selective approaches, through a loco-regional or tumour focused application (e.g. intra-arterial chemotherapy, radioimmunotherapy), still give poor results because they lack one of the two required selectivities (1,2). Besides, the liver is not removable or artificially replacable and cancer contraindicates liver transplantation (4,5).

In order to obtain a double selectivity of treatment the approach of autotransplantation and extracorporeal treatment, already proposed for bone marrow malignacies is being applied to the liver. The autotransplantation technique has been perfected on pigs; a pig was shown to survive without liver up to 10 hours (6). Some powerful therapies, normally excluded from in vivo application, could therefore be used. Among these BNCT was chosen as the best candidate and a BNCT project started in Pavia, where a suitable nuclear reactor is available.

BNCT developed mainly as a therapy for glioblastoma (7), chosen because the blood brain barrier could offer an anatomical base to obtain a favorable tumour/normal tissue boron concentration (T/N) ratio, at a time when tumour seeking compounds were not known. With the development of new tumour seekers, BNCT can be proposed for other targets.

Our first goal is therefore to investigate through pharmacokinetic screening, a tumour seeker suitable for liver cancers for a new application of BNCT. We first fulfilled the requirements of materials and methods for the screening by organizing two experimental oncology units for research with _in vivo_ and _in vitro_ models. The first experimental phase is now in progress, with the fol wing aims: to study and perfect materials and methods; to achieve in our

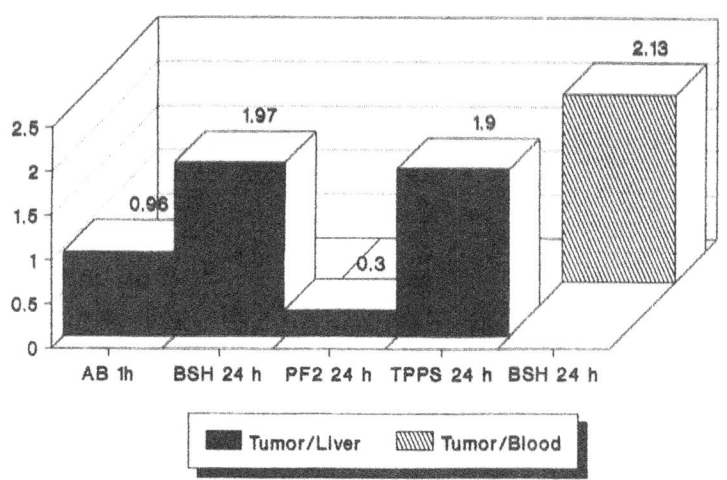

UPTAKE RATIO OF BORON COMPOUNDS
Walker carcinoma vs healthy tissues

Univ Pavia - Dpt Surgery - BNCT 90

Fig. 1

models pharmaceutical reference values of the most used compounds; to verify the reported capacity of some compounds to give a favourable boron tumour uptake versus both liver and blood. Our work will proceed with a second experimental phase of screening and a more detailed study of some compounds. We report here the results obtained with sodium borocaptate (BSH), the most used BNCT agent and tetraphenyl porphyrin sulfonate (TPPS), for which a positive tumor/liver distribution ratio is reported. These findings are compared with results obtained with boric acid, a simple boron compound and photofrin II, a widely used photodynamic agent, as reference compounds respectively for BSH and TPPS.

MATERIALS AND METHODS

Compounds

Na MERCAPTOUNDECAHYDRODODECABORATE - BSH (Callery/Centronics)
TETRAPHENYLPORPHINE SULFONATE - TPPS; (Porphyrin Products) BORIC ACID -
(Carlo Erba); PHOTOFRIN II - PF2 (QLT Phototherapeutics)

Experimental models

(i)   WALKER CARCINOMA 256 - Solid tumour implanted subcutaneously (tumour)
or in the liver (metastasis) in Sprague-Dawley outbred male rats of about 200
g, housed and fed conventionally (Charles River Italia), kindly provided by
Istituto M.Negri, Milano.

(ii)   LOVO - Human colonic carcinoma line, cultured in monolayer in Ham's
F12 + 10% FBS, kindly provided by Istituto Tumori, Milano.

(iii) CHANG - Human hepatocyte line, cultured in monolayer in Ham's F12 +
10% FBS (Istituto Zooprofilattico, Brescia).

(iv)   HEPG2 - Human hepatoma line, cultured in monolayer in RPMI + 10% FBS,
kindly provided by Ist Patologia Generale, Univ of Genova.

Compound determination

BORON ANALYSIS - ICP-AES at the wavelength of 249.67 nm (ICP 5000 Perkin
Elmer). Sample solubilization by wet digestion with perchloric and nitric
acid, in microwave furnace (CEM MDS-81D, Barletta Apparecchi Scientifici).
PORPHYRINS - Microspectrofluorimetry on frozen tissue sections.
Excitation=405 nm (HBO 100W lamp); spectra detection by microspectrograph
(Leitz) with optical multichannel analyzer (OMA Mod 1460) mounting an
intensified diode array detector (EG&G). Fluorescence intensity evaluated as
integrated area of selected emission bands: 630 ± 10 nm (Photofrin II), 665 ±
10 nm (TPPS).

EXPERIMENTAL RESULTS

Cytotoxicity

Boric acid and BSH were tested for cytotoxicity on Lovo, Chang and HepG2
lines, with various tests: proliferation inhibition, plating efficiency
inhibition, DNA synthesis inhibition (^{3}H Thymidine uptake), mitotic index. The
treatment for 2 hours at doses ranging from 10 to 200 µg B/ml medium shows a
dose-dependent effect. At useful doses for BNCT (between 10 and 100 µg/ml)
none of the three compounds showed significant toxic effects.

Distribution

Boric acid - 6 rats with Walker tumour, treated with 50 mg B/kg, body
weight, ip, sacrificed at 1 h (n=2), 3 h (n=2) and 5 h (n=2). Samples:
tumour, liver. Maximum boron uptake in tissues was seen at 1 h, with values
around 35 ppm. The T/N ratio was always around 1.

BSH - 4 rats with Walker metastasis, treated with 30 mg B/kg, body
weight, ip, sacrificed at 24 h (n=2) and at 48 h (n=2). Samples: tumour,
liver, blood. Maximum uptake was seen in the tumour at 24 h, with absolute
values below 10 ppm. The T/N ratio had decreased from a value around 2 at 24
h to a value below 1 at 48 h.

PF2 - 5 rats with Walker tumour, treated with 3 mg/kg, body weight, ip,
sacrificed at 24 h. Samples: tumour, liver.

TPPS - 3 rats with Walker tumour, treated with 3 mg/kg, body weight, ip, sacrificed at 24 h. Samples: tumor, liver. Fluorescence intensity shows a T/N ratio equal to 0.3 for PF2, while for TPPS this ratio is near 2.

DISCUSSION (Fig. 1)

Both TPPS and BSH show a tendency to localize preferentially in tumor tissue, as opposed to healthy liver tissue. This tendency is not manifest in the behaviour shown by the two reference compounds, PF2 and boric acid. These results are preliminary, but confirm our expectations that these two compounds, already suggested as tumor localizers in relation to other healthy reference tissues, can have a similar role also in relation to the liver. Taking into account the specific property of the liver in that it has a particular tendency to accumulate circulating compounds, we are encouraged by these data to continue the research in this same direction in more detail.

AKNOWLEDGEMENTS

The study is performed with the support of the European Collaboration for BNCT, Commission of the European Communities, 4th Medical and Health Research Project.

REFERENCES

1   De Vita V.T., Hellman S., Rosenberg S.A. (eds). Principles and practice of oncology. Philadelphia 1985, Lippincott.

2   Schiff L. and Schiff Er (eds). Diseases of the liver. Philadelphia 1982, Lippincott.

3   Zanetti R. and Rosso S. Incidenza dei tumori in Italia. Federazione Medica 1990,43:119-124.

4   Scharschmidt B.F. Human liver transplantation: analysis of data on 540 patients from four centers. Hepatology 1984,4:95s-101s.

5   Starzl T.E., Iwatsuki S., Shaw B.W.. Analysis of liver transplantation. Hepatology 1984;4:47s-49s.

6   Zonta A., Dionigi P., Del Ciotto N., Chiaraviglio D., Alessiani M., Bellinzona G., Ferrari C., Tibaldeschi C. Impiego sperimentale di un nuovo tipo di protesi vascolare in corso di autotrapianto ortotopico di fegato. Il Giornale di Chirurgia 1986;7:1631-1633.

7   Hatanaka H. and Sweet W.H. Slow-neutron capture therapy for malignant tumours. Its history and recent development. Vienna 1975, International Atomic Energy Agency. IAEA-SM-193/79.

TUMOUR LOCALIZATION OF BORONATED PORPHYRINS IN AN INTRACEREBRAL MODEL OF GLIOMA

J.S. Hill[1], S.B. Kahl[2], A.H. Kaye[1], M.F. Gonzales[1], N.J. Vardaxis[3], C.I. Johnson[4], S.S. Stylli[1], and Y. Nakamura[1]

1   Higginbotham Neuroscience Research Institute, Department of Surgery (Royal Melbourne Hospital), University of Melbourne, Parkville, 3052, Australia
2   Department of Pharmaceutical Chemistry, University of California, San Francisco, 94143-0446, California, U.S.A.
3   Department of Applied Science, Phillip Institute of Technology, Bundoora, 3083, Australia
4   Biorad Pty Ltd., Hawthorn, 3122, Australia

INTRODUCTION

Treatment of the most common cerebral tumour, cerebral glioma, is unsatisfactory as the tumour recurs due to inadequate local control (1). Photodynamic therapy (PDT) and Boron Neutron Capture Therapy (BNCT) offer some promise as adjuvant treatments for cerebral glioma. Several clinical trials have been reported utilizing PDT (for review see reference 1) and BNCT (2) to treat the high grade glioma, glioblastoma multiforme. We have investigated the pharmacokinetic tissue distribution of the photosensitizer Haematoporphyrin derivative (HpD), the nido carboranyl porphyrin, boron tetraphenyl porphine (BTPP) and the closo carboranyl monomeric protoporphyrin (BOPP) in CBA mice bearing the intracerebral C6 glioma xenograft (3).

MATERIALS AND METHODS

Intracerebral glioma xenograft: Adult CBA mice were injected with C6 glioma cells harvested from monolayer culture during the logarithmic phase of growth.   Each mouse was injected with 10 μl of a suspension of 1×10^6 cells suspended in RPMI 1640(2x) media containing 0.5% sea-plaque agarose as previously described (3).

Synthesis of sensitizers: HpD was synthesised and prepared for administration as previously described (1).   BTPP and BOPP were prepared as described previously (4,5) and suspended in sterile isotonic saline prior to administration.

Administration of sensitizers: Stock solutions of HpD, BTPP and BOPP were prepared in isotonic saline at a concentration of 5 mg/ml prior to either intraperitoneal (IP) or intravenous (IV) tail vein administration into tumour bearing CBA mice.   To study the kinetics of uptake, mice were injected with sensitizer at the appropriate time points such that all were sacrificed exactly 14 days post-implantation of tumour. To study the dose dependence of uptake, mice were injected with the appropriate dose of sensitizer 13 days post-implantation of tumour, and sacrificed 24 hours later.

Measurement of uptake: The uptake of HpD into tumour, normal brain and venous blood was determined as previously described (6). The uptake of BTPP and BOPP was determined using an adaption of this method (7), with the fluorescence emission of BOPP monitored at 625 nm and of BTPP at 657 nm.

Confocal laser scanning microscopy (CLSM): The sub-cellular distribution of the sensitizers in cells <u>in vitro</u> and tumours <u>in vivo</u> was determined by CLSM using a Biorad MRC500 or MRC 600 confocal microscope with an Argon ion laser excitation source. The excitation wavelengths were 488 nm and 514 nm and the emission was monitored above 600 nm.

RESULTS

Sensitizer pharmacokinetics: The uptake kinetics of BOPP following IP and IV doses of either 10 mg/kg body weight or 100 mg/kg body weight are shown in Fig 1. The BOPP levels in the tumour, normal brain and blood were determined by fluorescence assay following extraction from the tissue. This assay detects the porphyrin component of the carborane-porphyrin conjugate. Previous studies have demonstrated the <u>in vivo</u> stability of the bonds between the carborane cages and the porphyrin ring (8). Thus, since these molecules are approximately 30% Boron by weight, an estimate of the total Boron present in tissue can be made by measurement of total porphyrin content.

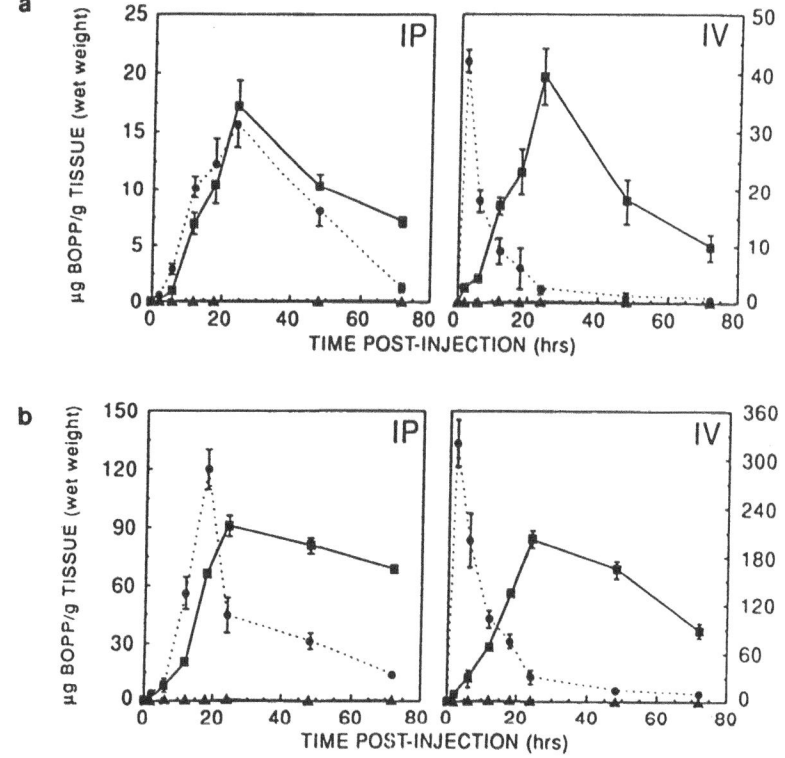

Figure 1. Kinetics of BOPP uptake following (a) 10 mg/kg or (b) 100 mg/kg body weight injection via IP or IV tail vein routes.
Tumour (—■—)   Normal brain (—▲—)   Venous blood (···●···)

502

It is apparent that BOPP is a highly selective tumour localizing agent when administered by either IP or IV route. Maximal tumour concentrations were observed at 24 hours at either low (10 mg/kg body weight, or high doses (100 mg/kg body weight). However, the uptake kinetics into blood were dependent on the route of administration. Maximum levels were detected 2 hours post IV injection for both low and high doses, whereas for IP injection maximum levels were noted at 24 and 18 hours post-administration for the low and high doses respectively. The rates of clearance from blood were also dependent on the route of administration with much more rapid clearance following IV injection. Tumour levels remained relatively high throughout the experimental time course following high dose injection by either route, indicating the retention of BOPP in the tumour, even though blood levels fell substantially. The tumour:normal brain and tumour:blood ratios for the data in Figure 1 are shown in Table 1. It is clear that BOPP is a highly selective tumour sensitizer. Ratios as high as 400:1 in tumour compared to normal brain were obtained 48 hours post IV injection of 100 mg BOPP/kg body weight, whilst at the same time point the tumour:blood ratio is 11:1. The tumour:normal brain ratios 24 hours post IV administration of BTPP and HpD which are also shown in the footnote to Table 1 demonstrate that BOPP exhibits more selective tumour localising properties than these compounds. BOPP was also far less toxic than BTPP when administered by single bolus injection, with doses of 200 mg BOPP/kg being tolerated with no death of animals. It was not possible to exceed a dose of 25 mg BTPP/kg due to death of a significant proportion of mice. The cause of this toxicity is as yet unknown.

Table 1.   Tumour:Normal Brain and Tumour:Blood Ratios following
            IP and IV administration of BOPP

| Time post-admin (hours) | 10 mg/kg | | | | 100 mg/kg | | | |
| | IP | | IV | | IP | | IV | |
	T:NB[a]	T:BL[b]	T:NB	T:BL	T:NB	T:BL	T:NB	T:BL
2	11[c]	0.21	138	0.12	16	0.15	43	0.05
6	47	0.32	64	0.25	51	1.1	31	0.15
12	87	0.68	124	1.8	74	0.36	40	0.67
18	116	0.85	124	3.7	158	0.55	113	1.8
24	157	1.1	136	15	203	2.0	238	6.5
48	114	1.3	203	15	253	2.6	402	11
72	90	5.9	253	14	215	4.9	287	9.7

a   Tumour:Normal brain ratio.
b   Tumour:Blood ratio.
c   All figures were calculated as the ratio of mean levels shown in Fig. 1.
     T:NB ratio 24 hours post IV dose of 20 mg/kg BTPP=180:1.
     T:NB ratio 24 hours post IV dose of 20 mg/kg HpD=50:1.

The dose dependence of BOPP uptake 24 hours post IP and IV administration was also studied (data not shown). In summary, these data showed that at doses greater that 100 mg/kg the tumour:brain and tumour:blood ratios decreased markedly suggesting that the circulating blood plasma levels of BOPP were so high that the apparent tumour selectivity was decreased. However, examination of these ratios at longer time points shows subsequent increases reflecting clearance of BOPP from plasma.

Sub-Cellular localisation: The *in vitro* sub-cellular distribution of these porphyrins in the human glioma cell line U251MG was determined using CLSM. None of the porphyrins were found in the nucleus although HpD, which is a mixture of oligomeric and monomeric porphyrins, was found to localise in both the cytoplasm and discretely into organelles in the perinuclear region, whereas BOPP localised almost exclusively in the same organelles and not the cytoplasm. BTPP localised in a similar manner to BOPP, and was also present in the nuclear membrane, but not within the nucleus itself. The *in vivo* distribution of BOPP and HpD were also determined in cryosections of the C6 tumour grown in CBA mice and confirm the results obtained *in vitro*. These results also show that in addition to selective localisation in the bulk of the tumour, BOPP was also selectively localised in isolated tumour cells infiltrating into the surrounding oedematous brain (Fig. 2). Density gradient ultracentrifugation studies showed that the sub-cellular organelles into which BOPP localised were mitochondria.

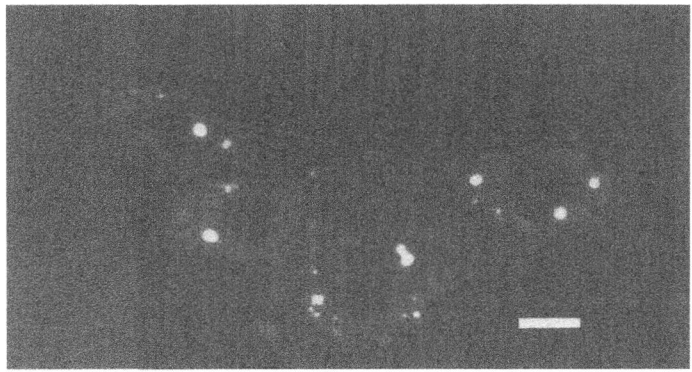

Figure 2.   CLSM image of BOPP in isolated nests of tumour cells invading into normal brain.   Bar = 5 μm.

CONCLUSIONS

The results presented in this study show that BOPP is a highly selective tumour localising agent. Since BOPP is 30% Boron by weight, then a BOPP concentration in tumour greater than 65 μg/g would result in Boron levels above the clinically suggested 20 μg/g threshold. The data in Fig. 1 show that 24 hours after a dose of 100 mg BOPP/kg body weight these levels are reached, with correspondingly low levels in blood and normal brain (Table 1). However, even more importantly the intracellular location of BOPP described in Fig. 2 has been calculated to result in a ten fold reduction in the amount of Boron required to achieve tumour necrosis since there is more efficient targeting of critical sub-cellular structures (9). Thus the tumour levels reported in this study are well above this threshold even at the low BOPP dose of 10 mg/kg body weight. Previous studies utilizing slow infusion of the sulfhydryl derivative of icosahedral borane, $Na_2B_{12}H_{11}SH$, in a patient with glioblastoma multiforme showed tumour concentrations of 2 to 6 μg boron/g, with parenchymal concentrations of approximately 1 μg/g (10). However, $Na_2B_{12}H_{11}SH$ has not been shown to localise intracellularly in glioma cells indicating that an alternative sensitizer is required since these levels are below the clinically useful threshold value. In contrast, tumour boron levels of approximately 12 µg/g and 63 µg/g using IV doses of 10 and 100 mg BOPP/kg body weight respectively are reported in this study. In addition, the selectivity of this uptake means that the levels in normal tissue and blood are very low, whilst the intracellular localisation suggests it will be extremely dose effective, and may offer great potential as a dual PDT/BNCT sensitizer.

REFERENCES

1. AH Kaye and JS Hill: Aust. N.Z. J. Surg. 58:767-780, 1988.
2. H Hatanaka in "Neutron Capture Therapy" (H Hatanaka Ed) Nishimura Co., 447-449, 1986.
3. AH Kaye, G Morstyn, I Gardner and K Pyke: Cancer Research. 46: 1367-1373, 1986.
4. SB Kahl and MS Koo: J. Chem. Soc. Chem. Commun. 1768-1771, 1990.
5. SB Kahl, DD Joel, M Nawrocky, PL Micca, KP Tran, GC Finkel and DN Slatkin. Proc. Natl. Acad. Sci. 87:7265-7269, 1990.
6. JS Hill, AH Kaye, WH Sawyer, G Morstyn, PD Megison and SS Stylli: Neurosurgery. 26: 248-254, 1990.
7. JS Hill, SB Kahl, AH Kaye, SS Stylli, MS Koo, MF Gonzales, NJ Vardaxis and CI Johnson. Proc. Natl. Acad. Sci. (in press).
8. RG Fairchild, SB Kahl, BH Laster, J Kalef-Ezra and EA Popence. Cancer Res. 40: 4860-4865, 1990.
9. D. Gabel, S. Foster and RG Fairchild. Radiat. Res. 111:14-25, 1987.
10. GC Finkel, CE Poletti, RG Fairchild, DN Slatkin and WH Sweet. Neurosurgery. 24:6-11, 1989.

ACUTE AND LATE REACTIONS FOLLOWING BORON NEUTRON CAPTURE EPITHERMAL-

NEUTRON THERAPY IN DOGS WITH SPONTANEOUS BRAIN TUMORS

P.R. Gavin,[1] C.E. DeHaan,[1] S.L. Kraft,[1] M.P. Moore,[1]
L.R. Wendling,[2] R.V. Dorn III[3]

[1]Veterinary Clinical Medicine & Surgery, Washington State
University, Pullman WA 99164
[2]Northwest Imaging, Spokane WA
[3]Mountain States Tumor Institute, Boise ID

INTRODUCTION

   Dogs have a relatively high incidence of primary tumors of the
central nervous system and have proven to be good models for new
therapeutic investigation.[1] The pharmacokinetics of borocaptate
sodium have been well documented in the dog.[2] Preliminary
investigations of the normal tissue tolerance to boron neutron capture
therapy have been performed utilizing normal laboratory dogs. This
study was an extension of the normal tissue tolerance and was designed
to ensure a therapeutic margin was present for the dogs with spontaneous
tumors; i.e., a measurable effect could be had on the tumor at doses
considered safe for the normal tissues.

MATERIALS AND METHODS

   Nine dogs were selected from a population of animals submitted to
the brain tumor referral network. These dogs all had evidence of
contrast enhancing lesions on computed tomography (CT) and/or magnetic
resonance (MR) imaging. Complete neurologic and physical examinations
were performed prior to treatment, including complete blood count, serum
chemistry evaluation, and cerebrospinal fluid analysis. Computed
tomographic guided biopsies were performed where feasible. A summary of
the patient profile is provided in Table 1. The dogs were transported
to Brookhaven National Laboratory and infused intravenously with 95%
B_{10} enriched borocaptate sodium at a dosage of 50 mg boron/kg bw,
dissolved in physiologic saline solution (11 ml/kg bw). The infusion
rate was 1 mg boron/kg bw/min. The irradiations were performed with a
target mean blood-boron concentration of 25 ppm. A single dorsal 10 x
10 cm portal was centered over the calvarium. The projected peak total
physical dose was 19 Gy to the blood. Post-treatment examinations were
scheduled at 3 weeks, 6 and 12 months following irradiation, or when
clinically indicated.

Acute Reactions

There were various causes of death for the 4 animals that lived less than 4 months. Dog 80 died of an anesthetic complication at the 3 week recheck. Dog 95 died within 24 hours following treatment. Dog 108 died within several weeks following treatment and was lost to further follow- up. Dog 100 did not improve following treatment and was euthanized.

All animals experienced epilation. Hair loss varied and was most noticeable starting at the third week post-treatment. Pigmentation reversal of the hair and skin occurred in all dogs. These changes were most visible within the incident beam region; however, the borders were not sharp and large portions of the head were involved.

Complete blood counts revealed a lymphopenia and a thrombocytopenia at the initial 3 week period or earlier. The lymphopenia was considered moderate in degree. Many of the animals had a thrombocytopenia with platelet counts in the 20-40,000 platelet/cu mm range.

On image analysis at 3 weeks post-irradiation, five of the animals had a significant decrease in the degree of contrast enhancement as seen on CT and MR imaging. There was a concurrent decrease in the region of peritumor edema and in mass effect. In three cases, there was no readily detectable change in the image parameters.

Late Reactions

The animals that lived beyond 3 weeks were all neurologically stable or improved. One animal (Dog 83) had a recurrence of seizure activity at 4 months following treatment with hemorrhage and MR contrast enhancement in the normal brain tissue on the contralateral side from

RESULTS

Four of the dogs lived less than the required 4 months needed to begin studying late effects of the central nervous system. Two animals lived between 3 months and 6 months, and 3 animals lived longer than 10 months (Table 1).

TABLE 1. Summary of initial dog brain
tumor treatments

Dog	Age	Breed	Tumor type	Days Surviving	Diagnosis
79	8 yrs	Boxer	Astrocytoma	348	Histo
80	4 yrs	Peke X	Astrocytoma	12	Histo
83	13 yrs	Doberman	Meningioma	170	Biopsy
87	11 yrs	Poodle X	Nasal Adenocarcinoma	140	Histo
93	7 yrs	Boxer	Oligodendroglioma	300	Histo
94	7 yrs	G. Retvr	Meningioma	>395	Imaging
95	8 yrs	Poodle X	Meningioma	0.5	Histo
100	8 yrs	GSD	Meningioma	43	Histo
108	5 yrs	Rottweiler	Choroid Plexus Papilloma	unknown	Imaging

the tumor. The animal was euthanized and ischemic necrosis was seen histologically in the abnormal areas on MR. Three of the 5 animals that lived longer than 3 months had moderate to marked tumor reduction as seen on CT and MR images. Two animals had no significant change in the tumor appearance. These 2 animals were euthanized and histopathologic examination revealed both viable and necrotic tumor. No significant change was seen in the surrounding normal brain tissue.

The 3 animals living beyond 10 months remained clinically improved for at least 6 months. At 6 months, Dog 79 had a return of its neurologic signs and a return of the contrast enhanced lesion. This animal continued to do relatively well on medication, and died at 11-1/2 months post-treatment of unrelated urinary tract disease. The majority of the contrast enhanced region corresponded to an inflammatory response to tumor necrosis. A small region of viable tumor was seen in association with the previous mass and there were intrathecal metastases.

Dogs 93 and 94 were both clinically normal at the 6 month post-treatment examination. There were areas of contrast enhancement indicative of cerebral necrosis in the gray and white matter. One of these animals subsequently died and there was malacia and demyelination in this area. The other dog is still alive 14 months after treatment and the lesion is diminished in size.

DISCUSSION

The epilation and hair color change was considered an acceptable normal tissue reaction. These changes are similar to those seen in normal tissue tolerance studies at 30 Gy total peak physical dose to the blood when the boron concentration was 50 ppm in the normal tissue tolerance studies.[3] The normal tolerance dogs were irradiated with a 5 x 10 cm incident beam while these dogs had a 10 x 10 cm incident beam. An increased field size would initially seem responsible for the decreased tolerance of the superficial tissues. However, increasing field size of the epithermal beam from the BMRR also changes the peak depth of the epithermal beam and the resultant effects should be largely offsetting. Therefore, this observed decrease in normal tissue tolerance in the tumor bearing dogs may be due to irradiation at a relatively lower blood boron dose (25 ppm vs 50 ppm).

Changes seen in the complete blood count may have been associated with one case of septicemia and two cases of urinary tract infection. The degree of lymphopenia could have been associated with immunosuppression. The degree of thrombocytopenia was insufficient to cause spontaneous hemorrhage; however, the thrombocytopenia was severe enough to have caused problems in surgery or if trauma had occurred. The blood counts were normal at the 6 month interval.

Three tumors were controlled for periods of about one year. Tumor control consisted of decreased contrast enhancement on CT and MR imaging, decreased peritumor edema, and decreased mass effect. Of the 6 dogs that lived longer than a few weeks post-treatment, one animal remains alive with apparent tumor control (18 months post-treatment). One animal died of central nervous system complications with no area of viable tumor detected (Dog 83). Four dogs (Dogs 79, 87, 93, and 100) all had viable tumors seen on histopathologic examination following their death. In 3 of the cases, considerable tumor necrosis was evident and the remaining tumor was considerably smaller than that initially seen on initial diagnosis.

Dog 83 died of CNS complications and seizures. Prior to euthanasia, magnetic resonance imaging revealed hemorrhage and contrast enhancement compatible with ischemic necrosis. These areas were in areas of the brain not associated with neoplastic invasion, but were involved with peritumor edematous changes on the pre-treatment MR examination. Previous studies have indicated peritumor edematous tissue contains levels of boron similar to those seen in neoplastic tissue.[2] The amount of boron that could have been present in this edematous tissue most likely contributed to a high dose and resultant changes.

Two of the animals (Dogs 93 and 94) had areas of contrast enhancement visible within the cerebral cortex compatible with vascular necrosis on the 6-month image examination. This change was similar to that visualized in the normal tolerance dogs at approximately 27 Gy total peak physical dose. Vascular sparing protects the endothelium to a large degree. Therefore, it is reasonable that as the boron concentration of the blood is decreased, the resultant proportion of non-boron related events could increase the apparent sensitivity of the normal tissues.

Dogs with spontaneous tumors have been treated with conventional radiation for several years and often have post-treatment survival periods long enough to study the development of late reactions of the central nervous system. The results from this study are encouraging. The dogs were treated close to tolerance (at 25 ppm blood boron) as evidenced by the change in the skin, hair, blood count, and vascular change in the cerebral cortex. At this level, most of the animals had an objective decrease in the size and appearance of their brain tumors. Control periods for the tumors was variable; however, the majority survived long enough post-therapy to study the appearance of late normal tissue reactions. Subsequent therapies will involve the use of higher mean blood boron concentrations in an attempt to increase the dose to the tumor while getting significant geometric sparing to the normal brain vasculature.

REFERENCES

1. J. Kornegay, "Central nervous system neoplasm," Contemporary Issues in Small Animal Practice 5:79 (1986).

2. S. L. Kraft, P. R. Gavin, C. E. DeHaan, and W. F. Bauer, "The biodistri- bution of boron in normal canine tissues following borocaptate sodium administration and its potential role in determining tissue tolerance to boron neutron capture therapy (BNCT)," Abstract and Presentation, Fourth International Symposium on Neutron Capture Therapy for Cancer, Sydney, Australia, December 1990.

3. C. E. DeHaan, P. R. Gavin, S. L. Kraft, C. W. Leathers, and F. J. Wheeler, "Quantitative dose response of the normal canine head to boron neutron capture therapy (BNCT)," Abstract and Presentation, Fourth International Symposium on Neutron Capture Therapy for Cancer, Sydney, Australia, December 1990.

TOLERANCE LIMITS OF THE NORMAL SKIN TREATED BY A SINGLE THERMAL NEUTRON CAPTURE THERAPY

H. Fukuda[1], K. Ando[1], C. Honda[2], M. Ichihashi[2], Y. Mishima[2], J. Hiratsuka[3], T. Kobayashi[4], and K. Kanda[4]

1. Division of Clinical Research, National Institute of Radiological Sciences, Chiba 260, Japan
2. Kobe University School of Medicine
3. Kawasaki Medical School
4. Kyoto University Research Reactor Institute

INTRODUCTION

In the treatment of malignant melanoma by BNCT, it is very important to estimate the damage to the skin, because we must eradicate the tumour within the tolerance limits of the normal tissues. In this paper, early and late skin reactions were observed in 8 patients treated by BNCT using ^{10}B-paraboronophenylalanine (^{10}B-BPA) and maximum neutron fluences to the skin were estimated. The RBE for the skin damage of high LET capture reaction from nitrogen-14 and boron-10 was also approximated.

METHODS

Boron-10 BPA fructose complex was used for the treatment except for case 1 and 2 in which ^{10}B-BPA.HCl was used. The compound was injected into the subcutaneous tissues of distant peri-tumoural region (4cm from the tumour edge) combined with systemic administration[1,2,3], the total boron-10 dose administered was 170 mg/kg body weight of the patients. The boron-10 concentration in the skin was evaluated by prompt gamma-ray analysis[4] in two cases or chemical assay[5] of the biopsy specimen in the other cases.

Musashi Reactor (MuITR) with power of 100 KW was used as a thermal neutron source. The neutron flux at the patient port was $1.0 - 1.2 \times 10^9$ n cm^{-2}s^{-1}. Total irradiation time was 139 - 223 minutes to yield neutron fluences of $9.6 - 12.5 \times 10^{12}$ n/cm^2. All the patients were treated by a single irradiation of thermal neutron. Gold foils or wire and small TLDs of Mg$_2$SiO$_4$(Tb) were used for the measurement of neutron fluences and gamma-rays, respectively. The patient was irradiated under slight sedation without anaesthesia, except for the first case.

For the quantification of skin damage after the treatment, skin score scales for the early and late reaction were used (Table 1, 2). For early skin reaction, score 2, 3 and 4 indicates dry reactions, moist reactions, and healing ulceration, respectively. Score 3 is considered to be a maximum tolerance limit. For late skin reactions, score 2 indicates slight pigmentation and atrophy of the skin and score 3 indicates severe atrophy of cutaneous tissues and hard fibrosis of sub-cutaneous tissues. Score 2 is considered to be a maximum limit. Early skin reactions were observed from day 1 to day 60 after the treatment. Late reactions of the skin were also observed from the 6th to 15th month. The maximum score during the observation was recorded and used for the evaluation.

RESULTS

Table 3 shows neutron fluences, absorbed doses (Gy), field size and skin reaction of each case. Neutron fluences varied from 9.6 - 12.5 x 10^{12} n/cm^2. Total absorbed dose was evaluated by summation of dose from $^{10}B(n,\alpha)^{7}Li$ and $^{14}N(n,p)^{14}C$ reaction and gamma-rays. Boron-10 concentration in the skin was measured as 3 to 5 $\mu g/g$ and as a value of nitrogen-14 concentration in the tissue, 3.52 % was used. The total absorbed dose varied from 7.6 to 14.9 Gy in each case. Field size varied from 6 to 250 cm^2.

Table 1
Early skin reaction score.

Score	Cutaneous	Subcutaneous
1	None	None
2	Erythema, pigmentation partial epilation	Moderate edema pigmentation
3	Brisk erythema, erosion moist desquamation	Complete alopecia severe edema
4	Confluent moist desquamation	Healing ulceration
5	Wide spread exfoliative dermatitis	Non healing ulceration or necrosis

Table 2
Late skin reaction score

Score	Cutaneous	Subcutaneous
1	None	None
2	Pigmentation Small telangiectasis	Slight fibrosis not interfering function
3	Extensive telangiectasis and skin atrophy	Hard fibrosis with symptom
4	Severe skin atrophy	Hard fibrosis with interfering function lymphedema of an extremity
5	Ulcer or necrosis	Necrosis

Table 3
Early and late reaction of the skin in the patients
treated by a single BNCT.

Case	Fluences (10^{12} n/cm^2)	Absorbed dose[a] (Gy)	Field size (cm^2)	Skin reaction Early[b]	Late[c]
1	9.4	10.8	34	2.0	2.0
2	12.5	13.8	36	3.0	d
3	11.0	12.1	20	3.0	2.0
4	11.0	10.4	16	3.0	2.0
5	9.3	7.6	6	2.0	2.0
6	12.0	10.7	16	3.0	2.0
7	12.3	14.6	250	4.0	d
8	11.7	14.9	50	4.0 - 5.0	d

a: Boron-10 concentration in the skin was 3-5 µg/g in all cases.
b: Score 3 is a maximum limit.
c: Score 2 is a maximum limit.
d: Evaluation of late reaction was not successful or not available.

As far as early skin reaction was concerned, case 1 to 6 showed scores
up to 3 which is considered to be a maximum tolerance limit. However, the
reactions in case 7 and 8 exceeded these limits. In case 7, severe erosion
and edema developed and lasted for a few months. Most of the lesion
recovered after 3 months, although it took several months to obtain a
complete cure (score 4). In case 8, severe moist reaction with ulceration
developed after the treatment and did not cure during the period of
observation (score 4 - 5). For the late skin reaction, 5 cases out of 8
were available for the evaluation. All showed a reaction score of 2 which
is within a tolerance limit.

DISCUSSION

The skin damage from case 1 to 6 was within the tolerance limits. On
the other hand, that of case 7 and 8 exceeded the limits, although neutron
fluences and boron-10 concentration in the skin were almost the same level.
One of the reasons might be larger radiation field size compared to that of
other cases. That may produce higher capture gamma-rays to yield higher
total absorbed dose. It is well known that a large radiation field reduces
the maximum tolerance dose to the skin in spite of the same absorbed dose[6].
From these observations, the maximum safe neutron fluence to the skin was
estimated as 11-12 x 10^{12} n/cm^2 for boron-10 concentration in the skin of 3
to 5 µg/g and radiation field size less than 50 cm^2. Although our
experience was limited, late reactions were not as serious as the early
reactions.

RBE of high LET capture reaction of ^{10}B(n, α)^{7}Li and ^{14}N(n,p)^{14}C to the
skin damage was estimated as follows. 1) RBE of both reactions are the
same and the effects are simply additive. 2) Maximum tolerance dose by an
X-ray for a single irradiation is 18 Gy[6] when the radiation field size is
less than 50 cm^2. The total RBE doses in 6 cases should be less than 18
RBE-Gy or Sv, because the skin reactions of these cases were within
tolerance limits. Then the following equation can be assumed-

$$\{Dose\ (n,p) + (n,\ \alpha)\} \times RBE + Dose\ (\gamma) < 18\ (Sv)$$

Solving the equation in each case, the RBE of high LET capture reactions was approximately 2.0.

CONCLUSIONS

   This paper has firstly described skin reaction in melanoma patients treated by BNCT. The maximum safe neutron fluence and RBE of high LET capture reaction to the skin were approximated. These values will be useful to determine the irradiation time for the treatment, although more cases are needed to confirm it. However, attention must be given to the fact that these values will be effective under limited conditions, such as single irradiation of thermal neutrons, boron-10 concentration in the skin of 3-5 μg/g, absorbed dose range of 10-13 Gy and field size of less than 40 cm^2. If a different treatment regimen is selected, the values will be different.

ACKNOWLEDGMENT

   This work was supported by a Grant-in-aid for Cancer Research from the Japanese Ministry of Science, Culture and Education.

REFERENCES

1. T. Kobayashi, S. Hatta, C. Honda, K. Yamamura, T. Akiyoshi, K. Kanda and Y. Mishima, Estimation of absorbed doses in human malignant melanoma treated by neutron capture therapy with special references to vertical direction, Pigment Cell Research, 2:361-364, (1989).
2. H. Fukuda, T. Kobayashi, J. Hiratsuka, H. Karashima, C. Honda, K. Yamamura, M. Ichihashi, K. Kanda, Y. Mishima, Estimation of absorbed dose in the covering skin of human melanoma treated by neutron capture therapy, Pigment Cell Research, 2:365-369, (1989).
3. Y. Mishima, C. Honda, M. Ichihashi, H. Obara, J. Hiratsuka, H. Fukuda, H. Karashima, T. Kobayashi, K. Kanda, K. Yoshino, Treatment of malignant melanoma by single thermal neutron capture therapy with melanoma-seeking ^{10}B-compound, The Lancet, Aug 12, 388-389, (1989).
4. K. Yoshino, K. Okamoto, H. Kakihana, T. Nakanishi, M. Ichihashi, Y. Mishima, Spectrophotometric determination of tracer boron in biological materials after alkali fusion decomposition, Analytical Chemistry, 56:839-842, (1984).
5. T. Kobayashi and K. Kanda, Microanalysis of ppm-order ^{10}B concentration in tissue for neutron capture therapy by prompt gamma-ray spectrometry, Nucl. Inst. Method, 204:525-531, (1983).
6. B. G. Douglas, Implication of the quadratic cell survival curve and human skin radiation "tolerance doses" on fractionation and super-fractionation dose selection, Int. J. Radiat. Oncol. Biol. Phys. 8:1135-1142, (1982).

QUALITATIVE DOSE RESPONSE OF THE NORMAL CANINE HEAD TO EPITHERMAL NEUTRON IRRADIATION WITH AND WITHOUT BORON CAPTURE

C.E. De Haan, P.R. Gavin, S.L. Kraft[1], F.J. Wheeler,
C.A. Atkinson[2]

[1]Veterinary Clinical Medicine & Surgery, Washington State
University, Pullman WA, USA
[2]Idaho National Engineering Laboratory, Idaho Falls, ID, USA

INTRODUCTION

Boron Neutron Capture Therapy is being re-evaluated for the treatment of intracranial tumors. Prior to human clinical trials, determination of normal tissue tolerance is critical. Dogs were chosen as a large animal model for the following reasons. Dogs can be evaluated with advanced imaging, diagnostic and therapeutic modalities. Dogs are amenable to detailed neurologic examination and subtle behavioral changes are easily detected. Specifically, Labrador retrievers were chosen for their large body and head size. The dogs received varying doses of epithermal neutron irradiation and boron neutron capture irradiation using an epithermal neutron source. The dogs were closely monitored for up to one year post irradiation.

METHODS

Animals

Twenty five adult, male Labrador retrievers were obtained from a United States Department of Agriculture licensed dealer. Ten dogs received epithermal neutron irradiation with peak doses at 10 Gy (n=5) and 15 Gy (n=5). Two dogs were sham irradiated and kept as controls. Eleven dogs received boron neutron capture irradiation with peak doses at 10 Gy (n=3), 20 Gy (n=3), 30 Gy (n=3) and 50 Gy (n=2). Two dogs received boron and sham irradiation and were kept as controls. Doses are calculated peak target doses at 3 cm depth.

Radiation Procedure

Epithermal Neutron Irradiation

Dexamethasone sodium phosphate (1 mg/kg) was administered intravenously one hour prior to irradiation. All dogs were irradiated under general anesthesia, positioned in right lateral recumbency with a 5 x 10 cm treatment field centered dorsally over the right cerebral hemisphere. Epithermal neutron energies ranged from 0.4 eV - 10 keV. Reactor power was 3 MW.[1] Dose rate was calculated at 6.36×10^{-2} Gy/min. Irradiation times were 156 and 237 minutes for 10 and 15 Gy.

Boron Neutron Capture Irradiation

Dexamethasone sodium phosphate (1 mg/kg) was administered

---

[1]Brookhaven Medical Research Reactor

intravenously one hour prior to irradiation. Borocaptate sodium ($Na_2B_{12}H_{11}SH$ or BSH) at a dose of 50 mg ^{10}B/kg was administered intravenously as an infusion in 11 mls/kg 0.9% saline over 50 minutes. Multiple blood samples were obtained following the BSH infusion and blood boron levels were determined using prompt gamma analysis. Irradiations were performed when mean blood ^{10}B levels were calculated to reach 50 μg/g. Blood samples were obtained prior to and following irradiation for definitive dose calculations. Irradiation protocol was the same as for epithermal neutron irradiations. Irradiation time was determined by the following formula:

Dose received =
(irradiation time)(reactor power)[(mean blood+^{10}B concentration)(D_B)+D_R]

D_B = 0.168 cGy/min-MW-μg-g^{-1} $\qquad$ D_R = 2.09 cGy/min-MW

<u>Monitoring</u>

Computed tomography (CT) and magnetic resonance (MR) imaging were performed pre-irradiation, 2-3 weeks, 6 months and 12 months post-irradiation and as indicated. All dogs were observed daily for dermal reactions and behavioral changes.

RESULTS

Grading systems for both dermal and neurological changes are summarized in Tables 1 and 2 respectively.

<u>Epithermal neutron irradiation</u>

Dose response of dermal tissues to epithermal neutron irradiation are summarized in Figure 1. Dose response of neural tissues are summarized in Figure 3.

Control group (6 month followup): No dermal reactions observed. Dogs remained neurologically normal and no abnormalities were seen on CT or MR images. At necropsy, brains were grossly normal.
10 Gy group (9 month followup & continuing): Severe dry and mild moist desquamation occurred at 2 wks with re-epithelialization, slow hair

Table 1 Dermal Tissues Grading

Grade	Dermal reaction
0	No reaction
1	Questionable reaction/erythema
2	Dry desquamation
3	Moist desquamation
4	Dermal necrosis

Table 2 Neural Tissues Grading

Grade	Neurological changes
0	No reaction
1	Imaging changes only
2	Neurological deterioration

516

Table 3 Boron Neutron Capture Irradiation Doses

Number of Dogs	Projected Dose	Calculated Dose
3	10 Gy	14.53 Gy
		12.58
		12.75
3	20 Gy	26.29
		25.45
		26.87
3	30 Gy	38.34
		38.00
		38.21
2	50 Gy	63.63
		63.74

regrowth and pigment reversal by 6 wks. Dogs have remained neurologically normal and no abnormalities have been seen on CT and MR images. Necropsy will be performed at 12 months post irradiation.
15 Gy group (12 wk followup): There was marked moist desquamation at 2 wks with incomplete re-epithelialization at 6 wks, progressing to dermal necrosis at 12 wks. Euthanasia was performed at that time. Dogs were neurologically normal and no abnormalities were seen on CT and MR images. At necropsy, brains were grossly normal.

Boron Neutron Capture irradiation

Following analysis of pre- and post-irradiation blood-boron levels, peak doses were recalculated (Table 3). Doses were higher than expected due to modifications in dosimetry calculations.
Dose response of dermal tissues to BNC irradiation is summarized in Figure 2. Dose response of neural tissues is summarized in Figure 3.

Control group (12 month followup): No dermal reactions were observed. Dogs remained neurologically normal and no abnormalities were seen on CT or MR images. At necropsy, brains were grossly normal.
10 Gy group (12 month followup): Dermal reactions were limited to questionable dry desquamation at 2 wks and mild pigment reversal by 10 - 12 wks. The dogs were neurologically normal and no abnormalities were seen on images of the brain or at necropsy.
20 Gy group (12 month followup): There was dry desquamation at 2 wks, slow hair regrowth and mild to moderate pigment reversal at 9 - 12 wks. No neurologic abnormalities were seen. At 6 months, there were changes on the MR images on 2 dogs characterized by focal edema and periventricular contrast enhancement. These changes were resolved at 9 months. At necropsy, all brains were grossly normal.
30 and 50 Gy groups (18 - 22 wk followup): In the 30 Gy group there was mild to moderate moist desquamation at 3 wks which re-epithelialized by 6-7 wks. Hair regrowth was slow and there was marked pigment reversal by 6 weeks. In the 50 Gy group, there was severe moist desquamation at 3 wks, incomplete re-epithelialization at 6 wks which progressed to dermal necrosis by 12 wks. All dogs suffered neurological deterioration 18 -22 weeks post irradiation and euthanasia was performed. Imaging prior to neurologic deterioration was normal. Images obtained at deterioration showed marked changes characterized by marked edema and periventricular contrast enhancement consistent with focal necrosis. At necropsy, the brains were grossly edematous. On cut section, there was focal necrosis and hemorrhage, primarily in the white matter.

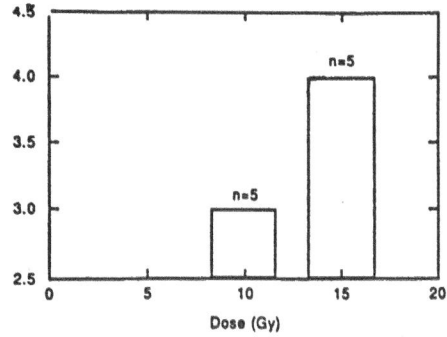

Figure 1

Qualitative dose response of dermal tissues to
epithermal-neutron irradiation.

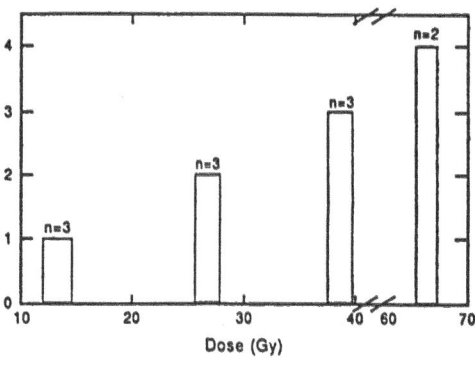

Figure 2

Qualitative dose response of dermal tissues to boron
neutron capture irradiation.

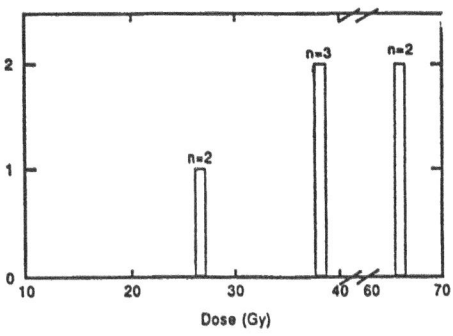

Figure 3

Qualitative dose response of neural tissues to boron
neutron irradiation.

CONCLUSIONS

Epithermal-neutron irradiation produced unacceptable dermal complications at 15-Gy peak dose. Neural complications have no yet been observed at 10 Gy. Boron neutron capture irradiation produced unacceptable neural complications at a dose than what was needed for unacceptable dermal complications (≥ 38 Gy vs ≥ 63 Gy). Due to the longer irradiations times required to reach the epithermal dose equivalent to a BNC dose, the incident fast neutron and gamma exposures were increased. This resulted in more damage to the dermis and less damage to the neural structures at the same dose.

COPYRIGHT

BORON NEUTRON CAPTURE THERAPY: THE RADIATION RESPONSE OF RAT SKIN AND

SPINAL CORD

G.M. Morris and J.W. Hopewell

CRC Normal Tissue Radiobiological Research Group
Research Institute (University of Oxford)
Churchill Hospital, Oxford. OX3 7LJ. U.K.

INTRODUCTION

In order to determine the full therapeutic potential of boron
neutron capture therapy (BNCT), more information is required on the
radiation tolerance of normal tissues. Investigations using animal
models, for example the rat spinal cord, can provide valuable
information on dose-effect relationships for normal tissue toxicity.

RESULTS AND DISCUSSION

All experimental procedures have been carried out on 12 week old
male Sprague Dawley rats. The neutron capture component used was 95%
^{10}B-enriched di-sodium mercaptoundecahydro-closo-dodecaborate (BSH).
The BSH was administered by intravenous infusion over a 10 minute period
and the boron content in blood and skin quantified using inductively
coupled plasma atomic emission spectrometry (I.C.P.A.E.S). Anaesthesia
was maintained with a flurothane (1.75%) and oxygen mixture.

(i) Pharmacokinetic Studies

Pharmacokinetic studies on the rat have examined the variation in
blood and skin boron concentration with time after the administration of
single doses of 50, 75, 100 and 200mg/kg of BSH (Fig. 1). After the
lowest dose of 50mg/kg BSH there was a progressive decline in the blood
boron content, with a biological half life ($t_\frac{1}{2}$) of 4.5h. Higher doses
of BSH resulted in slower clearance rates. After a dose of 75mg/kg of
BSH there was no significant reduction in the levels of boron in the
blood for the first 4h after infusion. The $t_\frac{1}{2}$ value was increased to
approximately 6h. Blood boron clearance times were further increased
after doses of 100 and 200mg/kg of BSH. After the highest dose
(200mg/kg) blood boron content remained essentially unchanged for the
first 8 hours after BSH infusion (Fig. 1). More rapid blood boron
clearance rates have been reported for the rat by other authors.
Clendenon et al (1990) obtained a $t_\frac{1}{2}$ value of 39 mins after the
administration of 50mg/kg of BSH; while Abe et al. (1986) indicated a $t_\frac{1}{2}$
value at 6h after the infusion of 100mg/kg of BSH. However, in the dog
(Gavin et al., 1989) a $t_\frac{1}{2}$ value of 5h was estimated after the infusion
of 55mg/kg of BSH.

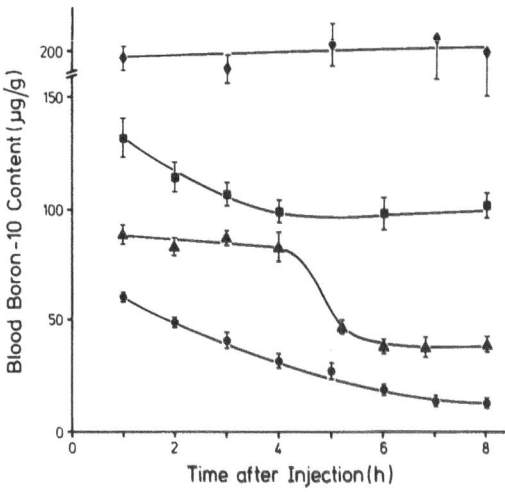

Fig. 1.   Time-related changes in blood boron concentration following the
intravenous infusion of 50 (●), 75 (▲), 100 (■) and 200 (◊)
mg/kg body weight of BSH.   (Error bars indicate ±S.E.).

Boron levels have been assessed in the skin of rats over an 8h
period after the infusion of 100mg/kg of BSH.   In common with the blood,
the boron content in the skin remained constant over the observation
period.   It was a factor of ~0.6 lower than that of the blood.   In a
previous study on the rat (Abe et al., 1986) boron levels in the skin
were found to be a factor of ~3 lower than in the blood at 12h after the
injection of 50mg/kg of BSH.   In dog skin after the infusion of 55mg/kg
of BSH, boron levels at 6h and 12h were 0.3 - 1.0 times those for the
blood (Gavin et al., 1990).

(ii)   <u>Radiobiological Studies</u>

The 20mm irradiation field encompasses vertebrae T12 to L2 of the
spinal cord.   At present, rats infused with 100mg/kg of BSH have been
irradiated for 3, 4, 4.5 and 5h with thermal neutrons (0.025eV) from the
H6 beam on the DIDO reactor (AERE Harwell), at a skin surface neutron
flux of 4.8×10^{8} n/cm^{2}/s.

Exposure times in excess of 3h resulted in marked skin reactions
that were analogous to those seen after single doses of $\geq$70Gy x-rays
(Hamlet and Hopewell, 1982).   Skin breakdown (moist desquamation) also
occurred over a similar time course to that seen after x-irradiation.
The time taken for the moist desquamation to heal was dependent on the
exposure time (Fig. 2).   In complete contrast to what was seen after
x-irradiation (Hopewell, 1985), there was a clear biphasic skin reaction
in the rat after thermal neutron exposure times of 4.5h (Fig. 2).   The
severity of the second wave response was dose dependent, with persistent
dermal necrosis in 60% of skin fields after a 5h exposure.   This result
indicates severe long term damage to the skin vasculature after thermal
neutron irradiation in the presence of BSH.

The estimated total doses to the skin at a depth of 1mm were 37Gy,
41Gy, and 46Gy for 4, 4.5 and 5h exposure times, respectively.   Possibly
due to an uneven distribution of boron in the skin these estimates must
be considered to be approximate.   However, there would appear to be an
appreciable enhancement in the radiosensitivity of the skin relative to
x-rays; by at least a factor of 2.   A similar conclusion has been
reported for pig skin (Archambeau et al., 1971).

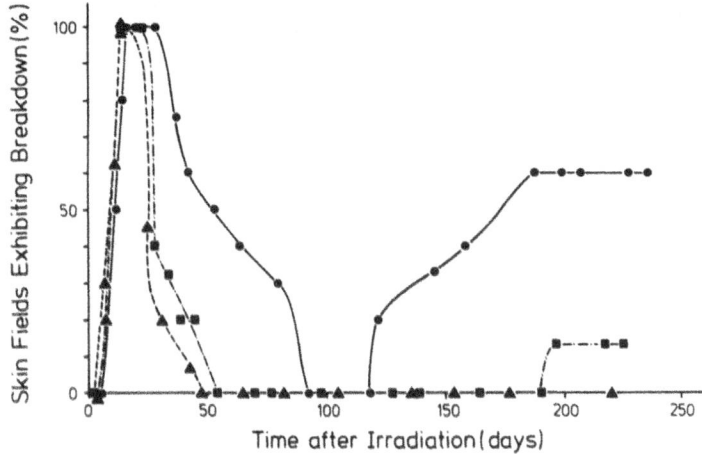

Fig. 2. Percentage of skin fields showing breakdown with time after
         thermal neutron exposure times of 4 (▲), 4.5 (■) and 5h (●)
         after the administration of 100mg/kg of BSH.

In a previous investigation (Hopewell et al., 1987) in which a
comparable length of spinal cord was irradiated to that of the present
study, a single dose of 21.5Gy of x-rays was sufficient to produce
paralysis in 50% of rats. In the spinal cord of rats which developed
paralysis within 30 weeks the most marked histological lesion was white
matter necrosis, while in rats which developed paralysis after >30 weeks
the predominant histological lesion was gross vascular abnormality
(Hopewell et al., 1987). The estimated absorbed doses at the centre of
the spinal cord, of rats used in the present schedule, assuming a blood
concentration of 100mg/kg of BSH, were approximately 22, 29, 33 and 37Gy
for 3, 4, 4.5 and 5h exposures, respectively. To date, rats have been
observed for up to 40 weeks after irradiation, with no evidence of
neurological changes. Observations are continuing to determine if
neurological effects related to gross vascular abnormalities develop
over a significantly longer latent interval.

REFERENCES

Abe, M., Amano, K., Kitamura, K., Tateishi, J., and Hatanaka, H., 1986,
        Boron distribution analysis by alpha-autoradiography, J. Nuclear
        Med., 27: 677.
Archambeau, J.O., Fairchild, R.G., and Brenneis, H.J., 1971, The
        response of the skin of swine to increasing absorbed doses of
        radiation from a thermal neutron beam a degraded fission neutron
        beam, and the $^{10}B(n,\alpha)$ Li reaction, Radiat. Res. 45: 145.
Clendenon, N.R., Barth, R.F., Gordon, W.A., Goodman, J.H., Alam, F., et
        al., 1990, Boron neutron capture therapy of a rat glioma,
        Neurosurgery, 26: 47.
Gavin, P.R., Kraft, S.L., Wendling, L.R., and Miller, D.L., 1989,
        Canine spontaneous brain tumors - a large animal model for BNCT,
        Strahlenther. Onkol., 165: 225.
Hamlet, R., and Hopewell, J.W., 1982, The radiation response of skin in
        young and old rats, Int. J. Radiat. Biol., 42: 573.
Hopewell, J.W., 1985, Effects of radiation on the skin, Radiological
        Protection Bulletin No. 62: 16.
Hopewell, J.W., Morris, A.D., and Dixon-Brown, A., 1987, The influence
        of field size on the late tolerance of the rat spinal cord to
        single doses of X-rays, Brit. J. Radiol., 60: 1099.

INFLUENCE OF BNCT RADIATIONS ON THE BLOOD-BRAIN BARRIER IN TERMS OF

BORON-10 UPTAKE

Yoshinobu Nakagawa[1], Tooru Kogayashi[2], Youri Ueno[2], Hiroshi Hatanaka[3], Maki Moritani[3], Kanji Mukai[4] and Keizo Matsumoto[4]

1. Dept. of Neurosurgery, National Kagawa Children's Hospital, Kagawa 765
2. Research Reactor Institute, Kyoto University, Osaka 590-04
3. Dept. of Neurosurgery, Teikyo University, Tokyo 173
4. Dept. of Neurosurgery, Tokushima University, Tokushima 770

INTRODUCTION

A key issue is to determine whether fractionated BNCT is a feasible proposition. This issue has been reviewed by Dorn et al[1], who call for further experimental investigation of BNCT induced changes in the blood brain barrier and investigated by Hatanaka et al[2]. In order to investigate the effect on BNCT, we measured ^{10}B concentration and water content in the normal brain which had been subjected to BNCT regimen.

MATERIALS AND METHODS

Wistar rats weighing 200-250mg were used in this study. Under anaesthesia with pentobarbital (50mg/kg), all animals received ^{10}B compound (50mg/kg) in the form of $Na_2B_{12}H_{11}SH$ by intravenous or intraperitoneal injection. Two hours (groups 1, 2, 3) or 3.5 hours (groups 4, 5, 6) after injection, irradiation was carried out at the Research Reactor Institute, Kyoto University (KUR) (Table 1). At 12 or 24 hours after irradiation the animals had a second injection of boron-10. The measurement of the ^{10}B concentration was performed at 60 minutes or 24 hours after the second injection. The animals were divided into 7 groups with 8 animals in the control group and 6 experimental groups of 5 animals each. Neutron exposure was given for 30 min. (group 1), 30 min. twice one day apart (group 2), 60 min. (groups 3 and 4), 90 min. (group 5), and 120 min. (group 6). Water content was measured by freeze-dry method (control, groups 1, 2, and 3). After decapitation, three brain specimens were obtained from each animal of groups 1, 2, and 3 (cerebral cortex, brain stem, and cerebellum). For groups 1, 2, and 3, ^{10}B concentration of the wet specimens were measured by prompt gamma ray spectrometry. For groups 4, 5, and 6, it was measured by chemical analysis of the brain specimens. For groups 1, 2, and 3, dried materials were also analysed by chemical method. Chemical analysis was done by chemists of the Shionogi Research Laboratories.

Table 1
EXPERIMENTAL METHODS

EXPERIMENT 1	EXPERIMENT II
1st ^{10}B compound injection (50mg/kg i.v)	1st ^{10}B compound injection (50mg/kg i.p.)
Time interval - 2 hours	Time interval - 3.5 hours

Neutron irradiation *
   Exposure time
     Control   0   min
     Group 1   30   min
     Group 2   30   min x 2
     Group 3   60   min
	Neutron irradiation *
	   Exposure time
	     Control 0 min
	     Group 4 60 min
	     Group 5 90 min
	     Group 6 120 min

Time interval : 12 hours	Time interval : 24 hours
2nd ^{10}B compound injection (50mg/kg i.v.)	2nd ^{10}B compound injection (50mg/kg i.p.)
Time interval : 60 min	Time interval : 24 hours
Blood & brain specimens **	Blood & brain specimens **

* Neutron flux: 3.7 - 4.5 x 10^9 (n/cm^2/sec)
** ^{10}B concentration was measured by prompt gamma-ray spectrometry before freezed dry method (wet brain tissue) in control animals and group 1, 2, & 3. In group 4, 5, & 6, ^{10}B concentration was measured by chemical analysis after freezed dry method (dry brain tissue).

Table 2
BORON-10 CONCENTRATIONS (PPM)

	B-10 concentration in blood at autopsy after second injection	B-10 concentration in wet brain after second injection
Control	1.26 ± 0.23	0.35 ± 0.14
Group 4	1.07 ± 0.47	0.48 ± 0.31
Group 5	1.18 ± 0.35	0.27 ± 0.18
Group 6	1.52 ± 0.49	0.62 ± 0.25

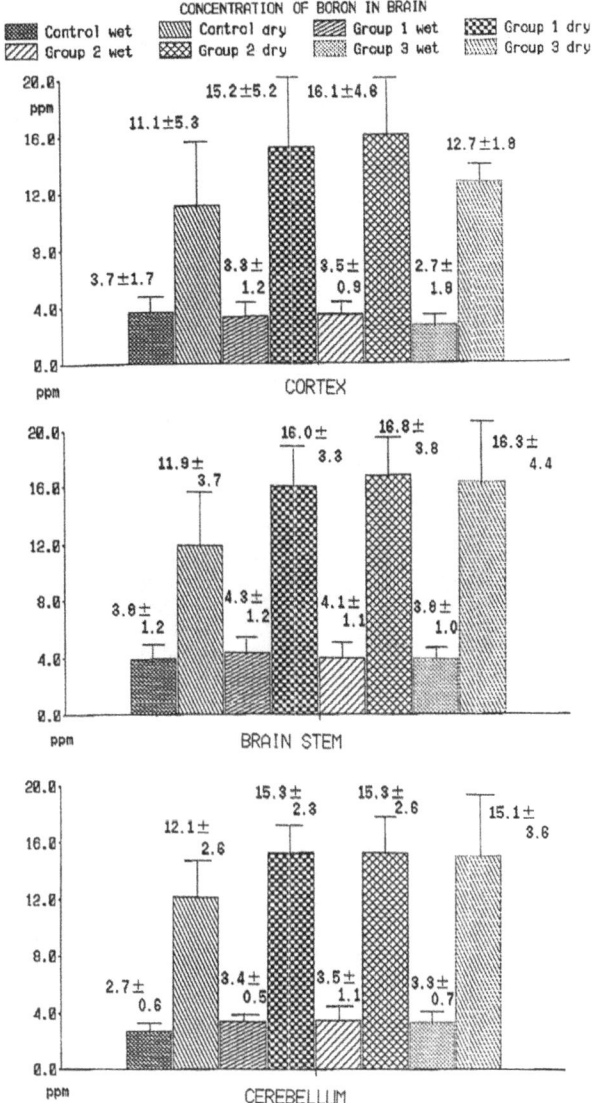

Figure 1. Boron-10 concentrations in the cerebral cortex, brain stem and cerebellum relative to unirradiated controls for wet and dry samples.

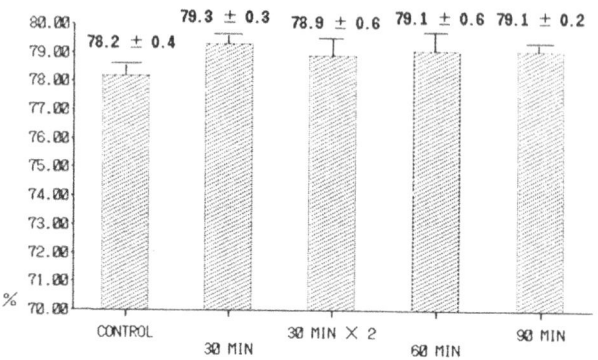

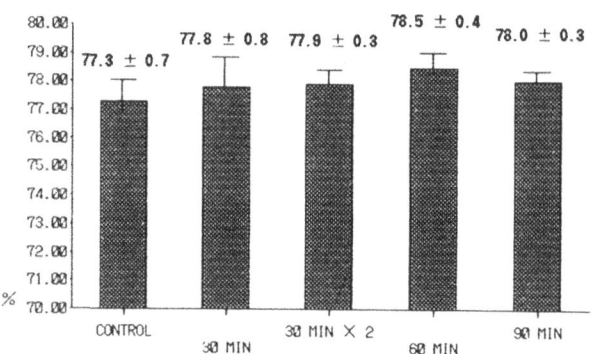

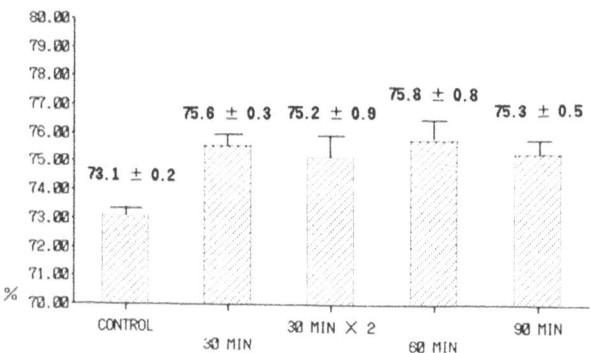

Figure 2. Water content in the cortex, cerebellum and brain stem after BNCT.

528

RESULTS

There was no significant difference in ^{10}B concentration in wet brain tissues between the control group and groups 1, 2, and 3. However ^{10}B concentration in dry materials after freeze-drying showed a significant difference between control and groups 1, 2, and 3 (fig. 1). Water content after BNCT radiation showed a mild increase in cortex (1 - 1.5%), brain stem (1.8 - 2.5%) and cerebellum (0.7 - 1.5%) 9 (table 2.) (fig. 2).

DISCUSSION

The average ^{10}B concentration in blood during BNCT radiation in patients with brain tumours was reported to be 10 - 20 ppm[2]. However, the effect upon the blood-brain barrier of various concentrations of blood boron is not yet clear. In a recent study using Wistar rats[3], the change of boron concentration in blood was continuously investigated by prompt gamma ray spectrometry. After the injection of boron compound, its concentration promptly rose and reached the peak in 10 min. In 60 min., the concentration rapidly decreased and then a gradual decline was noted. One to two hours after the injection, the concentration was 20 - 33 ppm and by 12 - 24 hours the concentration was below 5 ppm. In groups 1, 2, and 3 boron in blood was 20 - 40 ppm. These animals were used as a model of high boron-10 concentration. The other animals in groups 4, 5, and 6 were the models of low concentration. Although the boron-10 in the wet tissues of groups 1, 2, and 3 showed no significant difference from the control, there was a significant difference between the control (dry) and radiated brain (dry). it was noteworthy that there was a certain difference in water content between control and radiated brains. We postulate that in an acute stage after BNCT there may be a mild alteration of the blood-brain barrier which may allow the penetration of boron-10 as well as edema into the extracellular space of the brain matter.

CONCLUSION

The boron-10 concentration in the brain tissue after BNCT radiation should not be neglected because its presence in the brain will more or less increase the radiation dose to the normal brain matter and thus will decrease the selective advantage of boron-neutron capture therapy. This fact will thus decrease the value of a fractionated neutron irradiation schedule for BNCT.

REFERENCES

1. R. V. Dorn III, J. H. Spickard, M. L. Griebenow, The effect of ionising radiation on the blood-brain barrier; considerations for the application of boron neutron capture therapy of brain tumours, Clinical Aspects of Neutron Capture Therapy, Ed. R. G. Fairchild et al, Plenum Press NY, 145-152, 1989.

2. H. Hatanaka, M. Moritani, M. Camillo, Possible alteration of the blood-brain barrier by boron-neutron capture therapy, Acta Oncologica 30, 375-378, 1991.

BLOOD-BRAIN BARRIER AND ITS MANIPULATION:

IMPLICATIONS FOR NEUTRON CAPTURE THERAPY

Mary K. Gumerlock

Department of Neurosurgery
University of Oklahoma Health Sciences Center
Oklahoma City, Oklahoma

THE BLOOD-BRAIN BARRIER IN NORMAL BRAIN

The concept of the blood-brain barrier (BBB) dates from the early twentieth century when physiologists noted that administration of vital dyes stained tissues of the whole body with the exception of the central nervous system (CNS). Thus developed the concept that a barrier exists between the blood and the brain such that certain substances are excluded from access to brain parenchyma. Early studies showed that dye injection into the cerebrospinal fluid (CSF) space did allow brain tissue penetration. Initially, the anatomic location and morphology of this blood-brain barrier was felt to derive from a pial-glial sheath invaginating the vessels. Accumulating data has led to the conclusion that the blood-brain barrier resides at the capillary endothelial level.[1]

Brain capillary endothelial cells differ from those found systemically in that (1) the endothelial cytoplasm has high electron density, (2) there exists a thick basement membrane, and (3) the endothelial surface is covered by astrocytic endfoot processes and it appears that there is some effect of glial modulation on the intrinsic capillary endothelial properties, in a sense "tightening the blood-brain barrier." Brain capillary endothelial cells are also known for their tight junctions, increased mitochondria, and paucity of cytoplasmic vesicles. These cells demonstrate high electrical resistance and decreased hydraulic conductance. There also exists enzymatic localization, particularly with Na-K-ATPase at the abluminal surface.

Further studies have determined the selectivity of the BBB with CNS penetration limited by size, molecular weight, charge, and lipid solubility. These exclusionary properties in conjunction with the continuous production of CSF leads to the concept of the "sink action of the CSF".[2] Because the CSF circulates and extracellular tissue fluid of the brain does not, the CSF acts to sump solutes that may cross the blood-brain barrier. Thus, low levels of a substance in brain parenchyma are the result not only of slow penetration through the BBB, but also of the highly efficient sink action of the CSF where active removal by CSF bulk flow into venous blood prevents the establishment of a diffusional equilibrium.[2]

To circumvent this sink action, investigators have attempted to prolong infusion of various agents directly into the CSF. Such techniques allow for increased parenchymal concentration; however, this is limited to approximately 3mm beneath the subarachnoid space, even after prolonged perfusions. With direct intraventricular perfusion, there also results a ten-fold concentration difference between the ventricular and surface subarachnoid tissue.[3]

A number of physico-chemical properties determine CNS permeability. Lipid solubility heavily influences solute penetration across the BBB, as measured by plotting permeability against oil/water partition coefficient divided by the square root of the molecular weight.[4] In addition to bulk transport via simple diffusion, a number of specific transport mechanisms are operant in the CNS. These carrier-mediated transport systems may be defined as selective, stereo-specific, saturable, and subject to competitive inhibition. Physiologically important non-electrolytes which have demonstrable transport systems at the BBB include monosaccharides (D-glucose), monocarboxylic acids (L-lactate), neutral amino acids (L-leucine), basic amino acids (L-arginine), dicarboxylic amino acids (L-glutamate), amines (choline), nucleosides (adenosine), and purines.[5]

The role of pits, vesicles, and channels (microinvaginations of the endothelial plasma membrane) in cerebral transport is still being defined. Research has suggested that vesicles may be considered equivalent to large pores through which macromolecules may traverse the capillary endothelial cells.[6] Reese and Karnovsky have described the localization of horseradish peroxidase in lysosomes of cerebral endothelium in a graded fashion with less concentration at the abluminal side.[7] Some abluminal pits may actually be vesicles which can migrate from the abluminal to luminal side as well. While no series of pits or vesicles form a complete transendothelial channel, a single vesicle/pit may form and fuse temporarily with a transcellular channel, thus allowing solutes to rapidly traverse the endothelium.[8,9]

The BBB, well-developed by mid-gestation in humans, sheep, and pigs, is still open at birth in such species as the cat and rat. It is therefore important to take into account the age and species of animals studied when describing permeability across the BBB. For instance, it is after the second post-natal week that rats demonstrate a marked permeability decrease.[10] Any consideration of drug delivery to the brain must also take into account the physico-chemical properties of the drug: plasma protein interactions, drug administration frequency and route (intravenous, intra-arterial, intrathecal), and cerebral blood flow (CBF). Drug modification, by altering lipid solubility or coupling to carrier-transported substances, remains a potential method for increasing drug delivery across the BBB.

In addition to general drug behavior, it is important to keep in mind certain specifics of BBB pharmacology. One must consider the blood-to-brain transfer constant and not simply rely on permeability coefficients.[11] Permeability coefficients may be estimated and are somewhat dependent on CBF. Drugs cross primarily by simple diffusion or carrier-mediated transport, and the rate of CNS drug uptake varies. It is this extreme variability which limits the generalizability of a number of drug studies relative to the CNS. The rate of CNS uptake is also dependent on local CBF differences, capillary surface area, and capillary permeability. These three factors are themselves known to be quite variable from region to region and also from time to time, subject to the general physiologic state of the animal, and probable neural transmitter changes. Finally, because of the CSF sink effect, CNS drug uptake will vary depending on the proximity of parenchymal tissue to the CSF itself. Further drug distribution variables include plasma protein binding, drug plasma half-life, and endothelial or red blood cell sequestration of the drug in question.

THE BLOOD-BRAIN BARRIER IN BRAIN TUMORS

Brain tumors appear to grow in two stages: an initial pre-vascular stage, and a secondary phase, dependent on the release of tumor angiogenesis factor, stimulating the formation of new capillaries.[12,13] This relationship between blood vessels and tumor cells, particularly within the brain, remains an intriguing mystery of neuro-oncology. The blood vessels of brain tumor neovascularity differ from normal brain vessels in a number of respects.[14] In general, per volume of tissue, there is an increased number of capillaries, which in turn have an increased diameter. There is also an increase in the number of endothelial cells as well as the number of adventitial cells. The endothelial cells have an increase in the number of cytoplasmic vesicles. The basement membrane, so prominent a characteristic of normal brain, is variable. There is also an inconsistent amount of astrocytic investiture of the brain tumor capillaries. The perivascular space of brain tumors is increased with often more collagen and fibroblasts in comparison to the perivascular space of normal cerebral capillaries. Tumor capillary endothelial cells have open tight junctions, gap junctions, and fenestrae.[14]

What about the blood-brain barrier in tumors (blood-tumor barrier)? Much has been made of a lack of such barrier in tumors, thus suggesting that in tumors there is no limitation to drug delivery.[15] However, both experimental and clinical studies suggest evidence to the contrary.[16] Blasberg and colleagues have studied a variety of rat glial tumors, concluding that the amount of an intact barrier varied, both from tumor to tumor, and within any single given tumor type.[17] Their studies show that the BBB is not affected by tumor size or tumor location. Studies by Folkman and colleagues demonstrate that tumor neovascularity is not dependent on tumor size but rather on tumor angiogenesis factor. Their studies also seem to indicate that tumors may grow and remain viable up to a size of at least a 2mm sphere without requiring vascularity (and hence no BBB perturbation).[12,13]

Tumor pharmacology must also be taken into consideration. Tumor blood flow varies, thus drug delivery to tumor with or without a blood-tumor barrier will be variable. Blood flow is frequently reduced. There exists in general an increased intercapillary distance in most brain tumors, which therefore compromises diffusion of administered drugs. Because there is also a decrease in the diffusion of oxygen and nutrients, tumor cells often become quiescent, and thus unable to uptake drugs.[18] Capillary permeability in the peritumoral area is also usually less than that of normal brain. As described above, the CSF and normal brain surrounding a tumor may act as a diffusion sink for any drug that enters tumor. Thus, the increased permeability afforded to drugs in the tumor is rapidly reduced by diffusion. Additionally, brain tumors appear to have an efficient perivascular drainage system. Thus, the important factor in effective drug delivery, that of <u>sufficient concentration</u> over a <u>sufficient time period</u> may not be realized to any therapeutic advantage.

OSMOTIC OPENING OF THE BLOOD-BRAIN BARRIER

In addition to pathologic processes such as tumors, ischemia, infection, and trauma, BBB breakdown may result from hypercarbia, seizures, and hypertension. Most of these insults result in transient opening of the barrier. Research into the use of hyperosmolar solutions (arabinose, urea, lactamide, glycerol, sucrose, mannitol) has suggested that by rapid intracarotid infusion, these substances may also transiently disrupt the BBB.[1] Such methods have been used both experimentally and clinically as another method to increase the delivery of substances to brain parenchyma.[16,19] Through the work of various laboratories, it has become apparent that hyperosmolar disruption of the blood-brain barrier is a threshold event, depending on the osmolality, duration, rate, and volume of the infused solution.[19,20] The mechanism of reversible osmotic BBB opening remains to be elucidated, but theories range from osmotic shrinkage of the capillary endothelial cells with secondary disruption of the tight junctions to a theory of increased transendothial transport via vesicles and channels.[9,21]

Osmotic barrier opening has been accomplished in a number of animal species (rat, rabbit, dog, monkey) without producing significant cytopathologic changes or long-term behavioral or neurologic sequelae. This absence, however, does not preclude the possibility of subtle ultrastructural or chemical changes. It has been well-demonstrated that increased drug delivery occurs to tumor tissue and normal brain tissue through these changes.[22] A variety of agents, including chemotherapeutic drugs, enzymes, and monoclonal antibodies have been delivered with increased levels across the BBB. However, many agents from the vascular compartment to brain parenchyma may be associated with severe and unacceptable neurotoxicity, and this must be evaluated in preclinical trials.

While there has been some variability in the increased drug delivery to tumors and brain around tumor in animals with osmotic BBB opening,[17] it appears that in most patients, increased tumor radionuclide uptake is seen with mannitol infusion, and even in those cases without significant barrier opening (27/232), eleven procedures (41%) had increased enhancement of the tumor tissue itself, suggesting increased tumor drug delivery.[23]

THE BBB AND NEUTRON CAPTURE THERAPY

Given the principles outlined above regarding the BBB both in normal brain tissue and in tumors, several factors, some

534

perhaps cautionary, are worth considering. Work with boronated nucleic acids and olionucliotides as well as carboranyl nucleic acid precursors is promising from the perspective of specific carrier-mediated systems for delivery to the CNS. The penetration of gadolinium-labelled DNA ligands, as well as boronated dextrans and growth factors are likely to be limited because of their high molecular weight. Should delivery across an open blood-tumor barrier be achieved, these compounds, unless they demonstrate specific affinity to the tumor cells themselves, may well rapidly diffuse away (CSF sump/sink effect) due to poor concentration throughout adjacent brain tissue. Such makes the work of boronated monoclonal antibodies with selective binding properties particularly advantageous. Lysosomal and low density lipoproteins, while being of larger molecular weight and size, may be able to somewhat circumvent the CSF sink action. Boron complexed to oligosaccharides may be able to take advantage of the specific monosaccharide transport system across the blood-brain barrier. Boronated phenylalanine uptake and its use in BNCT remains controversial. Experimental work by Hawkins and Mans demonstrating ^{14}C-phenylalanine uptake by autoradiography shows a five-fold variation which correlated significantly with regional cerebral blood flow and capillary surface area.[24] Boronated porphyrins, with their ability to localize in mitochondria, have some targeting ability to tumor cells; however, the increased number of mitochondria in brain capillary endothelial cells may make the capillary endothelia particularly sensitive to uptake and subsequent radiation damage, perhaps even increased over the standard radiation vascular damage. Thus, with regard to the blood-brain barrier and its implications for NCT, the blood-brain barrier may be considered both friend and foe.

REFERENCES

1. Rapport SI: Blood-Brain Barrier in Physiology and Medicine. Raven, New York, 1976.
2. Davson H: The environment of the neurone. Trends Neurosci 1:39-41, 1978.
3. Rall DP, Oppelt WW, Patlak CS: Extracellular space of brain as determined by diffusion of inulin from the ventricular system. Life Sci 2:43-48, 1962.
4. Fenstermacher JD, Rapoport SI: Blood-brain barrier. In Renkin EM, Michel CC (eds): Handbook of Physiology. Microcirculation. American Physiological Society, Washington, DC, 1984, pp. 969-1000.
5. Bradberry NW: Transport across the blood-brain barrier. In Neuwelt EA (ed): Implications of the Blood-Brain Barrier and Its Manipulation. Volume 1 Basic Science Aspects. Plenum Publishing Corporation, New York, New York, 1989, pp. 119-136.
6. Brightman MW: The anatomic basis of the blood-brain barrier. In Neuwelt EA (ed): Implications of the Blood-Brain Barrier and Its Manipulation. Plenum Publishing Corporation, New York, NY, 1989, pp. 53-83.
7. Reese Ts, Karnovsky MJ: Fine structural localization of a blood-brain barrier to exogenous peroxidase. J Cell Biol 34:207-217, 1967.
8. Frokjaer-Jensen J: The plasmalemmal vesicular system in capillary endothelium. Prog Appl Microcirc 1:17-34, 1983.
9. Nagy Z, Peters H, Huttner I: Fracture faces of cell junctions in cerebral endothelium during normal and

hyperosmotic conditions. Lab Invest 50:313-322, 1984.

10. Woodbury DM: Distribution of nonelectrolytes and electrolytes in the brain as affected by alterations in cerebrospinal fluid secretion. Prog Brain Res 29:297-313, 1976.

11. Fenstermacher JD, Blasberg RG, Patlak CS: Methods for quantifying the transport of drugs across brain barrier systems. Pharmacol Ther 14:217-248, 1981.

12. Folkman J: Towards an understanding of angiogenesis: Search and discovery. Persp Biol Med 29:11-36, 1985.

13. Folkman J: How is blood vessel growth regulated in normal and neoplastic tissue? Cancer Res 46:467-473, 1985.

14. Greig NH: Brain tumors and the blood-tumor barrier. In Neuwelt EA (ed): Implications of the Blood-Brain Barrier and Its Manipulation. Volume 2 Clinical Aspects. Plenum Publishing Corporation, New York, NY, 1989, pp. 77-102.

15. Vick NA, Bigner DD: Chemotherapy of brain tumors: The blood-brain barrier is not a factor. Arch Neurology 34:523-526, 1977.

16. Neuwelt EA, Frenkel EP, Diehl JT, et al: Reversible osmotic blood-brain barrier disruption in humans: Implications for the chemotherapy of malignant brain tumors. Neurosurgery 7:44-52, 1980.

17. Blasberg R, Groothuis D: Chemotherapy of brain tumors: Physiological and pharmacokinetic considerations. Semin Oncol 13:70-82, 1986.

18. DeVita VT: The relationship between tumor mass and resistance to chemotherapy. Cancer 51:1209, 1983.

19. Gumerlock MK, Neuwelt EA: The effects of anesthesia on osmotic blood-brain barrier disruption. Neurosurg 26(2): 268-277, 1990.

20. Hardebo JE, Nilsson B: Hemodynamic changes in brain caused by local infusion of hyperosmolar solutions, in particular relation to blood-brain barrier opening. Brain Res 181:49-59, 1980.

21. Houthoff HJ, Go KG, Gerrits PO: The mechanisms of blood-brain barrier impairment by hyperosmolar perfusion: An electron cytochemical study comparing exogenous HRP and endogenous antibody to HRP as tracers. Acta Neuropathol (Berl) 56:99-112, 1982.

22. Neuwelt EA, Barnett PA: Blood-brain barrier disruption in the treatment of brain tumors: Animal studies. In Neuwelt EA (ed): Implications of the Blood-Brain Barrier and Its Manipulation. Volume 2 Clinical Aspects. Plenum Publishing Corporation, New York, NY, 1989, pp. 107-192.

23. Gumerlock MK, Belshe BD, Watts C: Chemotherapy with osmotic blood-brain barrier disruption in the treatment of high grade malignant gliomas. Submitted to J Neuro-Oncol, 1990.

24. Hawkins RA, Mans AM, Biebuyck JF: Amino acid supply to individual cerebral structures in awake and anesthetized rats. Am J Physiol 242:El-Ell, 1982.

THE BIODISTRIBUTION OF BORON IN CANINE SPONTANEOUS

INTRACRANIAL TUMORS FOLLOWING BOROCAPTATE SODIUM INFUSION

S. L. Kraft, P. R. Gavin, C. E. DeHaan, C. W. Leathers,[1]
W. F. Bauer,[2] and R. V. Dorn III[2,3]

[1]College of Veterinary Medicine and Surgery, Washington State
University, Pullman, WA   99164-6610
[2]INEL/BNCT Research Program, Idaho National Engineering
Laboratory, Idaho Falls, ID   83415-3519
[3]Mountain States Tumor Institute, Boise, ID   83712-6297

INTRODUCTION

Dogs with naturally-occurring, intracranial tumors were chosen as a
model for evaluating the pharmacokinetics and biodistribution of boron
using a single dose, intravenous administration of borocaptate sodium
($Na_2B_{12}H_{11}SH$ or BSH). Biologic variability was high with this model because
of differences in tumor type, stage, location, and size. However, the
natural behavior of these tumors provides results with a spectrum similar
to that of actual treatment conditions. The relatively large size of the
subject permitted extensive sampling of tumor, peritumor, and normal
tissues for boron analysis. The results from these biodistribution
studies have been applied toward related studies on boron neutron capture
therapy (BNCT), including canine dose tolerance studies and BNCT of canine
intracranial tumors.

MATERIALS AND METHODS

Dogs with naturally-occurring, intracranial tumors were obtained
through regional veterinary practitioners. Evaluation of tumor-bearing
dogs included complete blood count, serum biochemical profile, urinalysis,
and cerebrospinal fluid analysis. Diagnosis of intracranial tumors was
based on results of pre- and postcontrast magnetic resonance (MR) imaging
and computed tomography (CT) of the brain. Contrast media were intravenous gadolinium-DTPA and iothalamate meglumine, respectively.

The natural isotopic ratio (80% [11]B, 20% [10]B) of BSH (Callery Chemical
Company, Pittsburgh, PA) was administered intravenously at 10 (one dog),
30 (two dogs), or 55 mg boron/kg body weight (22 dogs), in 11 ml 0.9%
saline/kg body weight at a rate of 1 mg/kg-min[-1].

Serial venous blood and urine samples were obtained during and
following infusion. Euthanasia by an intravenous overdose of barbiturate
was performed two, six, or twelve hours following the end of BSH infusion.
Multiple samples of tumor, peritumor tissue (brain adjacent to grossly
visible tumor edges), standard regions of normal brain, and normal tissues
were obtained for boron and histologic analyses. Total boron (a summation
of [10]B and [11]B) concentrations for serum and tissues were derived by
inductively coupled plasma-atomic emission spectroscopy (ICP-AES).[(1)]

Size and number of tumor and peritumor samples were dictated by the
sensitivity of the boron analysis. Initial studies with dogs sampled at
12 hours postinfusion required 1-gram sample sizes. The higher tissue

boron concentrations found at 6-hour postinfusion allowed a reduction in sample size to 0.5 gram, and more recent increases in sensitivity permit analysis of 0.1-gram samples with at least 0.8 µg boron/g.

Region of interest analysis on CT images from six dogs sampled two hours post-BSH infusion was used to measure pre- and postcontrast CT density of intracranial tumors, and a contrast index value was calculated ((postcontrast tumor density - precontrast tumor density) ÷ (precontrast tumor density)). Tumor contrast index was then related to tumor boron concentration for each dog.

RESULTS

Twenty-five (25) dogs with intracranial tumors were sampled as shown in Figure 1 (graph excludes three dogs with diffuse astrocytomas). Extra-axial tumors, lacking a blood-brain-barrier, generally had higher boron concentrations than intra-axial tumors. Diffuse astrocytomas in three dogs had the same boron concentrations as normal brain. A positive relationship of boron concentration with contrast enhancement was observed (Figure 2). Mean tumor-boron concentrations were less than blood and declined at a similar rate. Tumor-to-blood boron concentration ratios were similar at all time periods, averaging 0.49 ± 0.3 SD. Normal brain had consistently low boron concentrations. Mean tumor-to-normal brain ratios were 8.6 ± 4.3 at two hours (n=10), 8.0 ± 4.5 at six hours (n=6), and 4.0 ± 1.9 at twelve hours (n=6). Peritumor boron concentrations were highly variable, but were greater than that of normal brain in half the dogs sampled.

DISCUSSION

Tumor-boron concentrations were in a range predicted to be adequate for tumor control using an epithermal beam for about six hours after BSH infusion.[2] The decline in mean tumor-boron concentration following infusion suggests that strong binding of boron to tumor tissue did not occur. This will be investigated further with temporal monitoring of tumor-boron uptake and decline using boron spectroscopy and imaging.[3]

Tumor-boron concentrations were associated with blood-brain-barrier integrity, resulting in a positive relationship with contrast enhancement. This represents a determinant of individual tumor-boron uptake, and may serve as a screening tool for identifying patients who may benefit the most from BNCT.

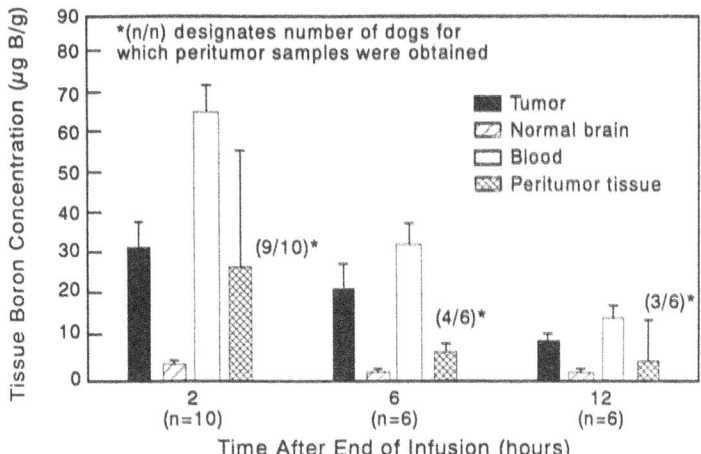

Figure 1. Boron concentrations of tumor-related tissues after five BSH infusions (n = number of dogs, n/n = number of dogs in which peritumor tissue was sampled).

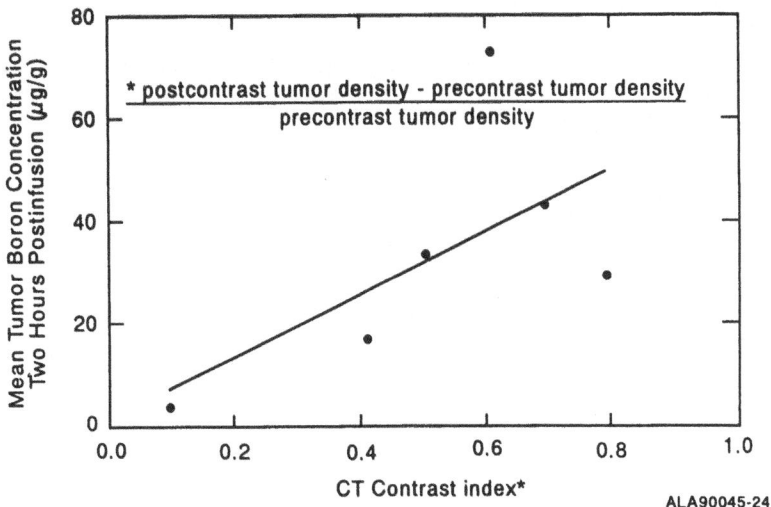

Figure 2. Relationship of tumor-boron concentration (μg boron/g) two hours post-BSH infusion with an index of contrast enhancement (n = 6).

The low boron concentration of normal brain is consistent with exclusion of boron by a normal blood-brain-barrier, indicating the potential dose sparing of normal brain parenchyma. The dose limitations imposed by the low tumor-to-blood ratios, which were almost always less than one, will depend upon the degree of geometric sparing of vascular endothelium.[4]

The elevated boron concentrations found in half of the dogs indicates the potential for affecting nests of invading tumor cells at tumor margins. In addition, peripheral neoplastic cells should be more susceptible than the tumor bulk to the low linear energy transfer (LET) radiation also produced during BNCT because of more normal oxygenation in marginal areas.

REFERENCES

1. Bauer, W. F., D. A. Johnson, S. M. Steele, K. Messick, D. L. Miller, and W. A. Propp, "Gross Boron Determination in Biological Samples by Inductively Coupled Plasma-Atomic Emission Spectroscopy," <u>Strahlen-therapie und Onkologie 165:</u> (2/3) 176-179 (February/March 1989).

2. Fairchild, R. G. and V. P. Bond, "Current Status of ^{10}B-Neutron Capture Therapy: Enhancement of Tumor Dose via Beam Filtration and Dose Rate, and the Effects of These Parameters on Minimum Boron Content: A Theoretical Evaluation," <u>Int. J. Radiat. Oncol. Biol. Phys. 11:</u> 831-840 (1985).

3. Bradshaw, K. M., T. L. Richards, and S. L. Kraft, "*In-Vivo* Chemical Shift Imaging of Canine Brain Tumors After Injection of $Na_2B_{12}H_{11}SH$," <u>Proceedings of Society of Magnetic Resonance in Medicine, Amsterdam, The Netherlands,</u> (August 1990).

4. Gabel, D., S. Foster, and R. G. Fairchild, "The Monte Carlo Simulation of the Biological Effect of the ^{10}B$(n,\alpha)^7$Li Reaction in Cells and Tissue and Its Implication for Boron Neutron Capture Therapy," <u>Radiation Research 111:</u> 14-25 (1987).

540

REGIONAL AND TOTAL BODY DOSE FOLLOWING BNCT EPITHERMAL HEAD IRRADIATION:

BIOLOGIC AND DOSIMETRIC EVALUATION

P.R. Gavin,[1] C.E. DeHaan,[1] S.L. Kraft,[1] Y.D. Harker,[1] P.D. Randolph,[1] F.J. Wheeler[2]

[1]Veterinary Clinical Medicine & Surgery, Washington State University, Pullman WA
[2]Idaho National Engineering Laboratory, Idaho Falls, ID

INTRODUCTION

Normal laboratory dogs received epithermal-neutron irradiation to the right cerebrum via a dorsal portal using a 5x10 cm incident field. The Brookhaven Medical Research Reactor (BMRR) power was 3 MW. Significant regional and total body radiation effects were noted. The reactions were of sufficient magnitude to reveal the need for additional shielding or other efforts to reduce these effects.

METHODS

Thirteen dogs were divided into 5 groups and given a total peak physical blood dose of 0-60 Gy with a mean blood-boron concentration of approximately 50 ppm. The boron compound was borocaptate sodium ($Na_2B_{12}H_{11}SH$ or BSH) administered intravenously at a dosage of 50 mg B/kg body weight in physiologic saline solution (11 ml/kg) at a rate of 1 mg B/minute.

Ten other dogs were given total peak physical doses of 10-15 Gy of epithermal irradiation alone. All dogs received systemic corticosteroid prior to irradiation (dexamethasone sodium phosphate 1 mg/kg intravenously). During irradiation, dosimeters (thermoluminescent and copper-gold alloy wire) were placed at varying locations on the dog, including the skin over the eyes, thyroid, thoracic spline, heart, and testicles. The dogs were placed in right lateral recumbency and the center of the incident radiation field on the right skull region was 1 cm from the exterior face of the beam delimiter and the dogs' bodies were covered with a sheet of Boroflex™.

Physical examinations, including complete blood counts and serum blood chemistries, were performed prior to irradiation several times in the initial weeks at 6 and 12 months postirradiation. Photographs of the dogs were obtained weekly.

RESULTS

Biologic

Changes observed in the hair and skin of the head and neck region indicated a superficial regional radiation much larger in size than the incident beam, and extended greater than 5 cm from the incident field. Observations were hair and skin depigmentation, epilation, and dry and moist desquamation. The severiy of the change was directly related to the peak radiation dose. When the radiation dose exceeded the skin tolerance, the area corresponding to the incident beam had dermal necrosis. The regional damage outside of the incident beam prevented successful skin grafts to the area.

Abnormalities were observed in the peripheral blood counts. The blood changes consisted of a transient leucopenia, predominately a lymphopenia (Figure 1). A thrombocytopenia occurred in 2 dogs in the 10-Gy epithermal only group and 3 dogs in the 15-Gy group. The thrombocyte counts ranged from 37 $\times$ 10^3/mm^3 to 90 $\times$ 10^3/mm^3 (normal range 100 $\times$ 10^3 to 250 $\times$ 10^3/mm^3). The thrombocytopenia generally occurred by day 8 postirradiation and persisted for about one week.

Dosimetric

Measured thermal-neutron fluences and gamma doses are presented in Table 1 for three dogs with boron and five dogs with no boron. Total scalp dose calculated for the boron dogs was nominally 1600 cGy, while that for the nonboron dogs was nominally 950 cGy. Total dose calculated at the central nervous system peak, was nominally 2700 cGy for the boron dogs and 1100 cGy for the nonboron dogs.

There was significant variation in measured dose for the different dogs. This is because of animal positioning, dosimeter placement, and sheilding. The boron dogs were irradiated with only a beam delimiter (25x25x4-cm thick) in place, while the nonboron dogs were irradiated with additional shielding placed at the wall.

DISCUSSION

Future irradiations will be performed with even more shielding at the wall and around the animal. Methods to reduce the regional and total body radiation include 1) increase the boron concentration during irradiation to decrease the relative hydrogen capture dose, 2) line the reactor wall with lithium carbonate to absorb neutron leakage, 3) utilize a flexible blanket containing lithium instead of boron, or 4) provide a collimated beam.

The major contributors to the regional and total body radiation effects were: 1) An isotropic beam, increasing the radiation scattered outside the incident field, 2) neutron leakage through the reactor wall outside of the beamport region, and 3) induced gamma radiation (boron and hydrogen capture).

The variations observed between dogs in each group in Table I were probably due to minor variation in patient positioning and dosimeter placement. The major variable between the two groups was the addition

Table 1. Measured Thermal-Neutron Fluence and Gamma Dose.

Location	Dogs with 45-60 ppm [10]B Thermal Fluence (n/cm^2)	Gamma Dose (cGy)	Dogs with no [10]B Thermal Fluence (n/cm^2)	Gamma Dose (cGy)
Top of skull			1.4E12 – 2.1E12	400 – 493
Eyes	1.1E12 – 4.7E12	129 – 165	3.8E11 – 5.5E11	249 – 332
Rear of skull	1.4E11 – 4.6E12	170 – 209	3.8E11 – 8.5E11	311 – 374
Spine at shldr	1.3E12 – 1.7E12	193 – 218	5.5E10 – 1.4E11	233 – 322
Trachea	2.0E12 – 4.1E12	176 – 230	7.2E11 – 1.3E12	307 – 358
External thyroid	3.8E11 – 5.4E11	98 – 143	5.9E10 – 1.2E11	179 – 202
Chest at heart	7.4E10 – 8.6E10	51 – 69	6.0E09 – 1.2E10	79 – 101
Testicle	1.5E10 – 3.4E10	15 – 17	2.4E09 – 4.1E09	24 – 38
Irradiation Time (MW-min)	222 – 270		470	

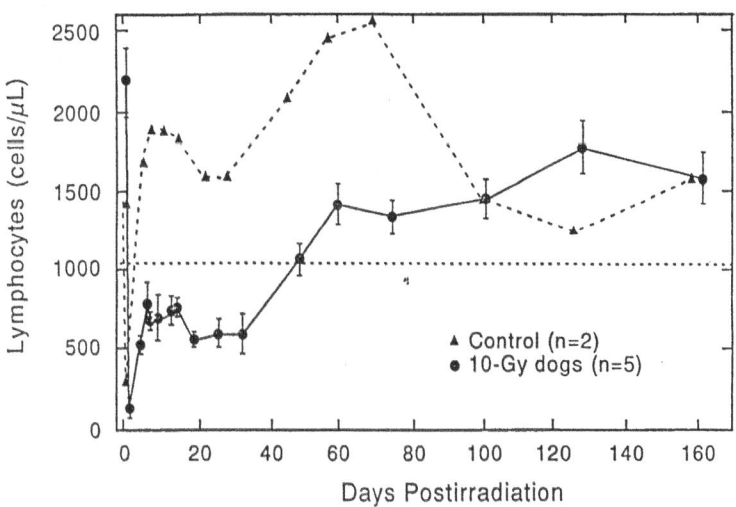

Figure 1. Average lymphocyte counts for dogs irradiated at 10 Gy (±SEM)

543

of lithium carbonate around the beam delimiter. This added shielding had a dramatic influence on the external thermal neutron flux. The dogs irradiated after the shielding was in place (dogs with no ^{10}B) had about twice the MW-min but less total thermal neutron fluence than dogs irradiated prior to the shielding modification. The influence on the external gamma dose was not so dramatic since the primary gamma source was from internal hydrogen capture caused by incident epithermal neutrons and the incident beam did not change between groups.

The regional and total body effects were not of a dose-limiting tolerance nature; however, the changes had clinical significance. The changes observed in the skin of the head outside of the incident field precluded typical skin grafting procedures when dermal necrosis occurred in the primary field.

The circulating lymphocyte depression was probably due to a combination of irradiation of blood flowing through the head in the primary field and total body effect. Obviously, the immediate depression was due to steroid administration. This degree of depression could indicate immune depression that may be of more significance in cancer patients. The platelet depression was not severe enough to cause spontaneous hemorrhage in a normal dog; however, surgery or other causes of hemorrhage could have been complicated by the degree of thrombocytopenia noted. Additional shielding placed on the wall near the beam caused a very substantial reduction in body dose. Even more shielding has become available and installed since the above-mentioned irradiations. There are significant variations in measured neutron fluxes and gamma doses because of animal positioning and local shielding placement.

BIODISTRIBUTION OF BORON SULFHYDRYL (BSH) IN HUMANS:

A QUALITY CONTROL OF ANALYTICAL METHODS[*]

G. Stragliotto[1], P. Zbinden[2], O. Pettersson[3], and H. Fankhauser[1]

[1]Department of Neurosurgery, CHUV, 1011 Lausanne, Switzerland
[2]Institute of Analytical Chemistry, University of Lausanne
1005 Lausanne, Switzerland
[3]Department of Radiation Sciences, University of Uppsala
751-21 Uppsala, Sweden

INTRODUCTION

Current methods for quantitative determination of boron in biological tissues include Inducticely Coupled Plasma-Atomic Emission Spectroscopy (ICP-AES) and Quantitative Neutron Capture Radiography (QNCR). These sophisticated techniques measure independent physical properties. Precise values of B-10 concentrations are reported in literature, even in the sub-ppm range. Nevertheless, convincing data on calibration curves and quality control are lacking. Furthermore, there are no reports on direct comparison of ICP-AES and QNCR. In order to obtain reliable data, we analyzed our specimens - whenever available - by both methods.

METHODS

Various tissue samples from 30 brain tumour patients injected with 10 mg/kg wt BSH were analyzed. Solid tissues and liquids were quick frozen; blood plasma was stored separately from sediment. Freeze-dried tissue sections of varying thicknesses (10-50 μm) were exposed on Kodak LR115 films to a neutron fluence of 5×10^{12} n cm^{-2} and 1×10^{13} n cm^{-2} (Studsvik-Reactor, Sweden). 0.5 μl droplets of liquids (plasma, urine, CSF) were dried on films and irradiated the same way. Liver homogenates and albumin solutions, supplemented with known amounts of boron, served as standards. Otherwise, liquid and solid samples were digested in $HNO_3 + H_2O_2$ in pressure resistent Teflon-bombs [1], then analyzed by ICP-AES (Perkin-Elmer 6000).

Standard calibration curves for tissue sections and droplets were obtained for 2 neutron fluences. Adjacent tissue sections were processed on different films and final quantifications compared. Irradiated films were etched according to the method of Gabel [2], and analyzed by automatic densitometry or by manual track counting.

---

*This work has been supported by the Fonds National de la Recherche Scientifique, the Ligue Suisse contre le Cancer, the Ligue Vaudoise contre le Cancer, and the Commission of the European Communities.

RESULTS

Calibration curves obtained with liquids and tissue standards ranged from 0.01 to 100 ppm B. Comparative curves were obtained with ICP-AES or QNCR for a cross calibration. A correlation factor of 1.0 was obtained by ICP-AES in comparison to the 0.93 factor obtained with the same specimen analyzed by QNCR automatic track analysis. Liquid standard curves by QNCR showed a correlation of 0.98 between predicted and measured track density. Identical tissue standards cut to increasing thickness yelded increasing track density, but the track density was stabilized at 50 microns thickness and over.

A number of intracerebral tumours were anlyzed both by ICP-AES and QNCR, these results are shown in table 1. Boron quantification found by QNCR ranged from an average of 2.6 to 4.2 ppm, and were constantly above the average of 2.2 ppm obtained by ICP-AES. These higher QNCR concentration represent an overestimation of 10-50% as compared to ICP-AES. Tissue samples were from the same location and of same size (1 x 1 cm cut area). Tumour to blood ratio was calculated using concentrations obtained only by ICP-AES.

Table 1. Details for Malignant Intracerebral Tumours analyzed by ICP-AES and QNCR.

Tumour	ICP-AES (ppm)	QNCR (ppm)	Blood (whole) (ppm)	Ratio* T/B	Time after injection (hrs)
Glioblastoma	1	2-3	0.6	> 1.5	17
Metastasis	4	4-5	1	> 1.5	19
Metastasis	3	3-6	1.5	> 1.5	17
Glioblastoma	0.7	1-3.5	3.1	< 1	17
Glioblastoma	2.7	3.5	1.3	> 1.5	23
Oligodendrogl.	0.2	1-1.5	1	< 1	27
Glioblastoma	2.2	2.5-5	1.6	> 1.5	18
Astrocytoma	0.3	0.3-1	0.5	< 1	19
Glioblastoma	3.9	5-7	3	> 1	12
Glioblastoma	3	3.5-8	3	= 1	13
Glioblastoma	7.5	5-7.5	2.6	> 1.5	23
Glioblastoma	1.3	1.5-2	1.3	= 1	19
Medulloblast.	1	1.5	1	= 1	18

*both values from ICP-AES

Image analysis of QNCR films yielded two kinds of standard calibrations depending whether automatic analyzer or manual counting was used. The number of tracks increased proportionally to the B density, yielding a linear segment from 0.3 up to 20 ppm B, thereafter, tracks became too dense and coalescent. Image analyzer showed a linear segment above 1-1.5 ppm up to 100 ppm B. Increasing the neutron fluence shifts the curve upwards, with no noticeable distorsion added; there is no gain in sensitivity of the useful segment.

DISCUSSION

In this work, we critically compared the quantitative techniques for low amounts of B in tissues, available in our laboratory. QNCR reproduces ideally a therapy procedure; in our initial experience we found inconstant and inconsistent values using this method without a number of preliminary studies. In our view, the factors influencing the final result are numerous. Only freeze-dried slices can be used, since conventional histological processing led to complete loss of B. The freezing process introduces artifacts, which cannot be completely predicted by current material. Small size tissue biopsies will inevitably crack, the amount of water evaporation will vary from one tissue to another. Our calibration using liquid and solid tissues show a lesser confident curve in the latter; 50 microns-thick sections minimize deformation and variations of water loss, but with this thickness, advantage of direct histologic correlation is largely lost. Processing of the irradiated films must be standardized by the user. The quantitative analysis of the films finally relies upon a detailed, reproducible calibration method. We did not find significant difference using brain or liver homogenates as tissue standards. Difficulties resulted mainly from the analytical technique choosed. Manual track count is more precise at low B concentration up to 10-20 ppm, but is slow and subjective. Automatic densitometry is highly influenced by film processing and is inprecise at low B concentration with which we had dealt with; however it is useful in concentration above 1ppm.

ICP-AES has been used recently for B detection in liquid samples. Preparation requires only digestion of solid tissue; with our specimen we needed at least 200 mg tissue (w/w) in order to overcome the detection threshold. Repeated measurements were easily reproducible. A series of samples processed and analyzed in 2 laboratories yielded maximal variations of 5-10% in tissue B concentration. Quantitative comparison of both methods yielded a constant overestimation by 15-50% of results obtained in tumour tissues with QNCR as compared to ICP-AES. Liquid specimen were also measured comparatively in selected cases; paradoxically, QNCR was relatively lower than ICP-AES. Significant variation not related to histologic features characterizes concentrations measured by QNCR. In the data shown, this variation was as high as 50%.

These considerations prompted us to consider QNCR as a quantitative technique only with caution However, we found it irreplaceable when the amount of tissue available was very small, and when correlation with histological features are of primordial importance. In our view, QNCR is not suitable for liquids.

REFERENCES

1.   Bauer WF, Johnson DA, Steele et al.: Gross boron determination in biological samples by inductively coupled plasma atomic emission spectroscopy. Strahlenther Onkol 165 :176-179, 1989

2.   Gabel D, Holstein H and Larson B : Quantitative neutron capture radiography for studying the biodistribution of tumor-seeking boron-containing compounds. Cancer Res 47:5451-5454, 1987

PHARMACOKINETICS OF BORON SULFHYDRYL (BSH) IN PATIENTS

WITH INTRACRANIAL TUMOURS *

G. Stragliotto[1], A. Munafo[2], J. Biollaz[2], and H. Fankhauser[1]

[1]Department of Neurosurgery, CHUV, 1011 Lausanne, Switzerland
[2]Division of Clinical Pharmacology, CHUV, 1011 Lausanne, Switzerland

INTRODUCTION

One prerequisite for successful BNCT is the determination of B-10 blood levels at the time of neutron irradiation, since the pharmacokinetics of BSH influences the optimal timing between injection of the boron compound and radiation. We collected extensive pharmacokinetic data from patients undergoing operation for intracranial tumours. This investigation is the corollary of the boron distribution study in tissues. We will also discuss these findings in perspective of comparable published studies.

METHODS

Four patients underwent a pharmacokinetic study over 7 days, consisting of repeated blood sampling and urine collection. BSH (95% B-10 enriched $Na_2B_{12}H_{10}SH$, Callery Chemicals, Pittsburg) at the dose of 10 mg/kg wt (=5 mg B/kg) was given as a constant rate 1 hour i.v. infusion. In a 5th patient, the dose was 10 mg B/kg. Blood was centrifuged, and plasma samples were kept frozen until analysis. Total urine collection (without catheter) was started simultaneously, divided into periods of 12 hours for the first day, and 24 hour thereafter. Laboratory values for haematology, electrolytes, creatinine and liver enzymes were obtained daily. Aliquots (0.5 g), diluted 10 times in de-ionised water, were analyzed in triplicates by Inductively Coupled Plasma-Atomic Emission Spectroscopy (ICP-AES). Half-lives and V_z were calculated by fitting a 3 exponential after zero-order input model to the data, by non-linear extended least square regression (Siphar). Clearance , V_{ss} and MRT were calculated by the classic model-independent method (trapezoidal rule for AUC).

RESULTS

Peak plasma values ranged from 30 to 50 $\mu g/g$ (ppm) for the 5 mg/kg dose, and 250 ppm for the higher dose patient, which correlates with the administered amount of 216-441 mg B. The data were best described (Akaike information criterion) by a 3 exponential-model, with $T_{1/2}$ alpha of 1.3 ($\pm$ 1.0), beta of 8.0 ($\pm$ 3.7) and gamma of 55.3 ($\pm$ 26.6) hours. V_z and Vss averaged 0.91 ($\pm$ 0.48) L/kg and 0.32 ($\pm$ 0.18) L/kg, respectively, and CL was 0.21 ($\pm$ 0.08) ml/min/kg. MRT averaged 29.9 ($\pm$ 18.6) hours. The detailed values are reported in table 1.

---

*This work has been supported by the Fonds National de la Recherche Scientifique, the Ligue Suisse contre le Cancer, the Ligue Vaudoise contre le Cancer, and the Commission of the European Communities.

Table 1

dose (mg B)	T1/2 (h)	MRT (h)	V_z (L/kg)	V_{ss} (L/kg)	CL (g/min/kg)
243	2.6 14.1 82.4	54.5	0.76	0.40	0.107
216	1.8 7.4 78.2	40	1.72	0.61	0.255
389	0.5 6.6 32.3	14.2	0.823	0.251	0.294
318	1.2 7.8 60.3	31.6	0.78	0.28	0.149
441	0.3 4.0 23.5	9.2	0.465	0.127	0.229

In urine, B excretion could be measured at least up to the 4th day after infusion. The total eliminated B during this period reached 50% of the injected dose in 2 patients, and 80 % of injected dose in 2 other.

DISCUSSION

Despite variable peak values in plasma at the end of BSH infusion, which did not correlate to tumour type, age, sex or weight, the decay of B-10 in all 5 patients appeared relatively similar. The second and third half-lives observed in our study are very close to those reported in the largest available pharmacokinetic study to date (ref. 1) in 12 patients receiving 1-34 mg B /kg intracarotid. However, the authors did not observe the very rapid distribution phase reported here, possibly because of the small number of samples in the early decay (about six points in the first 10 hours). In most patients, B was detected up to 8 days after the end of the infusion, even with our relatively low doses (detection limit : 0.1 ppm). Only in one patient with extensive intraoperative bleeding, could B no longer be detectable after 72 hours. In this latter patient, the fit to a 3 exponential-model was not as obvious as for the remaining four. Systemic clearance was low (13.1±7 g/min) and highly variable among the patients.
Despite a very high plasma protein binding - described by Sweet - the volume of distribution of B is relatively important. Together with the difference between the volume in the terminal phase V_z and V_{ss}, this could indicate a high affinity, slow releasing deep compartment. However, it should be emphasized that the reliability of V_z is highly dependent on the accuracy and precision of the later levels, and so upon the detection level and the length of sampling.
In 40 patients undergoing a biodistribution study (data not shown), B levels observed at discrete sampling times seem coherent with the pharmacokinetics in the five patients described here. We intend to pursue these studies at higher doses and repeated administration.

REFERENCE

1.   Sweet WH, Messer JR, Hatanaka H: Supplementary pharmacological study between 1972 and 1977 on purified mercaptoundecahydrododecaborate, in Hatanaka H (ed): Boron Neutron Capture Therapy for Tumours. Niigata, Japan, Nishimura, 1986, pp 59-76

BIODISTRIBUTION OF BORON SULFHYDRYL (BSH) IN PATIENTS WITH

INTRACRANIAL TUMORS*

Giuseppe Stragliotto, Heinz Fankhauser

Department of Neurosurgery
CHUV
CH-1011 Lausanne, Switzerland

INTRODUCTION

The therapeutic as well as the undesired effects of Boron Neutron Capture Therapy (BNCT) largely depends upon the absolute and relative ^{10}B concentrations in tumors and in normal tissues and body fluids. Our present work on BSH in patients with intracranial neoplasms has been prompted by crucial questions regarding : tumor levels, tumor-to-normal tissue ratios, variations between different tumors, variations inside the same tumor, correlation between histology and ^{10}B levels, time course of BSH uptake, pharmacokinetics of BSH, Temptative answers to some of these questions have been worked out for animals and experimental animal tumor models. For humans, Hatanaka et al. [2] have published boron concentrations measured at the time of re-operation and actual BNCT in 60 patients. Eleven to 17 hrs after intra-arterial or intravenous administration of 40 to 80 mg of $^{10}B/kg$ as BSH, 26 glioblastoma patients yielded a median ^{10}B concentration in the tumor of approximately 15 ppm and a median tumor-to-blood ratio of 1.1. In 13 cases of anaplastic astrocytomas the values were comparable with a median tumor concentration of approximately 22 ppm and a tumor-to-blood ratio of 1.4. In 4 cases of astrocytomas grade I-II, the median concentration dropped to around 5 ppm and the tumor-to-blood ratio remained always below 0.6. Beside Hatanaka's findings, the literature contains only anecdotal data on the situation in humans [1,4,5]. Finkel et al. [1] infused a patient over 25 hrs with 13.5 mg of ^{10}B as BSH 1 day before death and found tumor concentrations at necropsy of 4.5 to 6 ppm when measured with Quantitative Neutron Capture Radiography (QNCR). The same tumor analyzed with prompt gamma technique seemed to contain only 1.2 to 2.7 ppm. This latter observation attracts attention to the fact that analytical methods for boron are not routine procedures, especially when solid tissues are concerned. Definition of their precision and dynamic range and constant quality control retains high priority in this kind of work.

We have been using QNCR and Inductively Coupled Plasma-Atomic Emission Spectroscopy (ICP-AES) for tissue analysis. Our extensive work on validation of these methods and cross calibration, as well as pharmacokinetic data in a few patients are presented elsewhere in this volume. This paper reports the findings in 28 patients with intracranial tumors.

MATERIALS AND METHODS

Patients presenting with a likely intracranial neoplasm on Computed Tomography or Magnetic Resonance Imaging and scheduled for craniotomy gave their informed consent to participation in this study. They were infused intravenously over 1 hour with an intended amount of 10 mg of 95% ^{10}B enriched BSH/kg (Callery Chemical, Pittsburgh), diluted to a total of 50 ml. The infused dose of ^{10}B amounts to approximately 5 mg /kg. During craniotomy some 12 to 24 hrs later, tumor tissue, blood, and urine were collected in all cases. Additional normal tissues, including skin, periosteum, muscle, bone, dura, peritumoral normal brain, and CSF were obtained whenever possible. Solid tissues were immediately dip frozen in isopenthane and stored at -80° C. Blood was centrifugated and the plasma, urine, CSF and cyst fluids were stored at -80° C. Boron assessment was usually performed with ICP-AES. Some small samples unsuitable for this method were analyzed with QNCR. The technical details of these methods are described elsewhere in this volume [3]. For most tumors and some normal tissues, several fragments were analyzed and the mean concentration is given.

The patients included in this series harbored various intracranial neoplasms (table 1). For practical reasons they are subdivided into high grade intracerebral (13 patients), low grade intracerebral (5 patients), and low grade extracerebral tumors (11 cases). One patient with an ischemic infarct was excluded. The interval between injection and tissue harvesting was approximately 12, 18, or 24 h.

RESULTS

Table 1 lists the detailed results of ^{10}B analysis of tumor and various tissues in 29 patients and the approximate interval between infusion of BSH and tissue harvesting.

Tables 2, 3, and 4 summarize the results according to the histological category of the tumor and the approximate interval between infusion of BSH and tissue harvesting.

In the course of major intracranial operations it was not possible to take all the samples at exactly the same time, except for tumor and blood. The exact moment of tissue recovery has been recorded for each specimen. For the purpose of tables 1 to 5, this time interval has been rounded to ± 3 hrs, in order to get 3 categories analyzed around 12, 18 and 24 hrs after BSH infusion.

Heterogeneity of ^{10}B levels inside a single tumor was accounted for by taking average values when several samples had been analyzed. In some cases this heterogeneity was investigated further. The following are typical examples. In one glioblastoma case, 4 different areas of the same tumor were collected within the same hour and showed 9.5, 9, 6, and 4 ppm of B. Two blood samples analyzed at the beginning of this hour and 40 minutes later showed levels of 9.5 and 6 ppm.

In a second glioblastoma case 4 different areas collected within 1 hour gave values of 1, 3.5, 2, and 1 ppm. Three blood samples during the same hour each time contained 3 ppm of ^{10}B.

In a low grade astrocytoma case 3 specimen yielded 2, 0.5, and 2 ppm whereas 2 blood values remained at 2.5 ppm.

Table 1. ^{10}B concentrations in tumor and normal tissues and fluids of 29 Patients (ppm)

Histology	Time#	T	B	Sk	Du	Mu	Bo	No	Cs	Cf
1 Glioblastoma*	17	1	0.6	-	-	2	-	0.2	-	-
2 "	17	1	3.1	-	-	7	-	-	-	3.3
3 "	23	2.7	1.3	3	-	-	-	1	0.1	-
4 "	19	1.5	1.3	2.5	3	-	-	1	0.2	1.7
5 "	19	2.2	1.6	0.6	-	2	-	0.5	0.2	-
6 "	18	2.6	2.6	1	9	3	-	-	0	-
7 "	13	3.1	3	4.5	-	1	-	-	0.2	-
8 "	12	5	8.7	-	7	-	0.4	-	0.2	-
9 "	23	6	3	-	-	1.5	-	0.5	-	-
10 Medulloblastoma	18	1.1	1.3	-	-	1	-	0.3	0	-
11 "	18	2	1.5	6	-	2	-	-	-	-
12 Metastasis	17	3	1.5	-	-	-	0	0.3	0.2	-
13 "	19	4	1.5	1.7	6	3.1	-	0.1	-	-
14 Astrocytoma+	19	0.3	0.5	-	-	2	-	0.2	0	-
15 "	25	0.4	0.6	-	3	0.4	-	0.4	0	-
16 "	16	1.5	1.5	0.7	-	2	-	-	-	-
17 Oligodendroglioma	27	0.2	0.9	-	-	2.5	-	0.2	0.1	-
18 Hemangioblastoma	17	2	2.8	-	3	3	-	-	0	3
19 Meningioma	21	1.6	0.5	-	3	-	-	0.3	0.1	-
20 "	22	2	2.4	-	-	1.5	0	-	0.2	-
21 "	17	3	2.1	-	3.5	-	-	-	0.1	-
22 "	18	1	3.3	4	1.2	1	-	0.3	0.1	-
23 "	20	3	0.6	1.5	-	3	-	0.3	0.1	-
24 "	20	2.2	2.1	-	-	3.3	0.3	-	0.3	-
25 "	17	1.5	1.2	-	-	-	-	-	0	-
26 Schwannoma	18	1.2	1	-	3	-	-	-	0.1	-
27 "	19	2	1.6	-	4	-	-	-	0.2	-
28 "	12	7	7.7	4	-	3.5	-	-	0.3	-
29 Infarction	26	(1)	3.6	-	3	-	-	-	0.1	-

T = tumor, B = blood, Sk = skin, Du = dura, Mu = muscle, Bo = bone, No = normal brain, Cs = CSF, Cf = cyst fluid
#approximate interval between ^{10}B infusion and analysis (hrs)
*including anaplastic astrocytomas, +grades I and II

Table 2. ^{10}B concentrations and tumor-to-normal tissue ratios in 13 patients with high grade intracerebral tumors

		Time Interval		
		12 h	18 h	24 h
Maximum tumor levels (ppm)		5.0	4.0	6.0
Tumor/blood	> 1.5	0/2	7/9	2/2
	1 - 1.5	1/2	1/9	0/2
	< 1	1/2	1/9	0/2
Maximum brain level			1.0	1.0
Tumor/brain	> 2		6/6	2/2

Table 3. ^{10}B concentrations and tumor-to-normal tissue ratios in
5 patients with low grade intracerebral tumors

		Time Interval		
		12 h	18 h	24 h
Maximum tumor levels (ppm)			2.0	1.0
Tumor/blood	> 1.5		0/3	0/2
	1 - 1.5		0/3	1/2
	< 1		3/3	1/2
Maximum brain level			0.3	0.5
Tumor/brain	> 2		1/1	2/2

Table 4. ^{10}B concentrations and tumor-to-normal tissue ratios in
11 patients with low grade extracerebral tumors

		Time Interval		
		12 h	18 h	24 h
Maximum tumor levels (ppm)		8.0	3.0	3.5
Tumor/blood	> 1.5	0/2	3/7	0/2
	1 - 1.5	1/2	2/7	1/2
	< 1	1/2	2/7	1/2
Maximum brain level			0.3	
Tumor/brain	> 2		3/3	

Precise assessment of in vivo ^{10}B concentrations in tissues after parenteral administration of BSH encounters several obstacles. First of all, the amount of ^{10}B in the commercially available drug is not precisely defined due to water content which contributes up to 15% to the "dry" weight. Analytical problems further contribute to the uncertainty. In our experience, QNCR may give errors of 20 to 50%. When compared with our carefully established method of ICP-AES, QNCR constantly yields higher values. This stresses the importance to analyze tumor and blood by the same method in order to minimize wrongly elevated tumor-to-blood ratios.

Despite a considerable effort to optimize the methodology of ^{10}B determination, we still consider our results concerning solid tissues as approximate, especially those which had to be processed with QNCR due to small sample size. They need further validation.

The inclusion of intracranial tumors other than glioblastoma into this kind of study is justified by the fact that several intracerebral and extracerebral neoplasms, including benign forms, cannot or not always be totally extirpated during surgery and that there is usually no efficient alternative or adjuvant therapy. Furthermore, the exact histological diagnosis is often not known at inclusion into the study. Valuable information on normal tissue concentrations can be collected from any kind of patient.

Larger tumors analyzed for heterogeneity between several parts showed differences from one area to another. This heterogeneity was pronounced in high grade intracerebral, but not in low grade extracerebral tumors. Most significantly, tumor-to-blood ratios can vary from below to above 1 inside the same tumor. Heterogeneity was also present in low grade intracerebral tumors, but this is less significant since the absolute values were low, close to the background values of our methods.

^{10}B uptake in normal tissue was high in skin, muscle, periosteum and dura. When compared with tumor, the concentration was often similar, slightly above or below tumor values, without any systematic deviation, except for dura which tended to contain more ^{10}B than the corresponding high grade intracerebral or low grade extracerebral tumors. Cortical bone always contained less than 1 ppm and CSF always less than 0.3 ppm ^{10}B.

On the whole, BSH enters all tumors early, but initial tumor concentrations stay well below blood concentrations. Clearance from blood is slightly faster than from high grade intracerebral and some low grade extracerebral tumors. Between 15 and 18 hrs tumor-to-blood ratios rise above 1 in most high grade intracerebral tumors and Schwannomas. The best ratio nevertheless stays below 3.

Comparisons of our results with those of Hatanaka [2] are difficult, since the dose of BSH he used was 8 to 16 times higher than ours. On the other hand we have no detailed information about the performance of the chemical analysis method for boron as used by Hatanaka. In view of the problems encountered with QNCR and ICP-AES, comparison would be necessary. Hatanaka's patients were analyzed during re-operation. At that time the tumor bed may no longer have contained large amounts of actively growing tumor, but the blood-brain barrier might have been modified by the previous surgical manipulation. This situation comes of course closer to the one we have to deal with during actual BNCT. Median tumor-to-blood ratios in the two series are nevertheless comparable, although we did not observe ratios above 3, as has been the case in some of Hatanaka's patients. In many cases our findings are not as favorable as desired for BNCT. On the other hand, these bulk concentrations may not be relevant for the actual biological effect of BNCT which will depend to a large extend upon the micro-distribution of ^{10}B at the subcellular level. Theoretically, this is even true for low grade intracerebral tumors in which tumor-to-blood ratios were always below 1, supposing that ^{10}B may be selectively accumulated around or in isolated infiltrating astrocytoma cells. Our analysis of infiltrating astrocytomas with QNCR and histological correlation nevertheless did not show increased number of heavy particle tracks around these cells.

ACKNOWLEDGEMENTS

This work has been possible thanks to close collaboration with the Institute of Analytical Chemistry, University of Lausanne, Switzerland, the Studsvik Reactor, Sweden, the Division of Physical Biology in Uppsala, Sweden, the Department of Chemistry, University of Bremen, Germany, and the ECN in Petten, Holland.

REFERENCES

1.   Finkel GC, Poletti CE, Fairchild RG, Slatkin DN, Sweet WH: Distribution of ^{10}B after infusion of $Na_2{}^{10}B_{12}H_{11}SH$ into a patient with malignant astrocytoma: Implications for boron Neutron Capture Therapy. Neurosurgery 24: 6-11, 1989

2.   Hatanaka H, Amano K, Kanemitsu H, Ikeuchi I, Yoshizaki T: Boron uptake by human brain tumors and quality control of boron compounds, in Hatanaka H (ed): Boron-Neutron Capture Therapy for Tumors. Niigata, Japan, Nishimura, 1986, pp 77-106

3.   Stragliotto G, Zbinden P, Pettersson O, Fankhauser H: Biodistribution of boron sulfhydryl (BSH) in humans: A quality control of analytical methods. in this volume

4.   Sweet WH, Messer JR, Hatanaka H: Supplementary pharmacological study between 1972 and 1977 on purified mercaptoundecahydrododecaborate, in Hatanaka H (ed): Boron-Neutron Capture Therapy for Tumors. Niigata, Japan, Nishimura, 1986, pp 59-76

5.   Sweet WH: Medical aspects of boron-slow neutron capture therapy, in Fairchild RG, Bond VP (eds): Workshop on Neutron Capture Therapy. Upton, New York, Brookhaven National Laboratory, BNL-51994, 1986, pp 3-21

THE DISTRIBUTION OF BSH IN PATIENTS WITH MALIGNANT GLIOMA

Dietrich Haritz[1], Kurt Piscol[1] and Detlef Gabel[2]

[1] Department of Neurosurgery, Hospital St.-Jürgenstraße, Bremen, FRG
[2] Department of Chemistry, University of Bremen, Bremen, FRG

INTRODUCTION

One of the goals of the European Collaboration on Boron Neutron Capture Therapy is to treat gliomas, using $Na_2B_{12}H_{11}SH$ (BSH) as boron carrier. In order to treat these tumors with boron neutron capture therapy, it is necessary to accumulate sufficient amounts of boron in the tumor prior to irradiation, and at the same time ensure that healthy tissue unavoidably present in the neutron beam contains a minimal amount of boron. The concentration of boronated compounds in the tissues eventually exposed to the neutron beam is of utmost importance for the prediction of healthy tissue damage and tumor control. Within the European Collaboration, a study of the distribution of BSH has therefore been started.

In this study, detailed information about the possible toxicity of BSH will also be gathered.

We wish to report here on the distribution and pharmacokinetics of the first five patients.

PROTOCOL

For this study, a coordinated protocol has been established within the European Collaboration on Boron Neutron Capture Therapy. BSH is infused into patients during the course of 1 hour, and blood samples are taken at predetermined intervals. During the operation of the patients, tissue samples are obtained. These include: skin, muscle, bone, dura mater, galea, cerebrospinal fluid (CSF), normal brain and tumor tissue. Urine is collected.

In Bremen, the patients eligible to enter the study must have a preoperative diagnosis of a high-grade glioma. They are informed about the aim of the study and can participate on a voluntary basis, in accordance with the procedure authorized by the local Ethics Committee.

Patients with reduced liver, kidney, and cardio-vascular functions are excluded, as are those with major endocrinological disturbances.

The following clinical chemical parameters are among those measured prior to administration and following operation, in order to evaluate possible toxic effects of BSH: complete blood count and clotting, liver enzymes, creatinine, urea.

BSH is infused through the central venous catheter (placed there because of the needs of the scheduled operation), at a maximal concentration of 15 mg boron per kg body weight. The infusion lasts for one hour.

Blood is taken at the following intervals (post start of infusion) 5, 10, 15, 30 minutes, 1, 2, 4, 8, 12, 18, 24, 48, and 72 hours. Tissues are removed during the operation; it is aimed to get tissues at 3, 6, 12, 18, and 24 hours. Tissues are frozen rapidly.

BORON ANALYSIS

The concentration of boron in blood and tissues is measured by quantitative neutron capture radiography (QNCR) [1], that in urine and cerebrospinal fluid (CSF) by ICP-AES.

thickness of 50 μm. Sections are collected every 1 mm. Standards are prepared from chicken liver, calf brain, or human blood by adding known amounts of boric acid, and 50-μm sections are produced. The sections are mounted onto Kodak Pathé LR 115 Type 1 track detectors, and exposed to around $5 \cdot 10^{12}$ n cm^{-2} at the Studsvik Neutron Radiography facility. The detectors are etched at 60 °C in 10 % NaOH for around 50 minutes. The etched detectors are evaluated in an image analyzer, consisting of a microscope, a TV camera, a personal computer with appropriate hardware and software (Signum, München), and a TV monitor. Field sizes are 0.3 x 0.6 mm. With these conditions, boron-10 can be determined between around 0.5 and 200 ppm on the same film.

From the readings of the standards, a standard curve is constructed by fitting an exponential function to them. The sample readings are then converted to boron concentrations with a BASIC program.

Boron analysis by ICP-AES [2] was kindly carried out by V. Gregoire of the NKI Amsterdam at ECN Petten.

Precision of boron analysis by ICP-AES was found to be very good, with a standard deviation of less than 1 % of the mean. Precision of boron analysis by QNCR is inherently less good, with an estimated standard deviation of around 10-20 % of the mean. This less accurate precision stems from the small field size examined and artifacts from sectioning and freeze-drying of both samples and standards. Agreement between different types of tissue (blood, liver, brain) was, however, in the same range as the estimated standard deviation from the mean. Within the same margin, the results from QNCR agreed also with those from ICP-AES.

RESULTS

Results of the Toxicity Investigation

In none of the five patients that entered the study to date, could any measurable acute effects of the BSH administration be detected on cardio-vascular function, allergenic reaction, bone marrow depletion, and liver and kidney function.

Boron Distribution and Pharmacokinetics

Fig. 1 shows the boron concentrations in blood of three patients, normalized to an administered boron dose of 10 mg/kg.

For these patients, the boron decrease in blood after the end of the infusion follows a biphasic kinetics. The first component has a half time of around 10 hours, whereas the second shows a considerably longer half time (25 hours). From the limited observation time, the existence of still longer half times cannot be excluded. Differences between the patients were found both for half times and for distribution volumes.

The initial apparent distribution volume of BSH is considerably smaller than the total body water (which might be approximated to around 65 % of the total body weight). It is therefore probable that the compound distributes only into the plasma and interstitial spaces, at least during the first 24 hours. Boron is found in the urine already shortly after the beginning of the infusion. It is therefore unlikely that the second of the two half times corresponds to the elimination phase, and that the first half time would represent the distribution phase.

Boron concentration in healthy brain tissue is very low. Accumulation in the tumor is highly heterogeneous. Fig. 2 shows QNCR of tumor and brain tissue from patient VORM.

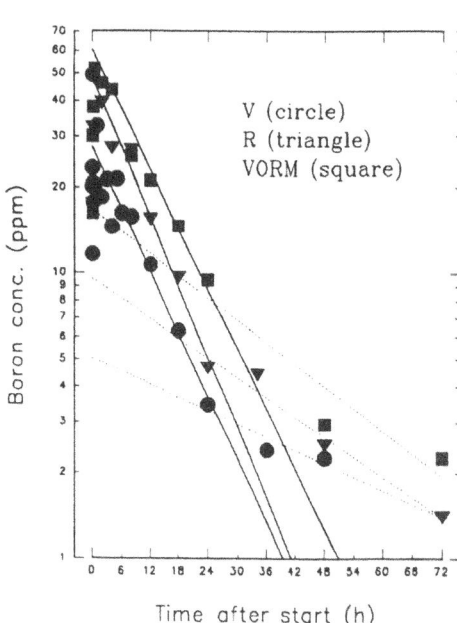

V (circle)
R (triangle)
VORM (square)

Time after start (h)

Fig. 1 Boron in blood of three patients. Solid lines are regression lines for t=1 to t=24 hours, dotted lines for t≥24 hours.

558

With the sections prepared, detailed histology is not possible. Therefore, it is not clear whether all tumor tissue accumulates boron, whether boron is present also in peritumoral edema, and whether local variations of boron concentrations reflect variations in uptake of similar tissue of local tissue type variations. These questions still await an experimentally feasible approach. Later experiments indicated that, by using a bone biopsy needle of 2.0 mm diameter, small samples can be obtained from the exposed surface of the tissue during microtomy. After fixation in formalin, these samples are well suited not only to determine the type of tissue, but actually to reconfirm the differential diagnosis.

Parts of the tumor tissue accumulate boron in concentrations greater than that in blood. Boron concentration in necrotic areas was found lower than that in adjacent tissue. It cannot yet be ascertained that the areas of brain and tumor tissue accumulating boron consist exclusively of tumor tissue, or whether any surrounding edema also contains boron.

For other tissues, boron concentration is low (bone, fat, cerebro-spinal fluid), or it reaches up to blood boron concentrations (skin, dura, galea). Here, care must be taken to remove excess blood from surgery by washing. This has been done only for patient RUP. In tissues from other patients, high boron concentrations were invariably associated with visible blood. Data for some tissues are compiled in Table 1.

Table 1

Summary of the first five patients

Patient	VORM	RUP	R	V	RK[a]
Operation time (h)	3	3	4.5	5.5	12
Diagnosis	G III-IV	G IV	Metastasis[b]	G IV	G IV
Sex,age,weight	M,61,81	F,55,75	M,71,66	M,50,74	F,70,70

Tissue	Boron concentration (ppm)				
Blood	30	12	32	12	74
Tumor (max)[d]	36	14	13	35	24
Brain	<1	<1	<1	<1	<1
Skin		<1			
Muscle		6			
Galea		4			
Bone	2	<1	1	3	5
CSF	<1	<1	.	<1	<1

Apparent Distribution Volume (% of body weight) for t=0

1st component	36%	24%	17%	21%	11%
2nd component	198%	277%	60%	95%	9%

$t_{1/2}{}^1 = 10.3 \pm 2.7$ hours[c] $t_{1/2}{}^2 = 25 \pm 8$ hours[c]

Footnotes to Table 1

a: Patient developed complications during operation and died within three days post operation.

b: Primary cancer: adenocarcinoma of the stomach.

c: Patient RK excluded from the average.

d: Delineation of tumor and surrounding edematous and healthy tissue could not be made; therefore, no minimal values for boron contents in tumor are given.

DISCUSSION

In this study, we showed that boron from BSH accumulates in brain tumor tissues. The boron concentrations are highly heterogeneous, with differences of one order of magnitude and more between adjacent parts separated by distances of a few millimeters and less. This again demonstrates the importance of boron determination with good spatial resolution.

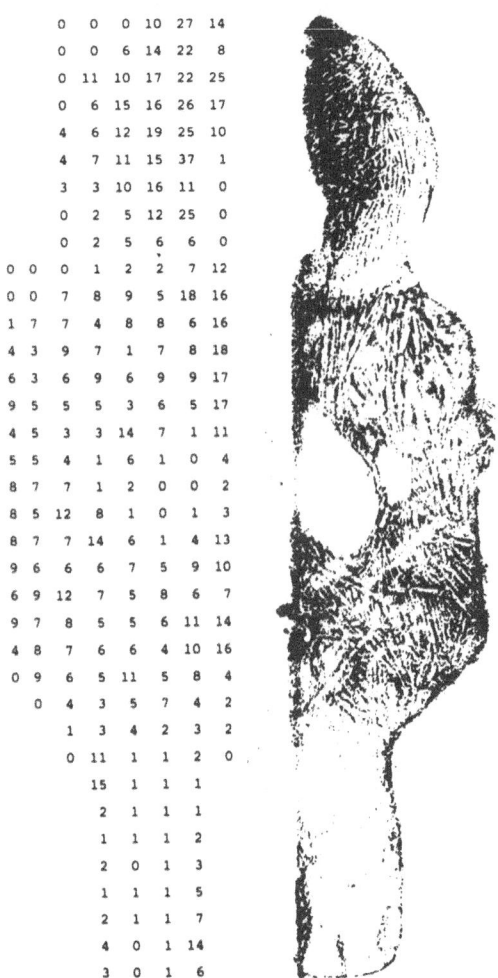

```
              0    0    0   10   27   14
              0    0    6   14   22    8
              0   11   10   17   22   25
              0    6   15   16   26   17
              4    6   12   19   25   10
              4    7   11   15   37    1
              3    3   10   16   11    0
              0    2    5   12   25    0
              0    2    5    6    6    0
    0    0    0    1    2    2    7   12
    0    0    7    8    9    5   18   16
    1    7    7    4    8    8    6   16
    4    3    9    7    1    7    8   18
    6    3    6    9    6    9    9   17
    9    5    5    5    3    6    5   17
    4    5    3    3   14    7    1   11
    5    5    4    1    6    1    0    4
    8    7    7    1    2    0    0    2
    8    5   12    8    1    0    1    3
    8    7    7   14    6    1    4   13
    9    6    6    6    7    5    9   10
    6    9   12    7    5    8    6    7
    9    7    8    5    5    6   11   14
    4    8    7    6    6    4   10   16
    0    9    6    5   11    5    8    4
         0    4    3    5    7    4    2
              1    3    4    2    3    2
              0   11    1    1    2    0
                  15    1    1    1
                   2    1    1    1
                   1    1    1    2
                   2    0    1    3
                   1    1    1    5
                   2    1    1    7
                   4    0    1   14
                   3    0    1    6
```

Fig. 2 Boron distribution in tumor and brain of patient VORM. Left: ppm values. Right: Neutron capture radiogram. The two sides are represented as mirror images of each other.

The outcome of clinical trials would greatly depend on the boron accumulation and retention not in the central parts of the tumor, but rather on boron concentrations in those parts that cannot be removed satisfactorily by surgery. With QNCR and the possibility to correlate histological status with a given boron concentration, such data can be collected.

ACKNOWLEDGMENTS

Financial support from the Senator for Health of Bremen and the Commission of the European Communities, and the gift of a cryomicrotome by Schering AG, Berlin, is gratefully acknowledged.

REFERENCES

[1] D. Gabel, H. Holstein, B. Larsson, L. Gille, G. Ericson, D. Sacker, P. Som and R.G. Fairchild, Quantitative Neutron Capture Radiography for Studying the Biodistribution of Tumor-Seeking Boron-Containing Compounds. Cancer Res. 47, 5451-5456 (1987)
[2] F. Stecher-Rasmussen, R. Huiskamp, M. Konijnenberg, V.G.A. Gregoire, B. Mijnheer, A.C. Begg, R.L. Moss and L. Dewit, Boron Detection for the Petten BNCT Project: Prompt-gamma, ICP-AES, Track Etch and ESI. These Proceedings.

CLINICAL RESULTS OF BORON NEUTRON CAPTURE THERAPY

H. Hatanaka[1], K. Sano[2], H. Yasukochi[3]

1 Professor of Neurosurgery, Teikyo University, Tokyo
2 Professor Emeritus of Neurosurgery, Tokyo University, Tokyo
3 Professor of Radiology, Teikyo University, Tokyo

INTRODUCTION

It is 22 years as of August 20, 1990 since Boron-Neutron Capture Therapy was revived by Hatanaka[1,4]. The authors have treated 107 patients by Boron-Neutron Capture Therapy (BNCT) as of the 20th August, 1990. These patients included malignant gliomas (grade III-IV), low grade gliomas (grade I-II), sarcomas, meningiomas, and cerebral metastases.

METHOD OF TREATMENT AND MATERIALS

Patients: Grade III-IV gliomas have traditionally been called "glioblastomas", but now there is a new tendency to call only grade IV a glioblastoma. Grade III gliomas are sometimes referred to as "anaplastic gliomas" and grade IV gliomas are termed "highly malignant tumours". To avoid confusion of nomenclature, the authors have made it a rule to use only the term "grade III-IV gliomas" in accordance with the World Health Organisation (WHO) standard. Between August 1968 and August 1990, there were 49 patients who had not been treated with conventional chemotherapy or radiotherapy out of a total of 107 patients. These patients can be easily compared with other people's statistics because grade III and IV glioma grouping is the most widely used grouping in European and American co-operative studies.

There is another reason for choosing grade III-IV gliomas for evaluation of efficacy. These are extremely malignant tumours that kill patients within a year or two, and thus can be used for a rapid assessment of the effect of a new therapy.

In the same period, one of the authors (H.H.) also treated 46 patients with grade III-IV gliomas by conventional therapies, including a combination of surgery, conventional radiotherapy, and chemotherapy. They could not be treated by BNCT because either a reactor or boron-10 was not available.

Group 1: This group consists of 46 patients treated by a combination of conventional treatments but not by BNCT. It is marked PHOTON because the most important part of the treatment was conventional radiotherapy with photons (Cobalt-60 or accelerator).

Group 2: This group consists of all 38 patients with grade III-IV tumours who were treated by BNCT between 1968 and 1985, excluding pre-irradiated cases. In this period all incoming grade III-IV glioma patients were treated without regard to location or depth of the tumour unless they could not be treated by BNCT due to the lack of a reactor or boron-10.

Group 3: This group is a subgroup of Group 2. It comprises the 12 patients sorted out from Group 2 because of the superficial location of their tumours. These tumours involved the cerebral mantle of the superficial layer of the brain; in other words, they were within 6 cm of the cortical surface. As will be noted, these tumours were within the limit of the maximum therapeutic depth[6] of the current regimen of BNCT.

Group 4: This group comprises all the 11 patients with grade III-IV gliomas who were treated after 1985 exclusively by BNCT alone. After 1985, patients with deep tumours were discouraged by the authors to apply for BNCT, but some patients with deep tumours who insisted on BNCT were accepted to be treated with the aid of deuterium water to partially replace the water content in the brain.

Reactors: Specifically-designed medical reactors have not been constructed in Japan. The Hitachi Training Reactor, 100 KW (HTR) was used for the initial 13 cases. The Japan Atomic Energy Research Reactor-3, 10MW (JRR-3) was used for a patient in 1969, and its kin JRR-2 (10 MW) was used most recently in August 1990 for one case. The Kyoto University Reactor (KUR) was used for a case in 1972, and again in 1990 for 4 cases before August 20th. In all these reactors, the thermal column or heavy water facility (KUR) was re-designed for BNCT purposes. The Musashi Institute of Technology Reactor was used from 1974 for the majority of cases, but the reactor has been temporarily closed for repairs since January 1990. The medical corps involved in the clinical activity were at first the neurosurgeons and radiologists of the University of Tokyo, but it moved to Teikyo University in 1974, and only since 1988 has it acquired some new members from Tokushima University/Kagawa National Hospital for Children and Kyoto University/Kishiwada City Hospital. The latter two groups have become semi-independent and started conducting BNCT for brain tumour patients in October 1990, in their own hospitals with the authors as advisors.

Procedure: the boron-10 compound dispensed by the authors since 1968 is mercaptoundecahydrododecaborate made from 95-97% enriched boron-10 (abbreviated to BSH or borocaptate). Its isotonic aqueous solution, diluted with an equal volume of physiological saline solution, is infused into the carotid (or vertebral) artery with a pressurised motor pump or by a simple intravenous drip. The boron-10 infusion is done 12-24 hours before neutron irradiation. There has been no single case which presented any untoward complication, although a mild flushing of the face may be seen if the infusion speed is too fast. Infusion usually takes 30-60 minutes. The patient whose tumour had been debulked in a craniotomy a week or two earlier, is taken to the reactor. Samples of blood and urine are collected for boron analysis by routine chemical quantification.

In the reactor the patient undergoes remote control anaesthesia and the skin flap is re-opened. The bone flap is usually removed during the procedure to obtain tumour tissue specimens for pathology and boron analysis. If further debulking is necessary, this is done. In cases in which heavy water replacement is carried out, physiological saline solution made of D_2O is instilled into the ventricles while the cerebrospinal fluid is drained. Gold wires and foils and simultaneous monitoring devices are placed where they are necessary for neutron monitoring. The whole head is covered with a sterilised plastic ^6LiF helmet except for the area to be radiated. The entire head is covered with a sterile plastic film to avoid contamination. The operating table is rolled into the radiation room to place the head against the beam. All the vital sign monitoring devices are connected. The door is closed, and the neutron beam irradiates the operating area. The irradiation time is calculated so that the deepest part of the tumour will be given <u>at least</u> 10 Gy (or 1000 rad) and that the superficial layer of the normal cerebral surface will be exposed to less than 20 Gy (or 2000 rad). After the radiation procedure, the head is closed as in any other craniotomy.

For intracerebral operations, anti-tumour agents such as methotrexate or ACNU solutions are used for irrigation to prevent tumour cell dissemination. A sufficient dose of prednisolone succinate is used intravenously to minimize cerebral edema arising from vascular wall radiation and surgical exposure of the brain.

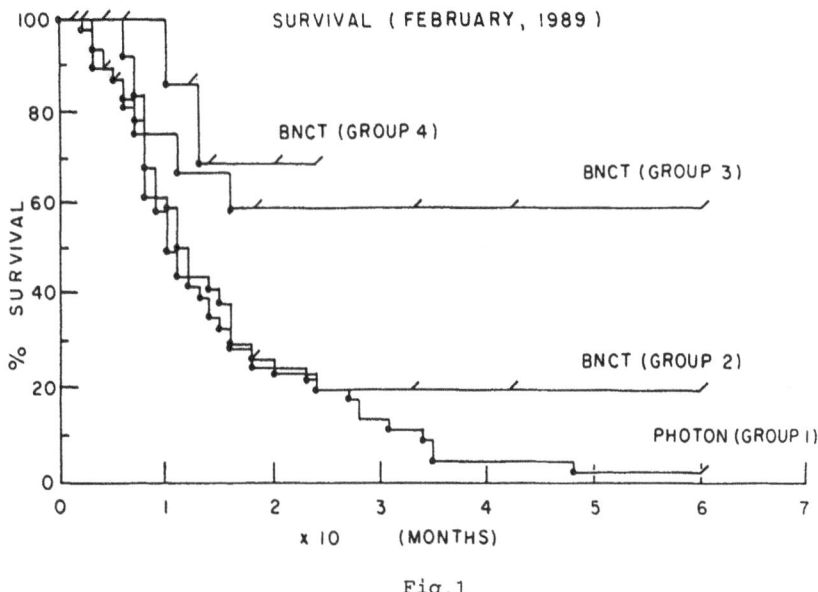

Fig.1

Photon (Group 1): All of the photon-plus-chemotherapy patients (linear accelerator or cobalt). BNCT (Group 2): All of the BNCT patients without regard to depth of the tumour, treated between 1968 and 1985 (38 cases). BNCT (Group 3): All of the BNCT patients with tumours found within 6 cm from the brain surface, treated between 1968 and 1985 (12 cases sorted out from 38 cases). BNCT (Group 4): All of the BNCT patients treated in the past 3 years (11 cases).

RESULTS

All of the 'photon' patients of Group 1 died within 7 years of their treatment. Their 5-year survival rate was less than 3% (Fig.1).

Group 2 patients, that is, all of the BNCT patients between 1968 and 1985, had a 5-year survival rate of 19%.

The Group 3 patients, a subgroup of Group 2, whose tumours were within the limits of maximum therapeutic depth, had a rate of 58% for 5-year survival.

Group 4 patients, who constitute all of the patients treated with thermal neutron capture but without photons for grade III-IV gliomas after 1985, have shown a tendency very comparable to Group 3.

Quality of survival has been excellent with all the long surviving patients. As of August 1990, seven patients have lived longer than 9 years (9-18 years) after BNCT. One of them (astrocytoma, grade II-III), who had been photon-radiated (Ca. 20 Gy) prior to BNCT, after working for 5 years as a postman, developed a contrast-enhanced mass which was recognised to be delayed cerebral necrosis around the original tumour site at 7 years. After necrotomy he continued to live, and it is now 12 years after BNCT. Although he has neurological deficits due to the necrotic mass, his mind is clear. In his case the pre-BNCT radiotherapy probably impaired the blood-brain barrier and thus allowed a certain penetration of boron-10 to the brain substance. Consequently the brain substance exposed to the neutron beam may have become necrotic after several years. All other six patients surviving 9, 10, 12, 12, 13 and 18 years have no new neurological deficits added to the pre-operative neurological deficits. Among them two had inexcisable benign meningiomas, one had chondrosarcoma, and three had grade III-IV gliomas. The 18-year survivor (then 50 years old) had a glioblastoma in the left motor cortex. His speech disturbance disappeared, and he had no neurological deficit except for a left eye cataract, probably related to gamma radiation contained in the neutron beam. He has worked as a farmer. The 13-year survivor (then 60 years old) had a grade III astrocytoma (also diagnosed as glioblastoma by a pathologist) in the right parietal area. The 9-year survivor had a huge (9 cm in size) astrocytoma, grade III in the right frontal lobe treated at the age of eleven (Fig.2). She went back to school two months after treatment. Nine years later she graduated from technical college and got a job as an architectural design assistant. The last two women were invited to the reception of the 2nd International Symposium on Neutron Capture Therapy to greet the participants in Tokyo in 1985, and have shown no deterioration whatsoever since then.

DISCUSSION

Clinical results as a whole clearly indicate the need to improve delivery of neutrons to the tumours [3]. From the authors' clinico-pathological experience it can be concluded that if some 17 boron-neutron capture nuclear reactions occur within a single tumour cell, the cell will be destroyed. To attain this goal, one has to deliver a minimum of 2.5 x 10^{12} neutrons per gram of tumour when the average concentration of boron-10 is 26 µg ^{10}B/g. There are three factors that can assist in achieving this objective. The first, epithermal neutrons, is already a well-known means to improve penetration of neutrons in the tissue. The second is a wide aperture for the neutron beam. If the aperture of the craniotomy bone window is large, the neutrons will reach deeper. A surgeon should bear this in mind before fashioning a skin and skull opening. The third is heavy (deuterium) water. When D_2O saline solution is used to replace tissue water or the cerebrospinal fluid in the spaces of the brain, it reduces attenuation of thermal neutrons and thereby facilitates a more satisfactory penetration of neutrons. The price of deuterium water is no longer prohibitively expensive as compared to anti-cancer drugs.

After 1985 the authors adopted a new strategy for treating patients with deep-seated tumours. It entails choosing patients with superficially located tumours or, in the case of deep tumours, using deuterium water to facilitate deeper penetration of thermal neutrons. It can be safely said that the results of this new strategy to treat deep tumours with the aid of heavy water are reinforcing the conclusion drawn from the Group 3 results.

When looking at these results, one must not be dismayed at the gloomy destiny of patients whose tumours are not within 6 cm of the surface, because, by now, we know that the replacement of water in the brain with deuterium water and/or the future use of epithermal neutrons will definitely increase the rate of survival of these patients.

(1)

(2)

(3)

(4)

(5)

(6)

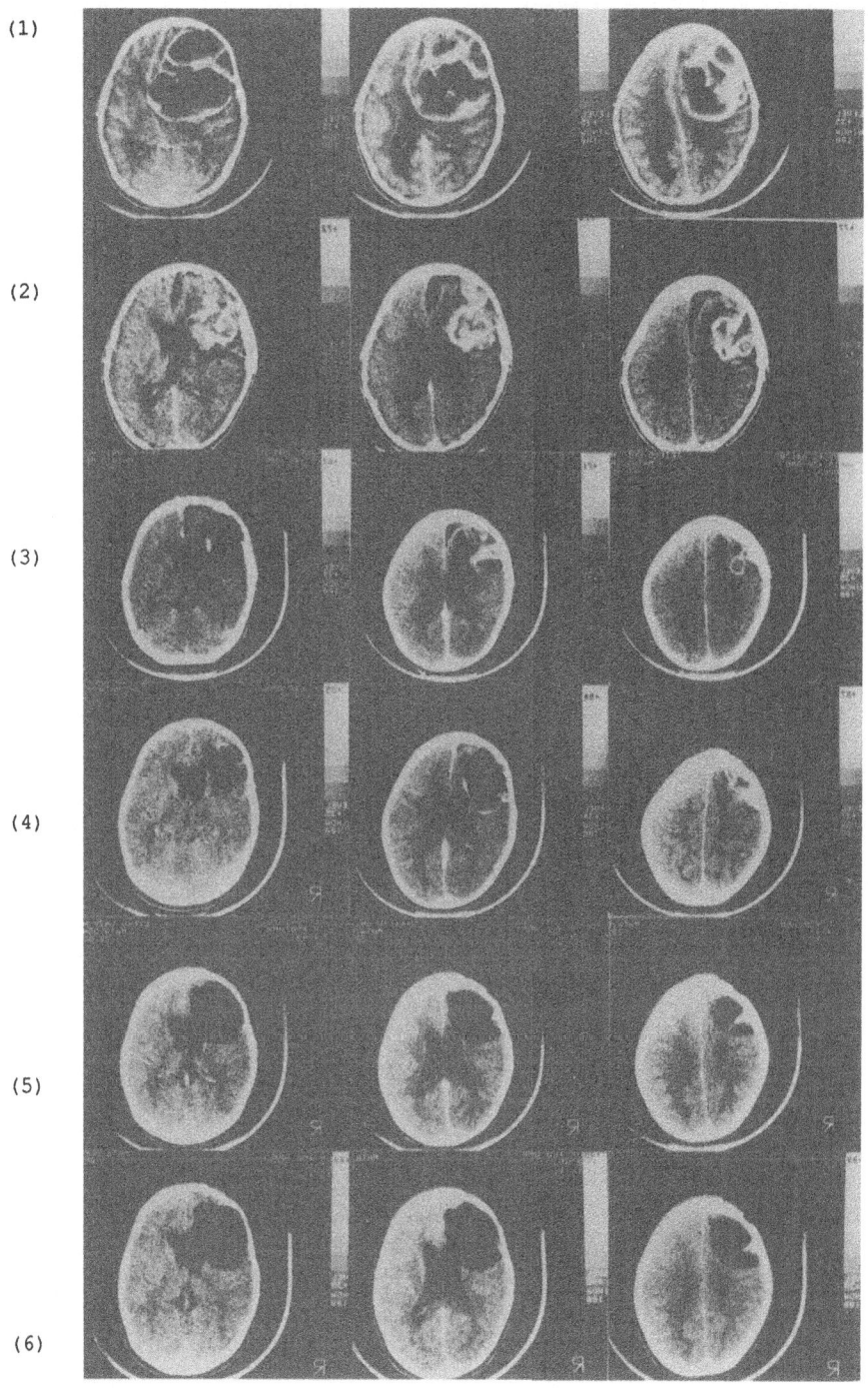

Fig.2   An 11 year old girl with a large juvenile glioblastoma in the right
frontal lobe. From top to bottom: (1) A week before surgery, a large
tumour 9cm in diameter. (2) 11 days after surgery the cystic content had
been removed, tumour parenchyma is mostly remaining. (3) 17 days after
BNCT, tumour is losing contrast-enhancement. (4) At 6 months, periphery of
the tumour is still visualised. (5) At 12 months, tumour is no longer
evidenced by CT. (6) CT scan at 18 months shows no alteration.

A randomised study is important and useful for testing drugs. The philosophical basis for it is the concept that the procedures of the therapy can be constant or, in other words, "standardised" without regard to differences among practicing physicians. However, it is inappropriate to apply randomisation to evaluate surgical efficacy. Boron Neutron Capture Therapy is essentially a type of surgery using radiological means as a tool. Surgical operations depend heavily not only on tools but also on individual surgeons. You cannot expect a reproduction of the same result from different physicians using BNCT because they may use the same means differently. We can standardise BNCT as to method, but the neutron dose and where and how to deliver the neutrons are entirely variable, depending on each tumour, as in surgery. The decision about how to deliver the neutrons depends on each surgeon's skill, experience, knowledge, and foresight. Even post-operative care influences the survival rate. Post-operative care and treatment also require utmost foresight and experience. This means that to make the best of BNCT, physicians have to be trained in BNCT.

Post-operatively, a BNCT patient should be followed only by a physician who can discard the prejudice that a glioblastoma is not curable [5]. This adamant misbelief among physicians providing follow-up care has caused the loss of more than a dozen patients who suffered from degenerating tumour tissue which gives some toxic effect to the surrounding brain matter. At this stage, dying tumours are often mistaken for recurrent tumours [3]. There was even a patient who committed suicide when he was told by a local radiologist that he had a recurrence. Some patients may require a surgical evacuation of the dead tissue. A case is presented whose post-BNCT tumour eventually required a second-look surgery. Fortunately in this case, after the second-look surgery, although the patient lost some normal motor cortex tissue and became hemiparetic, she remains well otherwise. The so-called "recurrent" tumour tissue turned out to be highly necrotic tumour tissue (Fig.2 and Fig.3).

The clinical results of the authors have been obtained using "make-shift" medical reactors which cannot yet yield epithermal beams which are not contaminated by fast neutrons and gammas. To evaluate the tumourcidal efficacy of the present BNCT with thermal neutron beams alone, which do not travel deep enough to treat all tumours everywhere in the brain, it is justifiable to limit the patient material to those with tumours located within the Maximum Therapeutic Depth [6] from the brain surface - 6 cm in the currently available regimen. These are the patients in Group 3.

As for the potential of BNCT, it is foreseeable that brain tumours beyond this 6 cm depth will be effectively treated with the aid of an epithermal neutron beam which could become available in the near future at large reactors like those in Tokai (Japan), Idaho, Cambridge (Mass.), Brookhaven (Long Island), Petten (Holland), and Lucas Heights (Australia).

At other small reactors which have no capacity to produce epithermal neutrons, replacement of cerebral water with heavy water (D_2O) will be useful to enhance the penetration of thermal neutrons. As discussed here, by sorting out tumours within the Maximum Therapeutic Depth of 6 cm from Group 2, we can see that BNCT is certainly effective and can be even curative.

Besides the survival rate, the low level of neurological deficit in BNCT patients is encouraging. The autopsy findings in "Boron-Neutron Capture Therapy for Tumours" reported by Hatanaka and Urano indicate that there were no viable tumour cells within the area to which neutrons of more than $2.5 \times 10^{12}/cm^2$ had been delivered. Given an average boron-10 concentration of 26 µg ^{10}B/gram, this neutron fluence gives approximately 10 Gy (or 1000 rad), and this estimated dose corresponds to 30 RBE Gy (3000

RBE rad). It is understandable that most of the long-term survivors did not develop any new neurological deficits, since their cerebral surface layer had received only less than 20 Gy (or 2000 rad).

After 1985, the brain tumours treated by the authors with thermal neutrons were either those in superficial layers of the brain or those in the brain stem region (thalamus, ventricles, pons, and medulla oblongata) which were treated by D_2O-assisted Boron-10 Neutron Capture Therapy. Occasionally if deemed necessary, 20 Gy - 30 Gy (2000 rad - 3000 rad) accelerator photons were given over 2 - 3 weeks either to the whole brain to take care of possible dissemination through the cerebrospinal fluid or to the brain stem, as a booster. A fuller evaluation of all these patients' clinical courses will have to wait for more time to pass. However, readers can see on the survival graph in Fig.1 the interim tendency of these cases - by excluding those treated with thermal neutrons plus a booster dose of photons.

We do need more information about heavy water[2]. However, three patients' glioblastoma specimens obtained for boron analysis during surgery for BNCT showed 33 - 80 μg ^{10}B/gram of tumour (57 on average) just before the tumours were going to irradiated. This extraordinarily high retention of boron-10 in tumour cells may well be related to some unknown biological mechanism of D_2O. It should be remembered that animals treated with barbiturates wake up late if D_2O has been given. The application of D_2O to BNCT has three advantages: 1) it facilitates deeper penetration of thermal neutrons, 2) it decreases gamma rays in the radiated field because D_2O replaces H_2O which produces more gamma when the tissue is exposed to thermal neutrons, and 3) it perhaps retains more boron-10 in the tumour cells - which is a great gift to BNCT clinicians. Other scholars are encouraged to investigate D_2O.

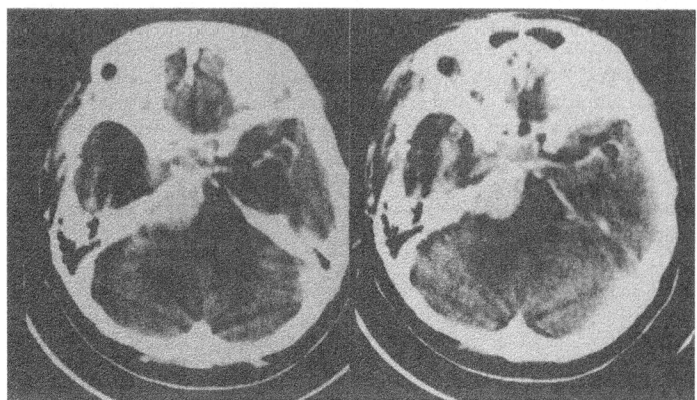

Fig.3 New dimension in the application of BNCT-benign but inoperable tumours. A meningioma surrounding the carotid artery was operated on at two different hopsitals unsuccessfully. Then the patient applied for stereotactic proton beam therapy but was not accepted. Then BNCT was conducted with the help of heavy water replacement of the brain water content. Four months later there is a tendency for the tumour to shrink. Left: before BNCT. Right: 4 months later.

CONCLUSION

The results presented in this paper support the immediate launch of clinical trials using thermal neutron beams which are easily available at many existing research reactors. A pure epithermal neutron beam which eliminates fast neutrons and gammas will require larger reactors, more sophisticated technology, and, above all, more biological studies. It is regrettable that many presently existing research reactors are being decommissioned because clinicians have been reluctant to apply sufficient political pressure on governments or institutions that subsidise these reactors. In the meantime, we have sadly lost enthusiasts like Dr Durrant, the Consultant Radiologist at Oxford, and Dr Fairchild, the Physicist at Brookhaven, due to heart stroke.

Physicians involved in malignant brain tumour treatment should start treating patients without waiting for the construction of an ideal epithermal beam because 500,000 people in the world are dying each year of brain tumours; at least one-third of them could be treated without waiting for the development and implementation of more more expensive epithermal beams.

REFERENCES

1. Hatanaka, H., 1986, "Boron-Neutron Capture Therapy for Tumours", Nishimura & Co., 1-754-39 Asahimachi-dori, Niigata.
2. Kadosawa, T., Takeuchi, A., Nakaichi, T., Matsumoto, T., Nozaki, T., Aizawa, O., Takagaki, M., Moritani, M., Amano, K., Hatanaka, H., Hayakawa, Y., and Inaba, T., 1987, Basic Research in Neutron Capture Therapy (Part 1) - Preliminary Study on the Use of D_2O for Boron-Neutron Capture Therapy, Annual Report of Joint Studies at Mushashi Institute of Technology Reactor, 12:9.
3. Hatanaka, H., 1988, Experience of Boron-Neutron Capture Therapy for Malignant Brain Tumours - with Special Reference to the Problem of Post-operative CT Follow-ups, Acta Neurochirurgica, Suppl., 42:187.
4. Brownell, G. L., 1973, A Re-assessment of Neutron Capture Therapy in the Treatment of Cerebral Gliomas, in: Proc. Seventh National Cancer Conf., p.827, American Cancer Society, Inc.
5. Hatanaka, H., Sano, K., Kitamura, K., Fujii, M., Mogami, H., Ushio, Y., Kuwabara, T., Kyuma, Y., Inaba, Y., Hiratsuka, H., Suzuki, J., Katakura, R., Takakura, K., Handa, H., And Yamashita, J., 1984, CT Findings in Patients with Gliomas, Surviving More Than 10 years, Acta Neurochirurgica, 27:106.
6. Hatanaka, H., 1991, Boron Neutron Capture Therapy for Tumours in Glioma - Principles and Practices in Neuro-Oncology, Ed. ABMF Karim & E.R. Laws, Springer Verlag (Heidelberg), 231-249.

CLINICAL EXPERIENCE OF BNCT FOR BRAIN TUMOURS AT JAERI

Eiji Sirai[1], Hidetake Takahashi[1], Masahiko Issiki[1], Kenji Arigane[1], Masao Iwaya[1], Hiroshi Hatanaka[2], Yoshinori Hayakawa[3] and Yoshinobu Nakagawa[4]

1 Japan Atomic Energy Research Institute (JAERI), Tokai
2 Dept. of Neurosurgery, Teikyo University, Tokyo
3 Proton Beam Medical Center, Tsukuba University, Tsukuba
4 Dept of Neurosurgery, Tokushima University, Tokushima

INTRODUCTION

BNCT in Japan was started at HTR (Hitachi Training Reactor) in 1968 and continued until 1975 when the HTR was closed permanently. After this, MuITR (Musashi Institute of Technology Research Reactor) was used for NCT in Japan[1]. However, MuITR was shut down in December 1989 because of reactor pool leakage. JAERI decided to collaborate at its research reactor, and began immediately to arrange the budget, contract, procedural minutes of the government, and investigate the experience in Japan for BNCT in order to implement it by the end of July. JRR-2 was chosen for BNCT. Modifications for BNCT proceeded uneventfully, except for optimizing the neutron flux and gamma ray dose which required more time than expected. The first BNCT at JRR-2 was conducted satisfactorily on the 10th of August, 1990. The specification of the modified facility and the first experience of BNCT at JRR-2 are reported in this paper.

OUTLINE OF THE FACILITY FOR BNCT AT JRR-2

JAERI has four research reactors in Tokai, and one in Oarai. The neutron beam can be used at JRR-2, JRR-3 and JRR-4, but JRR-2 was the only one to fit the needs for neutron flux, space and period for remodification for BNCT.

JRR-2 normally operate 13 cycles a year; each cycle consists of 2 weeks' operation and 1 week shut down. In 1990, there will be 8 cycles in order to allow a longer inspection period of 24 weeks as required every 10 years. Therefore, it was decided to conduct BNCT at the end of July just before the long shut down period.

The thermal column, which had been used for neutron radiography (NRG), was chosen for the high Cd cut off ratio of neutrons. The NRG facility had to be removed, and then the neutron flux and gamma dose were measured, and the configuration of the thermal column was designed. Then the irradiation room was constructed outside the thermal column. Parallel with the construction of the irradiation room, a surgical operating room was constructed outside the reactor hall. The irradiation room was designed as part of the reactor facilities in compliance with requirements

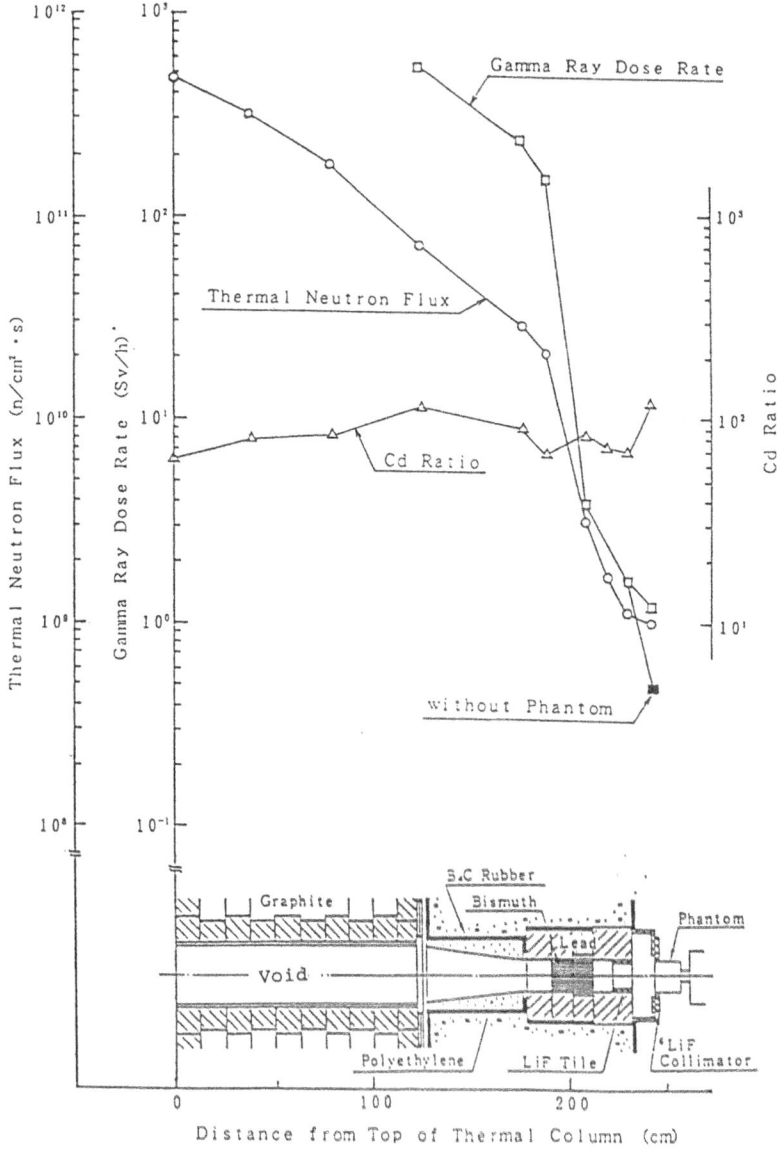

Fig. 1 Thermal Neutron Flux and Gamma Ray Dose Rate
of JRR-2 Thermal Column

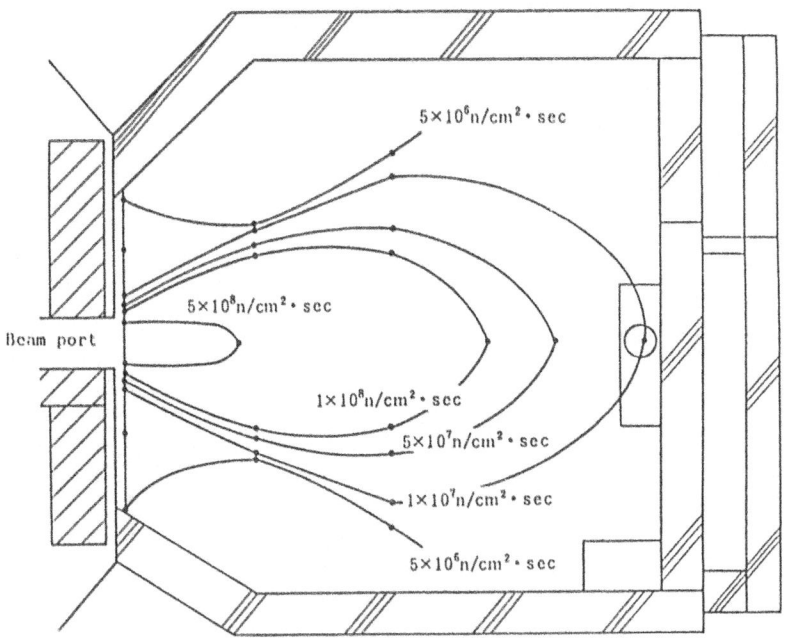

Fig. 2 Thermal Neutron Flux Distribution in Irradiation Room
(at 10MW of Reactor Power)

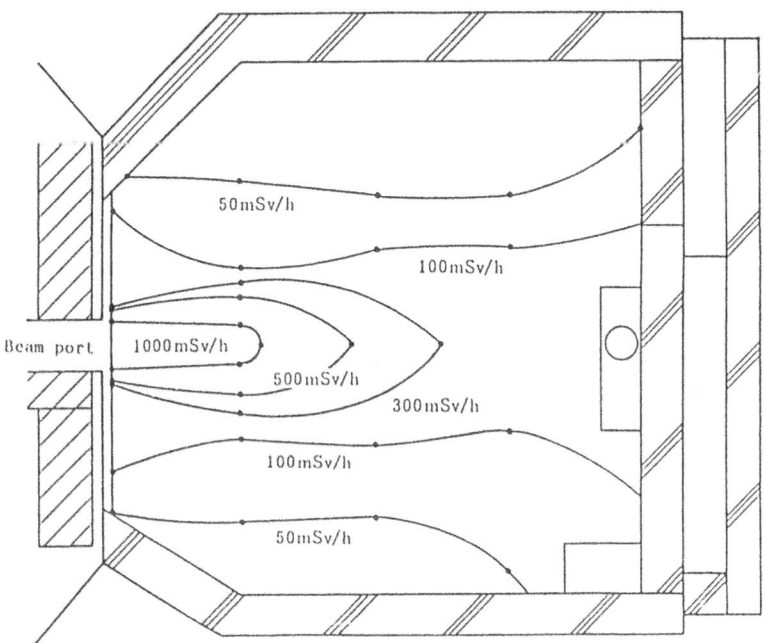

Fig. 3 Gamma ray dose Distribution in Irradiation Room
(at 10MW of Reactor Power)

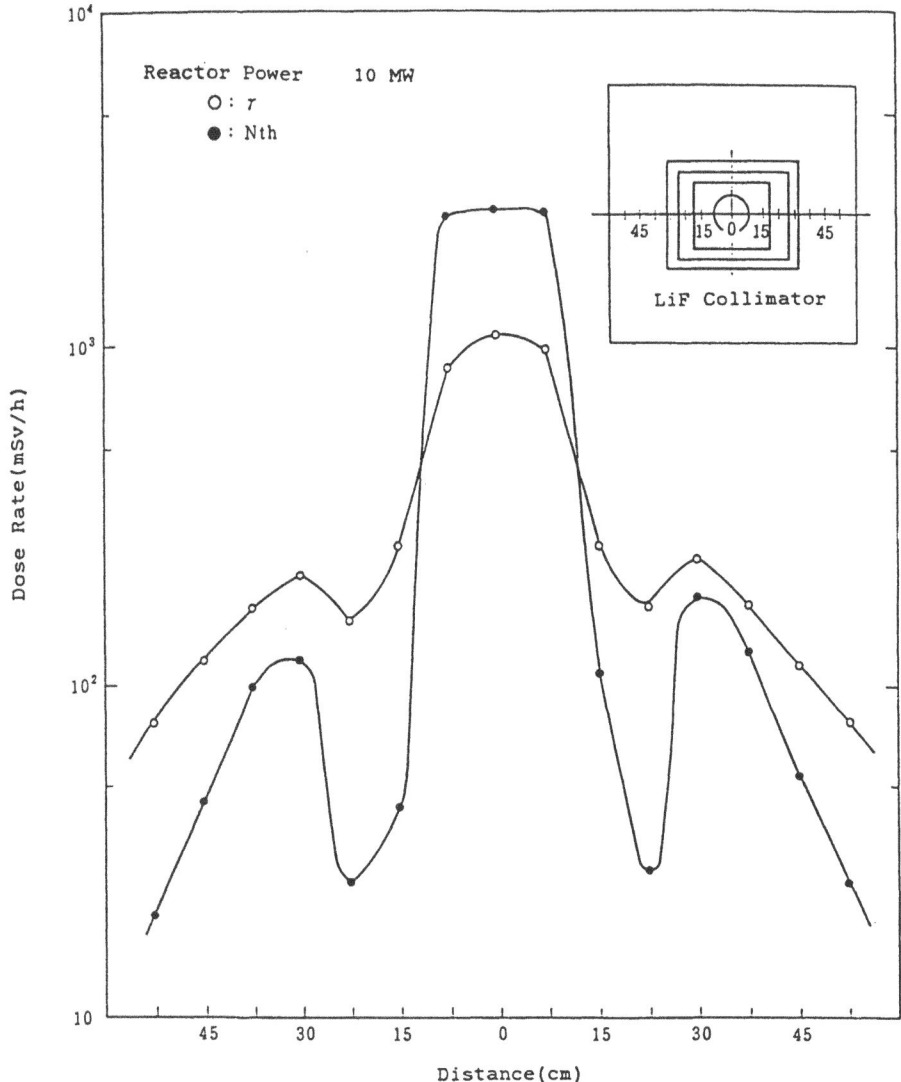

Fig. 4   Dose Rate of Gamma ray and Thermal Neutron at the
Surface of Thermal Column

Thermal Column

35°

⑤ ③ ① ② ⑥ ④ ⑦ ⑧

Phantom

^{6}LiF Collimator

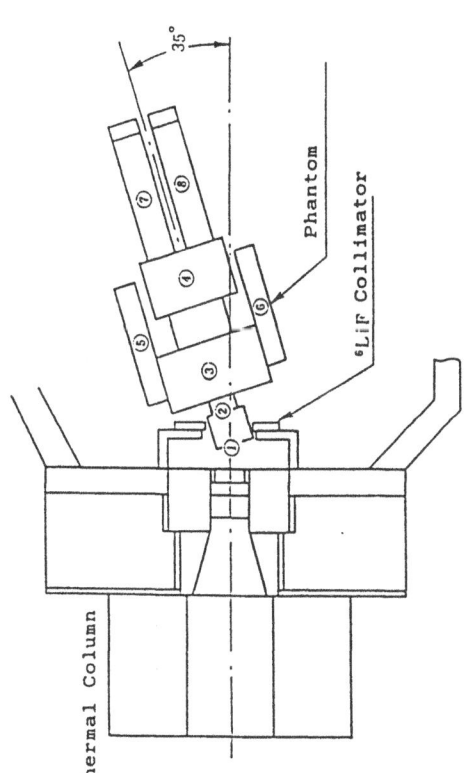

Measured date   1990.8.6

Reactor Power   10 MW

Irradiation Time   1 hr

		Measured Points							
Items		1	2	3	4	5	6	7	8
Gamma Ray Dose Rate	mSv/h	1825	285	142	33.8	84.5	44.2	15.3	6.0
Thermal Neutron Dose rate	mSv/h	2×10^3	129	7.5	3.7	15	3.4	1.4	1.2
Neutron Flux	n/cm²·s	1.1×10^9	8.3×10^6	5.0×10^5	2.4×10^5	9.8×10^5	2.2×10^5	8.8×10^4	8.0×10^4

Remarks: The gamma dose rate at the point 1 is 480mSv/h in the condition of "without phantom".

Fig. 5 Dose Rate of Gamma ray and Thermal Neutron on the Phantom

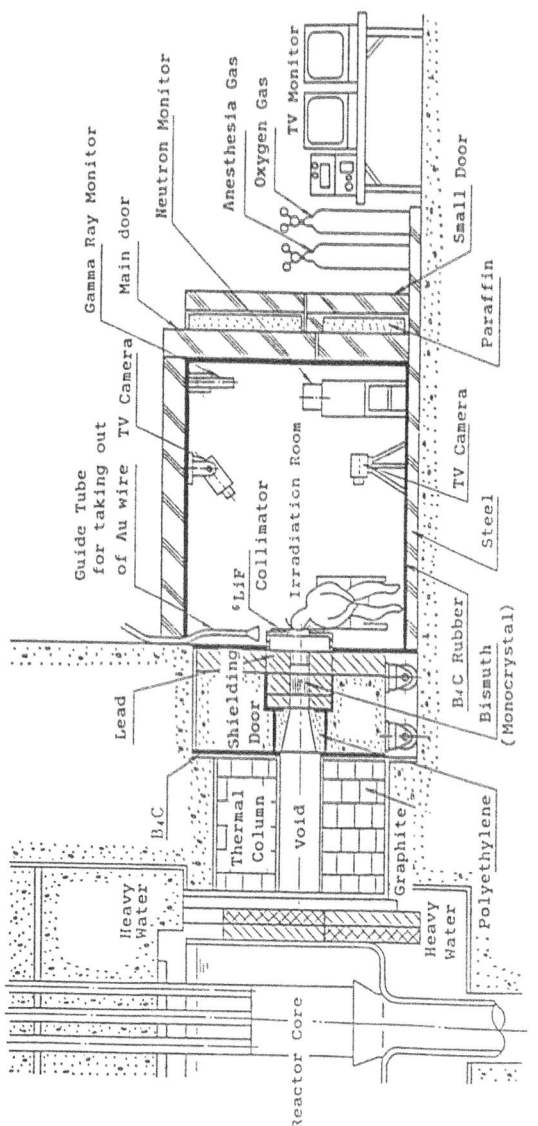

Fig. 6 Configuration of Facility and Instrumentations for BNCT in JRR-2

574

of the Science and Technology Agency (STA). The main points in designing the irradiation room were to have proper shielding ability and endurable tolerance to earthquakes. The dose rate at the surface of the irradiation room was limited to 0.03 mSv/h in the direction to the wall of the reactor hall, where the monitoring devices for the patient were placed. On the other hand, the space for the patient needed to be as wide as possible to allow free positioning of the patient so that any part of the head could be irradiated while avoiding direct exposure of the body to the beam from the port.

The steel wall thickness of the room was 200 mm for the side wall and ceiling, and for the door 200 mm of paraffin was sandwiched between two plates of 200 mm thick steel. Rubber plates containing B_4C developed in JAERI, were used to shield thermal neutrons. For seismic design, the grade of the irradiation room should be Class B, that is to endure 0.3 G of seismic intensity, but it was requested that the reactor shielding should not be affected in the irradiation room even for the Class A grade earthquake. Many braces to combine walls and ceiling plates and many bolts to fix the wall plates to the base plate were prepared to satisfy these requirements. As emergency counter measures, for electric power supply cut off, earthquakes, and sudden deterioration of patients, a small door was installed as an emergency exit. In the irradiation room, two TV cameras, monitoring devices for gamma and neutrons, and a guide tube to bring out Au monitors from the irradiation field of the patients were installed in the irradiation facility. Outside the irradiation room, TV monitors and other instruments were placed for monitoring the patient. A surgery room was also constructed in a separate area inside the JRR-2 reactor site.

SET-UP OF THE IRRADIATION CONDITION

Measurements showed that the neutron flux was much less than expected from calculation for a shortened length of graphite in the thermal column (shortened to one half). All the graphite in the thermal column was removed, and the thickness of monocrystalline bismuth was increased from 10 cm to 20 cm to reduce the increased gamma ray intensity caused by removing the graphite. The neutron flux as a consequence became sufficient to conduct BNCT (5×10^9 n/cm^2/sec), but the gamma ray intensity still increased to 34 Sv/h at the outlet. The high gamma ray intensity was interpreted to be caused mainly by secondary gammas from the capture of neutrons.

Then the Bi layer was removed backwards, replacing some graphite, to obtain a higher neutron flux and a lower gamma ray intensity be reducing the secondary gamma ray. Furthermore, LiF tiles of 10 mm thickness were applied to the surface of the irradiation port at the outlet of the Bi block. As a result, 1.1×10^9 n/cm^2/sec of neutron flux, 0.48 Sv/h of gamma dose rate were obtained as shown in Fig.1, and these specifications satisfied the request of the surgeons.

The dose rate in the irradiation room should be as low as possible to avoid unnecessary exposure to the whole body of the patient.

The gamma dose rate and neutron flux were measured in the irradiation room by using a human phantom which consisted of acrylic resin boxes with water in them, before the actual irradiation of patients. The measured distributions of gamma ray dose and neutron flux are shown in Fig.2-5 with/without phantom. Note that the radiation intensity measurements using a phantom may give higher values than those for human patient because of differences in composition.

1. Patient: 43 year old female with a deep-seated unexcisable brain tumour.

2. Course of the first BNCT at JRR-2

The 10th of August, 1990 was a stormy day with a typhoon pushing through the prefectures of Tokyo, Chiba and Ibaraki. The patient and the medical corps, however, arrived at JAERI at 8 a.m. The sterilized medical instruments were spread out, anaesthesia induced and the operation started. The main door was opened with the crane of the reactor hall, and the patient was rolled into the irradiation room. In place of a bed, a chair was used to place the patient as shown in Fig.6, to give better delivery of the beam. The reactor started to run up power at 14:44, and reached full power of 10 MW at 16:06. After half an hour at full power, Au wires that had been attached to the covered surface of the operative field were drawn out to estimate the neutron flux at the tumour. The patient was continuously observed by expert anaesthesiologists during the reactor operation using vital sign monitors and TV. The reactor was run at its full power for 4.5 hours. After irradiation, the patient was moved back to the surgical operation room and the head was closed. She was transported back to the hospital at 24:00. The irradiation and operation were conducted satisfactorily.

3. Irradiation condition
- Reactor operation time: 4.5 hours at 10 MW (corresponding to 4.9 hours of reactor full power).
- Radiation exposure: Maximum exposure at the brain surface is 1.8×10^{13} n/cm^2 of neutron, 3800 mSv of gamma ray dose.
- Exposure on doctors and nurses: Negligibly small (less than 0.1 mSv)

ACKNOWLEDGEMENTS

This work was done with the co-operation and support of many collaborators and many organisations in a relatively short time, in spite of difficulties caused by the lack of information which had been lost in the many years since construction of the reactor. The authors express their gratitude to Prof. O. Aizawa of Musashi Institute of Technology for his encouragement and suggestions to improve beam quality. We are also indebted to Director M. Kawasaki and Deputy Director K. Kanbara of the Research Reactor Dept. of JAERI, Assistant Prof. Y. Ito of Tokyo University, and all other colleagues for their support, effective discussion and constant encouragement.

REFERENCE

1. Hatanaka, H. & Seto, K.: Cancer Therapy Manual. Nippon Rinsho No. 46, 1988

ADVANCES IN THE CONTROL OF HUMAN CUTANEOUS PRIMARY AND METASTATIC

MELANOMA BY THERMAL NEUTRON CAPTURE THERAPY

Y. Mishima, M. Ichihashi, C. Honda, M. Shiono,
T. Nakagawa, H. Obara[1], J. Shirakawa[1], J. Hiratsuka[2],
K. Kanda[3], T. Kobayashi[3], T. Nozaki[4], O. Aizawa[4],
T. Sato[4], H. Karashima[5], K. Yoshino[6] and H. Fukuda[7]

Dept. of Derm. Special Inst. of Cancer NCT, [1]Dept. of
Anesth., [2]Dept. of Radiol., Kobe U. School of Med.,
Kobe, [3]Res. Reactor Inst., Kyoto U. Osaka, [4]Atomic
Energy Res. Lab., Musashi Inst. of Tech., Kawasaki,
[5]Dept. of Radiol., Hyogo Med. Center, Akashi, [6]Dept.
of Chem., Shinshu U., Matsumoto, [7]Div. of Clinical
Res., Nat. Inst. of Radiol. Sciences, Chiba, Japan

INTRODUCTION

Differing in principle from boron neutron capture therapy
(NCT) of brain tumors using passive accumulation of ^{10}B, since
1972 our idea[1] has been to develop a new ^{10}B delivery system
actively targeting cancers by utilizing their enhanced specific
metabolic activity. As a prototype, we have been working with
melanoma using $^{10}B_1$-p-boronophenylalanine ($^{10}B_1$-BPA), a ^{10}B-dopa
analogue, melanogenesis-seeking melanin polymer substrate[2].

Multi-disciplinary investigations were conducted in: I. In
vitro and in vivo radiobiological studies[3], II. Pharmacokinetics[4] of $^{10}B_1$-BPA compounds and their improvement of bio-
availability[5], III. Acute and sub-acute toxicity tests[6], IV.
Improvement of thermal neutron sources and radiation dosimetry[7]
V. In-situ ^{10}B assay by prompt-gamma spectrometry[8,9] and VI.
Pre-clinical NCT studies using naturally occurred melanoma-
bearing Duroc pig[10].

We first treated human melanoma by NCT in July, 1987 and
complete regression of a metastatic lesion on the scalp was
subsequently reported[11]. A comparative overview of our 6
treatments of primary and metastatic melanoma with local control
confirmed so far, is as follows:

1. *Metastatic melanoma of left occipital area in 66yr. old man.*
2. *Primary ALM in 80yr. old male on right sole of foot.*
3. *Nodular melanoma on left foot of 85yr. old female.*
4. *Subungual melanoma on right thumb of 50yr. old male.*
5. *Nodular melanoma on right sole of 59yr. old female.*
6. *Primary ALM on left sole of 79yr old male.*
   (Note : ALM is acral lentiginous melanoma)

Table 1. Tumor thicknesses fully regressed by single or once repeated application of our selective melanoma NCT. Irradiation fluence in neutrons/cm². Tumor thickness measured at maximum or center thickness.

Case	Tumor Thickness (mm)		Neutron Dose (nvt)
1	10.5	CT	0.95×10^{13}
2	3.0		1.00×10^{13}
3	6.0		1.00×10^{13}
4	8.5		1st NCT 0.97×10^{13} 2nd NCT 1.32×10^{13}
5	5.5	CT	1.05×10^{13}
6	4.0		1.08×10^{13}

Current immunochemosurgery of primary malignant melanoma has been shown to yield survival rates correlating to tumor thickness. This parameter indicates a tumor thickness above 3mm results in considerably poorer prognosis ranging from 22-55% for 5 year survival. Table 1 summarizes tumor thickness of our six successful melanoma treatments.

In this paper we will limit our description to case number four, our first NCT of subungual acral lentiginous melanoma, as an example. This melanoma occurred in the right thumb of 50-year-old male patient (Fig.1A) which presented in February 1989.

For final clinical dosimetry of absorbed radiation energy before actual treatment, collimation was done with Li-F sheet (Fig.2A) using a life-sized phantom cast from the lesion containing thumb.

^{10}B-dosimetry was based on a study of a different patient with a similar subungual melanoma on the right 1st toe which was treated by surgical removal. According to ^{10}B dosimetry obtained from this subungual melanoma, we gave a three-way administration of ^{10}B$_1$-BPA fructose complex (water soluble at pH=7, and less injurious to tissue than BPA·HCl) as 70% systemic and 30% distant perilesional. 1) *Systemic*: this was our first case using oral administration and we gave 2400mg, 30h prior to NCT, in addition to S.C. buttock injections at 7h and 3h prior to NCT (total 7200mg). 2) *4 and 8cm distant perilesional injections*: due to the restricted finger-tip area we gave repeated injections of 300mg beginning 63h before the first NCT (total 3000mg). Concentration of ^{10}B-BPA administered was 30mg/ml for all three administration methods.

The final ^{10}B-BPA dose was as usual 170mg/kg·BW, and an irradiation of 0.97×10^{13}n/cm² was given on April 13, 1989. Since only partial regression of the treated lesion was observed (Fig.1B), we scheduled a second NCT two and a half months later. In attempting to increase ^{10}B-BPA uptake into the lesion for this second NCT, we scheduled administration of ^{10}B-BPA fructose complex as follows: 1) *7-3 days prior* : non-distant perilesional injections of 60mg with 240mg oral doses (total 1,500mg), and 2) *2-0 days prior* : oral doses of 1,950mg with

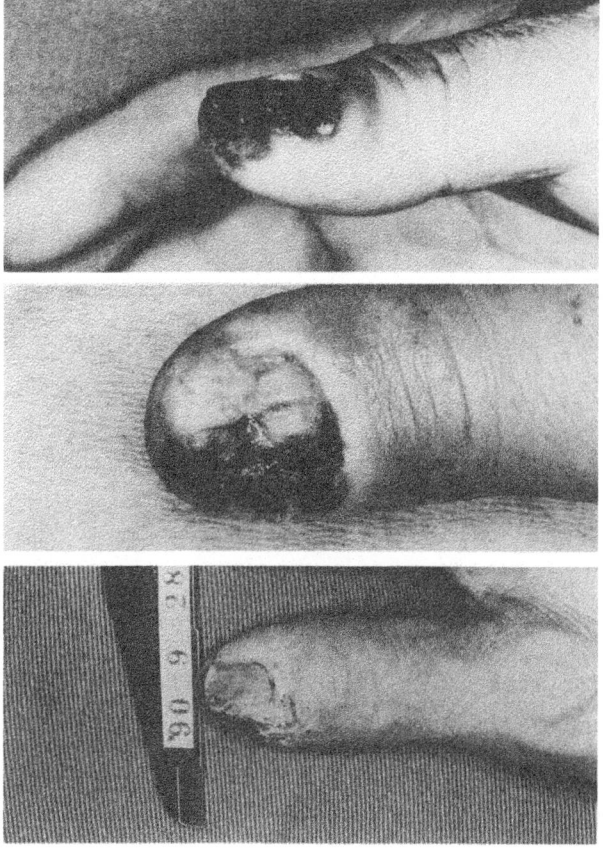

Fig.1 Subungual acral lentiginous melanoma on right
       thumb of 50 yr.old male. Top(A): just prior
       to first NCT. Middle(B): 2^1/$_2$ months later
       prior to second NCT. Bottom(C): 1 year
       3 months after second NCT.

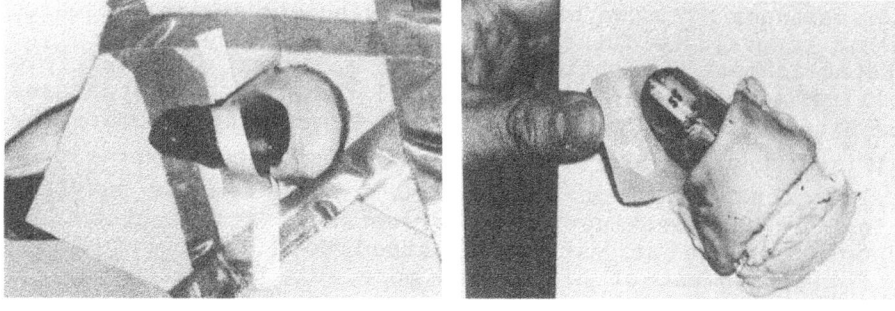

Fig.2 Lithium-Flouride sheet collimation. Left(A): phantom for
       dosimetry measurement cast from lesion containing thumb
       used for first NCT. Right(B): additional ^{6}Li-F colli-
       mation used for second NCT.

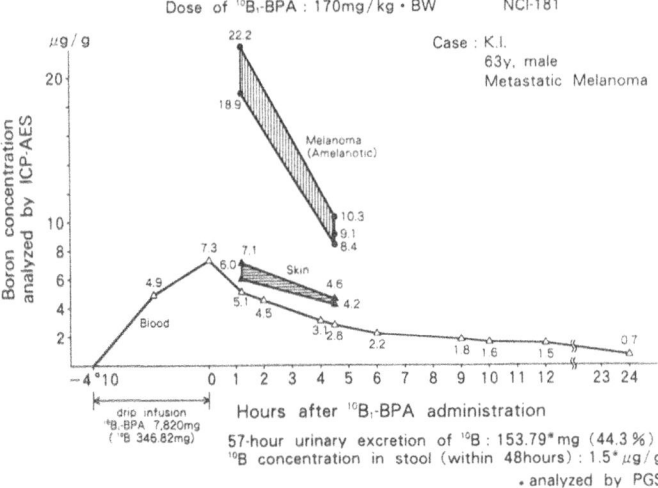

Drip Intravenous Infusion of $^{10}B_1$-BPA · Fructose Complex
to Human Melanoma Patient

Dose of $^{10}B_1$-BPA : 170mg/kg · BW   NCI-181

Case : K.I.
63y, male
Metastatic Melanoma

Melanoma
(Amelanotic)

Skin

Blood

Hours after $^{10}B_1$-BPA administration

drip infusion
$^{10}B_1$-BPA 7,820mg
(^{10}B 346.82mg)

57-hour urinary excretion of ^{10}B : 153.79*mg (44.3 %)
^{10}B concentration in stool (within 48hours) : 1.5* $\mu g / g$
. analyzed by PGS

Fig.3   Drip infusion of $^{10}B_1$-BPA in humans shows
higher uptake of ^{10}B compared to skin and blood
for amelanotic melanoma as measured by ICP-AES.

repeated 3cm distant perilesional injections of 150mg, given up
to $2^1/_2$ h before NCT to reduce edema around base of the thumb
(total 8,700mg).

The final ^{10}B-BPA dose of 170mg/kg·BW was supplemented with
1,950mg S.C. buttock injection given 5h before irradiation with
1.32×10^{13} n/cm². Further collimation was attempted by
placement of an additional ^{6}Li-F beam reflector sheet laterally
on the melanoma side of the lesion (Fig.2B).

By 3 months after the second NCT the melanoma had fully
regressed, leaving melanophage pigmentation, which clinically
further regressed to Fig.1C, taken 1 year 5 months after the
second and final NCT.

The successful treatment of the above six cases has led us
to our next phase in enlarging the applicability and precision
of our melanoma NCT. We have been carrying our further research
projects to evaluate future prospects on following:
I. Establishment of optimal NCT for melanoma with multiple
satellite metastases and/or regional lymph node metastases
through systemic administration of $^{10}B_1$-BPA·fructose complex by
i.v.(Fig.3) and $^{10}B_1$-BPA·cyclodextrin inclusion complex per oral
IIa. Fractionated NCT on complicated treatment areas has been
examined by pharmacokinetics of ^{10}B-uptake, skin reaction and
melanoma response at various absorbed dose following NCT.
IIb. For attainment of higher and more selective accumulation
of ^{10}B into malignant melanoma; 1) we have found dose-dependency
up to 500mg/kg·BW by systemic subcutaneous(s.c.) injection
(Fig.4), 2) increased efficacy of ^{10}B accumulation in Mm by
pulsed (s.c.) administration of ^{10}B-BPA (Fig.5).   L-isomer
^{10}B-BPA also appears to be promising.
III. In vitro/in vivo NCT study of $^{10}B_1$-conjugated MoAb[12].

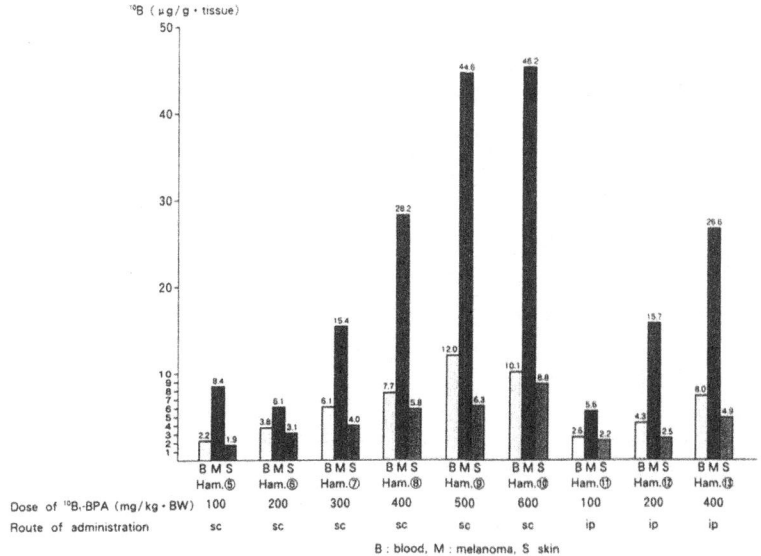

Fig.4 Increasing concentrations of ^{10}B in tumor relative to blood and skin are dose dependent as seen in subcutaneous and intraperitoneally ^{10}B-BPA injected hamster at 3 hours.

In vivo ^{10}B dynamics at Greene's melanoma site (●) and at normal skin (○) revealed by in situ assay using prompt gamma-ray spectrometry

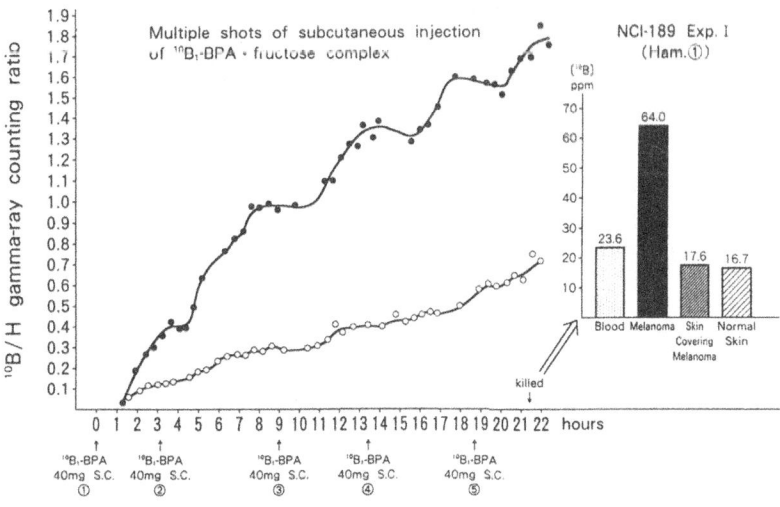

Fig.5 Pulsed administration of ^{10}B$_1$-BPA shows increasing concentration of ^{10}B in tumor relative to normal skin in s.c. injected hamster as measured by prompt-γ spectrometry

IV. Further improvement of in-situ $^{10}B_1$ assay for various types of human melanomas by prompt-gamma spectrometry in comparison with highly sensitive ICP-MS measurement of ^{10}B.
V. Design of Medical Reactor for NCT which is 2MW natural convection cooled, hospital-based and can treat 30,000 patients without needing refueling[13].

REFERENCES

1. Y. Mishima and T. Shimakage, Thermal neutron capture treatment of malignant melanoma using ^{10}B-dopa and $^{10}B_{12}$-chlorpromazine compound, in:"Pigment Cell", Vol.2:394, V. Riley, ed., S. Karger, Basel (1976).
2. Y. Mishima, C. Honda, M. Ichihashi, H. Obara, J. Hiratsuka, H. Fukuda, H. Karashima, T. Kobayashi, K. Kanda and K. Yoshino, Treatment of malignant melanoma by single thermal neutron capture therapy with melanoma-seekihg ^{10}B-compound, Lancet, II(8659):388 (1989).
3. T. Nakanishi, M. Ichihashi, Y. Mishima, T. Matsuzawa and H. Fukuda, Thermal neutron capture therapy of malignant melanoma:in vitro radiobiological analysis, Int. J. Radiat. Biol. 37:573 (1980).
4. K. Yoshino, M. Okamoto, H. Kakihana, T. Nakanishi, M. Ichihashi and Y. Mishima, Spectrophotometric determination of trace boron in biological materials after alkali fusion decomposition, Anal. Chem. 56:839 (1984).
5. Y. Mori, A. Suzuki, K. Yoshino and H. Kakihana, Complex formation of p-boronophenylalanine with some mono-saccharides, Pigment Cell Res. 2:273 (1989).
6. K. Taniyama, H. Fujiwara, T. Kuno, N. Saito, H. Shuntoh, M. Sakaue and C. Tanaka, Acute and subacute toxicity of ^{10}B-paraboronophenylalanine, Pigment Cell Res. 2:291 (1988).
7. K. Kanda, An overview: Radiation sources, beam quality, dosimetry and spectroscopy in neutron capture therapy, Strahlenther. Onkol. 165:67 (1989).
8. T. Kobayashi and K. Kanda, Microanalysis system of ppm-order ^{10}B concentrations in tissue for neutron capture therapy by prompt gamma-ray spectrometry, Nuclear Instruments and Methods 204:525 (1983).
9. C. Honda, Y. Mishima, M. Ichihashi and S. Hatta, In situ detection of cutaneous melanoma by prompt gamma-ray spectrometry using melanoma-seeking ^{10}B-dopa analogue, J. Dermatological Science 1:23 (1990).
10. Y. Mishima, M. Ichihashi, M. Tsuji, S. Hatta, M. Ueda, C. Honda and T. Suzuki, Treatment of malignant melanoma by selective thermal neutron capture therapy using melanoma-seeking compound, J. Invest. Dermatol. 92:321S (1989).
11. Y. Mishima, M. Ichihashi, S. Hatta, C. Honda, K. Yamamura and T. Nakagawa, New thermal neutron capture therapy for malignant melanoma: Melanogenesis-seeking ^{10}B molecule-melanoma cell interaction from in vitro to first clinical trial, Pigment Cell Res. 2:226 (1989).

12. A. Komura, T. Tokuhisa, T. Nakagawa, A. Sasase,
    M. Ichihashi, S. Ferrone and Y. Mishima, Specific
    killing of human melanoma cells with an efficient
    ^{10}B-compound on monoclonal antibodies, Pigment Cell Res.
    2:259 (1989).
13. Y. Mishima, Investigation of the nuclear reactor for cancer
    therapy (1) and (2), SINCT-REP-2 (1989) and SINCT-REP-4
    (1990).

A PROPOSAL FOR CLINICAL PILOT STUDIES FOR BORON NEUTRON CAPTURE THERAPY

L. Dewit[1], B. Mijnheer[1], R. Moss[2] and D. Gabel[3]

(1) Department of Radiotherapy, the Netherlands Cancer Institute (NL)

(2) Div. of High Flux Reactor, Joint Research Center (NL)

(3) Dept. of Chemistry, University of Bremen, Bremen (Germany)

INTRODUCTION

Boron neutron capture therapy (BNCT) has recently received renewed interest with the experience gained in Japan in malignant glioma patients (3). At present, the most promising compounds for clinical use are $Na_2B_{12}H_{11}SH$ (BSH) in malignant glioma patients and p-dihydroxyborylphenylalanine (BPA) in malignant melanoma patients. Within the European Collaboration on BNCT, research will be focussed, at first, on the treatment of malignant glioma patients. In a later stage, melanoma patients will be investigated and eventually patients with other tumors as well, if appropriate boron compounds become available.

STUDY DESIGN AND DISCUSSION

A. Pharmacokinetic study

In order to find the "optimal" tumor-to-blood ratio of ^{10}B, a time line study will be carried out. ^{10}B-enriched BSH will be administered in a dose of 25 $mg^{10}B/kg$ in a one hour infusion to subgroups of 8-10 patients at 3,6,12 or 18 hours prior to intraoperative tumor sampling for ^{10}B analysis. Blood samples will be obtained at short time intervals, whereas urine will be collected at 24 hour intervals ^{10}B concentrations will be determined using prompt gamma-ray spectroscopy (PGRS), inductively coupled plasma-atomic emission spectroscopy (ICP-AES) and quantitative neutron capture radiography (QNCR). The results of this study will determine the clearance pattern of BSH, e.g. whether it is monophasic, as observed in dogs (P. Gavin, pers. comm., 1990), or biphasic as found by a few investigators in patients (2,6,8). In addition, they will indicate at which time point the most favourable tumor-to-blood ratio will be obtained. It will be particularly interesting to see what ^{10}B concentrations are found at the boundary of the tumor, since for irradiation, only radically operated patients will be selected. The success of BNCT will therefore be determined by the ^{10}B concentration in this region, i.e. by the dose delivered to the remaining tumor cells.

Increasing doses of BSH will then be administered (e.g. 25,50,75 mg^{10}B/kg) at the "optimal" time interval, chosen from the previous study. Again, the pharmacokinetics of ^{10}B in serum and urine, as well as the ^{10}B concentration in various areas of the tumor will be determined. The aim is to determine the relationship between the administered dose of BSH and the observed ^{10}B concentrations in serum and in the tumor. In addition, eventual toxicity of BSH will be scored.

Next, the pharmacokinetics of BSH will be determined after repeated administration, e.g. 6 fractions at 48 hour intervals, presumably required for the proposed fractionated radiation treatment. Depending on the clearance of BSH after a single administration, the dose of the following BSH infusion might have to be adjusted in order to obtain the same ^{10}B concentration in the serum at each subsequent irradiation. Two assumptions are made here: one is that the ^{10}B concentration in serum determines the tolerance of the brain for BNCT, the other is that the blood-brain-barrier (BBB) is not affected by the previous irradiation. There is good evidence from experimental and clinical data that the first assumption is true (6, P. Gavin, pers. comm., 1990). The other, however, is an issue that remains to be investigated. Breakdown of the BBB has been shown at early time points after conventional doses of X irradiation (1,4,5).

It will be important, therefore, to assess the effect of prior irradiation on the distribution of a subsequent BSH administration in the brain in an appropriate animal model, for instance by a combination of histological examination and the QNCR technique in dogs. If a significant amount of BSH leaks through the BBB, cells other than the endothelial cells might become the critical target cells in the brain. Obviously, such information is of great importance prior to the start of treating glioma patients.

B. A Radiation dose escalation study

The aim of a radiation dose escalation study is to determine the "tolerance" of the human brain to BNCT. Patients with malignant glioma will receive postoperative irradiation with epithermal neutrons in 6 fractions at 48 hour intervals. Each fraction will be preceded by a BSH administration at a time interval chosen from the pharmacokinetic study. There are a number of logistical problems that need to be solved when performing such a dose escalation study. For instance, the dose range given to patients will be based upon the canine brain tolerance experiments to BNCT. Yet, due to the larger size of a human head compared with a dog head, there will be a larger contribution of the low LET component in the irradiated human brain, that is, more induced gamma rays in the human head from the $H(n, \gamma)^2H$ reaction. This difference needs to be taken into account, for instance with the use of Monte Carlo calculations. Other treatment parameters should be kept the same as much as possible in the human situation as in the canine model, the ^{10}B concentration in the serum at the time of irradiation, the number of radiation fields, and the fractionation schedule.

In order to determine normal brain toxicity for BNCT, a non-lethal endpoint should be used, such as contrast enhancement using computerized tomography or ^{157}Gd-DTPA magnetic resonance imaging. In dogs, contrast enhancement on ^{157}Gd-DTPA MRI was observed at lower radiation doses than lethal brain damage (P. Gavin, pers. comm, Dec. 1989). Using such a non-invasive assay, it should be possible to assess the normal brain tolerance for BNCT by gradually increasing the epithermal neutron exposure time per session without running too high a risk of causing life-threatening brain damage.

In this radiation tolerance study for the brain, presumably bilateral field irradiation will be used. The therapeutic ratio might be further improved by applying 3 or 4 beam portals, similar to what is routinely performed in conventional radiation therapy. This implies an extensive quality control study, in which a computer treatment planning system designed for BNCT will be used and verified by phantom and in vivo dosimetry. The various beam components will be displayed as well as the total absorbed dose distribution. We believe that this approach will be reliable and efficacious for a radiation tolerance study. It is well realized that the heterogeneity in energy deposition at the microscopic level in the tumor bed from the $^{10}B\ (n, \alpha)^7Li$ reaction is not taken into account.

Acknowledgements

The European Collaboration on Boron Neutron Capture Therapy is supported by the Commission of European Communities.

REFERENCES

1. Dorn III, R.V., Spickard, J.M. and Griebenow, M.L.: The effects of ionizing radiation and dexamethasone on the blood-brain-barrier and blood-tumor-barrier: implications for boron neutron capture therapy of brain tumors. Strahlenther. Onkol, 165: 219-221.

2. Haritz, D., Piscol, K. and Gabel, D.: The distribution of BSH in patients with malignant glioma. This volume.

3. Hatanaka, H.: Boron Neutron Capture Therapy for tumors, Japan, Nishimura, 1986.

4. Levin, V.A., Edwardo, N.S. and Byrd, A.: Quantitative observations of the acute effects of X-irradiation on brain capillary permeability : Part I. Int. J. Radiat. Oncol. Biol. Phys. 5: 1627 - 1631, 1979.

5. Qin, D.X., Zeng, R., Tang J., Li, J.X., Hu, Y.H.: Influence of radiation on the blood-brain barrier and optimum time of chemotherapy. Int. J. Radiat. Oncol. Biol. Phys. 19: 1507-1510, 1990.

6. Stragliotto, G., Munafo, A., Biollaz, J., Frankhauser, H.: Pharmacokinetics of boron sulphydryl (BSH) in patients with intranomial tumor. This volume.

7. Sweet, H.W.: Practical problems of the past in the use of boron-slow neutron capture therapy in the treatment of glioblastoma multiforme. Proceedings Int. Symp. on Neutron Capture Therapy, Brookhaven National Laboratory Report no. 51730: 376-378, 1983.

8. Sweet, W.: Supplementary pharmacological studies between 1972 and 1977 on purified mercaptoundecahydrododecaborate. Boron Neutron Capture Therapy for tumors, H. Hatanaka, Ed., Japan, Nishimura: pp. 59-76,1986.

PROPOSED CLINICAL APPROACH TO BNCT

R.A. Gahbauer,[1] R.G. Fairchild,[4] J.H. Goodman,[2] T.E. Blue[3]

[1]Div. of Radiation Oncology, [2]Div. of Neurosurgery, [3]Div. of Nuclear Engineering, The Ohio State University, Columbus, Ohio, USA; [4]Medical Department, Brookhaven National Laboratory, Upton, New York, USA.

INTRODUCTION

Assessing tolerance of normal tissues in BNCT is complicated by the mix of high LET and low LET radiations, the constituents of which vary rapidly as a function of depth in tissue. The known dependence of biological effects on the extra- or intracellular distribution of boron further complicates this assessment. First, a method is proposed to estimate the tolerance of normal tissue to low LET radiation for the numbers of fractions anticipated. Then an algorithm is suggested to estimate tolerance to mixed high and low LET radiations. From high LET trials, the CNS tolerance to high LET radiation is known for various beams. In animal tolerance studies, the ratio of observed tolerance to expected tolerance can provide a compound factor to account for the unknowns affecting biological efficacy, e.g., boron localization.

Experience using fast neutrons to treat brain tumors indicates efficacy in the control of glioblastoma multiforme that even very high doses of low LET radiation cannot achieve. Fast neutrons alone at levels above 1300 cGy[1] or mixed beam radiations above 600 cGy high LET show efficacy,[2] although not within the tolerance of normal CNS. The tolerance of the CNS to fractionated fast neutrons is generally thought to be below 1000 cGy. It is further well established that the iso-effectiveness of high LET radiation is quite insensitive to fractionation, especially when 4 or more fractions are employed.[3]

The RBE's of various high LET radiations vary significantly; however, this variation is probably small compared to the effects of insufficiently or imprecisely known parameters, such as cellular boron distribution, protective factors, etc. For these reasons, a compound factor (as proposed by Gabel) is needed. From our formula, this factor would be the ratio of observed effects to expected effects and would be unique to every combination of beam and boron compound.

MATERIALS AND METHODS

For reasons discussed extensively elsewhere,[4] we anticipate that BNCT with epithermal beams will be used with a fractionation scheme employing a minimum of 4 fractions. Therefore, our first objective is to establish the tolerance of normal brain to 4 fractions of low LET radiation. Pezner and Archambeau have used a modified version of the Ellis-NSD formula to more realistically reflect brain tolerance.[5]

Formula 1. $TD = BTU \times N^k \times T^l$

BTU = Brain Tolerance Unit	N = Number of Fractions	T = Time in Days
k = 0.45	l = 0.03	TD = Tumor Dose

In our discussion, we evaluate the formula for 4 fractions and a treatment time of 5 days, using a BTU of 1200 which would reflect the upper limit of acceptable risk to normal tissue. Evaluation of this formula suggests a maximum tolerated low LET dose of 2300 cGy in 4 fractions in 5 days.

Our second objective, to estimate the tolerance of normal brain to high LET radiations if only high LET radiations were used, is more difficult because the experience is more limited and because varying fractionations and beams with different RBE's have been used. The influence of fractionation on iso-effect is minimal if more than 4 fractions are used. From clinical information drawn from instances in which more than 4 fractions were used, we may infer that the tolerance of normal CNS is less than 1000 cGy of high LET radiations.[1,2] We apply this limit to any fractionation scheme with more than 4 fractions of only high LET radiation.

Using the 2 restrictions given above, the following formula represents the maximum normal tissue dose (MTD):

Formula 2. $MTD = D_\gamma + D_h \times 2.3 = 2300.$

Here D_γ = total dose in cGy for low LET components and D_h = total high LET or particle dose, including components from the $^{14}N(n,p)^{14}C$ and $^{10}B(n,\alpha)^7Li$ reactions and fast neutron dose. The factor, 2.3, is a number chosen to restrict normal tissue dose to levels of high LET radiations found acceptable in fast neutron therapy and can be viewed as taking the function of an RBE. In other words, in this case the estimated tolerance of normal tissue was used to determine RBE's rather than the reverse. The measured, single dose RBE of fast neutrons encountered in BNCT, as well as from the $^{14}N(n,p)^{14}C$ reaction, is around 2, while that from the $^{10}B(n,\alpha)^7Li$ reaction was found to be 2.3.[7,8] Increasing the number of fractions would effectively increase our factor (just as RBE's would) as the MTD increases (for 6 fractions MTD = 2800; 2800 = $D_\gamma + D_h \times 2.8$) [From Formula 2: The factor 2.8 limits D_h to 1000cGy, as the RBE would].

Sample Calculation (based on interptretation of BMRR data):

Brain, separation 16 cm, parallel opposed ports.

$MTD = D_\gamma + D_h \times 2.3$

Dose rate <u>midline</u> (8 cm):	D_γ = 22 cGy/min	D_h = 4.48 cGy/min
Dose rate <u>3 cm depth</u>:	D_γ = 18 cGy/min	D_h = 7.08 cGy/min

Midline:

$$Treatment\ Time = \frac{MTD}{D_\gamma + D_h \times 2.3} = \frac{2300\ cGy}{22\ cGy/min + 4.48\ cGy/min \times 2.3} = 71.2\ min$$

3 cm Depth:

$$Treatment\ Time = \frac{MTD}{D_\gamma + D_h \times 2.3} = \frac{2300\ cGy}{18\ cGy/min + 7.08\ cGy/min \times 2.3} = 67\ min$$

First Conclusion: Limiting normal tissue dose at 3 cm. Therefore, dose prescription to 3 cm depth.

Calculation of doses received by normal tissues at 3 cm:

$$D_\gamma \quad = 67 \text{ min x } 18 \text{ cGy/min} \quad = 1206 \text{ cGy}$$
$$D_h \quad = 67 \text{ min x } 7.08 \text{ cGy/min} \quad = 474 \text{ cGy (all high LET and 6 ppm } {}^{10}\text{B)}$$
$$\text{Tumor} \quad = 67 \text{ min x } 28 \text{ cGy/min} \quad = 1876 \text{ cGy + normal tissue dose}$$
$$(30 \text{ ppm B})$$

Using treatment time, dose can then be calculated at any other depth.

DISCUSSION

The biological efficacy of boron is known to be a strong function of intracellular distribution, which is generally unknown or imprecisely known for the compounds being investigated for possible use in BNCT. Problems associated with the application of dose and RBE to BNCT are discussed elsewhere.[6] To account for unknowns inherent to BNCT, Gabel has proposed a compound factor. From Formula 2, this compound factor would be the ratio of observed effects to expected effects. The formula should be evaluated for several depths, at the minimum: at surface, at 3 cm, and at midline. The complexity of mixed high and low LET radiation, rapidly varying beam composition with depth, and problems with the description of dose inherent to BNCT make the determination of a predictive RBE difficult. The proposed formula attempts to relate known information on tolerance to the experiment in BNCT.

REFERENCES

1. M. Catterall, H.J.G. Bloom, D.V. Ash, L. Walsh, A. Richardson, D. Uttley, N.F.C. Gowing, P. Lewis, and B. Chaucer, Fast neutrons compared with megavoltage X-rays in the treatment of patients with supratentorial glioblastoma: A controlled pilot study, Int. J. Radiat. Oncol. Biol. Phys. 6:261-266, (1980).

2. G.E. Laramore, M. Diener-West, T.W. Griffin, J.S. Nelson, M.L. Griem, F.J. Thomas, F.R. Hendrickson, B.R. Griffen, L.C. Myrianthopoulos, and J. Saxton, Randomized neutron dose searching study for malignant gliomas of the brain: Results of an RTOG study, Int. J. Radiat. Oncol. Biol. Phys., 14:1093-1102, (1988).

3. J.F. Fowler, "Nuclear Particles in Cancer Treatment," Adam Hilger, Bristol, England, (1981).

4. R. Fairchild, V. Bond, and A. Woodhead, "Clinical Aspects of Neutron Capture Therapy," Prodeedings of the Workshop on Boron Neutron Capture Therapy, Feb. 1-2, 1988, Brookhaven National Laboratory, Upton, NY, Plenum Press, New York, (1989).

5. R. Pezner and J. Archambeau, Brain tolerance unit: A method to estimate risk of radiation brain injury for various dose schedules, Br. J. Radiat. Oncol. Biol. Phys. 7:397-402, (1981).

6. D. Gabel, Approach to boron neturon capture therapy in Europe: Goals of a european collaboration on boron neutron capture therapy, preprint from: EPAC 90, European Particle Accelerator Conf., Inst. of Electrical and Electronics Engineers, New York, (in press).

7. D. Gabel, R.G. Fairchild, Börje Larsson, and H.G. Börner, The relative biological effectiveness in V79 Chinese hamster cells of the neutron capture reactions in boron and nitrogen, Rad. Res. 98:307-316, (1984).

8. R. Fairchild, J. Kalef-Ezra, S, Saraf, et al., "Installation and testing of an optimized epithermal neutron beam at the Brookhaven Medical Research Reactor," Proceedings of the Workshop on Neutron Beam Design, Development, and performance for Neutron Capture Therapy, Massachusetts Institute of Technology, Cambridge, MA, March 1989.

CLINICAL EXPERIENCE OF BNCT FOR BRAIN AND SKIN TUMOURS AT KYOTO UNIVERSITY REACTOR

Y. Ujeno[1], K. Akuta[1], H. Hatanaka[2], Y. Mishima[3], Y. Oda[4], Y Nakagawa[5]

[1] Department of Radiation Oncology, Research Reactor Institute, Kyoto University, Sennan-gun, Kumatori-cho, Osaka 590-04, Japan
[2] Department of Neurosurgery, Faculty of Medicine, Teikyo University, Kaga, Itabashi-ku, Tokyo 173, Japan
[3] Department of Dermatology, Faculty of Medicine, Kobe University, Kusunoki, Chuo-ku, Kobe 650, Japan
[4] Department of Neurosurgery, Faculty of Medicine, Kyoto University, Shogoin, Sakyo-ku, Kyoto 606, Japan
[5] Department of Neurosurgery, National Pediatric Hospital of Kagawa, Zentsuji-shi, Kagawa 765, Japan

INTRODUCTION

The research nuclear reactor of Kyoto University (KUR), which was established in 1963, has the power of 5 MW and has rendered services to scientists in various fields including biology and medicine. The first clinical application was carried out on a brain tumour patient by Professor Hatanaka in 1974. Ten patients were treated from 1987 to January of 1991. As no medical doctor had served in the KUR Institute and clinical facilities were not available, there were no treatments from 1975 to 1986. After two medical doctors arrived at their posts in the Institute, KUR opened its door for clinical activities again in 1987.

PATIENTS

Eight Japanese, 2 German and one American patients were treated. The ages of patients were 9 - 66 years and all were male. Skin tumours were irradiated at KUR to measure ^{10}B content in the tissues by Nickel Mirror Neutron Guide Tube (NMNGT) attached to KUR, before BNCT. Except in a few cases, patients had recurrent tumours after previous treatment by chemotherapy, radiotherapy or surgical treatments. The absorbed dose used in the previous radiotherapy before BNCT was a curative dose. The time intervals between previous radiotherapy and BNCT varied. The treated brain tumours included astrocytoma grades II and III and the treated skin tumours included various grades of melanoma. Some cases appeared to be astrocytoma grade IV.

PHYSICAL CONDITIONS OF BNCT

The neutron fluence and the absorbed dose of γ-rays were about 2×10^{13} n cm^{-2} and about 6 Gy at the deepest position of the brain tumours, and about 1×10^{13} n cm^{-2} and about 3 Gy for the skin tumours, respectively. In BNCT, the tumours were exposed to a single irradiation. Therefore, the absorbed dose in BNCT for a given effect corresponds to about 0.4 times the total photon dose for conventional fractionated irradiation for the same effect, which was the method for the dose evaluation in the intraoperative radiation therapy. Assuming the RBE value of 2 at the D_0 value, the curative absorbed dose of BNCT corresponds to about 0.2 times the total photon dose for conventional fractionated irradiation. The RBE value is used to approximate actual curative doses in BNCT in Japan. The exact estimation of absorbed dose of BNCT was very difficult, because we could not know the exact content of ^{10}B at a given point in the tumour immediately before BNCT. In the case of a skin tumour, we measured the content of ^{10}B in the tumour mass directly by NMNGT, without any surgical operation. Such a direct measurement cannot be carried out for brain tumours. Therefore, the absorbed dose was calculated with the experimental data on ^{10}B content of brain tumours. A computer technique was used for this calculation. The reliability of these measurements and calculations is not clear. In some cases of brain tumours, heavy water was given to increase thermal neutron penetration of the tissues. The content of heavy water administered in patients has not yet been reported by the physicians in charge.

^{10}B CARRIERS

The ^{10}B compounds used were sodium mercaptoundecahydroclosododecaborate (BSH) for brain tumours and p-boronophenylalanine (BPA) with/without fructose, which is used to make the boron compound soluble in the body fluid. The ^{10}B did not succeed to accumulate significantly in the skin tumour mass, though it had succeeded in animal experiments. The opinion of the physician in charge who did BNCT in spite of the lack of accumulation of ^{10}B in the tumour mass, was not completely consented by other doctors, but the authority to do BNCT belongs only to the physician in charge in Japan.

The lack of ^{10}B compounds and the difficulties in obtaining the compounds are disturbing the development of BNCT in Japan today. The doctors cast about for the ways to administer ^{10}B compounds and/or the time interval between the administration of compounds to patients and irradiation. The most suitable way to administer ^{10}B compounds, however, may be different for each patient.

SUPPORTING SYSTEM BY OTHER MEDICAL INSTITUTIONS

The supporting system for BNCT at KUR by other medical institutions in the adjacent area of KUR was important in achieving success in BNCT, because KUR Institute has neither a room for surgical operation, nor an intensive care unit (ICU), nor a bedroom. One national hospital (National Pediatric Hospital of Kagawa), one municipal hospital (Kishiwada Municipal Hospital) and one private hospital (Mukaiyama Hospital) supported KUR as the affiliated hospitals. The patients were treated surgically before and after BNCT at these hospitals and were transported to their home hospitals a few days later. The patients treated for skin tumours were transported to the home hospital directly. The transportation was carried out by ambulance. The use of a helicopter was considered but has not been carried out yet because flying near nuclear reactors is prohibited. Foreign patients were transported by passenger planes after a sufficient observation time of about two weeks following BNCT.

RESULTS OF BNCT AT KUR

The results of BNCT at KUR are not surveyed yet, because the time interval from each BNCT to the present time is less than 5 years, except for one case. The patient in this case died 6 days after NCT. The cause of death was bleeding in the irradiated region of brain. The cause of

594

Table 1. BNCT at Kyoto University Reactor

No.	date	patients sex age	disease	history before BNCT	prognoses
1	1974: 4 May	male 44	brain tumour		died at 6th day following BNCT
2	1987: 7 July	male 66	metastatic melanoma of the scalp [measurement of ^{10}B conc. by prompt gamma spectrometry]	onset of primary tumour in 1984; metastatic lesion after surgery with chemo and immunotherapies to the primary tumour	died at 11 May 1988 by distant metastases
3	1990: 10 Feb	male 64	glioblastoma	after partial resection (20%) of the primary tumour on 14 Dec 1989	dissemination to unirradiated part of the brain died at 21 Nov
4	1990: 10 Feb	male 45	astrocytoma grade III	biopsy was performed in Oct 1989	surviving
5	1990: 13 Feb	male 61	satellite lesions of the scalp melanoma [measurement of ^{10}B & BNCT]	onset of primary tumour in April 1989; BNCT was performed on 4 Oct 1989 at Musashi Reactor	died at 2 Jan 1991 by multiple distant metastases
6	1990: 9 June	male 9	recurrent astrocytoma grade III	surgery and radiation therapy in Jan 1989	died in Nov 1990 by intracranial dissemination
7	1990: 31 Aug	male 61	glioblastoma	no treatment (biopsy)	surviving
8	1990: 15 Oct	male 32	recurrent astrocytoma grade III	recurrence after 2nd surgery with full dose irradiation	died on 21 Dec 1990 by intracranial dissemination
9	1990: 19 Nov	male 57	melanoma of the sole; stage I (8mm depth) [measurement of ^{10}B & BNCT]	onset in 1988; rapid growth in 1990 inoperable	surviving
10	1991: 28 Jan	male 59	glioblastoma	onset in Sep 1990; conventional radiotherapy was interrupted by patient refusal (24kg)	surviving
11	1991: 28 Jan	male 30	recurrent astrocytoma grade II	onset in Feb 1990; recurrence after surgery in Feb 1990	surviving

bleeding has not been reported. The data on BNCT carried out till January 1990 at KUR are listed in the table. There is some lack of data in the table, because of the poor general management of BNCT in the period at the beginning of the therapy.

UNSOLVED PROBLEMS

Besides the medical aspect of BNCT, we should pay attention carefully to the design of the reactor for clinical use. This is mainly a problem for the nuclear reactor technologists at KUR. The only gantry for BNCT is horizontal and the size of the irradiation room is only 250×250 cm^2. Furthermore, there is no space, no fundamental medical instrumentation, no paramedical staff for the pre-irradiation treatment including surgical operation, nor our own ambulance to transport patients. Also, we do not have the system to control various medical wastes nor to control radioactive clinical instruments. Another problem is the very complicated administrative procedure for BNCT. The application of BNCT is examined in several committees before sending the documents to the government office responsible for BNCT. As KUR Institute is not a hospital, we cannot receive fees for BNCT. This is also a very important problem.

CONCLUSION

Our recent experience in BNCT is limited to only ten cases. Being in the first phase of BNCT and KUR, we have to face many difficulties. However, we believe we shall soon jump over these hurdles. The time for BNCT at KUR is tentatively allowed to one day per month and, in principle, to one patient per day, and is announced beforehand. Therefore, the applicants must select the patient for BNCT on the schedule of KUR. This does not mean that BNCT takes precedence over other experiments. KUR does not serve for therapy alone. The application for clinical research with BNCT must be examined in advance by the steering committee of KUR Institute and the researchers are requested to report their results orally and by papers for 5 years to gather and to analyse the data on BNCT.

THE STATE OF THE ART FOR RADIOTHERAPY FOR BRAIN TUMORS:

NONCONVENTIONAL FRACTIONATION, HEAVY IONS, AND FAST-NEUTRON THERAPY

Ronald V. Dorn III,[1,2]

[1]PBF/BNCT Research Programs, Idaho National Engineering Laboratory, Idaho Falls, ID
[2]Mountain States Tumor Institute, Boise, ID

INTRODUCTION

Radiation therapy has long played a vital role in the overall management of malignant brain tumors. Conventional photon irradiation, delivered with standard fractionation (1.8 Gy - 2 Gy/F, one fractionation per day, five days per week) to total doses of 60-66 Gy, has proven to be effective in the long-term control of low-grade gliomas and to provide prolongation of local control and median survival in high-grade tumors. However, local control and survival of patients with high-grade gliomas (Grade III-IV astrocytomas, glioblastoma multiforme) remains dismal and has not improved <u>significantly</u> for a number of years.

A variety of new radiation therapy approaches are under investigation in an effort to improve the therapeutic ratio (i.e., to increase the number of tumor cells killed with decreased normal tissue damage):

1. Nonconventional fractionation
2. Heavy ions and pions
3. Protons
4. Fast neutrons
5. Brachytherapy
6. Radiosurgery
7. Photodynamic treatment
8. Adjuvant chemotherapy
9. Targeted radionuclides
10. Hyperthermia

This paper reviews the rationale and presents the status of these techniques, concluding with a discussion of the limitations of these techniques and of the potential of Boron Neutron Capture Therapy (BNCT) in this setting.

NONCONVENTIONAL FRACTIONATION

<u>Rationale</u> The *in-vivo* setting of a malignant brain tumor exhibits a number of characteristics that influence radiosensitivity: (1) hypoxic, but viable tumor cells present, (2) more rapid cellular division and growth of tumor cells compared to normal tissue (i.e., glial cells), and (3) increased capability of sublethal repair by normal cells compared with tumor cells.

Hyperfractionation (increased number of radiation doses delivered each treatment day as compared with the standard one fraction per day) theoretically takes advantage of these characteristics by: (1) decreasing the oxygen effect through decreased dose per fraction, (2) permitting more sublethal repair in the normal tissues, and (3) increasing the probability of cell-cycle mediated damage in the more rapidly proliferating tumor cells. A number of research programs are investigating this effect on brain tumors, using 2-3 fractions per day to total doses at or above conventional radiation therapy.

Current Status A review of the referenced papers discloses mixed results. Though a few studies show little difference compared to conventional radiation therapy, a number of studies do suggest improved median survival with good overall normal tissue tolerance. As a result, interest remains high, and ongoing research is further addressing the question with randomization and escalation of the total radiation dose. Problems with the technique include increased time and expense (justifiable only if the results are better than with conventional treatment) and imprecise tumor definition (in common with conventional treatment) resulting in undertreatment of undetected microscopic extension.[6,7,11,13,41,43,44,46]

HEAVY IONS, PIONS, AND PROTONS

Rationale The use of the more exotic forms of ionizing radiation is intriguing for a number of reasons: (1) some of these radiations show an increase in Linear Energy Transfer (LET) compared to x-rays, resulting in a more densely ionizing tract through tissue, and an increase in Relative Biologic Effectiveness (RBE), (2) as a result, the relative lack of oxygen in the tumor cells provides less of a protective effect, and (3) certain of the particulate radiations (protons, heavy ions, pions) can be delivered more precisely to a specific treatment volume than x-rays can. Figure 1[19] illustrates the distribution of these ionizing particles with respect to the above characteristics.

Current Status Unfortunately, heavy ions, pions, and protons are difficult and expensive to produce. As a result, there have been few facilities capable of performing the necessary radiobiological and clinical research, and, accordingly, little data are available on the effect of these modalities on brain tumors. Ongoing programs continue at BEVALAC (heavy ions), TRIUMF and SIN (pions), and Harvard and Fermilab (protons). Much more extensiveinvestigation and application will be possible in the future at CHIBA (heavy ions), Loma Linda (protons), and, hopefully, a revised BEVALAC facility. Problems remaining to be overcome include the lack of facilities and expense (mentioned above), and again the potential for geographic miss of unimaged or subclinical viable tumor (particularly the more malignant glioblastoma multiforme) by these precision radiations.[4,12,14]

FAST NEUTRONS

Rationale The rationale behind the use of fast neutrons in the treatment of brain tumors includes the high-LET, increased RBE, and decreased oxygen enhancement ratio (OER) characteristics they have in

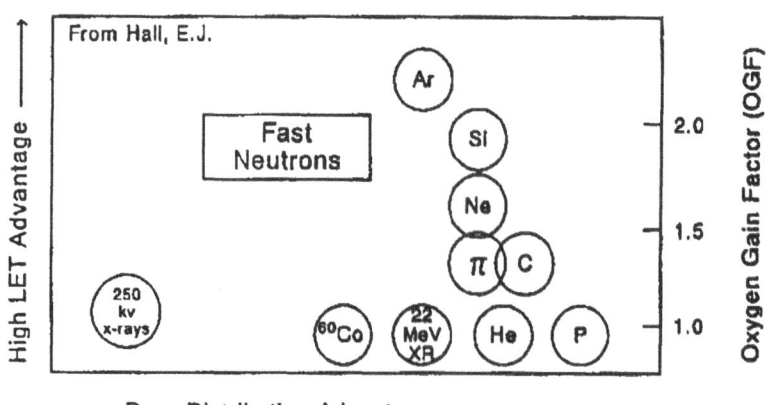

Figure 1. Distribution of ionizing particles.

common with the radiations discussed above. Fortunately, fast neutrons are much more readily produced permitting a far greater amount of research into their application. Several fast-neutron programs have been active for a number of years, including University of Washington (United States) and Hammersmith (United Kingdom), and a significant amount of data has accumulated with respect to brain tumors.

Current Status A synthesis of data from fast-neutron trials involving brain tumors reveals similar (but not improved) brain tumor survival when compared to conventional x-ray. This would appear to be due to two factors: (1) increased local tumor control, but at the same time (2) increased normal tissue (brain) damage because of the higher normal tissue RBE of the fast neutrons. (It is well to bear this fact in mind when discussing the need for reduced fast-neutron contamination in epithermal-neutron sources for BNCT.)

The disadvantages, then, of fast-neutron radiation for the treatment of brain tumors are several: (1) high normal brain RBE, (2) fast neutrons lack the precision-of-delivery characteristics of the other particulate radiations (Figure 1), and (3) lack of precise tumor-volume definition plagues this radiation modality in the same way as the others discussed above. [3,8,9,15-17,42,44]

BRACHYTHERAPY

Rationale As was mentioned in the introduction, brain tumors tend to recur locally rather than at a distant site. Implanted radioisotopes, because of their ability to deliver a more intense, localized dose to the tumor while delivering less dose to surrounding normal tissue, are an attractive modality for use in brain tumors. Additionally, the low dose rate inherent in "brachy"therapy should realize the same radiobiological benefits as hyperfractionation. A variety of isotopes has been investigated (^{125}I, ^{192}Ir, ^{60}Co, ^{198}Au), both afterloading and permanent, using stereotactic and intraoperative techniques.

Current Status A considerable amount of research continues in this area. Initial results are mixed (similar to hyperfractionation), though, again, some studies are showing early success with improved median survivals. Ongoing and proposed studies are investigating potential combination with chemotherapy, hyperthermia and external irradiation. Problems faced by this technique include the possibility of supralethal necrosis and the fact that the intensely localized irradiation can easily miss the more distant microscopic extensions seen in the most malignant tumors (i.e., glioblastoma multiforme). Additionally, the technique is invasive and not infrequently involves multiple surgical procedures, presenting both expense and quality-of-life concerns. [1,5,10,21,22,27-35,40,50,51]

OTHER APPROACHES

A number of other approaches are also being investigated that are beyond the scope of this review, including: (1) radiosensitizers and radioprotectors, [2,11,13,19,25,38] (2) radiosurgery (i.e., "gamma knife"), [24,35,36,47] (3) targeted radionuclides, [47,49] (4) hyperthermia, [37] and (5) photodynamic therapy. [20,23,26]

DISCUSSION - BNCT as a New Radiation Therapy Modality

A variety of new approaches to the application of ionizing radiation to the treatment of brain tumors has been reviewed. During the course of this review, several advantages and disadvantages of these approaches have been discussed including the need for more precise tumor definition (macro- and microscopically), the advantage of high-LET radiation, the relative radioresistance of hypoxic cells, and the advantage of precise dose delivery. Within the framework of these points, it is possible to review the potential of BNCT for brain tumors.

The theoretical advantages of BNCT for the management of malignant brain tumors include:

1.   Precise tumor definition (or visualization) is not as critical (ideally, a tumor-specific boron compound would localize to the tumor cells even when they are too small to "see");

2.	Therefore, microscopic disease would be treated;

3.	The (n,α) reaction, by definition, releases high-LET particles that are densely ionizing and lethal even to hypoxic tumor cells;

4.	Dose localization is precise at the cellular level; and

5.	BNCT treatment <u>could</u> be convenient, noninvasive, and fiscally reasonable (assuming it is nonsurgical, epithermal-neutron based and is delivered either in single dose or with relatively <u>few</u> fractions).

      As with the other radiation modalities discussed above, there are a number of specific problems with BNCT (assuming efficacy) that must be addressed to allow its full fruition as a viable treatment for brain tumors:

1.	More tumor-cell specific boron compounds must be developed;

2.	Epithermal-neutron sources must be developed that minimize as much as possible the fast-neutron component;

3.	The problem of supralethality may need to be addressed (perhaps requiring post-BNCT extirpation);

4.	The single dose <u>vs</u> fractionation question must be studied <u>in detail</u>. Not only may fractionation affect subsequent boron compound uptake, but fractionation would also markedly increase the per patient cost of BNCT treatment (possibly to a level not acceptable within the health care system).

SUMMARY

      The state-of-the-art of radiation therapy for brain tumors has been reviewed with a discussion of a variety of new treatment concepts. The advantages and disadvantages of BNCT for brain tumors have been reviewed within the context of the lessons learned from these modalities.

REFERENCES

1.	Bernstein, M., et. al., "Interstitial Brachytherapy for Malignant Brain Tumors: Preliminary Results," <u>Neurosurgery 26:</u> (3), 371-379; discussion 379-380 (1990).

2.	Bleehen, N. M., et. al., "A Randomized Study of Misonidazole and Radiotherapy for Grade 3 and 4 Cerebral Astrocytoma," <u>British Journal of Cancer 43:</u> 436-442 (1981).

3.	Breteau, B., et. al., "Fast Neutron Boost for the Treatment of Grade IV Astrocytomas," <u>Strahlentherapie Und Onkologie 165:</u> (4), 320-323 (April 1989).

4.	Castro, J. R., et. al., "Treatment of Cancer with Heavy Charged Particles," <u>International Journal of Radiation Oncology, Biology 8:</u> 2191-2198 (1982).

5.	Chun, M., et. al., "Interstitial ^{192}Ir Implantation for Malignant Brain Tumors. Part II: Clinical Experience," <u>British Journal of Radiology 62:</u> (734), 158-162 (February 1989).

6.	Deutsch, M., et. al., "Results of a Randomized Trial Comparing BCNU Plus Radiotherapy, Streptozotocin Plus Radiotherapy, BCNU Plus Hyperfractionated Radiotherapy, and BCNU Following Misonidazole Plus Radiotherapy in the Postoperative Treatment of Malignant Glioma," <u>International Journal of Radiation Oncology, Biology, Physics 16:</u> (6), 1389-1396 (June 1989).

7.	Douglas, B. G. and A. J. Worth, "Superfractionation in Glioblastoma Multiforme - Results of a Phase II Study," <u>International Journal of Radiation Oncology, Biology, Physics 8:</u> 1782-1794 (1982).

8.   Duncan, W., et. al., "Report of a Randomized Pilot Study of the Treatment of Patients with Supratentorial Gliomas Using Neutron Irradiation," British Journal of Radiology 59: 373-377 (1986).

9.   Duncan, W., et. al., "The Results of a Randomized Trial of Mixed-Schedule (Neutron/Photon) Irradiation in the Treatment of Supratentorial Grade III and Grade IV Astrocytoma," British Journal of Radiology 59: 379-383 (1986).

10. Etou, A., et. al., "Stereotactic Interstitial Irradiation of Diencephalic Tumors with ^{192}Ir and ^{125}I: Ten Years Follow-up and Comparison with Other Treatments," Childs Nervous System 5: (3), 140-3 (1989).

11. Fulton, D. S., et. al., "Misonidazole Combined with Hyperfractionation in the Management of Malignant Gliomas," International Journal of Radiation Oncology, Biology, Physics 10: 1709-1712 (1984).

12. Goodman, G. B., et. al., "Pion Therapy at TRIUMF. Treatment Results for Astrocytoma Grades 3 and 4: A Pilot Study," Radiotherapy and Oncology 17: (1), 21-28 (January 1990).

13. Green, S. B., et. al., "Randomized Comparisons of BCNU, Streptozotocin, Radiosensitizer, and Fractionation of Radiotherapy in the Postoperative Treatment of Malignant Glioma," Proceedings of ASCO 3: 260 (1984).

14. Greiner, R., et. al., "Anaplastic Astrocytoma and Glioblastoma: Pion Irradiation with the Dynamic Conformation Technique at the Swiss Institute for Nuclear Research (SIN)," Radiotherapy Oncology 17: (1), 37-46 (1990).

15. Griffin, B. R., et. al., "Neutron Radiotherapy for Malignant Gliomas," American Journal of Clinical Oncology 12: (4), 311-315 (August 1989).

16. Griffin, T. W., et. al., "Fast Neutron Radiation Therapy for Glioblastoma Multiforme," American Journal of Clinical Oncology 6: 661-667 (1983).

17. Hornsey, S., et. al., "Radiation Biologic Effectiveness for Damage to the Central Nervous System by Neutrons," International Journal of Radiation Oncology, Biology, Physics 7: 185-189 (1980).

18. Gutin, P. H., et. al., "Hypoxic Cell Radiosensitizers in the Treatment of Malignant Brain Tumors," Neurosurgery 6: 567-576 (1980).

19. Hall, E. J., in Radiobiology for the Radiologist, Lippincott, NY (1988).

20. Hill, J. S., et. al., "Selective Uptake of Hematoporphyrin Derivative into Human Cerebral Glioma," Neurosurgery 26: (2), 248-254 (1990).

21. Hirsch, J. F. et. al., "Stereotaxic Techniques with an Open Skull in the Treatment of Space-Occupying Brain Lesions," Neurochirurgie 35: (3), 164-168 (1989).

22. Jani, S. K., et. al., "Choice of Radioisotope in Stereotactic Interstitial Radiotherapy of Small Brain Tumors," Applied Neurophysiology 50: (1-6), 295-301 (1987).

23. Kaye, A. H., "Photoradiation Therapy of Brain Tumors," Ciba Found Symp 146: 209-221; discussion 221-224 (1989).

24. Kimmig, B., et. al., "Radiosurgery for Cerebral Angiomas (Meeting Abstract), Fourth International Conference on Advances in Regional Cancer Therapy, June 5-7, 1989, Berchtesgaden, FRG, Cyanamid Lederle, Arzneimittel GmbH and Co., C9 (1989).

25. Kinsella, T. J., et. al., "A Phase I Study of Intermittent Intravenous Bromodeoxyuridine (BUdR) with Conventional Fractionated

Irradiation, _International Journal of Radiation Oncology, Biology, Physics 10:_ 69-76 (1984).

26. Kostron, H., et. al., "Photodynamic Therapy of Malignant Brain Tumors: A Phase I/II Trial," _British Journal of Neurosurgery 2:_ (2), 241-248 (1988).

27. Kumar, P. P., et. al., "Intraoperative ^{60}Co Treatment of Glioblastoma Multiforme," _Radiation Medicine 6:_ (5), 219-228 (September–October 1988).

28. Kumar, P. P., et. al., "Survival of Patients with Glioblastoma Multiforme Treated by Intraoperative High-Activity ^{60}Co Endocurietherapy," _Cancer 64:_ (7), 1409-1413 (October 1989).

29. Larson, G. L., et. al., "Interstitial Radiogold Implantation for the Treatment of Recurrent High-Grade Gliomas," _Cancer 66:_ (1), 27-29 (July 1990).

30. Larson, D. A., et. al., "Stereotaxic Irradiation of Brain Tumors," _Cancer 65:_ (3) Suppl 792-799 (February 1990).

31. Leibel, S. A., et. al., "Survival and Quality of Life After Interstitial Implantation of Removable High-Activity ^{125}I Sources for the Treatment of Patients with Recurrent Malignant Gliomas," _International Journal of Radiation Oncology, Biology, Physics 17:_ (6), 1129-1139 (1989).

32. Leibel, S. A., et. al., "Interstitial Irradiation for the Treatment of Primary and Metastatic Brain Tumors," _Cancer: Princ Pract Oncol Updates 3:_ (7), 1-11 (1989).

33. Leibel, S. A., et. al., "The Integration of Interstitial Implanation into the Primary Management of Patients with Malignant Gliomas: Results of Phase II Northern California Oncology Group Trial," _American Journal of Clinical Oncology 10:_ 106 (1987).

34. Leibel, S. A. and P. H. Gutin, "Stereotaxic Insterstitial Implanation for the Treatment of Malignant Brain Tumors," _in_ Radiation Oncology, Vol. 2, T. L. Philips and W. M. Warea (editors), Raven Press, NY, 73-90 (1987).

35. Loeffler, J. S., et. al., The Treatment of Recurrent Brain Metastases with Stereotactic Radiosurgery," _J. Clinical Oncology 8:_ (4), 576-82 (1990).

36. Lunsford, L. D., et. al., "Stereotactic Gamma Knife Radiosurgery. Initial North American Experience in 207 Patients," _Arch Neurol 47:_ (2), 169-175 (1990).

37. Nelson, D. F., et. al., "Recent and Current Investigations of Radiation Therapy of Malignant Gliomas," _Seminars in Oncology 3:_ 46-55 (1986).

38. Nelson, D. F., et. al., "A Randomized Comparison of Misonidazole Sensitized Radiotherapy Plus BCNU for Treatment of Malignant Glioma After Surgery: Final Report of RTOG Study," _International Journal of Radiation Oncology, Biology, Physics 12:_ 1793-1800 (1986).

39. Nitta, T., et. al., "Astrocytic Tumors and Oligodendroglial Tumors, _Lancet 335:_ (8686), 368-371 (1990).

40. Ostertag, C. B., "Stereotactic Interstitial Radiotherapy for Brain Tumors," _Journal of Neurosurgical Sciences 33:_ (1), 83-89 (January–March 1989).

41. Packer, R. J., et. al., "Hyperfractionated Radiotherapy for Children with Brainstem Gliomas: A Pilot Study Using 7,200 cGy," _Ann Neurology 27:_ (2), 167-73 (1990).

42. Parker, R. G., et. al., "Fast Neutron Beam Radiotherapy of Glioblastoma Multiforme," _American Journal of Roentgenology 127:_ 331-335 (1976).

43. Payne, D., et. al., "Malignant Astrocytoma: Hyperfractionated and Standard Radiotherapy with Chemotherapy in a Randomized Prospective Clinical Trial," <u>Cancer 50:</u> 2301-236 (1982).

44. Saroja, K.R., et. al., "Failure of Accelerated Neutron Therapy to Control High-Grade Astrocytomas," <u>International Journal of Radiation Oncology, Biology, Physics 17:</u> (6), 1295-1297 (December 1989).

45. Schwade, J. G., et. al., "Small-Field Stereotactic External-Beam Radiation Therapy of Intracranial Lesions: Fractionated Treatment with a Fixed-Halo Immobilization Device," <u>Radiology 176:</u> (2), 563-565 (August 1990).

46. Shin, K. H., et. al., "Suprafractionation Radiation Therapy in the Treatment of Malignant Astrocytoma," <u>Cancer 52:</u> 2040-2043 (1983).

47. Smith, D. B., et. al., "Quantitative Distribution of ^{131}I-Labelled Monoclonal Antibodies Administered by the Intro-Ventricular Route," <u>Eur. J. Cancer 26:</u> (2), 129-136 (1990).

48. Stadler, B., et. al., "Misonidazole and Irradiation in the Treatment of Glioblastoma Multiforme: Preliminary Report of the Vienna Study Group," <u>International Journal of Radiation Oncology, Biology, Physics 10:</u> 1713-1717 (1984).

49. Stavrou, D., "Monoclonal Antibodies in Neuro-Oncology," <u>Neurosurgery Review 13:</u> (1), 7-18 (1990).

50. Weaver, K., et. al., "A CT-Based Computerized Treatment Planning System for ^{125}I Stereotactic Brain Implants," <u>International Journal of Radiation Oncology, Biology, Physics 18:</u> (2), 445-454 (1990).

51. Wowra, B. and H. P. Sturm, "Incidence of Late Radiation Necrosis with Transient Mass Effect After Interstitial Low Dose Rate Radiotherapy for Cerebral Gliomas," <u>Acta Neurochirurgica 99:</u> (3-4), 104-108 (1989).

COPYRIGHT

INCIDENCE AND SURVIVAL OF CANCERS FOR WHICH AVAILABLE

TREATMENTS APPEAR INEFFECTIVE

Dace Shugg 1, Michael Jones 1, Terence Dwyer 1, Anton
Bonett 2 & Anita Roberts 3.

1. Menzies Centre for Population Health Research,
   43 Collins St Hobart 7000 Australia.

2. Central Cancer Registry Unit PO Box 6 Rundle Mall
   Adelaide 5001 Australia.

3. Department of Geography and Environmental Studies,
   University of Tasmania, Sandy Bay Tasmania 7005 Australia.

INTRODUCTION

The prognosis for patients with some malignant neoplasms remains poor
despite all currently available treatment methods and the utilisation of the
latest diagnostic procedures. Incidence and survival data for brain, lung,
cutaneous malignant melanoma and pancreatic cancer are presented. We draw the
inference from these data that new treatment modalities may need to be sought
for patients with these malignant conditions which between them claimed 9,049
lives in Australia in 1988 alone.

MATERIALS AND METHODS.

Australian mortality data for the four sites covering a population of
nearly 17 million people have been obtained from the Australian Bureau of
Statistics. This data has been age standardised according to the World Health
Organization Population strata. Cancer incidence data for all of Australia is
only available for 1982.[1] To provide some indication of Australian incidence
trends we have combined data from the South Australian and Tasmanian State
cancer registries for the years 1978 to 1986, covering a population of
approximately 2 million people. Survival data from the Tasmanian cancer
registry is calculated by using the life table method. Survival was also
assessed for each site according to year of incidence to see if there had been
any improvement since 1978. Survival figures cover a population of just under
half a million people.

RESULTS AND DISCUSSION

Brain Cancer. Fig 1a shows Mortality and incidence rates are rising in
both men and women. Fig 1b shows survival of 236 brain cancer patients and 88
patients with glioblastoma or anaplastic astrocytoma diagnosed in Tasmania
between 1978 and 1987. The subset of cases was selected on the basis of ICDO
morphological codes 94013, 94403, 94413 & 94423.[2] These types have a very
similar prognosis [3] so they were combined for our analysis of glioblastoma
survival. The median survival was 5 months and the 5 year survival was 2%. A

Table 1. Summary of Incidence, Mortality and Survival trends.

SITES		INCIDENCE		MORTALITY		DEATHS	SURVIVAL		
		1982 ASR[a]	TREND[b]	1982 ASR	TREND[c]	1988 (N)	MEDIAN	5 YEAR	CHANGE[d]
BRAIN	M	6.3	rise	4.7	rise	848	7 mo	16%	NO
	F	4.1	rise	3.2	rise				
LUNG	M	54.0	fall	48.7	fall	6169	8 mo	6%	YES
	F	12.5	rise	10.5	rise				
MELANOMA	M	18.0	rise	4.5	rise	784	-	78%	NO
	F	17.6	rise	2.2	rise				
PANCREAS	M	8.0	fall	7.8	fall	1248	3 mo	1%	NO
	F	4.4	rise	4.4	rise				

a Age Standardized Rate / 100,000
b Incidence Trends showing rise or fall over the years 1978 - 86
c Mortality trends showing rise or fall over the years 1969 - 88
d Has survival changed since 1978?

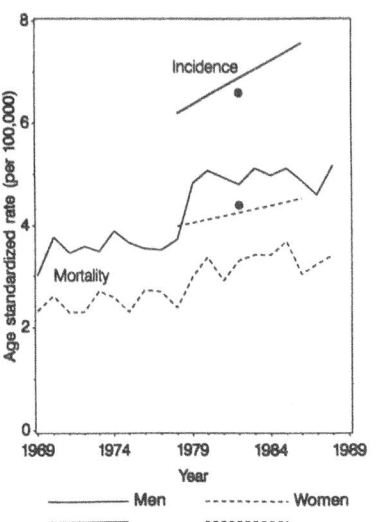 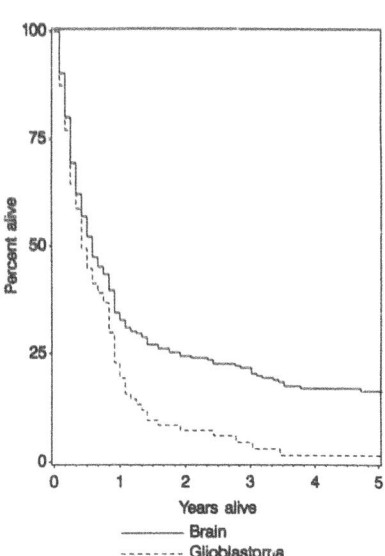

Fig 1a   Brain Cancer Incidence and Mortality. Black dot represents the 1982 age standardised incidence rate for Australia.

Fig 1b   Five year survival curves for 236 brain cancer patients and 88 glioblastoma patients.

recent survival analysis of patients with Grade III and Grade IV Astrocytomas in South Australia showed a median survival of 6 months [4]. There has been no improvement in survival for any of the brain cancers since 1978 in Tasmania.

Lung cancer. Mortality rates for men were rising till about 1980 but have levelled off and are now falling (Table 1). Female mortality rates continue to rise. Both male and female incidence rates follow the same trends as mortality in recent years. Lung cancer remains the most common cause of death from cancer in Australia. Survival for those patients diagnosed in 1985/86 is marginally better than for those diagnosed in 1978/79. However even in the improved group; survival is still less than 10% at 4 years.

Melanoma. Incidence and mortality rates are rising in both men and women (Table 1). Survival analysis of 101 Tasmanian patients with primary melanoma thicker than 3mm. but no distant metastases showed median survival of 5 years and five year survival of 50%. Patients with locally advanced disease and metastases in regional lymph nodes had a median survival of 21 months and five year survival was 29%. Median survival of patients with distant metastases was 8 months and five year survival was 16%. (Thickness of the primary lesion and loco-regional spread are important prognostic factors). These are the patients who are most likely to suffer local recurrence or distant metastases and die from the disease. The extremely poor prognosis and lack of effective therapy for recurrent melanoma, is also reported from the Sydney Melanoma Unit in 1988.[5] There is no evidence of improvement in survival for melanoma since 1978 in the Tasmanian data.

Pancreatic Cancer. Both mortality and incidence rates for men have decreased since 1980 and have increased slightly in women (Table 1). There has been no improvement in survival since 1978 for this most lethal cancer.

CONCLUSIONS

Clearly there is a need for more effective therapies for tumours in these four sites. Clinical trials in Japan have shown promising results with Neutron Capture Therapy for patients with advanced melanoma and glioblastoma [6,7]. Hopefully work will continue till we also have more effective therapies for the thousands of people who die of pancreatic and lung cancer every year.

REFERENCES

1. Giles GG, Armstrong BK, Smith LR, 1987, Cancer in Australia 1982, Australasian Association of Cancer Registries. National Cancer Statistics Clearing House Scientific Publication No 1.

2. International Classification of Diseases for Oncology 1st Ed. 1976 WHO Geneva.

3. McMenemey WH & Thomas Smith W, The Central Nervous System in: Systemic Pathology Ed: Symmers W.St.C, 2nd. ed. Churchill Livingstone New York 1979. 2208-2210.

4. North B, Reilly P, Blumbergs P, Roder D & Esterman A, Malignant Astrocytoma in South Australia:treatment and case survival.Med J Aust 1990;153,250-253.

5. Coates. A, Current Status of Clinical Trials of Therapeutic Modalities for Malignant Melanoma in Australia. Pigment Cell Research 2;370-371.

6. Allen BJ. The Potential of Neutron Capture Therapy in the Management of Uncontrollable Localised Tumours. Australas Radiol 1990;34 297-305.

7. Allen BJ, Epithermal neutron capture therapy: a new modality for the treatment of glioblastoma and melanoma metastatic to the brain. Med J Aust 153; 296-298.

LIMITATIONS IN THE CONVENTIONAL TREATMENT OF CEREBRAL METASTASES FROM MELANOMA

Graham Stevens

Department of Radiation Oncology and Sydney Melanoma Unit

Royal Prince Alfred Hospital, Camperdown, Sydney, 2050

Introduction

Cerebral metastases are a common diagnosis in patients with disseminated melanoma, giving rise to neurological symptoms that are frequently devastating for the patient and his family. Treatment options are often limited and in most series the median survival from diagnosis of cerebral metastases is 2-6 months[1-3] with death due to progressive intracranial disease. Therefore, the treatment of cerebral metastases is an issue of major concern for clinicians who manage patients with metastatic melanoma. This paper will summarise the current management of cerebral metastases from melanoma, based on a series of 129 patients treated in the Department of Radiation Oncology at Royal Prince Alfred Hospital from 1982 to 1990 (Stevens et al, Radiother. Oncol., 1991 submitted).

Management

Diagnosis

In most cases the diagnosis of intracranial metastases is made following investigation of neurological symptoms such as headache, changes in mental state or hemiparesis. A small number of patients are asymptomatic and are diagnosed as a result of routine or pre-treatment imaging. Histological confirmation of the cerebral lesions is not usually required if the patient has a past history of malignant melanoma.

Following diagnosis, high doses of corticosteroids are administered to reduce intracranial pressure. This leads to a marked improvement of the symptoms for most patients. Subsequent management depends on an inter-related set of factors, the most important being;

a) the number of cerebral lesions and their surgical accessibility for resection,

b) the general condition of the patient,

c) the presence and extent of extracranial metastases.

Solitary cerebral metastases

There is general agreement that complete surgical resection represents the optimal management of a single cerebral metastasis. This is particularly true if there is no evidence of extracranial disease, in which case craniotomy and resection provide the greatest chance for prolonged survival. In fact, most patients who survive two years or more following diagnosis of cerebral metastases have had complete resection of a solitary cerebral lesion[4]. Even in the presence of limited extracranial disease, resection of a single cerebral metastasis is warranted, as survival is improved and subsequent neurological symptoms can be prevented. However, as cerebral metastases are single in less than 50% of cases and as resection is usually restricted to patients with single cerebral lesions, this form of treatment is not applicable to the majority of patients.

Postoperative whole brain irradiation is indicated for all patients, as an en bloc resection of gross tumour is not possible in most cases and cerebral disease is often more widespread than suspected. Postoperative irradiation has been shown to reduce the incidence of further intracranial relapse, but does not have a significant impact on survival[5]. The usual dose schedule in this setting is 30Gy in 2 weeks.

If a single lesion is unresectable, due to its location in the brain, or the general condition of the patient is poor with widespread metastases, a course of palliative whole brain irradiation is indicated (see below). Survival for these patients with unresectable single lesions is similar to that of patients with multiple cerebral metastases. Also, survival following incomplete resection of cerebral metastases is similar to that of patients who have not had surgery. Therefore, unless the neurosurgeon believes that a complete resection of all intracranial disease is possible, it is doubtful that the surgery will be beneficial.

Multiple cerebral metastases

For the majority of patients, who have multiple or unresectable cerebral metastases, the only effective treatment is corticosteroids and radiotherapy, used with palliative intent. The most commonly used radiation schedule for whole brain irradiation is 30Gy in 10 fractions over 2 weeks, although higher doses and unconventional schedules have been investigated, due to the poor response to standard therapy. These unconventional schedules (listed below) have been based on a number of theoretical concepts;

a) high doses per fraction,[6-8] in an attempt to overcome the initial "shoulder" on the cell survival curve for melanoma,

b) accelerated fractionation,[9,10] to enable the dose of radiation to be delivered before tumour cell proliferation takes place,

c) chemotherapy used concurrently with radiation, eg the use of low-dose cisplatin to inhibit the repair of radiation-induced potentially lethal damage (Rosenthal et al, Europ. J. Oncol., 1990 submitted).

Unfortunately, none of these methods has led to a significant improvement in survival and most patients succumb to progressive cerebral disease. The most likely explanation for the failure of these strategies to control intracranial metastases is the inability to deliver a tumouricidal dose of radiation without exceeding normal brain tolerance.

Conclusion

The diagnosis of cerebral metastases from melanoma confers a very poor prognosis overall and usually is the terminal event in the disease. A better prognosis, with the possibility of long term survival, is found only for those few patients with no evidence of extracranial disease and a single cerebral metastasis that can be resected completely.

It is clear that current treatment options are inadequate for the majority of patients. If radiation is to be effective in controlling cerebral metastases from melanoma, much higher doses need to be delivered selectively to the tumour cells, avoiding damage to normal tissues. Boron neutron capture therapy (BNCT) offers this possibility of obtaining a therapeutic gain by selective uptake into melanoma cells of melanin precursors containing boron-10. Novel techniques, such as BNCT, have the potential to improve both survival and quality of life and should continue to be investigated actively.

References

1. Cooper, J.S. and Carella, M.D. Radiotherapy of intracranial malignant melanoma. Radiology 134: 735-738 (1980).

2. Gottlieb, J.A., Frei, E. and Luce, J.K. An evaluation of the management of patients with cerebral metastases from malignant melanoma. Cancer 29: 701-705 (1972).

3. Retsas, S. and Gershuny, A.R. Central nervous system involvement in malignant melanoma. Cancer 61: 1926-1934 (1988).

4. Madajewicz, S., Karakovsis, C., West, C.R. and Caracandas, J. Malignant melanoma brain metastases: review of Roswell Park Memorial Institute experience. Cancer 53: 2550-2552 (1984).

5. Hagan, N.A., Cirrincione, C., Thaler, H.T. and DeAngelis, L.M. The role of radiation therapy following resection of a single metastasis from melanoma. Neurology 40: 158-160 (1990).

6. Katz, H.R. The relative effectiveness of radiation therapy, corticosteroids, and surgery in the management of melanoma metastatic to the central nervous system. Int. J. Radiat. Oncol. Biol. Phys. 7: 897-906 (1981).

7. Vlock, D.R., Kirkwood, J.M., Leutzinger, C., Kapp, D.J. and Fischer, J.J. High-dose fraction therapy for intracranial metastases of malignant melanoma: a comparison with low-dose fraction therapy. Cancer 49: 2289-2294 (1982).

8. Ziegler, J.C . and Cooper, J.S. Brain metastases from malignant melanoma: conventional vs high dose fraction radiotherapy. Int. J. Radiat. Oncol. Biol. Phys. 12: 1939-1842 (1986).

9. Choi, K.N., Withers, H.R. and Rotman, M. Intracranial metastases from melanoma: clinical features and treatment by accelerated fractionation. Cancer 56: 1-9 (1985).

10. Choi, K.N., Withers, H.R. and Rotman, M. Metastatic melanoma in brain: rapid treatment or large dose fractions. Cancer 56: 10-15 (1985).

PHOTODYNAMIC THERAPY OF BRAIN TUMOURS

Andrew H. Kaye

Higginbotham Neuroscience Research Institute, Departments of Surgery
and Neurosurgery, Royal Melbourne Hospital, Victoria, Australia

Cerebral tumours are responsible for approximately 2% of all cancer
deaths and the high grade cerebral glioma is the most common cerebral
tumour in adults. At the present time there is no satisfactory treatment
for the malignant cerebral glioma. The best available treatment, using
surgery, radiation therapy and systemic chemotherapy results in a median
survival time of less than one year (Walker et al 1978; Walker et al 1980).
In most cases surgery only provides a histological confirmation of the
diagnosis and provides palliation of symptoms of raised intracranial
pressure. Radiotherapy prolongs the median survival to 37 weeks and at
present chemotherapy is of limited value when given by either conventional
or the intracarotid route. Most treatment failures occur because of local
recurrence of the tumour, indicating that a more aggressive local therapy
to the tumour could be beneficial for the treatment of gliomas.

Photodynamic therapy (PDT) is a technique that offers special
advantages as an adjuvant therapy for malignant brain tumours as it has
been shown to be an effective method of controlling local tumour growth in
other tumour types. The technique involves the selective uptake of a
photosensitizer, such as haematoporphyrin derivative, followed by radiation
of the tumour containing the sensitizer with light of a wave length that
will penetrate tissue and activate the sensitizer in the tumour cells (Kaye
et al 1988).

The use of light as a therapeutic agent goes back many centuries,
first being used by the Egyptians, Chinese and Indians in the treatment of
many diseases including vitiligo, Rickett's, psoriasis, skin cancer and
even psychosis (Daniell and Hill 1990). Photochemotherapy, or the use of
an exogenous sensitizer to absorb photons and then react for a therapeutic
effect also has a long history and psoralens were used in India as early as
1400 B.C. More recently psoralens have been used in PUVA therapy for
psoriasis, vitiligo and mycosis fungoid. The term photodynamic therapy was
used by von Tappeiner following his experience in the early 1990's with his
student Oscar Raab. He was the first to attempt phototherapy of tumours
with Jesionek when he applied a 5% solution of eosin topically to skin
tumours, and irradiated the area with light for several weeks (Daniell and
Hill 1990). In 1960 tumour fluorescence was reported using the
photosensitizer haematoporphyrin derivative (Lipson et al 1961) and this
was first used in 1966 to treat a patient with fungating breast tumour
(Lipson et al 1967). Diamond et al 1972 first investigated the use of PDT

on cerebral tumours and examined the effect of haematoporphyrin activated by white light on glioma cells in culture and on transplanted glioma tumours in rats. The experiments demonstrated death of cells in culture and considerable destruction of tumours in rats.

A clinical trial was commenced by Dougherty and his colleagues in 1976 and PDT has now been used in the treatment of several different tumour types, including tumours of the oesophagus, bladder and lung and has been demonstrated to be useful for the control of local disease (Kaye and Hill 1990). Perria et al (1980) reported the first attempts at PDT of human gliomas.

Laboratory Investigation of Photodynamic Therapy

PDT has been demonstrated to kill glioma cells in vitro (Diamond et al 1972, Laws et al 1981, Wharen et al 1986). Highly selective uptake of haematoporphyrin derivative into cerebral tumours in animal models has been demonstrated (Wharen et al 1983; Kaye et al 1985). The basis for the selective localisation to the tumour and its exclusion from normal brain is probably related to an intact blood brain barrier preventing the sensitizer entering the normal brain, and the relative lack of the barrier within the tumour allowing the sensitizer to penetrate into the tumour tissue. The evidence for this includes the fact that uptake of HpD into normal brain occurs only into areas known to be outside the blood brain barrier, or when the barrier is disrupted by mannitol (Kaye et al 1985).

The C6 glioma cell line has been used to develop a glioma model in adult rats and as a xenograft in both neonatal and adult mouse brains (Kaye et al 1986). These models have been used to investigate the use of PDT therapy for gliomas and to study the effect of PDT on normal brain to determine the most appropriate dose of light to obtain maximal kill with minimal damage to normal tissue (Kaye and Morstyn 1987).

PDT can achieve selective tumour kill of a cerebral glioma with sparing of normal brain using red light from either the gold metal vapour laser or the argon rhodamine pump dye laser (Kaye and Morstyn 1987). This selective destruction in the C6 glioma model occurred at doses of HpD at less than 20 mg/kg and light doses of less than 260 joule/cm^2. Using 20 mg/kg of HpD and 200 joule/cm^2 red light from the argon-dye laser, the mean depth of tumour kill was 4.5 mm and in 20% of animals the depth of tumour destruction was greater than 6 mm. Increasing the dose of HpD from 20 mg/kg to 60 mg/kg did not increase the depth of destruction but it increased both the likelihood of developing cerebral oedema and necrosis in normal brain. There was a significantly greater depth of tumour kill when higher doses of light (up to 600 joule/cm^2) were used in animals that had been pre-treated with either 20 to 40 mg/kg of HpD with destruction extending up to a depth of 1 cm. However, increasing the dose of red light above 260 joule/cm^2 significantly increased the likelihood and extent of necrosis in normal brain. Despite the relationship of depth of tumour destruction to dose of red light the dose rate effect with PDT was not evident.

Photodynamic Therapy in Clinical Neurosurgery

The first attempts of photoradiation therapy of human gliomas were reported in 1980. Table 1 shows series that have been reported since then. Most tumours have been adult high grade gliomas or recurrent gliomas. Light has been administered by either a Xenon arc lamp, argon-dye laser, helium neon laser of gold metal vapour laser. Although the early clinical studies of PDT were disappointing in their therapeutic effect, the studies

TABLE 1

SERIES REPORTING PRT OF CEREBRAL TUMOURS

Study	Number of patients	Power (watts)	Light dose	
			Total dose (joules)	Total dose to tumour (joules/cm^2)
Perria et al 1981	9	0.25	*	0.9-9
McCullouch et al 1984	16	0.280-0.460	1,620-2,520	*
Laws et al 1981	5	0.250-0.400	540-1,440	*
Wharen et al 1983	3	*	*	180**
Muller & Wilson 1985	8	*	439-3,888	8-68
Kostron et al 1986	20	*	*	25-200
Kaye et al 1987, 1990	85	0.75-5.0	3,360-10,613	72-260

* Information not available
** Derived from 100 mw/cm^2 for 30 minutes delivered by Xenon Arc Lamp

involved the treatment of recurrent gliomas and the doses or light were up to 100 times lower than used in systemic tumours.

The Royal Melbourne Hospital series consists of 85 patients with gliomas treated with PDT to the tumour bed following resection of the glioma. A gold metal vapour laser has been used with light intensity of up to 5 watt at the fibre tip and a tumour dose of up to 260 joule/cm^2. 0.5% intralipid is used as a diffusing agent. The temperature in the tumour bed is measured and kept below 37.5^{0}C with irrigating solution. Following surgery and PDT, a course of radiotherapy was administered (45 Gy in 20 doses).

Patients are instructed to remain out of direct sunlight initially for 4 weeks and then gradually to increase daily exposure to sun due to the skin photosensitization resulting from haematoporphyrin derivative infusion. Although increased cerebral oedema following photodynamic therapy has been reported this has not been a clinical problem in our series and the cerebral oedema is satisfactorily controlled with steroid therapy.

In the phase I-II Royal Melbourne Hospital trial the median survival time for glioblastoma multiforme is 18 months. Patients with recurrent glioblastoma multiforme have been treated by further tumour resection and PDT and the median survival time is 6 months.

Future Applications

The initial results using photodynamic therapy show a favourable trend, but the data are not sufficient to draw definite conclusions concerning the efficacy of the therapy. The major limiting clinical factors in treating cerebral gliomas are selectively of tumour uptake, particularly in the brain adjacent to tumour region, and the penetrating power of the laser light or other porphyrin activating systems. New sensitizers are being tested, particularly those that absorb light at a higher wavelength which would penetrate biological tissue better. There is a theoretical possibility of combining photodynamic therapy with boron neutron capture therapy if an appropriate sensitizer can be synthesized. This type of dual binary system treatment has particular theoretical advantages as it would maximise the local tumour kill in cancer where the basic clinical problem is that of local recurrence of the tumour.

Improved delivery systems by attaching sensitizers to monoclonal antibodies or tumour specific proteins may further increase the intracellular localization of the sensitizing compound.

Laser systems producing light of an appropriate wavelength to activate new sensitizers need to be developed. Advanced technology solid state lasers pumped by diode lasers have potential for producing a wide range of wavelengths at high power but the cost will be a major hurdle to their development for medical use.

References

Daniell M and Hill J. History of photodynamic therapy. Australian and New Zealand Journal of Surgery, 1990 (in press).
Diamond I, Granelli SG, McDonagh AF, Nielson S, Wilson CB and Janiecke R. Photodynamic therapy of malignant tumour. Lancet, 2: 1175-1177, 1972.
Kaye AH and Hill J. Photoradiation therapy of brain tumours; Laboratory and clinical studies. In Phototherapy of Cancer. Editors, Morstyn G and Kaye AH. Harwood Academic Publishers, New York, 101-118, 1990.

Kaye AH and Morstyn G. Photoradiation therapy causing selective tumour kill in a rat glioma model. Neurosurgery, 20: 408-415, 1987.

Kaye AH, Morstyn G and Apuzzo MLJ. Photoradiation therapy and its potential in the management of neurological tumours. J. Neurosurg., 69: 1-14, 1988.

Kaye AH, Morstyn G and Ashcroft RG. Uptake and retention of haematoporphyrin derivative in an in vivo/in vitro model of cerebral glioma. Neurosurgery, 17: 883-890, 1985.

Kaye AH, Morstyn G and Brownbill D. Adjuvant high-dose photoradiation therapy in the treatment of cerebral glioma: a phase 1-2 study. J. Neurosurg., 67: 500-505, 1987.

Kaye AH, Morstyn G, Gardner I and Pyke K. Development of a xenograft glioma model in mouse brain. Cancer Res. 46: 1367-1373, 1986.

Kostron H, Bellnier D-A, Lin C-W, Swartz MR and Martuza RL. Distribution retention and phototoxicity of haematoporphyrin derivative in a rat glioma:intraneoplastic versus intraperitoneal injection. J. Neurosurg. 64: 768-774, 1986.

Laws ER Jr., Cortese DA, Kinsey JH, Eagan RT and Anderson RE. Photoradiation therapy in the treatment of malignant brain tumours: a phase 1 (feasibility) study. Neurosurgery, 9: 672-678, 1981.

Lipson RL, Baldes EJ and Olsen AM. Haematoporphyrin derivative: a new aid for endoscopic detection of malignant disease. J. Thoracic. Cardiovasc. Surg. 42: 623-629, 1961.

Lipson RL, Baldes EJ and Gray MJ. Haematoporphyrin derivative for detection and management of cancer. Cancer, 20: 2255-2257, 1967.

McCullough GAJ, Forbes IJ, Lee See K, Cowled PA, Facka FJ and Ward AD. Phototherapy in malignant brain tumours. In: Doiron DR, Gomer CJ, Eds. Porphyrin localisation and treatment of tumours. New York, NY: Alan Liss Inc., 709-717, 1984.

Muller PJ and Wilson BC. Photodynamic therapy, cavitary photoillumination of malignant cerebral tumours using a laser couples inflatable balloon. Canc. J. Neurol. Sci. 12: 371-373, 1985.

Perria C. Photodynamic therapy in human gliomas by haematoporphyrin and He-Ne laser. IRCS Med. Sci. (Cancer), 9: 57-58, 1981.

Walker MD, Alexander E Jr., Hunt WE, MacCarty C, Mahaley MS Jr., Mealey J Jr. et al. Evaluation of BCNU and/or radiotherapy in the treatment of anaplastic gliomas: a co-operative clinical trial. J. Neurosurg. 49: 333-343, 1978.

Walker MD, Green SB, Byar DP, Alexander E Jr., Batzdorf U, Brooks WH et al. Randomized comparisons of radiotherapy and nitrosoureas for the treatment of malignant glioma after surgery. N. Engl. J. Med. 303: 1323-1229, 1980.

Wharen RE Jr., Anderson RE and Laws ER Jr. Quantitation of haematoporphyrin derivative in human gliomas, experimental central nervous system tumours, and normal tissues. Neurosurgery, 12: 446-450, 1986.

Wharen RJ Jr., So S, Anderson RE and Laws ER Jr. Haematoporphyrin derivative phototoxicity of human glioblastoma in cell culture. Neurosurgery, 12: 446-450, 1983.

CF-252 NEUTRON BRACHYTHERAPY, NEUTRON CAPTURE THERAPY

AND TELETHERAPY FOR MELANOMA AND MALIGNANT GLIOMAS

Yosh Maruyama and Jacek Wierzbicki

Radiation Therapy Oncology Center, University of Kentucky
Medical Center, Lexington, Kentucky   USA

INTRODUCTION

I review a few of our past and our projected clinical studies in this report. We began our work testing Cf-252 (Cf) neutron brachytherapy (NBT) for the treatment of bulky and advanced and localized cancers[1]. We used the brachytherapy method which is the direct placement of radiation sources into the tumor. When we began our studies other centers had tested but not discovered the great potential of Cf-252 neutrons for cancer therapy of radioresistant tumors. By our early studies we found that a very small radiation dose using Cf-252 produced a very marked effect compared to Cs-137[1] photon brachytherapy[1]. This effect is termed relative biological effectiveness (RBE)[1]. Tumors also regressed rapidly after treatment compared to photon therapy[2]. This led to the testing of a novel "early" or "up-front"[2] schedule for use of neutrons i.e., performed before photon beam therapy. In our trials we almost always combined Cf-252 implants with large doses of regional photon beam therapy[1]. These methods have led to highly successful trials based on local tumor control, patient survival and cure and absence of complications or significant late effects. This led to clinical trials testing feasibility, Phase I, Phase II, and Phase III trials, all conducted at a single institution. We have now entered into a phase aimed to test boron neutron capture therapy (BNCT) enhancement of brachytherapy[3] and the design and development of a Cf-252 teletherapy machine for hospital-based BNCT[4].

DISCUSSION

Cervix Cancer Therapy

We have studied cervix cancer for over 15 years and this was the first human cancer whose treatment we addressed in our studies[1]. We have treated over 500 patients and have treated all stages from bulky/barrel shaped IB to IV. We have cured all stages of disease successfully[5] even advanced Stage IVA disease where there was extensive bladder invasion, bilateral ureteral obstruction, and uremia[6]. The 5 year survival rates have been ~90% for Stage IB; ~65% for Stage II; ~55% for Stage IIIB disease treated by our early schedule[2]; ~35% for all patients treated, including feasibility and Phase I trials; and ~20% for Stage IV disease[5].

These results obtained mainly from feasibility and Phase I/II trials represent results that are already as good as the best that photon therapy (standard or experimental) experiences have reported to date. We are now focused on improving on the outcomes of those early trials in our Phase II, Phase III, and more advanced trials of cervix cancer therapy (e.g., combined Cf-NT and chemoradiotherapy).

The most important group of tumors we have studied is the Stage IB bulky/barrel shaped tumor[7]. We treated this group either with radiation alone or with combined radiation and surgery. Surgery provided specimens to study and with which to evaluate the effects of radiation therapy[8]. We evaluated the efficacy of radiation to completely eradicate a tumor from the hysterectomy specimen[9] and this allowed us to assess dose-response[9], RBE[10], dose survival curve shape[10], the low dose/high dose per session advantage[10], and the regenerative characteristics of cervix cancer during radiotherapy[11]. The second most important group was the Stage II tumors. This was based on the fact that combined radiation and surgery was possible with study of surgical specimens and also because the tumors are larger in volume than Stage IB disease but are still localized. The Stage III and IV tumors were used to develop our schedules and doses for neutron therapy and to recognize and evaluate the efficacy of neutrons for brachytherapy[12]. However, these are advanced tumors. They are poorly controlled locally by conventional[17] radiation or by chemoradiotherapy. We found that they were locally well controlled by neutrons. Although we have obtained good results with use of the early Cf-252 implant schedule, the 50% distant metastases and survival rate needs to be improved. We are now testing Cf-252 and chemoradiotherapy and believe we can improve our survival rates and cures. We have not had problems with the high complication rates reported by the external fast neutron beam studies.

Head and Neck Cancer

Our USSR[13] and Japanese colleagues[14,15] have studied the neutron brachytherapy of these tumors the most extensively. While survival rates are as good as photon radiotherapy, modern surgical oncology utilizes extensive radical surgery on these tumors with immediate reconstruction. Radiotherapy is used more as adjuvant therapy.

Malignant Glioma

We began the study of Cf-252 brachytherapy of malignant gliomas in 1980 in collaboration with Neurosurgery[16]. We have treated over 100 patients in this experience and the results have been very encouraging. We believe a Cf-252 BNCT (Cf-BNCT) trial is appropriate to enhance therapy[3]. Our initial trials combined Cf implant(s) with 50-60 Gy of whole brain photon therapy[17]. The results of those trials have been reported in detail by Chin et al[17] and Patchell et al[18] and led to our developing a Phase I dose-escalation trial which has been ongoing using Cf-NT only. Doses tested have increased from 9-13 Gy of neutrons and treated tumors approximately 4-5 cm in size after debulking. To date, we have seen little brain necrosis and with it have seen local tumor eradication[19]. We now recognize scalp necrosis as a problem for doses > 10 Gy of neutrons. This problem was also encountered by Sweet in his early trials of BNCT[20].
Our future trials will aim to test BNCT as a means of enhancing malignant glioma therapy in view of the encouraging results of Hatanaka[21]. To help select patients for trials, our brachytherapy staging system was developed based upon modern imaging methods[22].

Malignant Melanoma

Raju et al[23] reviewed our melanoma experiences and found that Cf was effective for destroying the local tumor. Unfortunately, these are highly malignant tumors and distant metastases led to the demise of most of these patients. Melanoma is one of the targeted tumors of our future Cf-BNCT trials using plaque Cf-NT. Mishima has been able to treat melanomas successfully using BNCT with ^{10}B-borono-phenylalanine[24].

Boron Neutron Capture Therapy

Beach, et al[3] presented evidence that Cf-252 neutron brachytherapy effects can be enhanced by use of neutron capture by administration of boron containing compounds i.e., elements with high capture cross section. Utsumi[25] has shown that selective agents specific for cancer

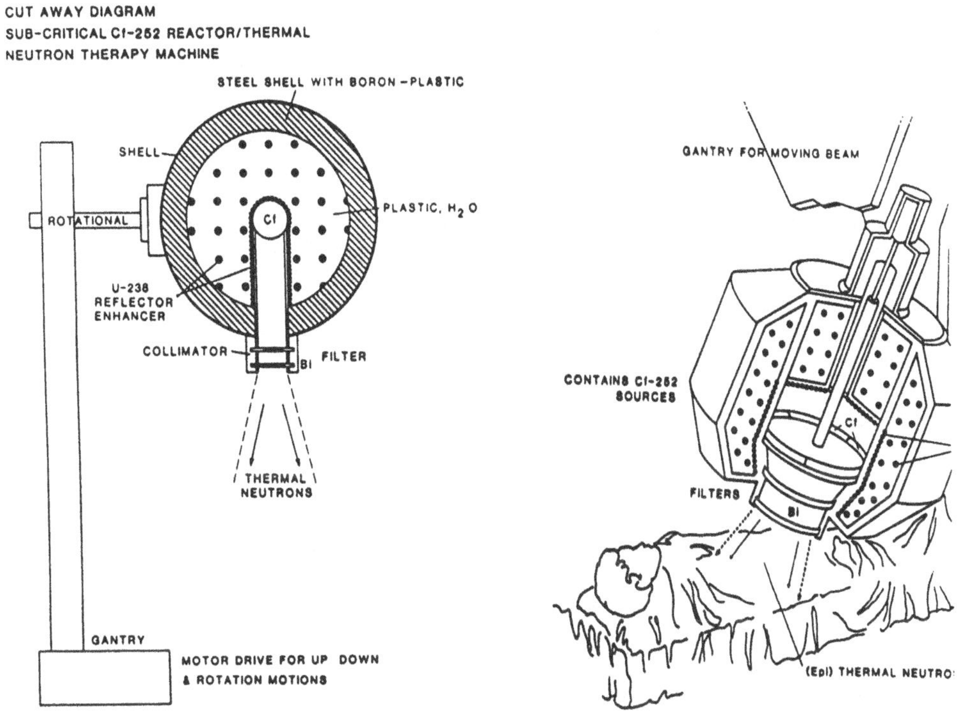

Figure 1. Proposed KY Cf-252 Teletherapy Machine for BNCT

cells can greatly enhance effectiveness of cell killing. The use of Cf-252 with drugs with better uptake into cells or the cell nucleus should be tested in the future. For malignant gliomas, only neutrons have shown efficacy in destroying tumor cells. In human cancer trials, Cf-252 has shown efficacy in eradicating tumor and in producing local control while avoiding the problems of brain necrosis. It has improved the duration and quality of survival of the brain tumor patient[17,18]. Further assessment of the potential of BNCT enhanced Cf-252 brachytherapy for human cancer therapy is planned at the University of Kentucky.

Cf-252 Teletherapy

There is a need for alternative neutron sources besides those from nuclear reactors. Nuclear reactors with portals that extend into the reactor core may be clinically usable for human cancer therapy but the public will be apprehensive about such facilities near urban areas. The development of hospital-based neutron capture therapy facilities would allow major cancer centers that are well equipped and staffed with medical specialists, qualified neutron radiation oncologists and physicists to undertake more sophisticated clinical studies of neutron capture therapy. Hence, alternative sources of neutrons are needed for neutron capture therapy, but these need to be safe and easily usable.

Cf-252 can easily be used as a source of thermal or epithermal neutrons[26] for the hospital-based facility by sealing a large Cf-252 source in an appropriately shielded head with an isocentric gantry and a treatment-suitable collimator like a Co-60 teletherapy machine. We recently proposed the development of a Cf-252 thermal neutron teletherapy machine for clinical therapy (Figure 1). Cf-252 as a source for thermal and epithermal neutrons for therapy was evaluated by Zamenhof, et al[26] and it was concluded that Cf-252 is an excellent source of neutrons for use in a hospital-based machine for thermal neutron teletherapy. The development of such a machine would advance clinical studies of BNCT for hemispheric malignant glioma.

Mishima's[24] results with BNCT of melanoma using ^{10}B-boronphenylalanine in recent human cancer clinical trials also indicates that it has potential for BNCT of many radioresistant body surface tumors. The hemispheric tumors of brain and body surface are excellent candidates for clinical trials for Cf-252 thermal neutron teletherapy BNCT. Still other tumors where BNCT may be useful with appropriate targeting pharmaceuticals or biologicals are advanced, or recurrent breast, recurrent head and neck, extremity and torso sarcomas, renal and bowel cancers. These are all poorly treated by current therapies available in cancer medicine.

CONCLUSION

Neutrons represent an important tool for the radiation therapy of cancer. Study of enhancing Cf-252 effects in tumor by using boron-loaded agents and neutron capture to increase effectiveness of brachytherapy is necessary. The building of a Cf-252 teletherapy machine would facilitate hospital-based neutron capture therapy. Cf-252 teletherapy would greatly reduce the problems and costs, and enhance the feasibility of conducting clinical trials.

REFERENCES

1. Maruyama, Y. Cf-252 Neutron Brachytherapy: An Advance for Bulky Localized Cancer Therapy. Nucl. Sci. Appl., 1:677-748, Harwood, London, (1984).

2. Maruyama, Y. Rapid Clearance of Advanced Pelvic Carcinomas By Low Dose Rate Californium Cf-252 Neutron Therapy. Radiol., 133:473-475, (1979).

3. Beach, J.L., Schroy, C.B., Ashtari, M., Harris, M.R., Maruyama, Y. Boron Neutron Capture Enhancement of Cf-252 Brachytherapy. Int. J. Radiat. Oncol. Biol. Phys., 18:1421-1427, (1990).

4. Maruyama, Y. Letter - Int. J. Radiat. Oncol. Biol. Phys. (to be published).

5. Maruyama, Y., van Nagell, J.R., Yoneda, J., Donaldson, E.S., Gallion, H., et al. Cure of Cervical Cancer Using Cf-252 Neutron Brachytherapy. Strahlenther. Onkol., 166:317-321, (1990).

6. Maruyama, Y., van Nagell, J.R., Yoneda, J., Donaldson, E.S., Gallion, H.H., Patel, P., Kryscio, R.J. Feasibility Study of Californium-252 for the Therapy of Stage IV Cervical Cancer. Cancer, 61:2448-2452, (1988).

7. van Nagell, J.R., Maruyama, Y., Donaldson, E.S., et al. Phase II Clinical Trial Using Californium-252 Fast Neutron Brachytherapy External Pelvic Radiation and Extrafascial Hysterectomy in the Treatment of Bulky, Barrel-Shaped Stage IB Cervical Cancer. Cancer, 57:1918-1922, (1986).

8. Maruyama, Y., Yoneda, J., van Nagell, J.R., Donaldson, E.S., et al. Tumor Response and Histological Clearance After Neutron Brachytherapy for Bulky Localized Cervical Cancers. Cancer, 50:2802-2809, (1982).

9. Maruyama, Y., van Nagell, J.R., Yoneda, J., Donaldson, E.S., Gallion, H.H. et al. Dose-Response for Californium-252 Neutron Brachytherapy by Histological Eradication of Bulky Stage IB Cervical Tumors. Endocuriether. Hypertherm. Oncol., 5:111-120, (1989).

10. Maruyama, Y., Feola, J.M., Wierzbicki, J., van Nagell, J.R., Powell, D., Yoneda, J. Clinical Study of Relative Biological Effectiveness For Cervical Carcinoma Treated By Cf-252 Neutrons and Assessed By Histological Tumor Eradication. Brit. J. Radiol., 63:270-277, (1990).

11. Maruyama, Y., Wierzbicki, J., Feola, J.M., Urano, M. Regeneration in Cervix Cancer After Cf-252 Neutron Brachytherapy. Int. J. Radiat. Oncol. Biol. Phys., 19:61-67, (1990).

12. Maruyama, Y., Kryscio, R.J., van Nagell, J.R., et al. Neutron Brachytherapy Is Better Than Conventional Radiotherapy in Advanced Cervical Cancer. Lancet, 1:1120-1121, (1985).

13. Vtyurin, B.M. and Tsyb, A.F. (1986), Brachytherapy With Cf-252 in the USSR: Head and Neck, GYN, and Other Tumors. Nucl. Sci. Appl., 2:521-538.

14. Tsuya, A. and Kaneta, K. Treatment of Cancers of the Tongue and Oral cavity and Lymph Node Metastases With Cf-252 at Cancer Institute Hospital, Tokyo, Japan. Nucl. Sci. Appl., 2:539-554, (1986).

15. Yamashita, H. Experience at Keio University Hospital for Cf-252 Radiation Therapy of Tumors of the Head and Neck and Other Sites. Nucl. Sci. Appl., 2:555-572, (1986).

16. Maruyama, Y., Chin, H.W., Young, A.B., Beach, J.L., Bean, J., Tibbs, P. Californium Cf-252 Neutron Brachytherapy for Hemispheric Malignant Glioma. Radiol., 145:171-174, (1982).

17. Chin, H.W., Maruyama, Y., Young, A.B., Beach, J.L., Tibbs, P., Markesbery, W. Cf-252 Brain Implantation for Malignant Glioma: Experiences of the University of Kentucky, Lexington. Nucl. Sci., Appl., 2:585-598, (1986).

18. Patchell, R.A., Maruyama, Y., Tibbs, P.A., Beach, J.L., Kryscio, R.J., Young, A.B. Neutron Interstitial Implant For Malignant Gliomas. 68:67-72, (1988).

19. Miller, J.P., Yaes, R.J., Young, A.B., Patchell, R., Tibbs, P., Chin, H., Brandenburg, W., Berner, B., Wierzbicki, J., Maruyama, Y. Californium Neutron Brachytherapy for Glioblastoma Multiforme. Int. J. Radiat. Oncol. Biol. Phys., 17:228, (1989).

20. Sweet, W.H. Personal Communication

21. Hatanaka, H. Boron Neutron Capture Therapy For Tumors. Nishimura, Niigata, Japan, (1986).

22. Maruyama, Y., Young, A.B., Chin, H.W., Markesbery, W. A Malignant Glioma Therapeutic Staging System For Cf-252 Neutron Brachytherapy at the University of Kentucky. Nucl. Sci. Appl., 2:727-732, (1988).

23. Raju, P.I., Maruyama, Y., Yoneda, J. Treatment of Melanoma Using Cf-252 Neutron Therapy at the University of Kentucky. Nucl. Sci. Appl., 2:695-702, (1986).

24. Mishima, Y. Melanoma Neutron Capture Therapy. A.R. Liss, N.Y., (1989).

25. Utsumi, H., Ichihashi, M., Kobayashi, T., Elkind, M.M. Sublethal and Potentially Lethal Damage Repair on Thermal Neutron Capture Therapy. Pigment Cell. Res., 2:337-342, (1989).

26. Zamenhof, R.G., Murry, B.W., Brownell, G.L., Wellun, G.R., Tolpin, E.I. Boron Neutron Capture Therapy for Treatment of Cerebral Gliomas. Theoretical Evaluation of the Efficacy of Various Neutron Beam. Med. Phys., 2:47, (1975).

1405/N/rmh

PROBLEMS OF DOSE FRACTIONATION IN BNCT

H. Rodney Withers

Director, Institute of Oncology,
Prince of Wales Hospital, High Street, Randwick, New South Wales,
Australia

Curative treatment of cancer with x-rays involves the administration of a high dose as a series of dose fractions spread over several weeks. This was discovered by early radiation oncologists to be more effective than administering a large single dose, which would be much more convenient and efficient. The total dose administered for an attempt at cure depends mainly upon the type of cancer and its size, although other clinical factors may "fine tune" the choice of dose. Usually dose fractions are of the order of 2 Gy but can range from about 1 Gy in newer approaches using "hyperfractionation" to about 3 Gy where logistic factors have in large part dominated treatment options.

It is now obvious that all cancers should not be treated with an identical dose fractionation regimen but we do not have the necessary technology to predict the best option for an individual patient. The best average option is still a matter of discussion but it seems likely that for an average tumour the best average treatment would involve the smallest dose per fraction given sufficiently often with interfraction intervals adequate to permit complete repair of sublethal damage but with the overall treatment given in the shortest time tolerated by the acutely responding normal tissues. In general, this principle would apply to BNCT.

For BNCT the choice of an optimal dose fractionation regimen is likely to be far more complex than it is for x-rays. Development of BNCT has an advantage over the development of x-ray therapy in that the basic phenomena influencing tissue responses to fractionated irradiation are now much better understood than even ten years ago. The four basic phenomenon involved in tissue responses to fractionated at irradiation are:-

*   Repair of sublethal injury.

*   Repopulation by surviving cells.

*   Reoxygenation.

*   Redistribution of survivors through the division cycle.

Reoxygenation: Because normal tissues are normally well oxygenated from a radiobiological viewpoint, reoxygenation only influences tumour responses. The extent of the influence of hypoxia depends upon the proportion of hypoxic cells in a particular tumour and the kinetics of their reoxygenation during fractionated radiotherapy. For most human cancers reoxygenation seems sufficiently rapid and extensive to minimise the influence of hypoxia as a determinant of radio-curability. Even if reoxygenation were inefficient, the importance of hypoxia in limiting radio-curability with BNCT would be predicted to be less than for x-ray therapy because hypoxia does not increase the radio-resistance of cells to densely ionising radiation such as alpha particles to the same extent as it does with the sparsely ionising electrons produced by x-rays.

Cell Cycle Redistribution: Division cycle related variations in radiosensitivity will be less of a factor in tumour responses to BNCT than to x-rays because the variation in radio-sensitivity is less with alpha particles than with x-rays.

Accelerated Regrowth: Clonogenic malignant cells and stem cells in acutely-responding normal tissues undergo an accelerated growth at some time after the start of radiotherapy. The lag time before it begins, and its rate varies between the various normal tissues and even more so among tumours. This accelerated regrowth is not a factor in the multi-fraction response of slowly responding normal tissues because of the slow turnover of their stem cells.   To a first order approximation, however, there should be no difference between the contribution to the therapeutic ratio of accelerated repopulation whether the patient is treated with BNCT and conventional x-ray therapy.

Repair of Sublethal Injury: This is the main biological phenomenon likely to contribute to difficulties in intercomparing the biological dosimetry of BNCT and conventional x-ray therapy. Operationally there are two mechanisms of x-ray induced cytotoxicity, single hit (non repairable) and multi-hit (repairable) injury. Single hit killing yields a simple logarithmic decline with increasing dose. The efficiency of multiple hit killing increases as the amount of injury accumulated by the cell increases, i.e. with increase in dose: to a reasonable approximation the dose survival relationship is a logarithmic function of the square of the dose over the range of doses of clinical interest. The co-existence of the two mechanisms of killing yields a downward bending survival curve, the product of both types of cell killing. The relative proportions of single hit and multi-hit killing determine the curviness of the dose survival relationship. If the co-efficients for single and multi-hit killing are alpha and beta respectively, the survival of cells is described by:

$$\text{Surviving fraction} = e^{-(\text{Alpha D} + \text{Beta D squared})}$$

and the curviness of the curve depends upon the alpha beta ratio. Importantly, sublethal injury accumulated in the cells can be repaired over a matter of hours and surviving cells respond to a subsequent dose as though they had not been irradiated previously. Since beta type injury is repairable a high alpha beta ratio is associated with less repair of sublethal damage, and therefore, with less change in the total dose required for a certain effect with change in dose per fraction. For x-rays, the alpha beta ratio for acutely responding tissues and most tumours is relatively high, whereas for late responding tissues the values are systematically lower. Thus, with x-ray therapy, late responding normal tissues are preferentially spared by dose fractionation. Such late responding normal tissues include spinal cord, kidney, liver, lung, muscle, bone and dermis.

With densely ionising radiations such as alpha particles most cell killing at doses of clinical interest is by a single hit mechanism, the alpha beta ratio being high for all tissues, both early and late responding. Thus there is little fractionation effect with alpha particles. This is a potential disadvantage for BNCT since the slowly responding normal tissues are often dose limiting, and it is the preferential sparing by fractionation of x-ray dose that has permitted some improvements in therapeutic ratio. If alpha particles were to predominate in the deposition of dose in the late responding tissues, those tissues would be disadvantaged relative to tumours and acutely responding tissues. This happened in early clinical trials of fast neutrons. Thus it is important to ensure as much as possible of the dose to late responding tissues in the incident path of the beam be from low LET events, that is, that the boron content be minimized and the neutron energy not be too high.

Obviously, with a changing gamma ray/neutron ratio as a thermal or epithermal neutron beam penetrates the tissues, as well as with variations in the relative boronation of the irradiated cells, the question of how to fractionate the dose optimally will be enormously difficult. The biological considerations will vary with the type of beam, the thickness of the patient (which determines not only the dose gradient but also the gamma neutron ratio) the relative boron affinity of the tumour and incidentally irradiated tissues, with time after administration of the boronated compounds and with the alpha beta ratios of the tissues in question.

These factors seem minor in the context of present preoccupation with maximising tumour to normal tissue ratios of boronated or gadalinium-laden molecules, and with achieving uptake by 100% of tumour cells. However, they will not be minor as BNCT approaches clinical reality. It is not always fully appreciated by biologists and physicists that both normal tissue sequelae and tumour control are steep functions of dose once the threshold for an effect has been exceeded. With such a threshold-sigmoid response, a 10% change in dose can mean a devastating change in either complications (with increase in dose) or tumour control (with decrease in dose). Achieving homogeneity, or an acceptable gradient of physical dose will be difficult. However it will be compounded in subtle but potentially significant ways by changes in biological dose. Biological dose changes with change in alpha beta value of the tissue, with change in size of dose fractions, with change in the level of dose at which changes in dose fraction occur, with variations in dose rate, with type and energy of beam, with factors that modulate neutron gamma ray ratios, as well as with boronation.

The importance of fine-tuning of "biological" dose, as distinct from just physical dose, was learnt with difficulty in early clinical trials of fast neutron beam therapy and with ^{252}Cf brachytherapy. Whilst we have a greatly expanded understanding of the relevant radiobiology now compared with when those clinical trials began, it is important to appreciate the complexity of the problems and expense of adequate animal research to avoiding errors in the calibration of biological dose.

ROUND TABLE REVIEW OF NEUTRON CAPTURE THERAPY -
THE CLINICIANS POINT OF VIEW

Barry Allen: Participating in this round table discussion are a number of leading Australian cancer clinicians. One could reasonably say that they are watching to see what NCT can do. Let me introduce them:

Professor Lester Peters - (Radiotherapy) - MD Anderson Hospital Texas
Assoc. Prof Alan Coates - (Chemotherapy) Sydney Melanoma Unit, Royal Prince Alfred Hospital
Professor Martin Tattersall - (Cancer Medicine) University of Sydney
Dr Andrew Kaye - (Neurosurgery), Royal Melbourne Hospital
Professor Rodney Withers - (Radiation Oncology) Prince of Wales Hospital

On my right hand side are representative proponents of NCT.

Professor Robert Zamenhof - (Medical Physics) Tufts University New England Medical Centre, USA
Professor Yutaka Mishima - (Dermatology) Kobe University, Japan
Professor Keiji Kanda - (Reactor Physics) Kyoto University, Japan
Professor Dr Detlef Gabel - (Chemistry) Bremen University, FRG
Dr Ralph Fairchild - (Medical Physics) Brookhaven National Laboratory, USA
Dr Ron Dorn - (Radiotherapy) Mountain States Tumour Institute Idaho, USA
Professor Hiroshi Hatanaka - (Neurosurgery) Teikyo University Hospital, Japan

Now, let me ask my colleagues on my left to say a few words about whether they believe that what we are doing is right or wrong, or where we should be putting more effort. From their collective experience as cancer clinicians perhaps they could say what they consider to be the weakness of Neutron Capture Therapy or perhaps what the strengths are. So I might ask Lester Peters to lead the discussion.

Lester Peters: Thank you Barry. There's always a plus and minus aspect to being the first to talk because you can be the Sally to be slapped down, but on the other hand you get a chance to put your point of view forward.

I believe that everyone who is here would agree that the concept of Neutron Capture Therapy is very appealing, as indeed is any binary therapeutic system, because in the perfect world you could decide whether it was appropriate to add the second element of the binary treatment system on an individual patient basis, and only apply it where it was indicated. Thus I think the real future of Neutron Capture Therapy hinges on the ability to be able to quantitate, on an individual patient basis, the uptake and the distribution of the capture element, before any thermal neutron or epithermal neutron exposure is given. For if there is not enough of the capture element the whole treatment would be wasted. Dr Dorn mentioned this morning about "geographic miss" as being a significant problem with conventional radiotherapy, but I submit to you that to irradiate, with an epithermal beam, a tumour whose every last cell has not taken up the capture element is tantamount to a "geographic miss". That seems to be the most limiting concern in my view. We can have reasonable confidence in where the <u>radiation</u> is going, but we have only a rough idea where the <u>capture element</u> is going, at the present time. The characteristic of radiotherapy that distinguishes it from most other cancer treatment modalities is that, with conventional radiotherapy techniques, it is very quantitative. We can state with great precision what the absorbed dose is in any tumour we would treat at the present time. With NCT, at least using present technology, we are talking in terms of administered doses, not absorbed doses. The administered doses can be a guide to what the absorbed doses are going to be, but it's certainly not an absolute criterion. That brings me back to my main point. The ultimate need is to develop a system of individual quantitation of uptake of the capture element before radiation is given. The other point I would like to bring up in a more generic sense is that the mere fact that a particular cancer has a bad prognosis doesn't justify treatment without some very good reason for expecting the treatment to work. So I think we ought not to rush into clinical trials with Neutron Capture Therapy unless we have a very good reason for thinking that the combination of capture element and beam is well enough optimised to give a good result, because it will undoubtedly damage the modality to have a bad clinical trial. It will set the whole subject back a generation until people forget the bad experience and then start again. I would urge that we don't necessarily rush into clinical applications now. There are many exciting new drug delivery systems on the horizon, so we should hold off until we have a better probability of success compared to the marginal gains that might be possible with present technology.

Detlef Gabel: Let me respond to these points by showing a couple of slides. This is a neutron capture radiogram of a mouse injected with boric acid, one of the compounds used clinically in the 1950's and 1960's. This mouse is lying flat on his back and you can see that most of the boron is in the brain and not in other healthy tissues. So the biodistribution does not appear to be optimal, to say the least. In the next slide we are looking at the distribution of BSH in a human tumour. To the right of the slide, on the neutron capture radiogram, some areas contain a lot of boron, some less. On the left side you see at 1mm spacings, a reading of all the boron concentration values in ppm. I would agree with Lester Peters that we do have to know how much of the neutron capture agents that we actually administered is distributed to the tumour. What we know, from the radiobiology of this therapy, is that we actually need to know this on a cell to cell basis. At present, and even at this symposium, I have not seen this capability demonstrated. We have no routine way of actually determining the boron concentration from cell to cell. You can see here from mm to mm there are huge variations. If you look at the upper part you go from 16 to 5 ppm ^{10}B. From 1 mm to the next this varies by factors of 2, 3 or 5 or even more in terms of boron concentration and this certainly is a problem. What is also a problem is that we do not know where those cells are that we need to reach. So I have advocated a cautious approach towards NCT but an approach that is an experimental approach because no matter how well we know on a macroscopic basis the uptake of boron, we also need to know this on a microscopic or subcellular level. Only then could we perhaps predict the outcome of a clinical trial. We might be asked, of course, whether BSH is the compound to start with now, or whether we should wait for BPA, or whether we should wait another five years perhaps for a porphyrin to be available for use in patients. But the question is whether a better compound would have a better chance of success. This is still open to experimental verification, and only with an experimental verification and not with any of these techniques, can we actually say NCT will work.

Robert Zamenhof: I would like to add to what Detlef said. I don't know what he defines as a "routine" technique for analysing cell to cell variations of boron-10. I agree there is no simple routine technique, but we do have a technique that we have demonstrated here in two or three of our presentations which does show in frozen tissue sections the variations of boron-10 on a cellular basis. So I think that the method does exist for screening and examining behaviour of various candidate boron compounds. I would also like to answer a point you have made which was very interesting, because it is mentioned by different Radiation Oncologists at different International Symposia. The question is whether it is necessary to kill every single cell in the tumour in order to assure the success of the technique. If that's the real goal, I think Neutron Capture Therapy is probably doomed to failure, although we know it isn't, because it works in animals, and that has been demonstrated. If you do a mathematical analysis using something quite simple like the Poisson distribution and you start off with the assumption that to get 1000 cGy (rads) of radiation dose to a tumour you need to have something of the order of ten boron captures reaction occurring within each cell, then simple statistics will show you that approximately 1 in 30 of those cells will receive less than 500 rads, and one in 10^5 of those cells will receive zero radiation, and that is just purely based on Poisson statistics. So, in the animals that we have treated and have shown that we can cure, I think there has to be some other kind of mechanism that is working that does not require the elimination of every single cell.

Lester Peters: The requirement is to exterminate every clonogenic cell. The clonogenic cell density would probably be quite small in many tumours, possibly on the order of 1 in 10^4 or 1 in 10^5 cells.   There is a major fallacy in extrapolating cure data from transplanted animal tumours especially when there is histoincompatability between those tumours and their hosts.   How many autochthonous spontaneous tumours can you cite that have been cured with NCT when they are not on the surface?   Another point that is relevant with the animal models is that if you look at a rat the distance from the surface of its head to a tumour in the brain is much more favourable than it is in a human.

Ron Dorn: Since in terms of speciality I'm the one on the panel with the same field as Dr Peters maybe I would like to address that question from a clinical point-of-view.   Maybe we are using the wrong end-point or I should say, too strict an end-point, in terms of deciding whether or not it is worth while to pursue BNCT in its present state or near future state with current compounds.   From your comment and those of other people about end points, you seem to be suggesting that we need to be as sure as we can that we are going to get boron in every tumour cell or every clonogenic tumour cell and successfully destroy that, before we proceed with BNCT.   In fact, that's a requirement that we really don't place on any other cancer treatment that I know of.   We certainly don't do that with conventional radiation.   We obviously don't do that with immunotherapy or chemotherapy. It seems to me that we should not look at whether we can absolutely guarantee cure or killing <u>all</u> those cells, but rather can we do better than what is currently available?   By that measure, it's going to be a lot easier to justify proceeding with BNCT.

Alan Coates: I should say I would like to talk about Melanoma and therefore about boronophenylalanine rather than BSH although I recognise that a lot more experience exists with the brain tumour but I have no expertise to comment on that.   I would agree with all that has been said about the fascinating application of technology that we are here to talk about.   If I wasn't interested in that I wouldn't be here and I am sure that many of my clinical colleagues would feel the same way.   However, I want to step back from that and, as a clinician, look at NCT as a black box.   Do I point this black box at my patients or not?   I think it's interesting to try to apply this to melanoma.   It has been shown by Professor Mishima that it can be applied.   About three years ago we attended the second Japan-Australian conference on Neutron Capture Therapy and agreed that, if a suitable patient came along, we would be willing to send a patient from the Sydney Melanoma Unit for treatment in Kobe.   Three years later we have not yet done so.   Why not?   Not because we are short of patients.   We have continued to see 800 or 900 new patients with new melanoma each year.   That's about 1/3 of all new patients occurring in the state.   Over 100 of those present with metastatic disease and die of their disease.   There are plenty of stimuli to try a new treatment.   I agree with

Lester Peters though, that just because things are going badly doesn't mean that you point this particular black box at the patients. One of the difficulties that has been alluded to by the speakers is practicality and the other difficulty, however, is the availability of alternative treatments. We are talking, with thermal neutrons, about a black box that goes a short distance into the body, and that means we are dealing with superficial melanoma, either in its primaries form, or where recurrent melanoma is near the surface and in a relatively limited anatomical location. Now, surgery is really good at dealing with primary melanoma. It has been pointed out by other speakers that most such patients are cured by their initial surgery and never require anything else. We in the unit would be most reluctant to abandon surgery as the primary treatment for primary malignant melanoma. I know there are cases that can be shown, and we have seen slides from Japan today, of very bad looking primaries and occasionally we see some of these as well. But I guess it is true to say the general spectrum of cutaneous melanoma in an Australian population is rather different from that seen in Japan, with far more cutaneous melanoma occurring on parts of the body other than the palms and soles. Most of the melanomas that we see are much smaller and much more amenable to primary surgery treatment. When we do get a bad one we have got a number of other techniques that can be used. The Unit is involved in one particular technique involving isolated limb-perfusion. It is a randomised international collaborative trial that is investigating the addition of that to primary surgery. Our commitment to that trial limits our number of bad primaries that we would be willing to assign to a competing investigational technique.

When it comes to recurrent disease, radiotherapy with conventional photons has been under-utilized, I believe, in the clinical treatment of melanoma, and probably that's not the fault of those in this room, but it has had a bad reputation. We have found, in fact, that it is a quite useful modality and we have been investigating the combination of photon radiotherapy with cisplatin, and in Kobe I presented some preliminary data which were updated recently at the ASCO meetings. We have been investigating therefore another means of dealing with the isolated troublesome metastasis similar in concept to the type of patient Professor Mishima first treated. All of these treatments are available here at a fraction of the dollar cost and more importantly at a fraction of the social dislocation that would be involved in transporting the patient to what would now be to Japan. But even in the best of all possible worlds if we had an NCT facility at Lucas Heights, it has been pointed out as an inconvenient place to treat patients.

I do see some glimmer of hope that maybe the box Mark II with an epithermal beam might offer something we really could use clinically. Then I would think in terms of brain metatases. Graham Stevens reviewed for us today the experience in our hospital with the treatment of brain metatases with

conventional radiotherapy and that is dismal. If a new modality came along
and enabled us to get the full depth of metastatic melanoma in the brain by
a non-invasive technique then certainly it would be worth looking at. So I
am watching the development of an epithermal beam at HIFAR with great
interest but until the black box Mark II comes along we won't be regarding
this as a routine treatment, but I wouldn't rule out the possibility of an
individual patient being sent for treatment at the Japanese facility. Let
us look on the other hand at the logistic implications if we took the other
view. We've heard of the progress of both the glioblastoma series and the
melanoma series and neither has put on huge number of patients in the last
three years. If we did have a stream of patients for whom this is a
regular treatment then I think the logistic implications for dedicated
reactors and the enormous amount of time and planning would pose problems
that may be insuperable, at least in the economy as we see it.

Yutaka Mishima: I would like to make many points. Among the audience
sitting here, who listened to my talk, I hope all will agree that our team,
including Kanda and many others, have no doubt that we can cure, in best
conditions melanotic malignant melanoma including all five types of
melanoma. The first case was of an inoperable patient with a metastatic
lesion that occured over the occiput, at the junction of the transverse and
sagital sinuses. The second patient could not proceed with an operation.
The surgeon put him on the operating table but in the beginning of general
anaesthesia this over eighty year old patient had heart trouble so they had
to stop the operation. With the finger melanoma (subungual) you lose a
finger and then you have a really great problem. Besides, statistics tell
us that in the best institute in the world, with a tumour more than 3mm in
thickness, you have a survival rate of less than 50% even if you apply the
best immuno and chemotherapy together with surgery. Now we should be
medical doctors as well as scientists, so we try to sort out the
fundamental science at the same time for the benefit of patients. I am
trying to prepare for the next step of treating metastatic satellite
lesions and lymph node metastasis by optimising NCT for the primary lesion.

Concerning the subcellular or cellular distribution I investigated this for
many, many years and we have also worked with Dr Takagaki and many others
with the α-track method. But please remember the total travelling range of
the α and ^{7}Li is 14 μm on average with random direction so the radiation
dose can also come from neighbouring cells. Besides this, we tried to
achieve uniform labelling or uniform accumulation as I have shown this
morning with pulsed administrations of BPA, because of considerations of
cell cycle, and the heterogeneity of cell lines, tyrosinase activity and
melanin synthesis. Usually homogeneous regression is observed in large
melanomas in spite of this heterogeneity, possibly because of nearest cell
effects.

Alan Coates: I think the concern you have about thick melanomas is one
that we would share. I don't believe however patients die of local
melanoma, they die of metatases which have been established before the

634

treatment of the primary and how you treat that primary really influences the local recurrence rate. I don't think it's easy to say that the local irradiation is going to be a systemic treatment. It is arguable, I suppose, that it might generate an immune response to the dying tumour cells but unless it does, you have just a different, maybe even a better, local treatment. The patient is still going to die of the cells that got away to the brain. What we need is an effective adjuvant therapy and that, in melanoma, is still lacking.

Andrew Kaye: I really just wanted to make the same point but to also emphasize that you cannot talk about curing melanoma by a local treatment. You can't use the word cure. All you can say is that you have controlled the local disease. I think that it is inappropriate and fallacious for us to talk about curing melanoma when you are talking about treating local disease.

Rod Withers: Can I ask you to explain that. If you have 50% survival for 25 years after excision of the primary, what more do you require to call somebody cured?

Andrew Kaye: I don't think that you can say that just by treating the local disease by a particular treatment that you actually cured the patient. You have to wait and see what actually happens in the long term, whether or not they are going to get metastases. I can't see how, as Alan said before, that NCT is not just another form of knife. It does not have any particular magical property. Alan suggested perhaps it may bring some sort of immune reaction. Well, I don't think that has been tested at all and I think he just put it forward to be kind, but it is just another form of knife.

Rod Withers: I would agree with that but the knife is pretty good.

Andrew Kaye: Absolutely!

Yutaka Mishima: Can I just reply please, as I think this is referring to me. I had the same discussion when I submitted my paper to Lancet. They advised me to change the word "cure" to the "complete regression" of treated regions. I have never used the term "the cure of the patient". I cautiously use "the cure of the NCT-treated lesions" when I have substantial evidence. I believe "complete regression of and cure of the NCT-treated lesions" are different terms and should be distinguished from one another in medical sciences. I have been working for more than a quarter of a century on melanoma treatment and I only use the term "cure of treated lesion" when I follow the patient for more than two years and find other supporting evidence. One might say that this is not enough time for the patient. but if you have treated a large number of melanoma patients, know the tumor thickness and type of melanoma, know the regression curve, and know other patterns as shown by MRI, ^{67}Ga scintigram, PET and also from a biochemical investigation such as detection of melanoma metastasis by measuring 5-cysteine dopa in the patient's urine, substantial evidence can show that the treated lesion has been cured. This is very sensitive as shown by the work that Professor Rorsman and our group reported. If the 5-cysteine dopa is below 100 ug/24h in urine for more than 2 years, we are quite confident that there are no internal melanoma metastases. I am very careful to use the term "cure" and I understand your point very well so that we use the term "local cure" but I am watching the patient as a total body.

I should add another point. I am not denying the contribution of the surgical treatment of malignant melanoma. However, the final objective of melanoma research is to obtain a non-surgical and biological melanoma therapy. In order to eradicate melanoma brain metastasis by NCT using epithermal neutrons, we have to establish all necessary prerequisite data by curing readily observable cutaneous melanoma by NCT.

Alan Coates: The matter of survival curves and their shape and how you can interpret them as cure has obviously generated a lot of discussion in the medical literature over the years. I think the simple fact remains that people can die of malignant melanoma after intervals from their primary treatment of 15, 20, 40 years. All of us have been treating melanoma for that length of time and have seen that happen, I don't believe that you can say an individual patient is cured with any certainty after a period as short as two years, and I would agree entirely with Andrew Kaye about that. I do think that individual patients are cured. They live out normal life spans and die of something else and so for that practical purpose, at the end of their life, you know that you have cured that patient. But there is certainly no period in the first two years where the expected force of mortality of any group of melanoma of patients equals the normal population, and groups of melanoma patients remain at risk of dying of melanoma well beyond two years.

Martin Tattersall: In talking to patients sometimes I say curing cancer is easy. It's keeping you alive which is the problem. What I mean by that is, we have a large number of poisons which will cure cancer, no problem, but the trouble is they will kill the patient as well. Now one of the great advantages of a binary approach is the idea that you may actually have an agent which, together with a local form of treatment, might achieve a rather special sort of knife with low toxicity. This is a possibility. I agree entirely with Lester Peter's view that now is the time to work with means of developing drug delivery systems because you don't have to get the same specificity of boron uptake into the tumour as we do with a poison such as a cytotoxic drug. We need a margin but it doesn't have to be anything like as tight a margin as if we are using diptheria toxin or one of these new magic bullets. So I really think with fine tuning of the delivery system, whether it is to be targeted by some other vehicle or whether boron attached to something is going to be the solution I don't know, but I certainly think there is a lot of mileage in that approach and I believe there are plenty of opportunities to study quantitation, of

636

seeing how much you can get the boron material, approximately, but without
an absolute specificity, to the tumour. But as Andrew has said we are
talking about a local therapy, and we are relying on the external agent to,
if you like, add the specifics to the treatment, and it is a knife. Which
tumours are locally controllable have obviously been discussed and Alan has
already indicated that there are often options for local treatments. Yet
even in spite of this fact a lot of people die with uncontrollable local
cancer. It would seem to me that it is in this setting that there is an
opportunity, when we have better refinement of the drug delivery system,
for reasonably evaluating this form of treatment.

Hiroshi Hatanka: As a surgeon who has produced some long surviving
patients with gliomas, I have one comment about the term "cure". In the
Japanese language there is a word "*naotu*" which means "to improve" but
quite often this also means "to be cured" and there is certainly a
confusion among the Japanese medical scientists about this word "cure". In
fact when I was younger, I had the same confusion but year by year I became
cautious in using the word "cure". I certainly have been avoiding the word
"cure", even to talk about a patient who had a glioblastoma 18 years ago,
but for practical reasons to explain to the layman, I sometimes use such as
expressions as "virtually cured patients" or "ex-glioblastoma patients".
As Dr Kaye pointed out, I completely agree with his warning and I tell you
I am pretty cautious in using the word "cure". However for practical
reasons it is sometimes necessary to use such a word in the Japanese
language. Thank you very much.

Ralph Fairchild: I would like to indicate the possibility, as we search
for more specific drug delivery systems, that we don't totally overlook the
ones we have in hand at this time. There are many who say that the
possibility exists that the drug delivery system that we have in hand at
the moment, and I will include in that the monomer (BSH) and the dimer
(BSSB) and BPA, are not adequate and we should wait for better things. I
think we want to be careful that we don't throw the BPA out with the bath
water before we discard these compounds. It is apparent with BPA and also
with the dimer form (BSSB) that there is indeed a physical differential of
about 4-5 times between what is in tumour and blood. If you are talking
about brain tumours, for example, and avoid the question of the problems
associated with metastatic melanoma, a ratio of 4:1 or 5:1 is obtained
between tumour and blood with BPA. If you take into account what has now
been demonstrated regarding the geometrical protection factor (for
capillaries) you get with the monomer and also I think with the dimer a 4:1
ratio. It is not at all clear that if we wait for a compound to have a
10:1 ratio that you gain anything of consequence because the improvement in
therapeutic gain is greatest up to about a 4:1, 5:1 and the rate of gain
decreases for therapeutic gains beyond about 4 or 5 to 1.

I think also, in view of the good results that we have had, and have been
reported here in the treatment of rat brain intracranial tumours with both

BPA and dimer, since we have roughly a 50% total regression rate, or what ever you want to call it with those tumour models, and since you cannot obtain that with comparable X-ray treatments, that indeed we may have demonstrated in an animal model that we have something that is indeed better than conventional radiation therapy. I think as you go to fractionation, and it is harder to do that, of course, in an animal tumour, that it would be on the side of Neutron Capture because with fractionation you ameliorate the dose to the normal tissues, but add up linearly with the boron reaction to achieve a better result.

Lester Peters: I think everything Ralph said is reasonable, and it is not necessarily in conflict with what I said is my opening position. We quantitate tumour to normal tissue ratios now in parts per million or whatever. What I wanted to bring forward was that the micro-distribution of the capture element is the big unknown at the present time. It is in many ways analogous to the treatment with labelled antibodies and internally administered radionuclides. It is of no use giving a radiolabelled nuclide if it doesn't hit the cell that you want it to kill, and if there is no capture element in any tiny part of a tumour, that tumour will not be cured by Neutron Capture Therapy. Given that limitation, I think if I were doing a clinical trial I would not put all my eggs in the neutron capture basket, but rather regard it as a way of augmenting the dose to at least a major part of the tumour, and giving a conventional dose to the tumour as well, which would at least be more likely to eliminate the parts of the tumour that haven't induced a new vascular system and therefore become protected by the blood brain barrier phenomenon. It is easy to have a geographical miss if there is no capture element there, and essentially no dose is given to the tumour, so it's too big of a risk, I think, with the present technology of quantitating where the capture element is located on a cellular basis.

The one other point I think that we really should not lose sight of was brought up in discussion earlier today. It was the need, if clinical trials are going to be done, to have them hospital based. The collapse of the Los Alamos Facility was the case that was brought up, and I think the people who were involved in research into the development of accelerators to produce epithermal neutron beams or perhaps the dedicated reactors that can be put into hospitals ought be strongly encouraged because it will never get above the level of an interesting but an esoteric line of research while it is out at the atomic energy agencies and reactors in the country side that have been mainly devoted to other concerns.

Detlef Gabel: I would like to make one comment on this and it is a comment we all, I think, might be aware of, but it has never been really put forward very out spokenly. What we are dealing with in NCT, no matter how well we design our beams, is always a mixed radiation therapy. As we give always a rather large dose of radiation actually to a healthy tissue other than that stemming from boron so we are kind of giving a background dose that can be quite high to healthy tissue. Now then the question is how do the boron compounds look that we actually want to synthesize? Should they be very specific and have tumour uptakes of what has been quoted as 100:1 or can we use other compounds as well? I think when you look at the background dose above which you have to raise your dose to the tumour in order to get an actual dose of 20% enhancement, you might actually do just as well with drugs that have much less specificity but much higher absolute uptake. I think those two parameters have to be seen in conjunction and so the search for improved drug delivery systems cannot have a single goal. I think you are all aware of the very specific uptake that has been accomplished in Nuclear Medicine. It is necessary there because you don't have any background radioactivity that you can image. We have to have a sufficiently high uptake and the absolute uptake will determine how specific the compound has to be in the tumour. I just wanted to bring this back to your attention.

Keiji Kanda: I want to discuss not this problem but the highlight of the Symposium at this time. That is the development of epithermal neutrons with several organisations presenting plans for clinical trials. Of course this kind of discussion is important and there are many physicists here. My simple question is, why do you insist on epithermal neutrons so much? The thermal neutrons are still so very beautiful. In Japan there are four reactors that are used for clinical purposes and if you have problems with our treatment then we can discuss it, but thermal neutrons are still working very beautifully. Of course, we have some limitations for some patients, so let's start a clinical trial first, then you can solve the many problems. Before the clinical trial we are working at one level, but in a trial we work at a higher level and suddenly we can solve the many problems and unexpected matters which occur when we treat patients. For example, we calculate phantom experiments with collimators, we did many things but once we see the patient, the conditions changed very much and we must suddenly adapt, for example, the collimator conditions, and so the science developed very much. I want to strongly recommend that you join the clinical trial first, then the many questions will be solved.

In the first stage we should treat the "advanced patients", I understand that this is the clinician's common sense and maybe Hatanaka or Mishima will make some comment. The common sense of medical doctors is very different from our common sense so we have many discussions and fight each other but after we treated the patients, many problems are settled. I want to emphasize that the development of this new field is also very exciting for the physicist. The thermal neutron is still beautiful and very easy to control, elimination of gamma rays is quite easy and also the field adjustment is easy but epithermal contamination by the fast neutrons and elimination of gamma rays are not easy problems. There are unknown factors but these are less than those keV neutrons. This is my personal opinion so please don't get angry. Join our clinical trial and you will understand more, that's my opinion. For example, we read Dr Sweet's papers published in the 1950's and 60's very carefully and we learned very much from them. Clinical trials are much more useful than the so called basic studies and sometimes I feel that this is not understood.

Rod Withers: I missed the opening discussions, but one important fact about Neutron Capture Therapy is that it has to be very much better, it just cannot be as good as conventional radiotherapy or as good as surgery or as good as chemotherapy, it has to be very much better to be worth the hassle and the expense. Talking about getting clinical responses is not sufficient justification of itself for continuing. You really need to look for significant therapeutic gains. Elaborating on the point that Lester Peters made: if for example 1% of the cells didn't have significant accumulation of boron then you might as well not bother treating at all because if you killed all those cells that had taken up the boron, you will produce two logs of cell kill rather than the maybe nine or ten logs necessary for tumour eradication. Therefore I think you will have to consider using BNCT with other modalities. I think the argument that you get some killing of the non-boronated cells from the neutron beam anyway is not sufficient. You have to get essentially 100% of the cells labelled with boron or taking up boron and you should be looking at multiple ways of getting the cells boronated, (e.g. antibodies and BOPP), not just one way.

I would also point out that very precise and specific dose delivery is getting easier and easier for conventional radiotherapy especially now that we have three dimensional planning and stereotactic beams. If you have a well defined localised lesion in the brain you can deliver dose ratios of 10:1 to the tumour compared with the normal brain with no problem. In fact you can get 100:1 for small tumours using stereotactic radio surgery, making it more difficult for boron capture therapy to provide an improved therapeutic gain.

Robert Zamenhof: I would like to answer a number of the points. First of all I know the requirements for clinical trials are different in the US than in Japan, and if I may I will review very quickly for those of you who don't know this difference. In the US if you have a therapeutic modality that you feel has a better theoretical basis than other modalities, or a different form of fractionation for an existing modality, what you do is try it out on animals, and if it shows a statistically significant improvement then you propose a "phase-one trial". The phase-one trial involves not a demonstration of efficacy but a demonstration of safety. With that in mind I don't understand why my colleagues on my left are being so unbelievably restrictive and biased towards Neutron Capture Therapy by saying that unless this technique, at the first crack, can provide complete cures then it's almost not worth initiating. I think that we should be afforded the luxury of enjoying the same criteria that other clinical trials enjoy in terms of being able to start clinical trials if we demonstrate efficacy in animals and if we then propose a clinical protocol in patients that everybody would agree would produce no harm. Then the evaluation of the results would determine whether this should be continued or not.

The second point I would like to make is, and I hoped Ron would respond to this but I will anyway, I think it is wrong to criticise a technique that is very very tedious, difficult and clumsy in the initial stages of its

application. If it is an experimental technique that hasn't yet been
proved I think one should tolerate a tremendous amount of inconvenience and
I think patients are in general willing to do that if there is some
promise. You have seen the papers that have been presented here. There
are the "foreground" papers, so to speak, which deal with the animal
studies and the physics of the reactor beams to try and bring them to a
useful condition. Then there are the "background" papers, and I don't mean
that in a perjorative way, which are working on the design of equipment for
Neutron Capture Therapy which could be placed in a hospital if NCT would
prove to be efficacious. I think that if this occurs in this country, it
would be a competing form of radiation therapy in terms of costs with many
other types of therapy. Clinac-25's as you know, can to be installed for
somewhere in the order of 1 million dollars today and there is a lot more
cost involved if you want to shield the rooms against neutrons. I think
some of the accelerator facilities that have been described could be, after
a little more research, installed for roughly the same cost; beyond that,
there would be no more extra cost to NCT. So I think you are being
unfairly restrictive to Neutron Capture Therapy in the sort of requirements
that you are placing upon it.

Yutaka Mishima: The Australian Government and our Government support NCT
in a bilateral agreement which has been running for the last four years.
The quality of regression after treatment by BNCT, as compared to the local
control you obtain by current radiotherapy and immunochemotherapy, is quite
different in quality. I hope soon you can come to Japan and see how the
quality of regression is really different from any other kind of current
non-surgical technique as far as melanoma is concerned.

Ron Dorn: Thank you, like Bob Zamenhof I have been saving a few points as
we have been going along, and I would like to address a couple of them.

First of all let me say as a preamble, to both Dr Peters and Dr Withers, I
am in general agreement in terms of clinical trials. The US, and it sounds
like from Dr Dewit's paper certainly the European collaboration as well, is
not about to embark on clinical trials tomorrow. While there are a couple
of additional questions we want to resolve, the requirements that are being
placed on BNCT are considerably more stringent than they are for other new
trials. For example, if I was looking at Interleukin and LAK treatment in
the US for malignancies, I would bet the house at this point in terms of
BNCT, already in the preclinical stage, being shown to be safer and more
effective for an individual treatment than Interleukin LAK which has been
out in the States for some time. My latest review indicated a 6.5%
complete response and a 6.5% fatality rate. That is just not morbidity
that is fatality. Already at this point I think BNCT is well beyond that
in terms of preparations for clinical trials. I think that there is some
middle ground in terms of being concerned about us starting clinical trials
tomorrow or waiting a judicious length of time like a year or two, to
establish the necessary baseline information.

Secondly, the "location problem" has been brought up a couple of times

today and I think it's about time we talked about reactors and their
location a little. I can't imagine which reactor is being referred to, but
since we have been talking about Los Alamos a couple of times today I have
the advantage of having been in both situations. You can consider both the
advantages and disadvantages, and having been Dr Kligerman's only resident
for three years, I was in Albuquerque during the pion trials. I can tell
you there is absolutely no comparison between the Los Alamos and INEL
situations. Certainly the pion trials in my experience, since I took care
of those patients, did not fail because the patients had difficulty in
coming there for treatment for their individual cancers.   Further, if we
were ever to get on with clinical trials at Idaho Falls, there is a big
difference between the transportation systems.   To people perhaps back
east and overseas, if you are out west you are out west and one thing is
the same as the other. But I can tell you that the transportation and the
referral situtations are entirely different.

Finally, just a comment because it may be a while before I get the
microphone back again. As we talk about and lead up to establishing the
clinical trials it certainly seems to me that the important task is to
continue the job of boron compound development. It is also an ongoing,
important task to develop the requirements that are necessary for building
the dedicated medical sources of neutrons that we need, and this goes back
to your point, Alan. I wouldn't say if, but when BNCT is successful, there
is not a neutron source that is available right now that's going to be able
to handle the patients or should be involved in handling a large number of
patients for treatment, no matter which reactor you are talking about. We
have to do the studies and we have to get the design requirements ready to
proceed with the construction of the appropriate neutron sources.

Lester Peters: I would like to come back to what Bob has said and maybe
Ron too. My comments were not meant to be restrictive, so much as to
outline what I think is the best strategy to follow. As a "fast
neutroneer" I can tell you that there is no sentiment what so ever in the
National Cancer Institute to support another round of improved clinical
trials of fast neutrons. We have had our go and it's finished. If you
embark on an NCT trial now, take a decade to do it (which is fairly likely)
and at the end of that time say, oops, we have used the wrong compound, we
would like to have another go, you can bet your most precious possessions
that the funding agencies won't let you have another go. So, I think in
that context and being aware of how much exciting new work is going on in
terms of drug delivery and knowing how much phase 1 and phase 2 toxicology
work with the neutron beams is yet to be done, it would behove us to hold
off a little bit before mounting "the trial" upon which the whole fate of
the strategy is going to rest, because if we flunk this one it will be a
whole generation before we have another chance.

Alan Coates: We are in some danger of comparing apples with oranges, when
we talk about phase 1 trials and compare it with the rules that apply in
the development of systemic therapeutic modalities. One of the things that
was not mentioned in the criteria that I applied in those trials is that

there is no better standard treatment available for this situation. I think that is the ethical imperative. How that would be interpreted and applied will differ from one situation to another and from one doctor to another, but I don't think there is any way we can use a treatment if we believe we have a standard effective treatment in that situation. Now, when you come into investigating a new treatment, there is no doubt that the best experimental animal is the human patient with the disease, no question about that. I am sure we will learn far more, quicker and faster about this modality by treating patients. I think the only difficulty is coming to some agreement about which are the suitable patients for treatment. I would take all the points that are made for making allowances for the clumsiness, costs and inconvenience in the developmental stage of a therapy, we will get past that if the treatment works. I am sure we will have shiny new machines in the departments that can develop the appropriate neutron source.

I think, on the other hand, my own personal responsibility is for patients who are beyond this sort of treatment. I personally treat patients with metastatic melanoma. Talking to my surgical colleagues in the unit and trying to find patients for our joint trial, the difficulty I have come up against and which I can't argue against either, is that they are confident that they have a surgical answer to the primary treatment and the only patients that are suitable for this investigational treatment would be patients strictly analagous to Professor Mishima's first patient with isolated, troublesome but incurable metastatic disease. Now, if that is a patient suitable for the phase 1 investigation for a new treatment modality, so be it. I would enthusiastically support that. Where I think we would part on emphasis, if not complete agreement, is whether it is appropriate to start treating primary melanoma at this stage, and in the Australian setting the answer of the past three years is that we have not come across such a patient.

Ron Dorn: I got the microphone back Barry! Just a quick comment and I know perhaps, Alan, you were speaking specifically of melanoma, but it seems to me the comment you just made applies to one of the primary tumours that we were thinking of doing phase 1 clinical trials on and that is glioblastoma. I think that as far as I know essentially everywhere, people would recognize there is no alternative, viable treatment for glioblastoma at this point, so it would satisfy that particular criterion in terms of being very worthwhile doing the phase 1 trial. Going back to the discussion about how long it will take to do a trial, I think the comment was 10 years or so for the phase 1 trial. For a tumour that has a median survival of less than a year, I suspect that, if there is a big difference, you are going to see an answer long before 10 years.

Andrew Kaye (added in proof)

The concept of Neutron Capture Therapy offers a very real chance of an effective adjuvant therapy, especially for those tumours where the major problem is one of local control. The classical tumour in this situation is the cerebral glioma as this tumour usually recurs locally, indicating that the present treatments have failed to control the local disease. Neutron Capture Therapy is a binary treatment system that might be used as an adjuvant therapy. Theoretically it offers the possibility of a highly selective treatment system in which the tumour cells are killed and the local brain spared. At this symposium it was apparent that considerable advances have been made to optimize Neutron Capture Therapy. New forms of boron and methods of delivery have been described as well as new types of neutron sources. Whilst it is my opinion that the therapy is not yet ready for a formal patient trial, I do think that improved boron compounds and neutron sources offer a very really possibility for treatment in the future.

Lester Peters (added in proof)

As I see it, one of the biggest problem for NCT in the future will be to overcome the negative image it now has in the United States as being costly and impractical. The only way to overcome this negative image is to demonstrate that real progress is being made in the delivery of capture elements and the feasibility of producing epithermal neutron beams in a hospital environment. A delicate balance needs to be struck between maintaining the enthusiasm of researchers in the field while avoiding the criticism of unfounded claims for success. My own attitude is based on these principles. Please do not interpret it as being negative to the science.

Barry Allen: I think probably a feature of this symposium has been that in the main we kept on time, and another interesting feature is that most of the participants are still here, perhaps in anticipation of the on-coming trial which is scheduled to commence in a couple of minutes. So with your permission, I'd like to have the last word on all of this. The first point I would like to make is that NCT in Australia and everywhere depends very much, not only on the skills and enthusiasm of the physicists, chemists and biologists, it requires very much the moral support of clinicians as well. Continually, and I think this is probably true all over the world, we have to compete for research grants for boron chemistry and for pharmacological and NCT experiments. I would have to say that in Australia, and I don't think this will be any different to anywhere else in the world, it's an uphill battle. But ultimately, when we have to move or approach the trial stage to prove the efficacy of this method, it very much requires input from the medical community. As I worked towards this symposium, I thought surely one of the big rewards for Australia might be that no longer could our cancer clinicians ask, "what is Neutron Capture Therapy and how does it work?" I hope that is the case and that we will be able to attract further support. I must say in my own case, I have received this support from some close collaborators and this has been vital to maintain my own enthusiasm, and I think that is probably true elsewhere around the world.

We have seen a lot of results here today and during this conference. The technology, skills, the growing support, the results with all the different animal models, the development of new neutron beam facilities, new improved analytical techniques; all this is pointing one way and I believe, as I think Al Soloway has said, it is just a matter of time.

So with that last word I would like to make a couple of announcements. First, I would like to mention Doug Moore. Doug has been of enormous assistance to me and I would like you to thank him very much. Secondly, I would like to mention Al Soloway who, for reasons best known to himself, has assumed this burden in two years time. Al, you are trapped there in your seat.

Al Soloway: I think this has been a great conference, and it has been very healthy to have the panel here. I think this has been one of the highlights of the whole program, because we want to hear the criticism and not just hear ourselves pat ourselves on the back. If this is going to be a truly useful modality, then in the ultimate it is the clinician who is going to have to use it and people have to be convinced this is a good way of going, but I don't want to make this a long speech. I thought, Barry, as the outgoing president, I should give you something that you would be able to remember. Bill Sweet said it should have been Robert's Rules of Order, but I thought I will give you something to wear. Why don't you put it on for me, because that is where the next meeting is going to be in two years and I would like all of you to come and I hope you that you will. Also there are some fliers here, I would be very happy if people would take these off my hands so I don't have to drag them back to the US.

Barry Allen: With those words I would like to declare the symposium closed and thank you very much for your attendance and contributions.

AIZAWA Otohiko
Musashi Institute of
Technology
Ozenji Asao-ku
Kwasaki/shi
Fax No: 81-44-955-6071

AKABOSHI Mitsuhiko
Research Reactor
Institute
Kyoto University
Kumatori-cho Osaka
590-04, Japan

AKINE Yasuyuki
Dept of Radiation
Therapy
The National Cancer
Centre
5-1-1 Tsukiji, Chuo-Ku
Japan

AKUTA Keizo
Research Reactor
Institute
Kyoto University
Kumatori-cho, Osaka
590-04 Japan

ALLEN Barry
Biomedicine & Health
Program
Ansto PMB 1, Menai
Australia
Fax No: 61-2-543-9262

AMOLS Howard I.
Dept of Radiation
Oncology
Columbia University,
Oxford
622 West 168 St,
New York, NY 10032, USA
Fax No: 1-212-305-5935

ANDERSSON Annelie
Dept of Radiation
Sciences
Uppsala University, Box
535, S-75121
Uppsala Sweden

ANTHES Janet
39 Hope Street
Seaforth NSW 2092,
Australia

ARONEY Rodney S.
Dept of Medical Oncology
Repat General Hospital,
Concord 2139
Australia

BALDAS John
Australian Radiation
Laboratory
Lower Plenty Road,
Yallambie VIC 3085,
Australia

BALLAGNY Alain
CEA - Centre d'Etudes de
Saclay
91191 Gif-Sur-Yvette
France
Fax No: 33-1-69-08-80-15

BARKLA David
Dept of Anatomy
Monash University
Wellington Road
Clayton VIC 3168,
Australia

BARTH Rolf F.
Ohio State University
Department of Pathology,
4170 Graves Hall
333 W. 10th Avenue
Columbus, Ohio 43210,
USA
Fax No: 1-614-292-7072

BARTLE, Murray
DSIR, Physical Sciences
PO Box 31312 Lower Hutt
New Zealand

BAUER Bill
INEL, EGG Idaho Inc
PO Box 1625
Idaho Falls, ID
83415-2208, USA
Fax No: 1-208-526-0528

BENARY Vili
Medical Department
Brookhaven National
Laboratory
Upton, NY 11973, USA
Fax No: 1-516-282-3000

BILEK Marcela
14 Stephen Road
Engadine NSW 2233,
Australia

BLAGOJEVIC Ned
Biomedicine & Health
Program
Ansto PMB 1, Menai
Australia
Fax No: 61-2-543-9262

BLUE Jim
NASA Lewis Research
Centre
Cleveland Ohio 44135
USA
Fax No: 1-614-292-3163

BROOMHEAD John
Chemistry Department
Australian National
University
Canberra ACT 2601,
Australia

BROWN Keith
Biomedicine & Health
Program
Ansto PMB 1, Menai
Australia
Fax No: 61-2-543-9262

BROWNELL Anna-Liisa
Medical Physics
Salem Ma USA

BROWNELL Gordon
Director, Physics
Research Laboratory
Massachusetts General
Hopsital
Professor, Nuclear
Engineering
and Whittaker College,
MIT
Boston MA 02114
Fax No: 1-617-726-5123

BRUGGER Robert M.
University of
Missouri-Columbia
Nuclear Engineering
333 EE Bldg
Columbia MO 65211, USA
Fax No: 1-314-882-0397

BURIAN Jiri
Nuclear Research
Institute
CSSR 250

68 REZ Near Prague
CZECHOSLOVAKIA
Fax No: 42-2-896-255

CAROLAN Martin
University of Wollongong
Wollongong NSW 2500,
Australia

CHIARAVIGLIO, Dino
Via Scarpa 5
27100 Pavia Italy

COATES Alan
Special Unit Level 9
Royal Prince Alfred
Hospital
Camperdown NSW 2050,
Australia

CODERRE Jeffrey A.
Medical Department
Brookhaven National
Laboratory
Upton NY 11973, USA
Fax No: 1-516-282-5311

CONSTANTINE Geoff
Biomedicine & Health
Program
Ansto PMB 1, Menai
Australia

CORDEROY-BUCK, Sue
Nuclear Medicine
St Vincents Hospital
Victoria Street
Darlinghurst NSW 2010

CRAWFORD John F.
P.S.I Villegan
CH-5232 Villigen
Switzerland
Fax No: 41-56-99-3294

D'CUNHA Glenn
Peter MacCallum Cancer
Institute
481 Little Lonsdale
Street
Melbourne VIC 3001,
Australia

DAVIS Sidney
1 Lane St
Blackburn, North Vic
3130

DELANEY Ian
Biomedicine & Health
Program
Ansto PMB 1, Menai
Australia
Fax No: 61-2-543-9262

DEWIT L
Nederlands Kanker Inst.
Amsterdam
Plesmanlaan 121
1066 CX Amsterdam (Nl)
Fax No: 31-20-669-1101

648

DORN Ron
INEL, EGG Idaho Inc
PO Box 1625
Idaho Falls, ID
83415-3519
USA
Fax No: 1-208-526-0528

DOUGAN Don
Johnson & Johnson
Research
154 Pacific Highway
ST Leonards, NSW 2065,
Australia

DUIGAN Gwynne
46 Swanston Street
Geelong, Vic 3220,
Australia

ELLISTON Peter
School of Physics
University of NSW
Kensington NSW 2033,
Australia

FAIRCHILD Ralph
Medical Department
Brookhaven National
Laboratory
Upton 11973, USA
Fax No: 1-516-282-3000

FANKHAUSER Heinz
Department of
Neurosurgery
CHUV 1011 Lausanne
Switzerland
Fax No: 41-21-314-4873

FRANKLIN Ian
36 Woodland Street
Ansgrove, 4060
Queensland

FUKUDA Hiroshi
Department of Radiology
and Nuclear Medicine
The Research Institute
for Cancer, Tohoku
University
4-1 Seiryocho, Aoba-ku
Sendai 980
Japan
Fax No: 81-22-275-7324

GABEL Detlef
Department of Chemistry
University of Bremen
Box 330440, D-2800
Bremen 33
FRG
Fax No: 42-1-218-2871

GAHBAUER Reinhard A
Radiation Oncology
Arthur James Cancer
Hospital & Research
Institute
300 W 10th Ave.,

Columbus Ohio 43210
USA
Fax No: 1-614-293-4044

GAVIN Patrick
Washington State
University
Pullman WA 99164-6610
USA
Fax No: 1-509-335-0880

GOODMAN Joseph H
Ohio State University
Hospital
410W West 10th Ave Rm
950-N
Columbus, Ohio
43210-1228 USA

GRIEBENOW Merle
INEL, EGG Idaho Inc
PO Box 1625
Idaho Falls, ID
83415-3515
USA
Fax No: 1-208-526-0528

GRUSELL Erik
Department of Radiation
Scinces
Uppsala University,
Uppsala,
Sweden
Fax No: 46-18-18-38-33

GUMERLOCK Mary Kay
University of Oklahoma,
Health Sciences Center,
Division of
Neurosurgery, South
Pavillion, 4SP200
Post Office Box 26901,
Oklahoma City, Oklahoma
73190-3048, USA

HARITZ Dietrich
2800 Bremen 33, Germany
Oberneulander Landstr
195
Bremen

HARLING Otto
MIT Nuclear Reactor
Laboratory
138 Albany Street
Cambridge MA 02114 USA
Fax No: 1-617-253-7300

HARRINGTON Baiba
Nuclear Technology
Ansto PMB 1
Menai, NSW 2234,
Australia
Fax No: 61-2-543-5097

HATANAKA Hiroshi
Dept of Neurosurgery
Teikyo University,
2-11-1 Kaga
ITABASHI-KU Tokyo 173
Japan
Fax No: 81-3-5375-1716

HAWTHORNE Frederick
UCLA Dept of Chemistry
and Biochemistry, 405
Hilgard Ave Los Angel,
California 90024 USA
Fax No: 1-213-206-7197

HILL John
Department of Surgery
Royal Melbourne Hospital
Parkville, VIC 3052,
Australia
Fax No: 61-3-347-8332

HILTUNEN Jukka
Technical Research
Centre of Finland
Finland Reactor
Laboratory
Otakaari, 02150, Finland
Fax No: 358-046-1085

HOLECEK Milan
Royal North Shore
Hospital
St Leonards, NSW 2065,
Australia

HONDA Chihiro
Department of
Dermatology
Kobe University School
of Medicine
5-1 Kusunoki-cho
7-chome, Chuo-Ku
Kobe 650, Japan

HUISKAMP René
Netherlands Energy
Research Foundation
ECN PO Box 1
1755 ZG Petten, The
Netherlands
Fax No: 31-2246-4480

HUNT W.E.
Ohio State University
Hospital
N935 Dean, Columbus,
Ohio 43210 USA

ICHIHIHASHI Masamitsu
Kobe University School
of Medicine
5-1 Kusunoki-cho
7-chome, Chuo-Ku
Kobe 650, Japan
Fax No: 81-78-382-2497

JAMES Steven
Ohio State University
Hospital
410 W 10th Ave., Rm.
950-N
Columbus, Ohio 43210 USA

JONES Robert
Prince of Wales Hospital
Randwick, NSW 2031,
Australia

JONES Robert M.L
Department of Medical
Biochemistry
Centre Medical
Universitaire
9 Avenue De Champel,
Geneva, Switzerland

JONSSON Olle
The Svedberg Laboratory
Uppsala University

KABALKA George
Chemistry Department
University of Tennessee
Knoxville TN USA
Fax No: 1-615-544-8888

KAHL Stephen B.
Department of Pharm.
Chem.
University of California
San Francisco,
94143-0446
USA
Fax No: 1-415-476-0688

KANDA Keiji
Kyoto University
Kumatori-cho,
Sennan-gun, Osaka 590-04
Japan
Fax No: 81-724-53-0360

KASAMO Shizuya
Takeoka 1 Chome
5-6 Kagoshima, 890 Japan

KAYE Andrew
Dept of Neurosurgery
Royal Melbourne Hospital
Melbourne VIC 3050,
Australia

KINOSHITA Yasuhiko
Department of Chemistry,
Faculty of Science,
Shinshu University,
ASAHI, Matsumoto 390,
Japan
Fax No: 81-724-53-0360

KOBAYASHI Tooru
Kyoto University
Kumatori-cho
Sennan-gun Osaka 590-04,
Japan
Fax No: 81-724-53-0360

KOMURA Atsuko
Kobe University

KRAFT Susan
Washington State
University
Pullman WA 99164-6610
USA
Fax No: 1-509-335-0880

LAMBRECHT Richard
Biomedicine & Health
Program
Ansto PMB 1
Menai, NSW 2234,
Australia
Fax No: 61-2-543-9262

LARSSON Bengt S.
Dept of Toxicol, BMC
Uppsala University
Box 594, S-75121
Uppsala, Sweden
Fax No: 46-18-551-759

LARSSON Börje
Strahlenbiologisches
Institut
der Universitat Zurich
August Fore-str. 7
CH-8029 Zurich
SWITZERLAND
Fax No: 41-1-385-6204

LENNOX Arlene
Fermi National
Accelerator Lab.
PO Box 500 MS301 Batavia
Il
60510-0500 USA
Fax No: 1-708-840-4552

LIDDELL John
29 Kirksway Place
Hobart 7004, Australia

LINDSTRÖM Peter
Department of Chemistry
Uppsala University,
Box 531, S-75121,
Uppala, Sweeden

MADOC-JONES Hywell
750 Washington St
Boston MA 02111 USA

MAMEGHAN Hedy
Oncology & Radiotherapy
Prince of Wales Hospital
Randwick, NSW .2031,
Australia
Fax No: 61-2-399-0111

MARTIN Roger
Peter MacCallum Hospital
481 Little Lonsdale
Street
Melbourne, VIC 3001,
Australia
Fax No: 61-3-641-5489

MARUYAMA Yosh
University of Kentucky
Lexington KY
40536 USA
Fax No: 1-606-257-4931

MASON Rebecca S.
Pharmacy Department
University of Sydney
Sydney, NSW 2006,
Australia

MATSUMOTO Tetsuo
Musashi Institute of
Technology
Ozenji Asao-ku
Kwasaki/shi

McCALMONT Samuel A.
Callery Chemical Company
Division of Mine Safety
Appliances Company,
Pittsburgh, Pennsylvania
USA

McCARTHY William
Sydney Melanoma Unit
Royal Prince Alfred
Hospital
Camperdown, NSW 2050,
Australia
Fax No: 61-2-550-6316

McGREGOR Brian
Nuclear Technology
Ansto, PMB 1
Menai, NSW 2234,
Australia
Fax No: 61-2-543-5097

MERIATY Harry
Biomedicine & Health
Program
Ansto, PMB 1
Menai, NSW 2234,
Australia
Fax No: 61-2-543-9262

MISHIMA Yutaka
Department of
Dermatology
Kobe University School
of Medicine
5-1 Kusunoki-cho
7-chome, Chuo-ku
Kobe 650, Japan
Fax No: 81-78-382-2497

MONGER Carmela
Peter MacCallum Cancer
Institute
481 Little Lonsdale
Street
Melbourne, VIC 3001,
Australia

MOORE Douglas
Pharmacy Department
University of Sydney
Sydney, NSW 2006,
Australia
Fax No: 61-2-552-3760

MORRIS Gerard M.
Research Institute,
University of Oxford and
Oxfordshire Health
Authority, The Churchill
Hospital, Headington,
Oxford OX3 7LJ
Fax No: 44-865-741-756

MORRIS John H.
Department of Pure &
Applied Chemistry
University of
Strathclyde
Glasgow U.K.
Fax No: 44-041-552-5664

MORRISON George
Cornell University,
Department of Chemistry,
Baker Laboratory,
Ithaca, New York
14853-1301, USA
Fax No: 1-607-255-9930

MOSS Ray. L
Joint Research Centre
Postbus 2, 17557G,
Petten, Netherlands
Fax No: 31-2246-1449

MUKHERJEE Bashkar
Ansto PMB 1
Menai, NSW 2234,
Australia
Fax No: 61-2-543-5097

NAKAGAWA Yoshinobu
Manigema Kagewa 765
National Kagawa
Children's Hospital
Japan
Fax No: 81-87-762-5384

NARAYAN Kailash
Peter MacCallum Cancer
Institute
481 Little Lonsdale St
Melbourne, VIC 3000,
Australia

NEMOTO Hisao
Department of Chemistry
Tohoku University
Sendai 980 Japan

NIGG David
INEL, EGG Idaho Inc
PO Box 1625, Idaho
Falls, ID 83415-3519,
USA
Fax No: 1-208-526-0528

PAGE Jonathan
39 East Esplanade
Manly, NSW 2095,
Australia

PAPASPYROU Manfred
Institute of Medicine
Research Centre
Julich 5170, Julich FRG
Fax No: 24-616-4770

PETERS Lester J.
UT MD Anderson Cancer
Ctr
Division of Radiotherapy
Box 97
1515 Holcombe Blvd
Houston Texas 77030, USA

PETTERSSON C-B
Scanditronix AB
Husbyborg, S-752 29
Uppsala

PETTERSSON Orn-Anong
Department of Radiation
Science
Uppsala University, Box
555 S-75121, Uppsala,
Sweden
Fax No: 46-18-183-833

POPE Jim
School of Physics
University of NSW
Kensington, NSW 2033,
Australia

RADOMSKI Richard A.
Callery Chemical Company
Division of Mine Safety
Appliances Company,
Pittsburgh, Pennsylvania
USA

RALSTON Anna
54 Tennyson Avenue
Tranmere, SA 5073,
Australia

RAMSAY Eric B.
Dept of Radiation
Oncology
State University of
N.Y., Stony Brook, NY
11794-7028, USA
Fax No: 1-516-689-8801

RENDINA Lou
Department of Chemistry,
Faculty of Science,
Australian National
University
Canberra, ACT 2601,
Australia

ROBERTSON James S.
US Dept of Energy
ER-73 Washington DC
20585

ROSE Michael
Chemistry Department
Melbourne University
Parkville, NSW 3052,
Australia

ROSS David
89 Bristol Road
University of Birmingham
B57Tu, England
Fax No: 44-21-414-6709

SAKAKI Seigo
Vearata-Cho 761
Kagoshima-City Japan

SAKURAI Yoshinori
Kyoto University
Kumatori-cho
Sennan-gun Osaka 590-04,
Japan
Fax No: 81-724-53-0360

SALFORD Lief
Associate Professor,
Dept of Neurosurgery,
Lund University Hospital
S-221 85 Lund, SWEDEN
Fax No: 46-46-104-711

SAUERWEIN Wolfgang
Unversitaisklinikum
Essen
HufelandstraBe 55, 4300
Essen 1
Germany
Fax No: 49-201-723-5908

SCHOFIELD Peter
AEA Technology, Harwell
Laboratory Oxon OX11 ORA
UK
Fax No: 0235-436-579

SHANI Gad
Nuclear Engineering
Ohio State University
Columbus, Ohio 43210,
USA
USA
Fax No: 1-614-292-3163

SHELLY K.
UCLA Dept of Chemistry
and Biochemistry
405 Hilgard Ave Los
Angel
California 90024 USA
Fax No: 1-213-206-7197

SHIONA Masahiro
Department of
Dermatology
Kobe University School
of Medicine, 5-1
Kusunoki-cho 7-chome,
Chuo-ku, Kobe 650, Japan
Fax No: 81-78-382-2497

SHUGG Dace
Menzies Centre
43 Collins Street
Hobart 7000, Australia
Fax No: 002-300-816

SJOBERG Stefan
Uppsala University
Inst of Chemistry, Box
531
S-75121, Uppsala Sweden

SMEE Robert
Prince of Wales Hospital
Randwick, NSW 2031,
Australia

SOLOWAY Albert
500 W. 12th Avenue
Columbus OH 43210
Fax No: 1-614-292-2435

SPIELVOGEL Bernard
Boron Biologicals Inc
2811 O'Berry St
Raleigh N.C. 27607 USA
Fax No: 1-919-832-5980

STECHER-RASMUSSEN Finn
Netherlands Energy
Research Foundation
ECN PO Box 1, 11755 ZG
Petten, The Netherlands
Fax No: 31-2246-3490

STENING Warwick
Neurosurgery
Prince of Wales Hospital
Randwick, NSW 2031,
Australia

STEVENS Graham
Radiotherapy Department
Royal Prince Alfred
Hospital
Camperdown, NSW 2050,
Australia
Fax No: 61-2-516-8057

STORR Greg
Nuclear Technology
Ansto PMB 1
Menai, NSW 2234,
Australia
Fax No: 61-2-543-5097

STRAGLIOTTO Giuseppe
Department of
Neurosurgery
CHUV 1011 Lausanne,
Switzerland

STROUF Oldrich
Institute of Inorganic
Chemistry
Chemistry, Majakovského
24, Prague 6
Fax No: 42-268-57567

SUNDSTRUP Bertel
WPH Holman Clinic
Launceston General
Hospital
Tasmania 7250, Australia

SWEET William
Massachusetts General
Hospital
Boston, MA 02114, USA
Fax No: 1-617-726-7546

TAKAGAKI Masao
Department Neurosurgery
Kyoto University
54 Kawara-machi, Shogin,
Sakyo-kyu, Kyoto 606
Japan
Fax No: 81-75-771-6415

TAKEUCHI Akira
Department of Veterinary
Surgery
Faculty of Agriculture,
Bunkyo-Ku, Tokyo 113,
Japan
Fax No: 81-3-3813-2776
or
81-3-5684-5194

TAYLOR Doris D
One Second St
South Fargo, Northdakota
5-104
USA

THOMAS Geoffrey Wayne
15 Cliff Way
Claremont, WA 6010,
Australia

TJARKS Werner
OSU College of Pharmacy
Ohio State University
500 Cannon Drive
12th Avenue Columbus OH
43210 USA

UJENO Yowrie
Research Reactor
Institute
Kyoto University
Kumatori-cho Osaka
590-04, Japan

WHITTAKER Anthony
Chemistry Department
Melbourne University
Parkville, VIC 3052,
Australia

WHITTEMORE William L.
General Atomics
San Diego, California
USA
Fax No: 1-619-455-4169

WIERZBICKI Jacek G
University of Kentucky
Lexington KY, 40536 USA
Fax No: 1-606-257-4931

WILSON Gerald
Biomedicine & Health
Ansto PMB 1
Menai, NSW 2234,
Australia
Fax No: 61-2543-9262

WITHERS Rodney
Radiation Oncology
Prince of Wales Hospital
Randwick, NSW 2031,
Australia

WOOTON Peter
Department of Radiation
Oncology
University of Washington
Medical Centre, Seattle,
Washington, 98195 USA
Fax No: 1-206-548-6218

YAMAMOTO Yoshinori
Department of Chemistry
Faculty of Science,
Tohoku University Sendai
980
Japan
Fax No: 81-022-263-9207

YANAGIE Hironobu
400 Brookline Ave. #21-E
Boston MA 02215, USA

YANCH Jacquelyn
Massachusetts Institute
of Technology
45 Carleton Street
Cambridge MA 02139
Fax No: 1-617-253-8000

YOSHINO Kazuo
Department of Chemistry
Faculty of Science,
Shinshu University,
ASAHI, Matsumoto 390,
Japan
Fax No: 81-263-33-5323

ZAMENHOF Robert G
129 Clinton Road
Brookline MA 02146, USA
Fax No: 1-617-956-5353

654

INDEX

665

The manufacturer's authorised representative in the EU is Springer
Nature Customer Service Centre GmbH, Europaplatz 3, 69115 Heidelberg,
Germany. If you have any concerns regarding our products, please
contact ProductSafety@springernature.com

Printed and bound by CPI Group (UK) Ltd, Croydon, CR0 4YY
23/04/2026
02095629-0018

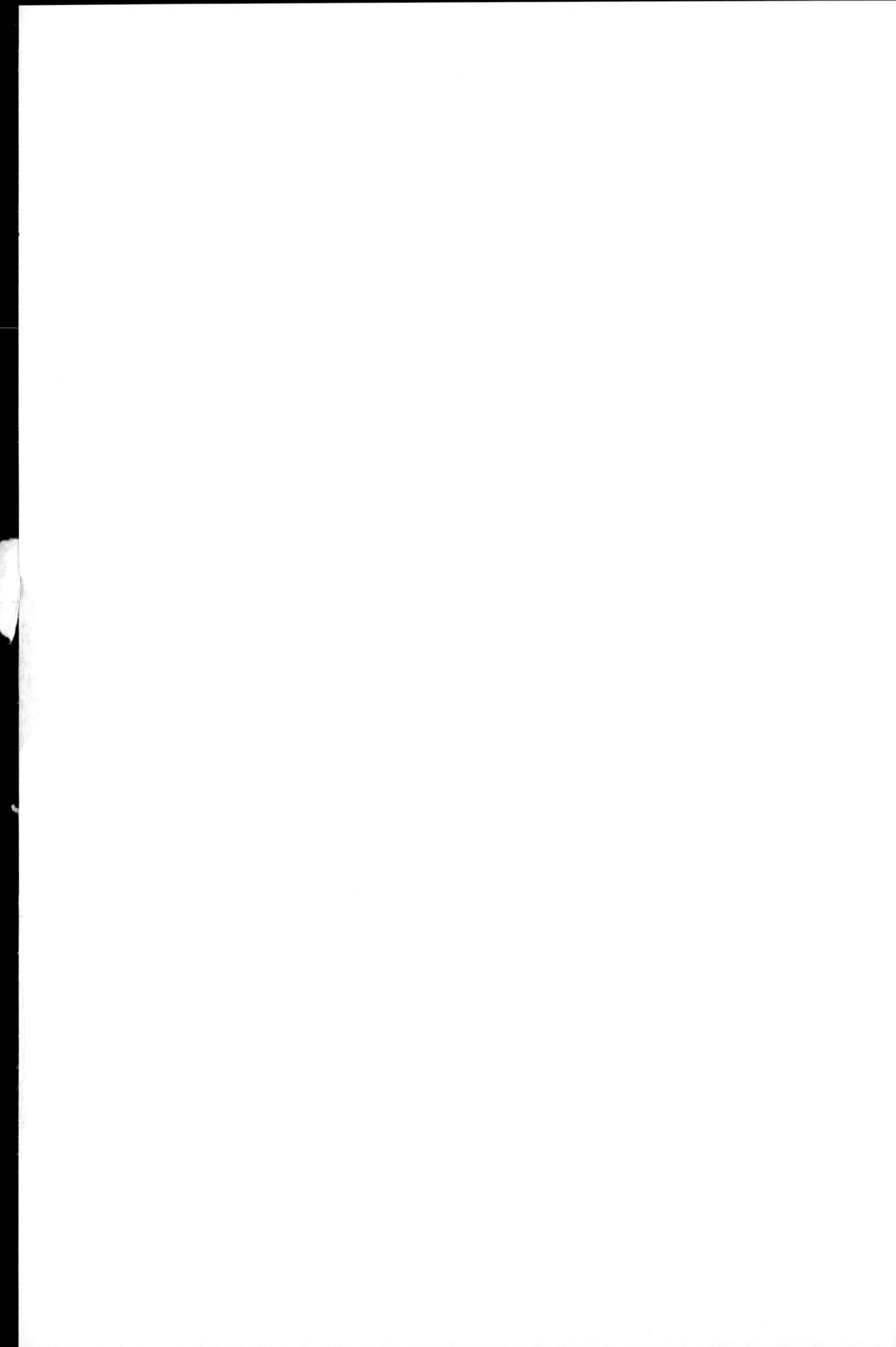